The Comprehensive Manual of

Therapeutic Exercises

• Orthopedic and General Conditions •

The Comprehensive Manual of

Therapeutic Exercises

• Orthopedic and General Conditions •

Elizabeth Bryan, PT, DPT, OCS
Doctor of Physical Therapy
Boone Hospital Center
Boone Therapy Outpatient Clinic
BJC Healthcare
Columbia, Missouri

Former Instructor
State Technical College
Department of Physical Therapist Assistant Program
Linn, Missouri

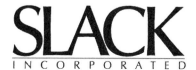

SLACK
INCORPORATED

www.Healio.com/books

ISBN: 978-1-63091-164-5

The procedures and practices described in this publication should be implemented in a manner consistent with the professional standards set for the circumstances that apply in each specific situation. Every effort has been made to confirm the accuracy of the information presented and to correctly relate generally accepted practices. The authors, editors, and publisher cannot accept responsibility for errors or exclusions or for the outcome of the material presented herein. There is no expressed or implied warranty of this book or information imparted by it. Care has been taken to ensure that drug selection and dosages are in accordance with currently accepted/recommended practice. Off-label uses of drugs may be discussed. Due to continuing research, changes in government policy and regulations, and various effects of drug reactions and interactions, it is recommended that the reader carefully review all materials and literature provided for each drug, especially those that are new or not frequently used. Some drugs or devices in this publication have clearance for use in a restricted research setting by the Food and Drug and Administration or FDA. Each professional should determine the FDA status of any drug or device prior to use in their practice.

Any review or mention of specific companies or products is not intended as an endorsement by the author or publisher.

SLACK Incorporated uses a review process to evaluate submitted material. Prior to publication, educators or clinicians provide important feedback on the content that we publish. We welcome feedback on this work.

Published by: SLACK Incorporated
                  6900 Grove Road
                  Thorofare, NJ 08086 USA
                  Telephone: 856-848-1000
                  Fax: 856-848-6091
                  www.Healio.com/books

Contact SLACK Incorporated for more information about other books in this field or about the availability of our books from distributors outside the United States.

Library of Congress Cataloging-in-Publication Data

Names: Bryan, Elizabeth (Doctor of Physical Therapy), author.
Title: The comprehensive manual of therapeutic exercises : orthopedic and
   general conditions / Elizabeth Bryan.
Description: Thorofare, NJ : Slack Incorporated, [2018] | Includes
   bibliographical references and index.
Identifiers: LCCN 2017048155 (print) | LCCN 2017049621 (ebook) | ISBN
   9781630911652 (epub) | ISBN 9781630911669 (web) | ISBN 9781630911645 (pbk.
   : alk. paper)
Subjects: | MESH: Exercise Therapy--methods | Musculoskeletal
   Diseases--therapy
Classification: LCC RM700 (ebook) | LCC RM700 (print) | NLM WB 541 | DDC
   615.8/2--dc23
LC record available at https://lccn.loc.gov/2017048155

Printed in the United States of America.

Last digit is print number: 10 9 8 7 6 5 4 3

DEDICATION

I dedicate this book to my students who inspired me to write this book; to my late mother who loved and supported me the best she could; and to my sister, my son, and Britta, who encouraged me to keep working through the tedious process of completing this project.

Contents

ACKNOWLEDGMENTS

This book would not have happened without the following students, educators, friends, and colleagues who gave their knowledge, time, and bodies to help create this textbook:

- Marlene Medin, PT, MEd, PT, who mentored me as an educator and through the beginning stages of this process.
- Katherine Berry, MS, PTA, who assisted with editing and reviewing the text.
- Pamela Gwin Coleman, yoga instructor, for contributions to Section 7.04 Yoga and Tai Chi.
- Natasha Kremer, Maura Mudd, Phillip Wilkinson, John Schibi, Chris Bruce, Kara Carr, Emma Brown, Paul Salierno, Hilary Matney, Brad Russell, Lois Bennett (Kay), Taylor Fick, Kayla Schanuth, Jason Woody, Mikala Green, Spencer Collins, Haley Musick, Juliette Jaegers, Melissa Thoenen, Britta Simpson, Isaac Holzer, Stephanie Schumacher, Tricia Dietrich, Merissa Turner, Rachel Ann Penn, Megan Hall, and Sharon Quinn for the donation of their time and bodies to be photographed for the book.
- Tony Schiavo, Acquisitions Editor at SLACK Incorporated, who helped to support and guide me through the process of writing my first textbook.

ABOUT THE AUTHOR

Elizabeth Bryan, PT, DPT, OCS received her BA in Biology in 1995 from Missouri Valley College in Marshall, MO and her BHS in Physical Therapy from the University of Missouri in Columbia in 1998. She went on to work in the outpatient Orthopedic setting at Fitzgibbon Hospital in Marshall, MO before moving to Colorado Springs, where she managed a spine specialty clinic for the next 4 years. After having her son, she moved back to Columbia and practiced full time in an orthopedic clinic. She completed her Board Certification in Orthopedics through the American Physical Therapy Association in 2008, at which time she entered into the teaching profession. She then completed her Doctorate in Physical Therapy from A.T. Still University in Kirksville, MO in 2010 in addition to 12 credit hours in Education at the University of Missouri. Liz was a lead instructor and Academic Coordinator of Clinical Education in the Physical Therapist Assistant Program at Linn State Technical College of Missouri for 6 years. Her teaching responsibilities included teaching subjects such as orthopedics for the PTA, Principles of Therapeutic Exercise, Human Anatomy and Physiology, Medical Terminology, Functional Anatomy and Kinesiology, PTA Trends and Issues, Documentation, and Medical Terminology, and she was a lab assistant for Basic Patient Care and Neurological Interventions and coinstructor for Health and Disease. She helped to develop and coordinate clinical education internship sites for the entire body of students, perform assessment of clinical education, and manage the clinical education of her students.

It was in this realm of her career Liz became compelled to create this textbook. She felt there was a great need for a comprehensive manual of exercises geared toward educating students and clinicians on how to properly implement clinically relevant exercises. She also wanted to provide a wide range of appropriate exercises for clinicians and students to choose from in accomplishing their physical therapy goals. She began the process of compiling exercises from every source she could find, including many of the clinics she worked in. She utilized many of her own smaller versions that she had compiled in her own practice. In using these for teaching, she started to see how helpful these manuals would be for clinicians and students. The detailed table of contents and the proposal took over 2 years to complete as she strived to incorporate thousands of exercises she had used and had seen used in the clinic—truly striving for it to be comprehensive in nature. Since the book has been completed, Liz has returned to her calling in clinical work. She currently works in the outpatient setting in Columbia and focuses much of her treatment on manual therapy and exercise. Her experience in the clinical setting—although very heavy in the outpatient settings—also includes experience in acute care orthopedics and extended care in skilled nursing facilities.

Liz also has a strong second career as an artist. She has been drawing and sculpting the human form even at a young age, part of where her interest in physical therapy was derived. She continues to express herself through art of many forms, including painting and large-scale art installations.

PREFACE

The purpose of this book is twofold. Primarily, its purpose is for instruction in the classroom and lab for student physical therapists (PT, MPT, DPT), physical therapy assistants (PTA), occupational therapists (OT, OTD), occupational therapy assistants (OTA, COTA), chiropractors (DC), exercise physiologists, athletic trainers (ATC), and personal trainers. In this realm, the book is a helpful supplement to a primary textbook on exercise theory and techniques and written to be used at the postsecondary education level. It provides a comprehensive resource of clinically effective and therapeutic exercises. Students can utilize the text to visualize, understand, design, and implement appropriate exercise programs for learning purposes. The second purpose of the book is for use in the clinical setting as a reference for the previously named professions to help design exercise programs for clients/patients. It is an essential reference for clinicians in assisting them to find the most appropriate exercises for their clients'/patients' needs as they expand their knowledge. It also assists in proper application, as the descriptions accompanying each exercise are geared toward the clinician rather than the patient.

The book utilizes a detailed table of contents and index, and an introductory chapter that includes discussion on the importance of form, muscle soreness, exercise parameters, exercise progression, and descriptions of body positions to serve as a reference for terms used in the exercise chapters. The following chapters are organized by body area and cover a large majority of the clinical exercises in use today. The following sections delve into protocols and specialty exercises. Each of the exercises has photographs that illustrate the exercise, a list of the target muscles or systems that will be affected, detailed student/clinician directed instructions, and detailed substitutions.

In the spirit of evidence-based practice, this textbook provides "Where's the Evidence?" boxes where substantial evidence is available. The supporting evidence is briefly discussed, with references available at the end of each section. An effort was made to include up-to-date, relevant, sufficient, valid, and reliable studies.

The book offers a practical approach to instruction and implementation of a clinically relevant exercise prescription and may be utilized throughout the students' education in the more advanced stages once they have their foundational knowledge of human anatomy and physiology, kinesiology, and exercise theory. It is a new approach in that it is a comprehensive manual of the current exercises used clinically in addition to instruction for the student/clinician on how to implement the exercise. This book takes all of the information that is spread out amongst multiple texts and websites and packages it into one very useful manual.

Chapter 1
THE BASICS

Bryan E. *The Comprehensive Manual of Therapeutic Exercises:*
Orthopedic and General Conditions (pp 1-26).
© 2018 SLACK Incorporated.

Section 1.01

INTRODUCTION

Therapeutic exercise has been used for centuries to address deficits in the neuromuscular and musculoskeletal systems and can affect the muscular, skeletal, circulatory, lymphatic, endocrine, digestive, and neurological systems. Goals of therapeutic exercise are by and large geared towards improvement of one or more of the following:

- Strength/force production
- Power
- Coordination
- Flexibility
- ROM
- Neuromotor communication
- Balance
- Posture
- Static and dynamic stability
- Functional mobility
- Cardiac function
- Pulmonary function
- Lymphatic function
- Pain

Thorough assessment of the patient is the first component of proper exercise prescription. This entails identification of the overall health condition of the patient by a review of systems and health history and a physical assessment of the patient's current status. Once the deficits have been established, the clinician or trainer will utilize all pertinent information to develop an exercise prescription that best suits the patient or client to optimize overall health, physical performance, and function. Critical thinking in the prescription process involves consideration of health history, risk factors, orthopedic and/or neurological conditions, psychosocial issues, personal goals, and accessibility of exercise equipment.

Section 1.02

THE IMPORTANCE OF FORM

Identification of deficits is the first step in exercise prescription. Exercises are then chosen to address these deficits. Equally important is the technique with which the exercise is implemented. Many exercises can worsen musculoskeletal conditions or cause injuries if not implemented correctly. Persons performing exercises can often cause themselves harm when utilizing incorrect postures and substituting with incorrect movements and accessory muscles. During the instruction, focus on correct form is imperative. This involves paying close attention to the patient's technique, recognizing signs of possible harm, and modifying until optimal form is demonstrated. Correct performance will result in the patient achieving the best possible outcome.

There are 5 main factors to consider when implementing proper form with patients and clients:

1. Posture
2. Substitution
3. Pain
4. Fatigue
5. Breath

Posture is defined as the position of the body in sitting or standing. Many patients will present with faulty postures and bad habits most easily observed in weightbearing positions such as seated and standing. It is important to address these postural deficits as each exercise is implemented. The body will be more efficient when good posture is maintained, thus minimizing the chance of injury. Addressing posture involves visual inspection of the entire body at the start of each exercise and constant monitoring during the exercise. Clinicians should look for neutral spinal alignment and maintenance of the normal spinal curves during activities (A through C).

Additionally, with respect to implementing exercises to the extremities, a strong stable base in the lumbopelvic or scapulothoracic regions is imperative. This is accomplished through activation of core and scapulothoracic muscles prior to UE and LE movements respectively.

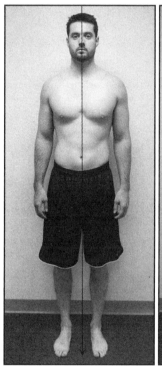 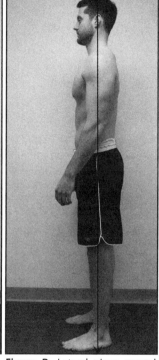

Figure A. Anterior view: normal posture.

Figure B. Lateral view: normal posture.

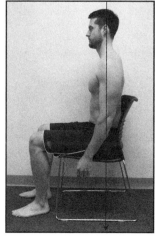

Figure C. Lateral view: normal posture, seated.

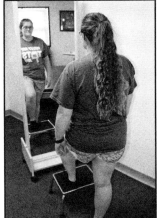
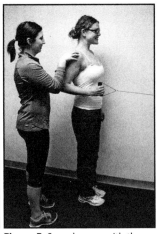

Figure D. Forward step-up in front of mirror.   **Figure E.** Scapular row with therapist manual cue.

Clinicians may choose to use a mirror with the patient to offer the patient visual feedback and help the patient become more aware of their body mechanics and posture (D). *Manual cues* involve using the hands to guide the patient's movements (E). Using the hands to assist with scapular retraction or tapping on the scapular retractors to facilitate contraction are examples of manual cues. *Verbal cues* require the use of words directed towards the patient to help them understand errors and help guide them towards correction. Constant monitoring is crucial, especially in the early stages of teaching new exercises. Performing a prone scapular "T" exercise for middle trapezius strengthening is more effective when doing 5 repetitions correctly rather than 15 repetitions done improperly. The primary goal is quality not quantity. It is vital to encourage the patient to move slowly at the start until they can do the exercise correctly before progressing to the goal speed.

When noticing the patient, losing good form, shaking, grimacing, or holding their breath, consider lessening the amount of resistance or allow the patient to rest before resuming the exercise. Knowing how to challenge the patient or client appropriately can be difficult. If the patient is unable to maintain the proper form, this can be one of the primary indicators of fatigue. Discerning what is the limiting factor is key in being able to modify the exercise appropriately. Discussing with the patient what they feel is limiting them is a good place to start. With prompting, the patient may reveal that they are experiencing pain during the activity. Patients may describe the pain as tiredness, burning or cramping, which may indicate fatigue. Other types of pain can be sharp, stabbing, shooting, or aching which suggest irritation of anatomical structures. Knowledge of anatomy and pain types is important in making the correct modifications. Once the patient is completing the desired repetitions and continues to demonstrate good form, then the patient may be ready to advance.

Substitution in exercise describes the use of an unwanted movement or muscle activity that may be used by patient to assist the target movement or muscle activity. One of the

TABLE 1.02-A	
MUSCLES PRONE TO WEAKNESS	*MUSCLES PRONE TO TIGHTNESS*
• Gastrocnemius/soleus • Tibialis posterior • Hip adductors • Hamstrings • Rectus femoris • Iliopsoas • TFL • Piriformis • Thoracolumbar extensors • Quadratus lumborum • Pectoralis major • Upper trapezius • Levator scapulae • Scalenes • SCM • Upper limb flexors	• Peroneus longus, brevis • Tibialis anterior • Vastus medialis, VL • Gluteus maximus, medius, minimus • RA • Serratus anterior • Rhomboids • Lower trapezius • Deep neck flexors • Upper limb extensors

primary goals in exercise prescription is to correct muscle imbalances. *Muscle balance* refers to the normal amount of opposing forces acting around a joint that keeps the joint centered during movement. This requires a balance of muscle length and strength between antagonistic muscles. *Muscle imbalance* describes a condition in which opposing muscles create pulling of the joint out of proper alignment. This can be a result of one or more muscles being tight (pulling too much) or weak (not pulling enough). An incorrect resultant force occurs, causing undue stress to the joint and surrounding structures. When a muscle imbalance is present, the muscular system fails to support the body region in the most efficient manner.

Most muscle imbalances are an imbalance between muscles anterior and posterior to a joint or region, but an imbalance from the right to left side of the body can also occur. Generally, the cause is due to one of two things, biomechanical or neuromuscular. Shirley Sahrmann and Florence Kendall both detailed how biomechanical issues refer to an imbalance resulting from repeated movements or prolonged postures (Kendall, McCreary, & Provance, 1993; Sahrmann, 2002). Vladimir Janda and Moshe Feldenkrais elaborated that neuromuscular causes are described as a muscle's predisposition to be either tight or weak based on movement patterns that evolved from birth (Feldenkrais, 1981; Page, Frank, & Larcher, 2010). Whatever the reasoning behind it, the agreement is muscle imbalances cause dysfunction. Knowledge of which muscles are commonly tight and/or weak in the body can help to guide assessment and treatment (Table A).

TABLE 1.02-B			
POSTURAL SYNDROME	*TIGHTNESS*	*WEAKNESS*	*RESULTS*
LCS	Thoracolumbar extensors Iliopsoas Rectus femoris	Deep abdominals Gluteus maximus Gluteus medius	• L4 to L5, L5 to S1, SIJ, and hip dysfunctions • APT • Increased lumbar lordosis • Lateral lumbar shift • Lateral leg rotation • Knee hyperextension
UCS	Upper trapezius Levator scapulae Pectoralis major Pectoralis minor	Deep cervical flexors Middle trapezius Lower trapezius Serratus anterior	• Atlanto-occipital joint, C4 to C5, cervicothoracic joint, glenohumeral joint, and T4 to T5 dysfunction • Forward head posture • Increased cervical lordosis • Increased thoracic kyphosis • Elevated and protracted shoulders • Abduction and winging of scapula
Layer syndrome	Combination of LCS and UCS—often seen on older adults		

Three common postural presentations have been identified by Janda. Although these have not been rigorously tested or advanced, they can offer some guidance for the new clinician. These are the LCS, UCS, and layer syndrome. In LCS, tightness of the thoracolumbar extensors on the dorsal side cross with tightness of the iliopsoas and rectus femoris. Weakness of the deep abdominal muscles ventrally cross with weakness of the gluteus maximus and medius. This imbalance creates joint dysfunction, particularly at the L4 to L5 and L5 to S1 segments, SIJ, and hip joint. Postural deviations include APT, increased lumbar lordosis, lateral lumbar shift, lateral leg rotation, and knee hyperextension. In UCS, also referred to as *proximal* or *shoulder girdle crossed syndrome*, tightness of the upper trapezius and levator scapula on the dorsal side cross with tightness of the pectoralis major and minor. Weakness of the deep cervical flexors ventrally cross with weakness of the middle and lower trapezius. This imbalance creates joint dysfunction, particularly at the atlanto-occipital joint, C4 to C5 segment, cervicothoracic joint, glenohumeral joint, and T4 to T5 segment. Postural deficits that are seen in UCS include forward head posture, increased cervical lordosis and thoracic kyphosis, elevated and protracted shoulders, and rotation or abduction and winging of the scapulae. These postural changes decrease glenohumeral stability as the glenoid fossa becomes more vertical due to serratus anterior weakness leading to abduction, rotation, and winging of the scapulae. This loss of stability requires the levator scapula and upper trapezius to increase activation to maintain glenohumeral centration. *Layer syndrome* is a combination of

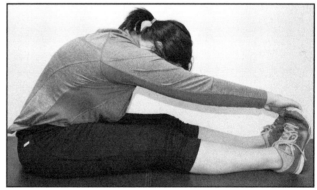

Figure F. Incorrect form for long-sitting hamstring stretch (notice kyphotic spine).

UCS and LCS and is often seen in older adults (Page, Frank, & Larcher, 2010; Table B).

Many times, when attempting to target specific muscles with exercise, poor habits and muscle imbalances become apparent. The patient will substitute in an effort to "do more." For example, a person attempting to stretch the hamstrings in long-sitting will often substitute with lumbar flexion in order to reach their toes. However, in many cases, the combined excessive lumbar flexion when performing a hamstring stretch can aggravate a low-back problem (F). When a person is stretching the hamstrings, the lumbar spine should be maintained in a neutral position. This can be done by cueing the patient to "lead with the chest" and to monitor the ability to maintain the lumbar lordosis (G). Let's look at another example with resisted elbow flexion or

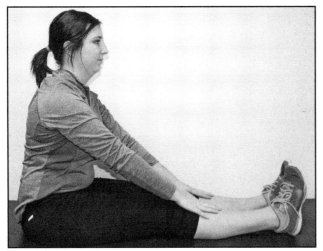

Figure G. Correct form for long-sitting hamstring stretch (notice neutral spine).

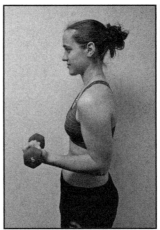

Figure H. Incorrect bicep curl (notice anterior humeral head).

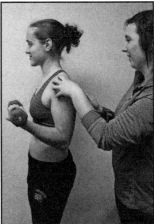

Figure I. Correct bicep curl (notice humeral head centered in glenoid fossa with scapular retraction).

bicep curls in seated or standing. A common substitution noted with this exercise is excessive forward movement of the humeral head and shoulder shrugging. The ideal posture consists of scapular and shoulder retraction during the entire exercise. Proper cueing and correction is often needed as clients or patients will try to increase power by throwing trunk forward. Additionally, without proper stabilization of the scapula, the scapula will elevate and tip anteriorly as the person curls the weight due to the biceps pull on the origin. The upper trapezius will also attempt to compensate for weakness of the biceps brachii, brachialis and/or brachioradialis resulting in a shrugging shoulder during the exercise (H). Many patients with shoulder problems have a significantly tight and overused upper trapezius with correlating weak middle and lower trapezius. These weaker muscles cannot stabilize the scapula well enough to create a stable base while the weight is being lifted. This improper form therefore accentuates the problem as the humeral head is moved forward, creating poor biomechanics and injurious forces to the shoulder joint and long head of the biceps tendon. These substitutions may be observed during the initial repetitions and should be promptly corrected. Correction of the form involves education, visual monitoring, and verbal and manual cueing during the exercise (I). Additionally, the patient may return to poor form when fatigue sets in. Close observation can alert the therapist or trainer when the patient is fatiguing. Inability to maintain a neutral or retracted shoulder with cueing during the activity would indicate the patient needs to stop and rest. These examples illustrate how substitution can be detrimental and correction beneficial to the overall physical well-being of the patient.

As muscles grow fatigued, performance decreases. At the onset of fatigue, the patient begins to demonstrate subtle substitutions that gradually worsen as they continue with the exercise. Common substitutions will be outlined with each exercise presented in this manual. When the substitutions are noticed, the clinician should attempt to correct the form using manual, verbal, and visual cues. If fatigue is a factor, the patient will either be unable to correct their form or only for brief moment before returning to the incorrect pattern. At this point, the exercise should be halted and the patient should be allowed to rest and recover before continuing on to performing another set. The clinician should take note of the number of repetitions performed correctly and utilize that number to establish goals in the next set. Repetitions performed correctly in each set may decrease as cumulative fatigue occurs.

Pain is another factor to consider during exercise prescription. Patients may complain of pain during exercises. The type, intensity, and location of the pain are all factors to consider when determining which modifications need to be made. Is there an acceptable level of "pain"? How does the clinician and/or patient know when an exercise should be stopped or when the patient should "push through" the pain? Normal "pain" during exercise can be described as mild "burning" in the target muscle(s) with strength training or mild "pulling" sensation in the target muscle(s) with stretching. A mild "pull" or pressure in the joint with activities designed to increase joint range can also be considered a normal and expected response. The patient should be guided during these sensations by educating them that the "burn" they are feeling is the sensation of muscle fatigue and the "pulling" is the stretch on the muscle or tendon. A "pull" or "pressure" in the joint at end ROM is explained as a stretch to the joint capsule. Any other pain complaint with exercise would not generally considered normal. Modifications to the exercise should be made to eliminate any pain beyond what has been described here as normal. The "no pain, no gain" rule is based on the theory that exercise induced muscle soreness means the inflammatory response has been triggered, which will result in hypertrophy of the muscle tissue. However, this does not apply when the "pain" is something other than normal burning fatigue or acute muscle soreness. Patients' facial expressions need to be monitored for grimacing as patients will often try to push through "pain" during exercises. This stoic exercise performance can result in further injury. Frequent reminders are often necessary to prompt the patient to communicate their pain complaints during activities. Therapists should ask the patient how they "feel" with every exercise they are implementing and monitor the patient's sensation of pain during all activities. If abnormal pain is presenting during an exercise, the first step would be to attempt to modify the exercise so that it can be performed without pain. Modifications could include posture correction, correction of compensatory muscle patterns, position change, or decreasing the resistance. If all attempted modifications do not alleviate the pain, the exercise should be removed from the patient's program. The clinician would then choose a different exercise that meets the same goals but can be performed without pain.

Breathing properly is a key component with every exercise and should be monitored closely. Smooth and efficient breathing is crucial for delivering oxygen the body needs during exercise. Proper breathing can also help a person exercise longer with less effort and anxiety. During running and walking, developing a tempo with the breath is important. A 2:2 rhythm is recommended in which the patient breathes in for two steps (right then left) and breathes out for two steps (Daniels, 2014; McConnell, 2011). Nasal and mouth breathing are both fairly similar, as far as oxygen delivery, with mouth breathing offering less resistance and improved oxygen delivery (Wheatley, Amis, & Engel, 1991; Yamamoto, Miyashita, Takaki, & Goto, 2015). However, nasal breathing can help warm the air entering the lungs during cold weather exercise. Generally, what is most effective for each patient will be individualized based on these factors as well as what feels right for the patient. For resistance training, it is recommended the patient exhale on the exertion phase. Active exhaling also helps contract muscles that stabilize the lumbar spine during heavier lifting (Lamberg & Hagins, 2010). Holding the breath will increase intrathoracic pressure, impede blood flow to the coronary muscles, and raise the blood pressure which are all negative results. Encouraging the patient to breath with exercise is fundamental in implementing safe exercise.

REFERENCES

Daniels, J. (2014). *Daniels' running formula*. Champagne, IL: Human Kinetics.

Feldenkrais, M. (1981). *The elusive obvious or basic Feldenkrais*. Santa Cruz, CA: Meta Publications.

Kendall, F. P., McCreary, E. K., & Provance, P. G. (1993). *Muscles testing and function: With posture and pain* (4th ed.). Baltimore, MD: Williams and Wilkins.

Lamberg, E. M., & Hagins, M. (2010). Breath control during manual free-style lifting of a maximally tolerated load. *Ergonomics, 53*(3), 385-392.

McConnell, A. (2011). *Breathe strong perform better*. Champage, IL: Human Kinetics.

Page, P., Frank, C., & Larcher, R. (2010). *Assessment and treatment of muscle imbalance: The Janda approach*. Champagne, IL: Human Kinetics.

Sahrmann, S. (2002). *Diagnosis and treatment of movement impairment syndromes*. Maryland Heights, MO: Elsevier.

Wheatley, J. R., Amis, T. C., & Engel, L. A. (1991). Influence of nasal airflow temperature and pressure on alae nasi electrical activity. *Journal of Applied Physiology, 71*(6), 2283-2291.

Yamamoto, N., Miyashita, T., Takaki, S., & Goto, T. (2015). Effects of breathing pattern on oxygen delivery via a nasal or pharyngeal cannula. *Respiratory Care, 60*(12), 1804-1809.

DELAYED ONSET MUSCLE SORENESS

When implementing a strengthening program, the patient may experience muscle soreness for up to 3 days afterward. Acute muscle soreness is pain that develops in muscles during and immediately after strenuous physical activity and is caused by an accumulation of hydrogen ions in the muscle cells, edema in the muscle tissue, and fatigue. DOMS happen later, with the onset beginning 12 to 72 hours after the activity and resolving within 96 hours. This soreness is a result of microscopic damage to the muscle fibers inside the muscle cells. The muscles may be swollen, stiff, and tender to touch and have less force production during this period. During this time, the muscle is repairing itself. Using a general warm-up, one that uses large muscle groups to increase overall core temperature, and a specific warm-up, which mimics the actual exercises, are advised to minimize muscle damage by increasing muscle elasticity. Eccentric exercise also tends to result in more DOMS than concentric exercise. It is recommended that concentric exercises be implemented prior to eccentric exercises (Szymanski, 2001). During the repair phase, the muscle will demonstrate decreased strength and activity should be modified. Strength training should be resumed only after DOMS has resolved. Lower intensity exercise can assist to increase circulation to the area and provide a temporary analgesic effect but has little effect on recovery time (Zainuddin, Sacco, Newton, & Nosaka, 2006). The best advice may be to perform light exercise and simply wait for the symptoms to resolve. Therapeutically, efforts should be made to avoid DOMS as treatments may be stalled for up to a week after intense eccentric training. A more gradual and steady increase in exercise is desired when rehabilitating from an injury. It should be emphasized that exercise-induced muscle damage is a normal response that will in itself provide protection against damage from repeated exercise bouts (Connolly, Sayers, & McHugh, 2003).

Where's the Evidence?

Aminian-Far et al. (2011) found that *whole body vibration* administered before eccentric exercise may reduce DOMS via muscle function improvement and may be a good addition to a warm-up. Massage may also be effective in alleviating DOMS by up to 30% and reduce swelling but it does not have an effect on muscle function (Zainuddin, Newton, Sacco, & Nosaka, 2005). Traditionally, *cryotherapy* was thought to decrease DOMS if applied after exercise; however, a 2015 systematic review of the literature revealed no evidence that cooling affects any objective recovery variable in a significant way during a 96-hour recovery period (Hohenauer, Taeymans, Baeyens, Clarys, & Clijsen, 2015).

REFERENCES

Aminian-Far, A., Hadian, M. R., Olyaei, G., Talebian, S., & Bakhtiary, A. H. (2011). Whole-body vibration and the prevention and treatment of delayed-onset muscle soreness. *Journal of Athletic Training, 46*(1), 43-49.

Connolly, D. A. J., Sayers, S. P., & McHugh, M. P. (2003). Treatment and prevention of delayed onset. *Journal of Strength and Conditioning Research, 17*(1), 197-208.

Hohenauer, E., Taeymans, J., Baeyens, J. P., Clarys, P., & Clijsen, R. (2015). The effect of post-exercise cryotherapy on recovery characteristics: A systematic review and meta-analysis. *Public Library of Science, 10*(9), e0139028.

Szymanski, D. (2001). Recommendations for the avoidance of delayed-onset muscle soreness. *Strength & Conditioning Journal, 23*(4), 4-7.

Zainuddin, Z., Newton, M., Sacco, P., & Nosaka, K. (2005). Effects of massage on delayed-onset muscle soreness, swelling, and recovery of muscle function. *Journal of Athletic Training, 40*(3), 174-80.

Zainuddin, Z., Sacco, P., Newton, M., & Nosaka, K. (2006). Light concentric exercise has a temporarily analgesic effect on delayed-onset muscle soreness, but no effect on recovery from eccentric exercise. *Applied Physiology, Nutrition and Metabolism, 31*(2), 126-134.

Section 1.04

CHOOSING THE RIGHT PARAMETERS

For every exercise given to a patient, parameters are also prescribed. Parameters are the values given to an exercise to outline the quantity or dosage. Generally, these are measurable factors such as time, repetitions, or weight. There are differing parameters for exercises dependent on the type of exercise (i.e. progressive resistive, stretching) and the goals of the exercise.

In order to stimulate adaptation toward specific training goals, progressive resistance training protocols are necessary. The optimal characteristics of strength-specific programs include the use of concentric, eccentric, and isometric muscle actions and the performance of bilateral and unilateral single- and multiple-joint exercises. In addition, it is recommended that strength programs sequence exercises to optimize the preservation of exercise intensity; large before small muscle group exercises, multiple-joint exercises before single-joint exercises, and higher-intensity before lower-intensity exercises (American College of Sports Medicine, 2009).

Strengthening exercises are designed to increase the force production of a muscle or muscle group. The mode or method of exercise can vary greatly from free weights to closed kinetic chain activities. Specific strengthening exercises are usually given in multiple sets of a predetermined number of consecutive repetitions (reps). Rest periods are allowed between each set. *Duration* may refer to the amount to time the exercise takes, the length of the sets, and/or the rest periods, or a combination. With strength training, the objective is to overload the muscle so that the body will respond with an adaptation. This overload causes fatigue and requires time for recovery and adaptation to reach a new level of increased strength. The specific adaptations to imposed demands principle (SAID) states that if a human body is placed under stress of varying intensities and duration, it attempts to overcome the stress by adapting

specifically to the imposed demands (Kent, 2017). In short, to affect the performance of an activity, the training must be geared towards mimicking that specific activity. For example, to improve speed with jogging, the patient would need to train by jogging. The cross-training principle states that there are also some crossover benefits from training in another mode of exercise to the specific exercise that is trying to be improved upon. Adding swimming to improve endurance in long distance running is an example of this (Bandy & Sanders, 2012). Most of the effects seen in cross-training are due to improved physiologic measures and less due to improved specific performance of the target activity.

The strength endurance continuum describes strength and endurance as being in competition and states that it is impossible to maximize both at once in strength training (Kent, 2017). Decreasing resistance or weight during a strengthening exercise will result in completion of repetitions in a set before fatiguing, thus carrying over to improve muscle endurance. Increasing resistance or weight during a strengthening exercise will result in completion of fewer repetitions in each set before fatigue, resulting in larger increases in force production or strength. In summary, lower weight with higher repetitions provides the best endurance gain with little hypertrophy. Higher weight with lower repetitions provides the best strength gain and hypertrophy.

There are several evidence-based progressive resistance training protocols that have demonstrated improvement in strength. Delorme and Oxford both identify the patient's 10 repetition maximum (also called *rep max* or *RM*). This is determined by finding the maximum weight that the patient can properly lift 10 times consecutively. Both protocols use this number to determine the training dosage. Other protocols use a 1 RM or a 6 RM found by determining how much the patient or client can maximally lift 1

TABLE 1.04-A	
STRENGTH-TRAINING PROTOCOL	*PROTOCOL DETAILS*
Delorme	• Set 1: 10 reps at 50% 10 RM • Set 2: 10 reps at 75% 10 RM • Set 3: 10 reps at 100% 10 RM
Oxford	• Set 1: 10 reps at 100% 10 RM • Set 2: 10 reps at 75% 10 RM • Set 3: 10 reps at 50% 10 RM

Daily adjustable progressive resistive exercise	• Set 1: 10 reps at 50% 6 RM
	• Set 2: 10 reps at 75% 6 RM
	• Set 3: maximum reps at 100% 6 RM *(use this number of reps to calculate how much to increase set 4)*
	• Set 4: use number of reps in set 3 to decide:
	  ◦ If 0 to 2 reps in set 3—decrease by 5 to 10 lbs
	  ◦ 3 to 4 reps—decrease by 0 to 5 lbs
	  ◦ 5 to 7 reps—keep weight the same
	  ◦ 8 to 12 reps—increase by 5 to 10 lbs
	  ◦ 13+ reps—increase by 10 to 15 lbs
	• *Do as many reps as you can for the weight determined by set 3*

TABLE 1.04-B	
ACSM PROGRAM (2009)	*GENERAL GUIDELINES*
Novice Training Program (untrained individuals)—Strengthening	• 8 RM to 12 RM loads recommended • 2 to 3 days week • Increase 2% to 10% per week
ACSM Endurance	• Use 40% to 60% 1 RM loads for high reps (> 15 reps) and short rest periods (< 90 seconds) • Increase 2% to 10% per week
ACSM Power	• Use multiple joint activities • 0% to 60% 1R M loads for LE • 30% to 60% 1 RM loads for UE • Fast contraction velocity • 3 to 5 minutes of rest between 3 to 5 sets • Increase 2% to 10% per week
ACSM Hypertrophy	• 1 RM to 12 RM loads emphasis on 6 RM to 12 RM zone • 1 to 2 minutes of rest between sets • Moderate velocity • Higher volume, multiple sets • Increase 2% to 10% per week
Strengthening Intermediate and Advanced Frequency	• Intermediate 3 to 4 days/week • Advanced 4 to 5 days/week

Adapted from American College of Sports Medicine. (2009). American College of Sports Medicine position stand. Progression models in resistance training for healthy adults. *Medicine and Science in Sports and Exercise, 41*(3), 687-708.

or 6 rep(s). Eccentric to concentric ratio is also important to consider when implementing resistance exercises. The eccentric contraction should be generally twice as long as the concentric contraction in a 2:1 ratio.

Some examples of protocols that have been used for progressive resistance exercises are provided here (Table A). The American College of Sports Medicine (2009) also published guidelines for strengthening protocols and these are also provided (Table B).

General recommendations for strengthening patients in the clinical setting are as follows:

- Select a mode of exercise that feels comfortable throughout the ROM. There is very little evidence to support the superiority of free weights or machines for increasing muscular strength, hypertrophy, power, or endurance.
- Choose a repetition duration that will ensure the maintenance of consistent form throughout the set. Consider the eccentric to concentric ratio of 2:1 (i.e. 2s/4s, 3s/6s, 4s/8s).
- Choose a range of repetitions between 3 and 15. There is very little evidence to suggest that a specific range of repetitions (e.g., 3 to 5 vs 8 to 10) or time-under-load (e.g., 30s vs 90s) significantly impacts the

increase in muscular strength, hypertrophy, power, or endurance.

- Perform 1 to 3 sets of each exercise. The preponderance of resistance-training studies shows no difference in the gains in muscular strength, hypertrophy, power, or endurance as a result of performing a greater number of sets.
- After performing a combination of concentric and eccentric muscle actions, terminate each exercise at the point where the concentric phase of the exercise is becoming difficult, if not impossible, while maintaining good form. There is very little evidence to suggest that going beyond this level of intensity (e.g., supramaximal or accentuated eccentric muscle

actions) will further enhance muscular strength, hypertrophy, power, or endurance.

- Allow enough time between exercises to perform the next exercise in proper form. There is very little evidence to suggest that different rest periods between sets or exercises will significantly affect the gains in muscular strength, hypertrophy, power, or endurance. Depending on individual recovery and response, choose a frequency of 2 to 3 times a week to stimulate each targeted muscle group. One session a week has been shown to be just as effective as 2 to 3 times a week for some muscle groups. There is very little evidence to suggest that training a muscle more than 2 to 3 times a week or that split routines will produce greater gains in muscular strength, hypertrophy, power, or endurance (Campos et al., 2002).

Graded exercise therapy is a physical activity that starts very slowly and gradually increases over time. Following the principles of graded exercise therapy may be more appropriate for the patients with fatigue-related diagnoses such as multiple sclerosis and chronic fatigue syndrome. Graded exercise therapy starts with active stretching followed by ROM activities starting for 5 minutes per day for an inactive individual or at the level that is comfortable to the individual. Gradually, the exercise program is increased in frequency, duration, and intensity. Grading gradually is an important factor in all exercise programs as it allows the body time to make the necessary adaptations to the imposed demands. Gradual increase of an exercise program will render maximum positive effects while limiting negative effects such as pain, soreness, and tenderness.

The beginning of an exercise program should begin with gentle exercises such as walking, riding a stationary bike, swimming, stretching, and low-level yoga. Some recommendations for patients performing graded exercise therapy are:

- *Slow and Steady Wins the Race*: Have patient start and gradually increase exercise at their own pace. What is most important to an exercise program is the completion of the activity.
- *Gradual Increases*: It is possible for the patient or client to over-extend themselves. Gradually increase the frequency, duration, and intensity of the workout program. Slow down if necessary and only complete what is scheduled. Patients may feel as if more exercise is possible on a "good" day, but this may only serve to hinder overall progress if injury/strain/pain occurs.
- *Track Progress*: Have the patient keep an exercise diary, writing down their daily activities and schedule upcoming activities. Encourage them to make goals, write feelings, and be proud of their accomplishments.
- *Take Time Off*: If the patient is experiencing pain or muscle strain, it is ok to take some time off from

exercising. Stretching may serve as a possibility to relieve some muscle stress caused by exercising. Time off does not mean quitting; it is simply a short break. Be sure the patient resumes the exercise program as soon as the patient is comfortable. The more time spent away from a scheduled exercise program, typically the harder it is to begin again.

Graded exercise therapy was developed for chronic fatigue syndrome based around the patient's deconditioned state and poor exercise tolerances. It was theorized that the syndrome was perpetuated by physiological changes as a response to avoidance of activity and the resultant deconditioning, thereby maintaining the fatigued state. The aim of treatment is to assist the patient and condition them back to appropriate physical activities. Utilization of target heart rates can help the patient to avoid overexertion. The end goal is 30 minutes of light exercise 5 times a week. Once the goal is achieved, the intensity of the exercise is gradually increased within participant's tolerance. The most commonly chosen exercise is walking, but other alternatives include swimming and bicycling.

Flexibility programs are aimed at increasing muscle length. To effectively stretch a muscle, the clinician must design a program that effectively utilizes the responses of the sense receptors in the muscle and tendon. These are the muscle spindle and the GTO. Muscle spindles are located in the muscle bellies and respond to changes in the length of the muscle. When a muscle is stretched, the muscle spindles send sensory information to the spinal cord which results in a reflexive muscle contraction of the target (or agonist) muscle. This is a protective mechanism that resists a quick stretch. The muscle spindle also causes a reflexive inhibition of the opposing muscle (antagonist) known as reciprocal inhibition (Table C). Therapists may use this to their advantage by having the patient actively contract the muscle that opposes the target muscle they want to stretch. For example, the therapist applies a stretch to the hamstrings. After a brief 10 to 15 second hold, the therapist asks the patient to actively engage the rectus femoris and bring the leg further into the stretch. The therapist then takes up the slack and holds the stretch in the new range. This can be repeated 3 to 5 times with a final 30 to 60 second stretch (depending on age) at the end range (A through C). In upper motor neuron injuries, such as stroke or SCI, the muscle spindles can become overactive resulting in increased muscle tone. GTO are sensory structures located in the musculotendinous junction and offer a reverse effect. The GTO likewise responds to the changes in muscle/tendon tension caused by contraction or stretch and stimulate a reflexive inhibition or relaxation of the target muscle (agonist) known as autogenic inhibition and a reflexive contraction of the opposing muscle (antagonist). The GTO can also override the muscle spindle. The GTO is stimulated after approximately 7 to 10 second of static stretching (Table D). One can also use these sensory organs to his or

TABLE 1.04-C		
	MUSCLE SPINDLE	*HAMSTRING STRETCH EXAMPLE*
LOCATION	Muscle bellies	Hamstring tendon
SENSES	Changes in length of the muscle (stretch)	Hamstring being stretched
RESPONSE	Responds by reflexive contraction of muscle being stretched *Reciprocal inhibition*: Reflexively inhibits opposing muscle	Causes reflexive contraction of the hamstrings to resist stretch and a relaxation of the opposing muscle quadriceps
REACTION TIME	Immediate	Muscle spindle action dampens down after 7 to 10 seconds

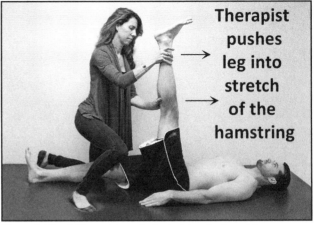

Figure A. Step 1: Therapist passively stretches the hamstring.

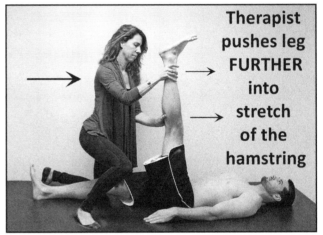

Figure C. Step 3: Therapist passively holds the leg in the new range.

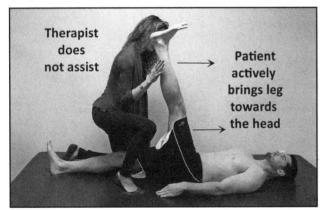

Figure B. Step 2: Patient actively brings the leg further toward him or her using the muscle spindle in the quadriceps to assist in reciprocal inhibition of the hamstrings.

her advantage when stretching. For example, a therapist may passively stretch the hamstring of a patient. When they reach the point where the patient feels the stretch, the therapist will need to hold the stretch long enough to bypass the muscle spindle "guarding" and stimulate the GTO to assist in relaxing the hamstrings. This is often followed by an isometric contraction of the hamstrings holding 7 to 10 seconds at end range. This results in increased stimulation of the GTO and a further reflexive relaxation after the contraction stops allowing hamstring to be stretched further (autogenic inhibition) (F).

Static stretching is a method in which the muscle is taken to the length in which a mild "pull" is felt and held for a prolonged period of time. The stretch should avoid ranges in which pain or excessive discomfort is felt. Evidence has supported the optimal time to hold a stretch is 30 seconds for adults and 60 seconds for individuals over the age of 65. Researchers found that holding a stretch for less than 15 seconds resulted in no change in muscle length. Therefore,

a static stretch should be held at least 15 seconds up to 60 seconds depending on age (Bandy & Sanders, 2012).

Dynamic stretching involves gentle movement of the muscle towards the end range and can focus on several different muscle groups at one time. It is designed as a warm-up and is more favorable to utilize before a competitive event. In dynamic stretching, the clinician and/or patient does not hold the stretch at the end range for a predetermined amount of time. It is slow, continuous motion into end range and back out, repeated in such a manner as to increase heart rate and blood flow. The movements should occur in a similar manner as to what will be performed in the workout or sport. Dynamic stretching during warm-ups as opposed to static stretching is most effective in preparing for high speed sports such as soccer. Evidence suggests that shortening the duration of the stretches will minimize the decrements to power-based sports and when performed during the warm-up may be the most effective preparation for subsequent high-speed performance (Little & Williams, 2006).

Ballistic stretching involves a repetitive bouncing movement when stretching the muscles and has fallen out of favor in treating non-athletic populations. Bouncing into and beyond the end range of muscles extensibility can lead

TABLE 1.04-D		
	GOLGI TENDON ORGAN	*HAMSTRING STRETCH EXAMPLE*
LOCATION	Tendon	Hamstring tendon
SENSES	Changes in length of the muscle (by contraction or stretch)	Hamstring being stretched
RESPONSE	• Autogenic inhibition: Responds by reflexive relaxation of muscle being stretched (inhibits muscle spindle action) • Reflexive contraction of opposing muscle (antagonist to the muscle being stretched)	Relaxing the hamstring (by dampening down the muscle spindle action) and causing reflexive contraction of the quadriceps
REACTION TIME	7 to 10 seconds before relaxation occurs	Stretch must be held at least 7 to 10 seconds before GTO will affect relaxation of the hamstrings and allow lengthening

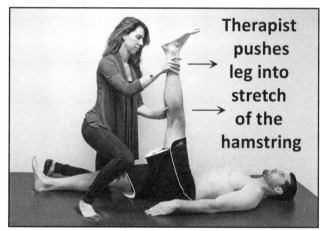

Figure D. Step 1: Therapist passively stretches the hamstring.

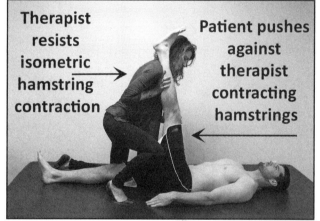

Figure E. Step 2: Patient actively contracts the hamstrings pushing against the therapist as the therapist resists. Active contraction of the hamstrings for > 7 to 10 seconds will activate the GTO resulting in autogenic inhibition of the hamstrings.

to microtrauma of the muscle tissue. This type of stretching should be avoided in most patient populations.

Recommendations for flexibility exercises are summarized in Table E.

Facilitation and inhibition techniques can also be utilized to increase or decrease muscle fiber recruitment and performance during strengthening activities. PNF techniques are used to elicit or inhibit motor responses to improve neuromuscular control and function. Manual tapping over the muscle belly can stimulate a quick stretch sensation in the muscle spindles and cause a reflexive muscle contraction. Deep pressure over the muscle belly can result in the opposite, decreasing muscle fiber recruitment. Cueing the patient verbally with words like "push" or "pull" as well as having them watch the limb being moved during the activity can help to increase force production. Using the muscle spindle by giving the muscle a quick stretch at the beginning of the ROM will facilitate a reflexive contraction at the start of the exercise movement. A quick stretch can be performed at any point in the range to facilitate contraction. Approximation of a joint via weight-bearing can also increase muscle fiber recruitment. Use of functional patterns (D and E) in the extremities and the

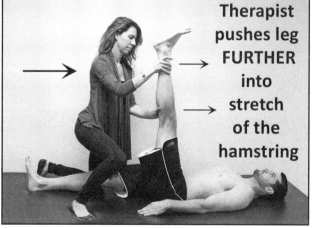

Figure F. Step 3: Therapist passively holds the leg in the new range.

trunk is also beneficial to improving strength production and increased movement. These functional patterns are summarized in Table F. Timing specific movements to

TABLE 1.04-E	
TYPE OF STRETCHING	*PARAMETERS*
Static stretching	Minimum hold 15 seconds Optimal hold 30 seconds for adults Optimal hold 60 seconds for persons >65 years of age
Dynamic stretching	Continuous slow repeated movement into the stretch and out without holding—effective for stretching before high-speed sports such as soccer
Ballistic stretching	Repetitive bouncing movements into stretch—not recommended

TABLE 1.04-F				
LOWER EXTREMITY	*LOWER EXTREMITY D1 FLEXION* "Up and in"	*LOWER EXTREMITY D1 EXTENSION* "Down and out"	*LOWER EXTREMITY D2 FLEXION* "Down and in" to "fire hydrant"	*LOWER EXTREMITY D2 EXTENSION* "Fire hydrant" to "down and in"
Pelvis	Anterior elevation	Posterior depression	Posterior elevation	Anterior depression
Hip	Flexion Adduction External rotation	Extension Abduction Internal rotation	Flexion Abduction Internal rotation	Extension Adduction External rotation
Ankle	Dorsiflexion Supination Inversion	Plantarflexion Pronation Eversion	Dorsiflexion Pronation Eversion	Plantarflexion Supination Inversion
Toes	Extension	Flexion	Extension	Flexion
UPPER EXTREMITY	*UPPER EXTREMITY D1 FLEXION* "Grab ear" to "toss tissue"	*UPPER EXTREMITY D1 EXTENSION* "Toss tissue" to "grab ear"	*UPPER EXTREMITY D2 FLEXION* "Unsheath sword" to "tada!"	*UPPER EXTREMITY D2 EXTENSION* "Tada!" to "sheath sword"
Scapula	Anterior elevation	Posterior depression	Posterior elevation	Anterior depression
Shoulder	Flexion Adduction External rotation	Extension Abduction Internal rotation	Flexion Abduction External rotation	Extension Adduction Internal rotation
Forearm	Supination	Pronation	Supination	Pronation
Wrist	Radial deviation	Ulnar deviation	Radial deviation	Ulnar deviation
Fingers	Flexion	Extension	Extension	Flexion
UPPER EXTREMITY COMBINATION PATTERNS	*REVERSE CHOP*	*CHOP*	*LIFT*	*REVERSE LIFT*
Affected arm	D1 extension to D1 flexion	D1 flexion to D1 extension	D2 extension to D2 flexion	D2 flexion to D2 extension
Unaffected arm	Holding wrist palm down follows affected arm	Holding wrist palm down follows affected arm	Holding wrist palm up follows affected arm	Holding wrist palm up follows affected arm
Trunk associated movement	Trunk rotation toward affected side	Trunk rotation toward unaffected side	Trunk rotation toward affected side	Trunk rotation toward unaffected side

TABLE 1.04-G	
RANGE OF MOTION	*DESCRIPTION*
PROM	Performed completely by external source (therapist, machine)—patient is fully relaxed
AAROM	Patient performs the movement, and therapist assists only at the end to achieve further ROM
AROM	Performed solely by the patient with no assistance

happen in sequence during the exercise can also help to develop proper coordination of muscle contractions.

ROM describes the osteokinematic movement of a bone resulting from the movement of the joint surfaces arthrokinematically with or without assistance. AROM is a voluntary movement performed by the individual. AAROM is performed by the individual until they reach their end range and then, is assisted by the therapist to achieve an even greater ROM within their tolerance. PROM is done solely by the clinician or a machine/device and the individual is relaxed throughout. There are no formal parameters found in the literature regarding ROM activities. Clinically, it is thought that ROM activities should be done 1 to 3 times per day to maintain and improve joint ROM, capsular pliability and promote circulation and lubrication in the joint. Repetitions should be determined based on patient's response and goals of treatment. Speed is also dependent on treatment goals, but generally the speed should be slow and controlled with proper attention to form.

Summary of types of ROM exercises are summarized in Table G.

It is important to keep in mind that recommended protocols for types of exercises can vary depending on the patient's status, the goals of the exercise program, and the individual response to the exercise. The therapist should be flexible in application of exercises, allowing variances as needed. The information in this chapter is designed to give the therapist a guide of where to start. A general exercise program should include a warm-up and a cool-down when possible. A warm-up should consist of an activity that works the large muscle groups for 5 to 10 minutes while increasing the heart rate. A cool down is also 5 to 10 minutes and should allow the heart rate and core temperature

to recover. Stretching can be done after the warm-up as muscles are more prepared for stretching.

The following chapters of the book illustrate a large body of exercises that can be applied to the patient's exercise program. Choosing the right exercise is important in helping the patient reach their goals while not causing harm to them or worsening any condition they may have. Understanding any underlying pathology or injury can help the clinician to prescribe the proper exercises. Physicians may have put the patient on restrictions or precautions based on injuries or conditions. In selecting the proper exercises, incorporating these restrictions is imperative. Also, when choosing activities, knowledge of how the exercise might affect injured or healing tissues should be well thought out.

REFERENCES

American College of Sports Medicine. (2009). American College of Sports Medicine position stand. Progression models in resistance training for healthy adults. *Medicine and Science in Sports and Exercise, 41*(3), 687-708.

Bandy, W. D., & Sanders, B. (2012). *Therapeutic exercise for physical therapist assistants* (3rd ed.). Philadelphia, PA: Wolters Kluwer/ Lippincott, Williams & Wilkins.

Campos, G. E., Luecke, T. J., Wendeln, H. K., Toma, K., Hagerman, F. C., Murray, T. F., . . . & Staron, R. S. (2002). Muscular adaptations in response to three different resistance-training regimens: Specificity of repetition maximum training zones. *European Journal of Applied Physiology, 88*(1-2), 50-60.

Kent, M. (2017). *The Oxford dictionary of sports science & medicine* (3rd ed.). Oxford, UK: Oxford University Press.

Little, T., & Williams, A. G. (2006). Effects of differential stretching protocols during warm-ups on high-speed motor capacities in professional soccer players. *Journal of Strength and Conditioning Research, 20*(1), 203-207.

Section 1.05

EXERCISE PROGRESSION

How does the clinician or trainer know when to progress the exercise? This is usually determined by the following factors:

- Does the patient feel the exercise is easy?
- Is the patient able to do the entire exercise with proper form and low to medium effort?
- Does the patient's muscle soreness resolve in less than 24 to 48 hours after the exercise was performed?

If the clinician is able to answer yes to all of the above questions, then most likely the patient is ready to progress. Progression can be in the form of adding repetitions, sets, modifying the intensity via increasing resistance, or modifying the speed of the activity depending on the goals of their program. When training at a specific resistance load, it is recommended that 2% to 10% increase in load be applied when the individual can perform the current workload for 1 to 2 repetitions over the desired number (American College of Sports Medicine, 2009).

Progression in power training entails two general loading strategies: 1) strength training and 2) use of light loads (0% to 60% of 1 RM for lower body exercises; 30% to 60% of 1 RM for upper body exercises), performed at a fast contraction velocity with 3 to 5 minutes of rest between sets for 3 to 5 sets per exercise. It is also recommended that emphasis be placed on multiple-joint exercises, especially those involving the total body. For local muscular endurance training, it is recommended that light to moderate loads (40% to 60% of 1 RM) be performed for high repetitions (>15) using short rest periods (<90). Recommendations should be applied in context and should be contingent upon an individual's target goals, physical capacity, and training status (American College of Sports Medicine, 2009).

REFERENCE

American College of Sports Medicine. (2009). American College of Sports Medicine position stand. Progression models in resistance training for healthy adults. *Medicine and Science in Sports and Exercise, 41*(3), 687-708.

Section 1.06

How to Use This Manual

The following pages include a comprehensive listing of clinically therapeutic exercises. Each exercise will give the information needed to properly implement the exercise in the practice. A thorough description of the exercise is presented along with what muscles or systems the exercise will affect. Detailed instructions that can be used to teach the exercise to the patients are also provided for each exercise. Each description will also include common substitutions to look for so that modifications can be made to ensure proper form. Lastly, parameters will be suggested that will help guide the clinician in developing the proper prescription. The exercises are grouped by body area, but there is some cross-over for multiple body areas that the exercise may target. The manual also includes specialized exercises for targeting specific structures and systems such as vestibular or pelvic floor. The manual also includes various protocols and treatment ideas for different diagnoses for use in creating programs for injured and healing individuals. Important precautions and restrictions will be highlighted as well, but as previously noted, follow any additional precautions or restrictions ordered by the physician. Using the knowledge gained from other texts on exercise principles and patient diagnoses, this book will help the clinician find exercises that best fit the patient's needs.

Section 1.07

POSITIONS, DESCRIPTIVE TERMS, AND SPECIAL EQUIPMENT

1.07.1 NAMING OF POSITIONS

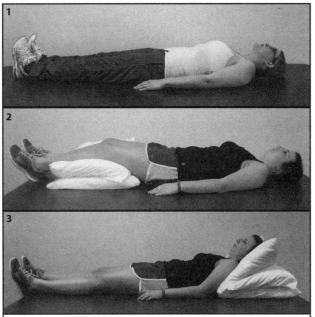

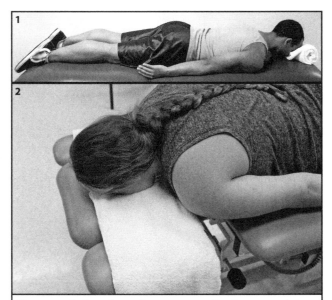

SUPINE: Lying face up, therapist may place a small towel roll under the neck and/or lumbar regions to increase comfort as needed (1). Use of a pillow under the knees may relieve low-back discomfort and allow for a modified supine position (2). Patients with extreme thoracic kyphosis may require pillows under the upper back and head for comfort (3). If a patient is unable to tolerate supine, it is recommended to move to hook-lying to decrease stress on the lower back.

PRONE: Lying face down, generally in prone-lying, the spine should be in neutral. Use of a small rolled up towel under the forehead is helpful to avoid cervical rotation (1). Patients should not be allowed to lie prone with the cervical spine rotated to one side or another for prolonged periods of time. Use of a table with a hole for the face is optimal when performing prone exercises and should be utilized if available. Often padding the sides of the face hole with towels increases patient's comfort (2).

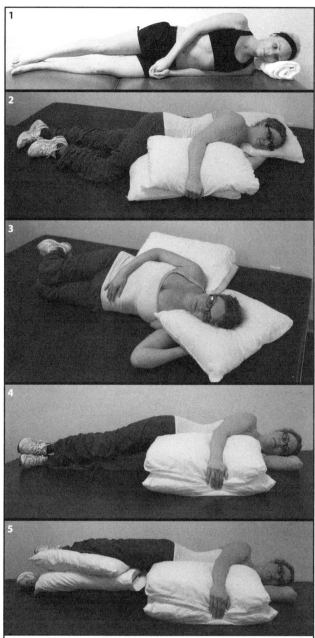

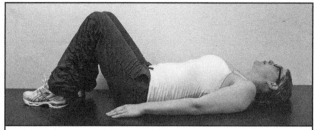

HOOK-LYING: Face up with knees bent and feet planted on surface. This position relieves pressure on the lumbar spine and can be more comfortable for the low-back than supine.

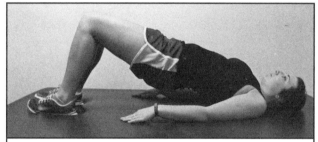

BRIDGE: Face up with knees bent. Hips are lifted off table with hips at 0 degrees of flexion. Pelvis is level with ASIS in same horizontal plane.

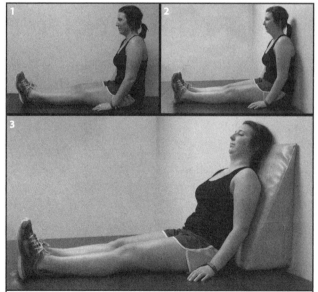

SIDE-LYING: Lying on the right or left side (1). Patients may have poor tolerance for this position due to hip and shoulder pressures. Modified side-lying can be used in which pillows are placed either in front of the patient (2) or behind the patient (3), allowing the patient to rotate slightly either direction and relieve straight downward pressure on the hip and shoulder. Hugging a pillow can also decrease discomfort in the top shoulder (4). Placing a pillow between the knees and ankles can also increase comfort by neutralizing the hip, sacroiliac, and lumbar joints (5).

LONG-SITTING: Seated with legs in front, knees extended (1). This position requires normal hamstring length. If the hamstrings are restricted, the lumbar spine will flex to compensate. Having the patient perform long-sitting against a wall may help to stabilize the lower spine alignments and can be used as a modification (2). Allowing patient to lean back slightly on a wedge may allow this position to be used with a patient who has tight hamstrings (3).

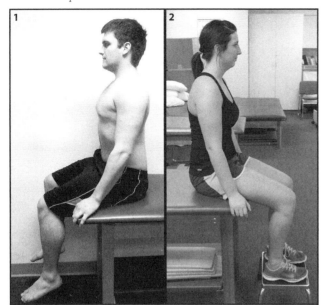

SHORT-SITTING/SITTING: Sitting can be performed with feet hanging off the edge of the table (1) or with feet planted on the ground or a stool (2). Allowing the patient's feet to be in contact with a surface is less demanding on balance and should be used for patients with poor sitting balance.

"W" SITTING: Generally, not a desirable position due to the pressure on the medial knee structures.

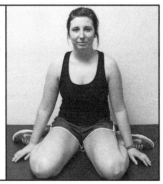

HALF-KNEELING: Tall-kneeling with one knee bent in front. This is a slightly more stable position than tall-kneeling.

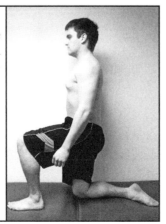

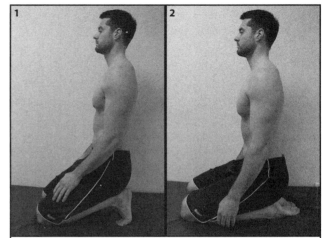

HEEL-SITTING: Sitting with heels underneath the buttocks and knees fully flexed. Feet can be dorsiflexed (1) or plantarflexed (2).

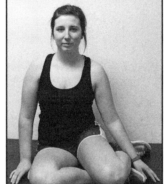

SIDE-SITTING: Sitting in heel-sit position with lower trunk and buttocks situated to one side of the lower legs.

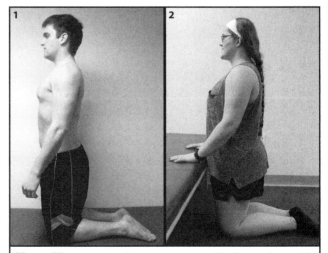

TALL-KNEELING: Erect posture with knees bent (1). Consider using a softer surface for the knees such as an exercise mat, pillows, or folded towels. Monitor neutral pelvic position, rectus femoris tightness may pull the pelvis into an anterior tilt and should be monitored and corrected. This is an effective position to work on trunk stability. Patient may hold onto a surface to increase stability when beginning this position (2).

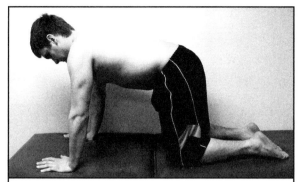

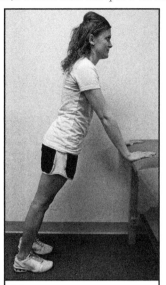

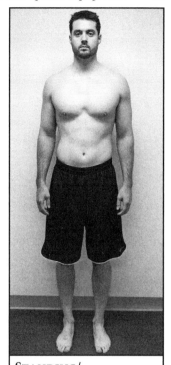

QUADRUPED: Prone on all fours. Wrist creases are placed directly below the shoulders and knees directly below the hips. This is a very active position throughout the body. Patient should distribute weight through the fingertips, pulling up and cupping through the palm of the hand to avoid excessive wrist pressures. Scapula should be depressed and retracted. The humeral head should not be jammed into the glenoid fossa. Encourage the patient to push away from the floor. Neutral spine is maintained by active contraction of the lower abdominal muscles and hips should be at 90 degrees of flexion. Patient should also maintain a slight chin tuck. This can be an uncomfortable position for the knees. Padding under the knees with towels or a pillow may relieve pressure and discomfort.

MODIFIED PLANTIGRADE: Standing with UE supported using table or counter. This position can be useful when needing UE for balance or to un-weight the LEs.

STANDING/ PLANTIGRADE: Fully erect posture with full weight on LEs.

1.07.2 EXERCISE BALL

An exercise ball is a useful tool in the clinic. The exercise ball has gone by many names: Swiss ball (TheraGear), physioball, stability ball, and fitness ball to name a few.

Where's the Evidence?

Utilization of the exercise ball has been shown to be more effective at stimulating the lumbar multifidi than a stable surface in patients with LBP. Use of a less stable surface can be quite effective in spinal rehabilitation (Scott, Vaughan, & Hall, 2015). Sedentary office workers have utilized them as an alternative to an office chair. A 2006 study by Gregory, Dunk, and Callaghan (2006) measured activation of lumbar stabilizers while sitting on an exercise ball as compared to an office chair and found slight improvements in muscle activity. Another study revealed that, although sitting on an exercise ball did result in more trunk motion and more variation in lumbar muscle activation, participants on the ball reported higher levels of discomfort and concluded that the ball did not significantly alter the manner in which a person sits and may even worsen their symptoms. Also, there was more spinal shrinkage noted than when sitting an office chair. The study concluded that the benefits of sitting on an exercise ball may not outweigh the disadvantages (Kingma & Dieën, 2009).

TABLE 1.07.2-A		
EXERCISE BALL DIAMETER	*PERSON'S HEIGHT (FEET/IN)*	*PERSON'S HEIGHT (CM)*
30 cm/12"	Less than 4'6"	Less than 137 cm
45 cm/18"	4'6" to 5'0"	137 to 152 cm
55 cm/22"	5'1" to 5'7"	155 to 170 cm
65 cm/26"	5'8" to 6'2"	171 to 188 cm
75 cm/30"	6'3" to 6'7"	188 to 200
85 cm/34'"	6'8" and taller	200+ cm

APPROPRIATE BALL SIZING:
Choose the appropriate size ball for the patient based on their height and the activity (Table A). If the patient is close to a cut-off height, try testing both sizes above and below and see which works best. The patient should be able to sit on the ball with the knees and hips at 90 degrees of flexion, thighs parallel to the ground and feet flat on the floor (A).

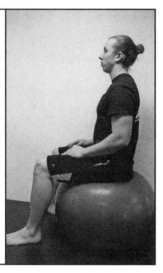

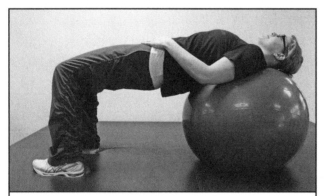

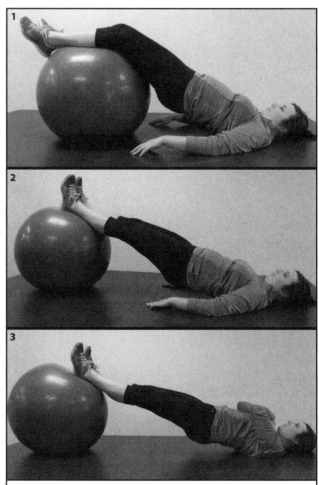

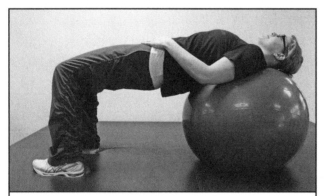

REVERSE BRIDGE/TABLE TOP ON BALL: Start in sitting and roll the ball down along the back towards the head until it is situated at the level of the scapulae. The knees should be at approximately 90 degrees. An active hip extension must occur to keep the hips in neutral. Feet and knees should be at the same distance apart as the hips (relatively inches or 15 cm distance between feet).

BRIDGE ON BALL: Patient is supine with the ball under the knees (1) or ankles (2). Active hip extension is needed to hold the hips in neutral position. Patient must control arching of the lower back with active abdominal control. Hands may be placed on the floor for added support. Activities in this position can be advanced by placing the hands across the chest (3).

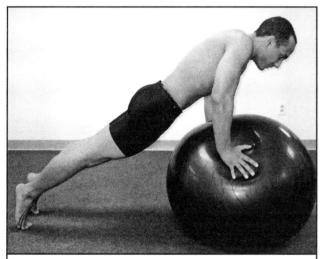

PRONE PLANK ON BALL: Patient is prone with knees on ball (1) or progression to ankles on ball (2). As with quadruped, patient should distribute weight through the fingertips, pulling up and cupping through the palm of the hand to avoid excessive wrist pressures. Scapula should be depressed and retracted. The humeral head should not be jammed into the glenoid fossa. Encourage the patient to push away from the floor. Neutral spine is maintained by active contraction of the lower abdominal muscles and hips should be at 90 degrees of flexion. Patient should also maintain a slight chin tuck.

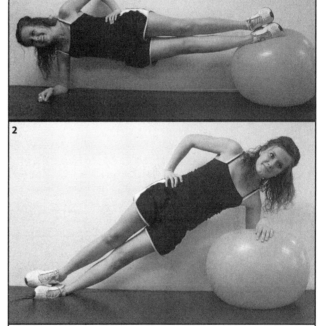

PRONE PUSH-UP ON BALL: This is a plank position in which the toes are in contact with the floor and the UEs are bearing weight on the ball. Hand positions can be modified depending on the exercise goal by varying distances apart. Active contraction through the scapular muscles is important in avoiding shoulder compression. Instructing the patient to push away from the ball is helpful.

SIDE PLANK ON BALL: The patient is in a side-lying position using the ball in three variations. The ball can be placed under the ankles (1) or the elbow (2). Advanced side plank can be done bearing weight on ball through hand and extended elbow (not shown).

1.07.3 EXTREMITIES

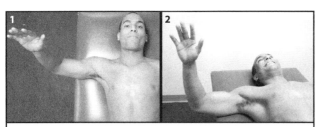

UPPER 90/90: Supine or standing, shoulder abducted 90 degrees and elbow flexed 90 degrees (1 and 2).

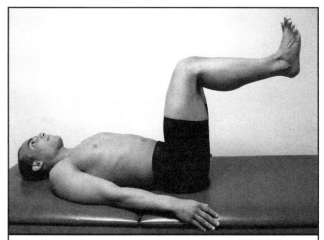

LOWER 90/90: Patient is lying supine with hips and knee both flexed 90 degrees.

1.07.4 PLANES OF MOVEMENT

The body can be divided into three main planes used to describe the direction of movements. The sagittal plane is a vertical plane passing through the standing body from front to back. The mid-sagittal, median or sternal plane splits the body into left and right halves. It is perpendicular to the coronal plane. Movement in this plane includes flexion and extension movements.

A coronal plane (also known as the frontal plane) is any vertical plane that divides the body into ventral and dorsal (belly/back or anterior/posterior) sections. It is perpendicular to the sagittal plane. Movement in this plane includes abduction and adduction movements.

The transverse plane (also called the horizontal plane, axial plane, or transaxial plane) is an imaginary plane that divides the body into superior and inferior parts. It is perpendicular to the coronal and sagittal planes. Movement in these planes included spinal, hip, and shoulder rotational movements and horizontal abduction/adduction.

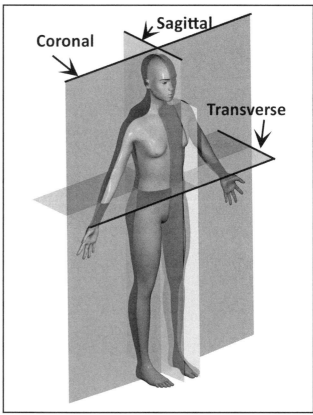

Figure 1.07.4. Planes of movement. (Reprinted from Richfield, D. (2014). Medical gallery of David Richfield. *WikiJournal of Medicine, 1*(2). doi:10.15347/wjm/2014.009. ISSN 2002-4436.)

1.07.5 RESISTANCE BANDS

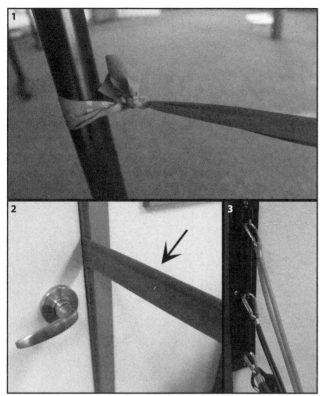

Figure A. Resistance band and tubing anchoring options.

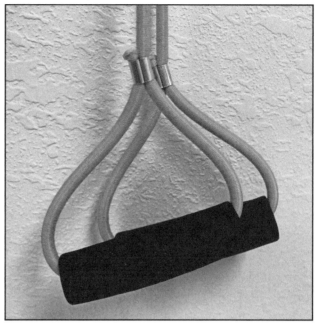

Figure B. Resistance tubing handles.

Resistance bands are large rubber bands that can be used to increase exercise intensity. There are several brands and colors to choose from depending on your preferences. Color-coding is used to identify the amount of resistance the band provides.

How to Use Safely

Resistance bands are a way to apply resistance and progress strengthening exercises. They can also be used for balance, cardiopulmonary, sport-specific and gait training. Patients can also use them at home, which allows for more options in developing a progressive home exercise program. There are some important things to consider when using resistance bands. Always inquire if the patient has any latex allergies. Most resistance bands offer a latex-free version. Before each use, examine the resistance band or tube to make sure there are no small tears, nicks, or punctures.

These can lead to the resistance band breaking during use. Also, the resistance band should not be stretched more than 3 times its resting length. For example, a 12-inch (30-cm) band should not be stretched to more than 36 inches (91 cm). This can help determine the length of band needed for any given exercise. The band should be wrapped around the hand at least once to avoid slipping out during use.

To affix the band to a stationary object for anchoring, make sure the object is heavy enough to resist the pull. A knot can be tied on one end and then placed in a doorway, closing the door to secure the band (A1 and A2). Bands may also come with attachments built in for use with wall units. These bands often have handles attached as well for ease in use (B). Bands should be positioned to allow for resistance through the full range when possible. Some exercises may require repositioning of the bands in the middle range to allow for optimal strengthening throughout the range. Most bands will come with detailed instructions for further information. Always read the safety precautions when using bands and tubes.

1.07.6 OTHER KEY TERMS AND ACRONYMS

<u>UNILATERAL</u>: On one side (right or left)

<u>BILATERAL</u>: On both sides (right and left)

<u>IPSILATERAL</u>: Relating the same side of the body; i.e. when contracting unilaterally the SCM performs ipsilateral lateral flexion.

<u>CONTRALATERAL</u>: Relating the opposite side of the body; i.e. when contracting unilaterally the SCM performs contralateral rotation.

AAROM—Active assistive range of motion

ACL—Anterior cruciate ligament

ADL—Activities of daily living

AIIS—Anterior inferior iliac spine

APT—Anterior pelvic tilt

AROM—Active range of motion

ASIS—Anterior superior iliac spine

ATFL—Anterior talofibular ligament

BAPS—Biomechanical ankle platform system

BPPV—Benign paroxysmal positional vertigo

BPTB—Bone-patellar tendon-bone

CPM—Continuous passive motion

CROM—Cervical range of motion

CTS—Carpal tunnel syndrome

DASH—Disability of arm, shoulder, and hand

DIP—Distal interphalangeal joints

DKTC—Double knee to chest

DOMS—Delayed onset muscle soreness

DVT—Deep vein thrombosis

EMG—Electromyography

FWB—Full weight bearing

GTO—Golgi tendon organs

ITB—Iliotibial band

LAQ—Long arc quad

LBP—Low back pain

LCS—Lower crossed syndrome

LE—Lower extremity

MCP—Metacarpophalangeal joints

MD—Doctor of medicine

MRI—Magnetic resonance imaging

MIVC—Maximal involuntary contraction

MVC—Maximal voluntary contraction

MWM—mobilization with movement

NDI—Neck disability index

NSAIDs—Nonsteroidal anti-inflammatory drug

PCL—Posterior cruciate ligament

PIP—Proximal interphalangeal joints

PNF—Proprioceptive neuromuscular facilitation

PPT—Posterior pelvic tilt

PROM—Passive range of motion

PWB—Partial weight bearing

QL—Quadratic Lumborum

RA—Rectus abdominis

RC—Rotator cuff

ROM—Range of motion

RNT—Reactive neuromuscular training

SAQ—Short arc quad

SCI—Spinal cord injuries

SCM—Sternocleidomastoid muscle

SIJ—Sacroiliac joint

SKTC—Single knee to chest

SLR—Straight leg raise

TA—Transverse abdominus

TFL—Tensor fascia latae

THA—Total hip arthroplasty

TKA—Total knee arthroplasty

TKE—Terminal knee extension

TOS—Thoracic outlet syndrome

TSA—Total shoulder arthroplasty

UBE—Upper body ergometer

UCL—Ulnar collateral ligament

UCS—Upper crossed syndrome

UE—Upper extremity

VAS—Visual analogue scale

VL—Vastus lateralis

VMO—Vastus medialis oblique

WBAT—Weight bearing as tolerated

1 RM—One-repetition maximum

REFERENCES

Gregory, D. E., Dunk, N. M., & Callaghan, J. P. (2006). Stability ball versus office chair: Comparison of muscle activation and lumbar spine posture during prolonged sitting. *Human Factors, 48*(1), 142-153.

Kingma, I., & van Dieën, J. H. (2009). Static and dynamic postural loadings during computer work in females: Sitting on an office chair versus sitting on an exercise ball. *Applied Ergonomics, 40*(2), 199-205.

Richfield, D. (2014). Human anatomy planes. *Wikimedia Commons.* Retrieved from https://upload.wikimedia.org/wikipedia/commons/7/79/Human_anatomy_planes.jpg

Scott, I. R., Vaughan, A. R., & Hall, J. (2015). Swiss ball enhances lumbar multifidus activity in chronic low back pain. *Physical Therapy in Sport, 16*(1), 40-44.

Chapter 2
CERVICAL EXERCISES

Bryan E. *The Comprehensive Manual of Therapeutic Exercises:*
Orthopedic and General Conditions (pp 27-54).

Section 2.01

CERVICAL RANGE OF MOTION

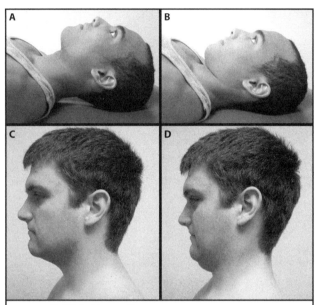

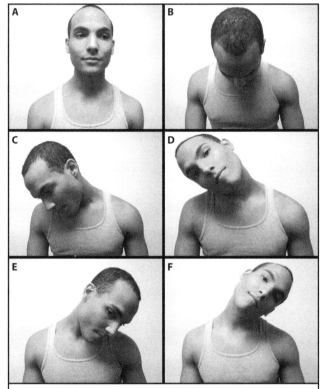

2.01.1 ROM: CHIN TUCK

<u>POSITION</u>: Supine progressing to seated; supine is the best place to start with patients with severe weakness in the deep neck flexors.

<u>TARGETS</u>: Stretch upper cervical extensors, correct forward head posture, recruit deep neck flexors

<u>INSTRUCTION</u>: In supine, instruct patient to flatten neck, decreasing the space between neck and table making a double chin (A and B). Therapist may place hand underneath the neck and instruct patient to "smash" the therapist's hand. If patient is seated, check for proper posture, depression, and retraction of the scapula before beginning. Patient may sit with back and shoulders against a wall if this is difficult. In seated the instructions are the same. Use the "smash" my hand trick if patient is seated against a wall. Patient should keep the eyes level when tucking the chin (C and D).

<u>SUBSTITUTIONS</u>: Monitor patient's head to avoid looking down while keeping the eyes level; pushing back with the head will result in recruitment of the neck extensors which is not the goal; eyes should be kept level, looking up or down is incorrect.

<u>PARAMETERS</u>: Hold for 1 to 2 seconds, 10 to 30 repetitions, 1 to 3 times per day; can be increased to hourly.

2.01.2 ROM: CERVICAL ANTERIOR SEMICIRCLES

<u>POSITION</u>: Seated

<u>TARGETS</u>: Lubricates facet and intervertebral joints, facet opening

<u>INSTRUCTION</u>: Check for proper posture, depression, and retraction of the scapula before beginning (**2.01.5**). Instruct patient to look down, flexing the neck (A and B). Have the patient roll right ear toward the right shoulder (C and D), followed by the left ear to the left shoulder while maintaining forward flexion of the neck (E and F). Have the patient keep chin tucked in throughout the ROM.

<u>SUBSTITUTIONS</u>: Avoid jutting the chin out, slouching, shoulder shrug

<u>PARAMETERS</u>: Move slowly and rhythmically, 10 to 30 repetitions, 1 to 3 times per day

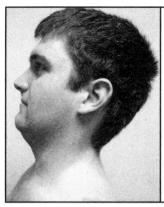

2.01.3 ROM: CHIN TUCK WITH CERVICAL EXTENSION

POSITION: Seated

TARGETS: Lower cervical and upper thoracic mobilization for extension

INSTRUCTION: Check for proper posture, depression and retraction of the scapula before beginning. Instruct patient to tuck the chin as shown in **2.01.1-D**. Maintaining this chin tucked position, instruct the patient to extend neck, looking up towards the ceiling. A double chin should be maintained during the entire movement. Patient should proceed until they feel this in the lower neck and upper thoracic spine.

SUBSTITUTIONS: Avoid jutting the chin out, slouching, posterior trunk leaning

PARAMETERS: Move slowly and rhythmically, 10 to 30 repetitions, 1 to 3 times per day

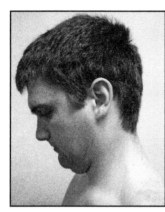

2.01.4 ROM: CHIN TUCK WITH CERVICAL FLEXION

POSITION: Seated

TARGETS: Lower cervical and upper thoracic mobilization for flexion

INSTRUCTION: Check for proper posture, depression and retraction of the scapula before beginning. Instruct patient to tuck the chin as shown in **2.01.1-D**. Maintaining this chin tucked position, instruct the patient to flex neck, looking down towards chest. A double chin should be maintained during the entire movement. Patient should proceed until they feel this in the lower neck and upper thoracic spine.

SUBSTITUTIONS: Avoid jutting the chin out, slouching, shoulder shrug

PARAMETERS: Move slowly and rhythmically, 10 to 30 repetitions, 1 to 3 times per day

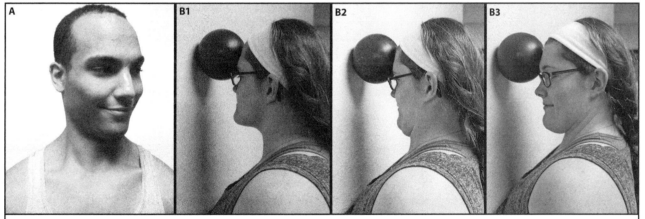

2.01.5 ROM: CHIN TUCK WITH CERVICAL ROTATION

POSITION: Supine, seated (with and without ball); starting in supine is recommended for more acute neck injuries.

TARGETS: Lubricates facet and intervertebral joints of C1 to C7; targets upper cervical primarily C1 to C2 where most rotation occurs.

INSTRUCTION: Instruct patient to tuck the chin as shown in **2.01.1-D**. Maintaining this chin tucked position, instruct the patient to rotate to the right, bringing the chin toward the right shoulder. Repeat to the other side. A double chin should be maintained during the entire movement (A). A ball placed on a wall at forehead height can be used to add support and maintain proper alignment. The ball rolls along from temple to forehead to temple while rotating towards each side (B1 through B3).

SUBSTITUTIONS: Avoid jutting the chin out, slouching, shoulder elevation or forward movement

PARAMETERS: Move slowly and rhythmically, 10 to 30 repetitions, 1 to 3 times per day

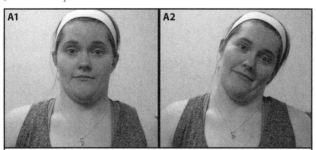

2.01.6 ROM: Chin Tuck With Cervical Lateral Flexion

<u>Position</u>: Supine, seated; starting in supine is recommended for more acute neck injuries.

<u>Targets</u>: Lubricates facet and intervertebral joints of C1 through C7; opens facets on opposite side.

<u>Instruction</u>: Check for proper posture, depression and retraction of the scapula before beginning. Instruct patient to tuck the chin as shown in **2.01.1-D**. Maintaining this chin tucked position, instruct the patient to side bend, head bringing the right ear to the right shoulder and repeat to the other side. A double chin should be maintained during the entire movement (A1 and A2).

<u>Substitutions</u>: Avoid jutting the chin out, slouching, posterior trunk leaning

<u>Parameters</u>: Move slowly and rhythmically, 10 to 30 repetitions, 1 to 3 times per day

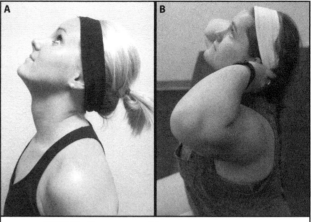

2.01.7 ROM: Cervical Extension

<u>Position</u>: Seated with and without UE support; initially the patient may want to self-assist in the return motion for acute injuries.

<u>Targets</u>: Cervical spine mobility

<u>Instruction</u>: Check for proper posture, depression and retraction of the scapula before beginning. Instruct the patient to extend neck and look up at the ceiling, allowing the chin to come up toward the ceiling (A). If the patient has severe weakness or pain in the anterior cervical muscles, have the patient place the hands behind the head, locking the fingers and cradling the posterior head in palms (B). Instruct patient to keep the shoulders and upper trapezius relaxed.

<u>Substitutions</u>: Posterior trunk lean, loss of proper posture in shoulders and thoracic spine; if they are using the arms for support, pay close attention to avoid shrugging the shoulders during the activity.

<u>Parameters</u>: Move slowly and rhythmically, 10 to 30 repetitions, 1 to 3 times per day

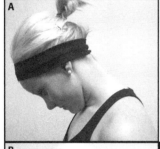

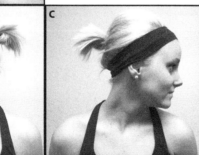

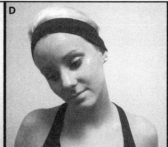

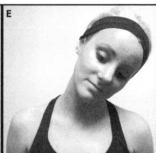

2.01.8 ROM: Cervical Flexion, Rotation, and Lateral Flexion

<u>Position</u>: Seated; starting in supine for rotation and lateral flexion is recommended for more acute neck injuries; flexion is seated.

<u>Targets</u>: Lubricates facet and intervertebral joints of C1 through C7

<u>Instruction</u>: Check for proper posture, depression and retraction of the scapula before beginning. Instruct patient to look down, allowing chin to come towards the chest (A). Follow with patient, then looking over each shoulder (B and C) and then bringing the ear towards each shoulder (D and E).

<u>Substitutions</u>: Avoid jutting the chin out, slouching, shoulder elevation or forward movement

<u>Parameters</u>: Move slowly and rhythmically, 10 to 30 repetitions, 1 to 3 times per day

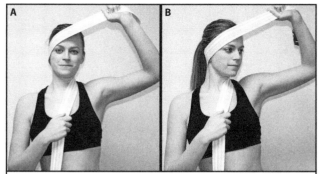

2.01.9 ROM: CERVICAL ROTATION, SELF-ASSISTED WITH STRAP

POSITION: Seated

TARGETS: Lubricates facet and intervertebral joints of C1 through C7; allows patient to apply assistance/overpressure to increase ROM.

INSTRUCTION: Check for proper posture, depression and retraction of the scapula and ear should be directly over the acromion process for cervical alignment. Cue patient to perform a slight chin tuck to ensure this. Position the strap or belt as shown (A). The patient will pull inferiorly on one end of the strap and pull across the ear and temple with the other end rotating the head towards the shoulder (B). Switch hands and repeat to the opposite side.

SUBSTITUTIONS: Avoid jutting the chin out, slouching, shoulder shrug

PARAMETERS: Move slowly and rhythmically, 5 to 10 repetitions; allow the patient to hold at the end of the range a few seconds as tolerated, 1 to 3 times per day.

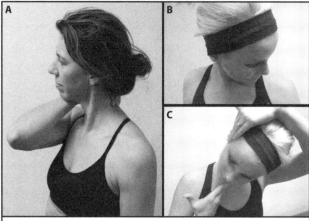

2.01.10 ROM: CERVICAL ATLANTO-AXIAL SELF-MOBILIZATION IN NEUTRAL AND WITH FLEXION

POSITION: Seated

TARGETS: Upper cervical spine mobility

INSTRUCTION: In seated, check for proper posture, depression, and retraction of the scapula before beginning. Patient may sit with back and shoulders against a wall if this is difficult. *In neutral*: Have the patient hold the lower spine as shown as they slowly rotate the head, looking over the forearm until a gentle stretch is felt. Repeat to other side (A). *In flexion*: Have the patient flex the neck as far as they can comfortably as they bring the chin towards the chest. Slowly rotate the chin towards the right and up towards the ceiling (B). Repeat to the left. Primary focus should be towards the direction of the restriction. Overpressure may be lightly applied by the patient's use of hands (C).

SUBSTITUTIONS: Slouching, shoulder shrug, thoracic rotation

PARAMETERS: Hold for 1 to 10 seconds, 5 to 10 repetitions, 3 times per day

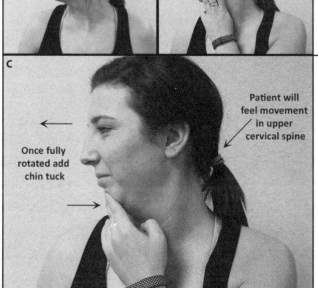

Once fully rotated add chin tuck

Patient will feel movement in upper cervical spine

2.01.11 ROM: CERVICAL ATLANTO-OCCIPITAL SELF-MOBILIZATION WITH CHIN TUCK

POSITION: Seated

TARGETS: Upper cervical spine mobility

INSTRUCTION: Check for proper posture, depression and retraction of the scapula before beginning. Have the patient rotate the neck fully with slight overpressure using the fingertips as shown. At the end of the range, have the patient perform a chin tuck until feeling a stretch in the opposite upper cervical region (A through C).

SUBSTITUTIONS: Slouching, shoulder shrug, thoracic rotation

PARAMETERS: Hold for 1 to 10 seconds, 5 to 10 repetitions, 3 times per day

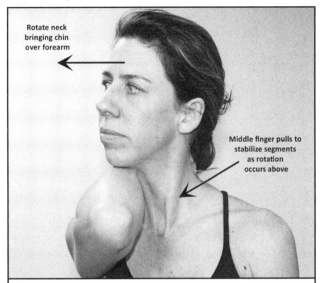

Rotate neck bringing chin over forearm

Middle finger pulls to stabilize segments as rotation occurs above

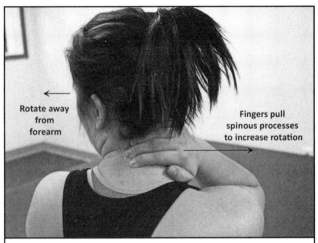

Rotate away from forearm

Fingers pull spinous processes to increase rotation

2.01.12 ROM: Cervical Facet Opening, Self-Mobilization

POSITION: Seated

TARGETS: Mid- to lower-cervical mobilization and lubrication of facet joints; facet capsule stretching.

INSTRUCTION: Check for proper posture, depression and retraction of the scapula before beginning. Have patient reach across neck as shown, placing the fingers across the posterior aspect of the neck. Have the patient rotate the head towards the *same*-side shoulder and instruct the patient to stabilize one segment of the cervical spine with middle finger as they rotate the segment above. Therapist may guide patient as to which segment needs to be mobilized.

SUBSTITUTIONS: Slouching, shoulder shrug, thoracic rotation

PARAMETERS: Hold for 1 to 10 seconds, 5 to 10 repetitions, 3 times per day

2.01.13 ROM: Cervical Facet Closing, Self-Mobilization

POSITION: Seated

TARGETS: Mid- to lower-cervical mobilization and lubrication of facet joints; facet capsule stretching.

INSTRUCTION: Check for proper posture, depression and retraction of the scapula before beginning. Have patient reach across neck as shown, placing the fingers across the posterior aspect of the neck. Have the patient rotate the head towards the *opposite*-side shoulder and instruct the patient to pull with the middle finger at the cervical spine to increase the rotation in the cervical spine.

SUBSTITUTIONS: Slouching, shoulder shrug, thoracic rotation

PARAMETERS: Hold for 1 to 10 seconds, 5 to 10 repetitions, 3 times per day

2.01.14 ROM: Self-Cervical Traction, Towel Roll

POSITION: Seated

TARGETS: Lower cervical and upper thoracic mobilization for extension

INSTRUCTION: Check for proper posture, depression and retraction of the scapula before beginning. Have patient use a towel and wrap it at the base of the head just below the occiput. The patient should look up just slightly, keeping the upper trapezius relaxed, use the triceps to pull the head up while simultaneously pulling down on the scapula using the lower trapezius.

SUBSTITUTIONS: Pay close attention to the unwanted contraction of the upper trap as it will prohibit traction from occurring.

PARAMETERS: Pull for 10 seconds, repeat 5 to 10 repetitions, 2 to 3 times per day as needed for pain, headache

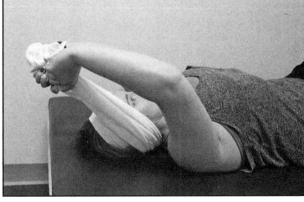

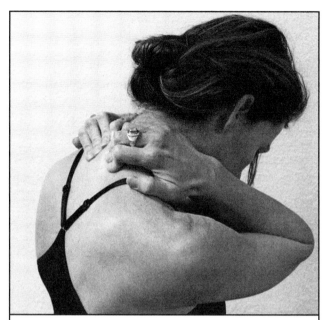

2.01.15 ROM: Cervicothoracic Flexion and Extension, Self-Mobilization

<u>Position</u>: Seated

<u>Targets</u>: Lower cervical and upper thoracic mobilization

<u>Instruction</u>: Check for proper posture, depression and retraction of the scapula before beginning. Instruct patient to place ring and middle fingers below the most prominent vertebra (generally C7 or T1). Patient flexes the neck while pulling upward with the fingers at the base of the neck. Patient should proceed until they feel this in the lower neck and upper thoracic spine.

<u>Substitutions</u>: Avoid slouching and lumbar extension; abdominals stay engaged to maintain neutral pelvis.

<u>Parameters</u>: Hold end range 3 to 5 seconds, repeat 5 to 10 repetitions, 2 to 3 times per day

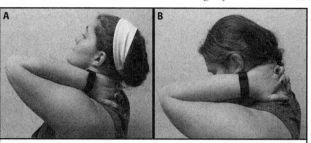

2.01.16 ROM: Upper Cervical Flexion and Extension, Nodding With Hands Clasped Behind Neck

<u>Position</u>: Seated

<u>Targets</u>: Upper cervical atlanto-occipital primarily

<u>Instruction</u>: Check for proper posture, depression and retraction of the scapula before beginning. Have the patient interlock the four fingers of both hands behind the neck to minimize movement below C2 (A). Have the patient flex forward in the upper cervical region only and then extend over the locked hands for an upper cervical nodding motion (B). Hold at the end of range for several seconds as tolerated.

<u>Substitutions</u>: Avoid jutting the chin out, slouching, posterior trunk leaning

<u>Parameters</u>: Move slowly and rhythmically, hold end range 3 to 5 seconds, repeat 5 to 20 repetitions, 2 to 3 times per day

2.01.17 ROM: Cervical Neural Self-Mobilization/Nerve Glides/Nerve Flossing

<u>Position</u>: Seated

<u>Targets</u>: Improves and maintains nerve root mobility in the intervertebral foramen

<u>Instruction</u>: Refer to **5.17**

Section 2.02

CERVICAL STRETCHING

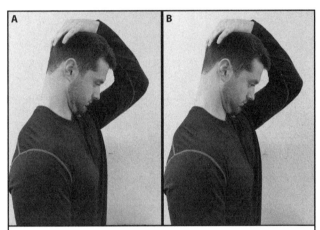

2.02.1 STRETCH: SUBOCCIPITAL MUSCLE

POSITION: Seated

TARGETS: Stretch upper cervical and suboccipital extensors

INSTRUCTION: In seated with proper posture, depression, and retraction of the scapula before beginning, instruct patient to tuck the chin in towards superior chest (sternal notch), adding slight overpressure at the chin to increase the chin tuck (A). Patient uses other hand to pull forward from the top of the head, causing a stretching sensation in the upper cervical region (B). A slight rotation to one side or another will target the opposite site.

SUBSTITUTIONS: Slouching, loss of chin tuck, tensing the upper trapezius

PARAMETERS: Hold for 15 to 30 seconds, 3 to 5 repetitions, 1 to 3 times per day

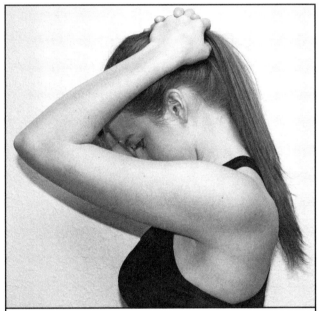

2.02.2 STRETCH: SELF-ASSISTED CERVICAL FLEXION, HANDS BEHIND HEAD

POSITION: Seated

TARGETS: Stretch cervical extensors: splenius cervicis, splenius capitis, semispinalis capitis, semispinalis cervicis, longissimus capitis, longissimus cervicis, multifidus cervicis, iliocostalis cervicis, spinalis cervicis

INSTRUCTION: Check for proper posture, depression and retraction of the scapula before beginning. Instruct patient to look down, flexing the neck while patient places hands behind the head, locking fingers. Patient should pull down on the head gently until a stretch is felt in the posterior neck.

SUBSTITUTIONS: Avoid jutting the chin out, slouching, shoulder shrugging

PARAMETERS: Hold for 15 to 30 seconds, 3 to 5 repetitions, 1 to 3 times per day

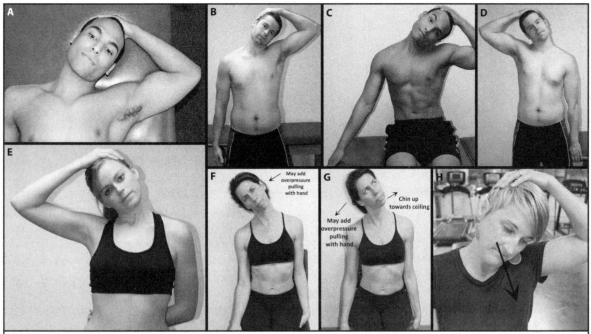

2.02.3 STRETCH: SELF-ASSISTED CERVICAL LATERAL FLEXION

<u>POSITION</u>: Supine, seated, standing with variations in arm position

<u>TARGETS</u>: Stretch upper trapezius

<u>INSTRUCTION</u>: *Supine* should be utilized first for more acute patients. With one arm at side, have the patient reach over the head with the other arm as shown and pull ear towards the shoulder until a stretch is felt in the contralateral upper trapezius (A). In *seated* or *standing*, the affected side arm can be in the lap, reaching towards the floor (B), holding onto a chair or table edge (C and D), behind the back (E), or tucked under the thigh (F) to enhance the pull down of the affected shoulder and increase the stretch. Slight rotation of the chin towards the ceiling targets the clavicular portion (G) whereas slight rotation down towards the axillary region targets the scapular portion (H). Have the patient perform these additional motions depending on where the stretch is felt to be most effective.

<u>SUBSTITUTIONS</u>: Avoid jutting the chin out, slouching, lateral trunk leaning, shrugging

<u>PARAMETERS</u>: Hold for 15 to 30 seconds, 3 to 5 repetitions, 1 to 3 times per day

Where's the Evidence?

Yoo (2013) monitored EMG activity of muscles during shoulder elevation in patients with forward shoulder posture. The results showed a significant increase in activation of the upper trapezius and the clavicular portion of the pectoralis major in symptomatic patients as compared to asymptomatic patients. The activity of the middle trapezius and serratus anterior in the symptomatic group were also significantly decreased compared with those in the asymptomatic group.

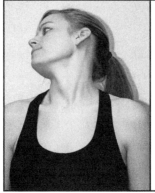

2.02.4 STRETCH: CERVICAL EXTENSION AND ROTATION

<u>POSITION</u>: Seated

<u>TARGETS</u>: Stretch anterior, middle, and posterior scalenes

<u>INSTRUCTION</u>: In seated with proper posture, depression and retraction of the scapula before beginning, instruct patient to gently extend neck to a comfortable, slight pulling sensation on the opposite side of the neck, followed by rotating the chin upwards towards the ceiling until a stretch in felt in the scalenes region just above the mid-clavicle and anterolateral neck. An active scapular retraction and depression will increase the stretch. The patient may also use hand to pull down on the clavicle to increase the stretch.

<u>SUBSTITUTIONS</u>: Slouching, tensing the upper trapezius

<u>PARAMETERS</u>: Hold for 15 to 30 seconds, 3 to 5 repetitions, 1 to 3 times per day

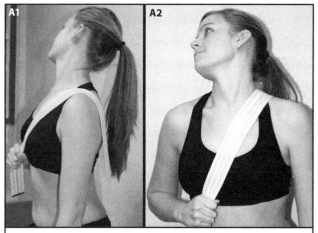

2.02.5 Stretch: Cervical Rotation and Extension, First Rib Stabilization With Belt/Strap

Position: Seated

Targets: Stretch anterior, middle, and posterior scalenes with first rib depression

Instruction: In seated with proper posture, depression and retraction of the scapula before beginning, have the patient place a belt, towel, or sheet across the clavicle and first rib region. Patient may sit on one end of the belt and pull down on the belt in the front with the hand on the opposite side (1). Have the patient then extend the neck and rotate the chin upwards towards the ceiling until a stretch is felt in the scalenes region just above the mid-clavicle and anterolateral neck (2). By depressing the first two ribs, the scalenes are pulled from both origin and insertion.

Substitutions: Slouching, loss of chin tuck, tensing the upper trapezius

Parameters: Hold for 15 to 30 seconds, 3 to 5 repetitions, 1 to 3 times per day

2.02.7 Stretch: Cervical Flexion and Rotation

Position: Seated or standing

Targets: Stretch levator scapula

Instruction: Check for proper posture, depression and retraction of the scapula before beginning. Instruct patient to look down, flexing the neck, while patient places opposite hand behind the head and pull the head gently bringing the nose down towards the opposite hip. The arm can be behind the back (A), behind the neck (B), or down by side or in standing grasping a table or chair seat (C and D). Have the patient place the arm behind the back or grasp a chair or table to help stabilize the scapula for an improved stretch.

Substitutions: Avoid jutting the chin out, slouching, shoulder shrugging; avoid upper trapezius contraction when placing the hand behind the neck if using that variation.

Parameters: Hold for 15 to 30 seconds, 3 to 5 repetitions, 1 to 3 times per day

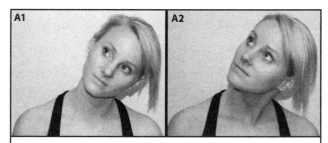

2.02.6 Stretch: Cervical Lateral Flexion and Contralateral Rotation

Position: Seated

Targets: Stretch SCM

Instruction: In seated with proper posture, depression and retraction of the scapula before beginning, instruct patient to gently grasp top of head and pull the ear towards the shoulder. Once patient reaches a slight pulling sensation on the opposite side, patient rotates the chin upwards towards the ceiling until a stretch is felt in the scalenes region just above the mid clavicle and anterolateral neck (A1 and A2).

Substitutions: Slouching, loss of chin tuck, tensing the upper trapezius

Parameters: Hold for 15 to 30 seconds, 3 to 5 repetitions, 1 to 3 times per day

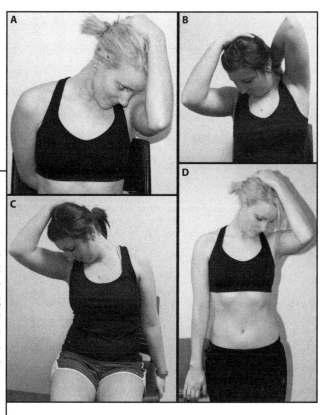

Reference

Yoo, W. (2013). Comparison of shoulder muscles activation for shoulder abduction between forward shoulder posture and asymptomatic persons. *Journal of Physical Therapy Science, 25*(7), 815-816.

Section 2.03

CERVICAL STRENGTHENING

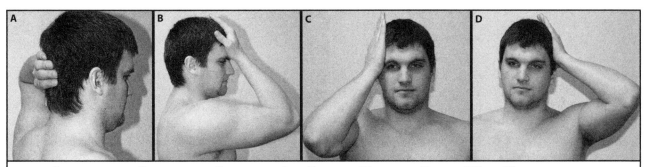

2.03.1 STRENGTHEN: ISOMETRIC; CERVICAL ALL PLANES NEUTRAL RESIST WITH HAND

<u>POSITION</u>: Seated

<u>TARGETS</u>: Strengthening of the cervical muscles all planes

<u>INSTRUCTION</u>: With proper posture, depression, and retraction of the scapula before beginning, the patient should maintain a slight chin tuck for proper cervical alignment. *Extension*: Place the fingertips behind the head (A). *Flexion*: Place the fingertips on the forehead (B). *Rotation*: Place the fingertips on the temporal bone slightly above and lateral to the eyebrow (C). *Lateral flexion*: Place the fingertips at the temporal bone above the ear. For each exercise, patient's neck should be in neutral alignment (D). Instruct the patient to move head towards the direction of the hand for each motion, but do not allow any movement by resisting with the hand. For more acute patients, have patient contract only slightly at less than 25% of maximum strength. For subacute and chronic patients, instruct patient to push at 50% to 75% of maximum strength. It is very important that the contraction is ramped up to the target intensity for 1 to 2 seconds and ramped down at the end of each repetition for 1 to 2 seconds. This will assist in preventing injury. Watch carefully that shoulder muscles are not tensing particularly the upper trapezius.

<u>SUBSTITUTIONS</u>: Slouching, loss of chin tuck, tensing the upper trapezius

<u>PARAMETERS</u>: Hold for 6 to 10 seconds, 1 to 3 sets, 8 to 12 repetitions with 1 to 2 second ramp up and down, 1 time per day or every other day

2.03.2 STRENGTHEN: ISOMETRIC; CERVICAL ALL PLANES MULTI-POSITIONAL RESIST WITH HAND

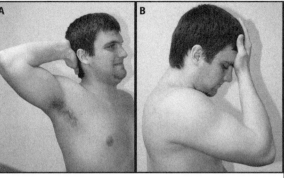

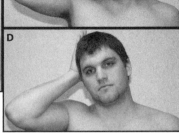

POSITION: Seated

TARGETS: Strengthening of the cervical muscles all planes

INSTRUCTION: With proper posture, depression, and retraction of the scapula before beginning, the patient should maintain a slight chin tuck for proper cervical alignment. *Extension*: Patient extends neck to desired range for strengthening. Patient places the fingertips behind the head and resists isometric extension (A). *Flexion*: Patient flexes neck to desired range for strengthening. Patient places the palm at the forehead and resists isometric flexion (B). *Rotation*: Patient rotates neck to desired range for strengthening. Patient places the palm on the temporal bone slightly above and lateral to the eyebrow and resists isometric rotation (C). *Lateral flexion*: Patient side bends neck to desired range for strengthening. Patient places the palm on the temporal bone just above the ear and resists isometric side-bending (D). For each motion, you will have the patient's neck in differing degrees of the motion. *Avoid isometrics at the end range of any motion in the neck staying approximately 15% away from the end of available range.* Instruct the patient to move head towards the direction of the hand for each motion, but not to allow any movement by resisting with the hand. For more acute patients, have patient contract only slightly at less than 25% of maximum strength. For subacute and chronic patients, instruct patient to push at 50% to 75% of maximum strength. It is very important that the contraction is ramped up to the target intensity for 1 to 2 seconds and ramped down at the end of each repetition 1 to 2 seconds. This will assist in preventing injury. Watch carefully that shoulder muscles are not tensing particularly the upper trapezius.

PARAMETERS: Hold for 6 to 10 seconds, 1 to 3 sets, 8 to 12 repetitions with 1 to 2 second ramp up and down, 1 time per day or every other day

2.03.3 STRENGTHEN: ISOMETRIC; CERVICAL BI-PLANAR NEUTRAL RESIST WITH BALL ON WALL

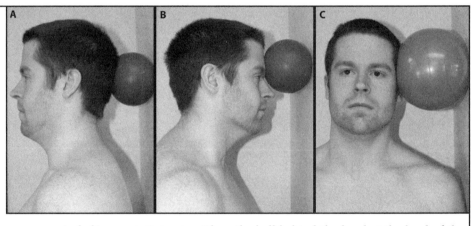

POSITION: Seated

TARGETS: Strengthening of the cervical muscles sagittal and transverse planes

INSTRUCTION: With proper posture, depression, and retraction of the scapula before beginning, the patient should maintain a slight chin tuck for proper cervical alignment. *Extension*: Place the ball behind the head at the level of the occipital protuberance (A). *Flexion*: Place the ball at the forehead (B). *Rotation*: Place the ball at the temporal bone slightly above and lateral to the eyebrow (C). *Do not do lateral flexion with the ball.* The hand technique works better as the ball will slide down the wall. Instruct the patient to move head towards the direction of the ball for each motion, but not to allow any movement by resisting with the hand. For more acute patients, have patient contract only slightly at less than 25% of maximum strength. For subacute and chronic patients, instruct patient to push at 50% to 75% of maximum strength. It is very important the contraction is ramped up to the target intensity for 1 to 2 seconds and ramped down at the end of each repetition 1 to 2 seconds. This will assist in preventing injury. Watch carefully that shoulder muscles are not tensing, particularly the upper trapezius. Use of the ball eliminates the need to have the arm held up and can work better for patients who have difficulties keeping the upper trapezius silent.

SUBSTITUTIONS: Slouching, loss of chin tuck, tensing the upper trapezius

PARAMETERS: Hold for 6 to 10 seconds, 1 to 3 sets, 8 to 12 repetitions with 1 to 2 second ramp up and down, 1 time per day or every other day

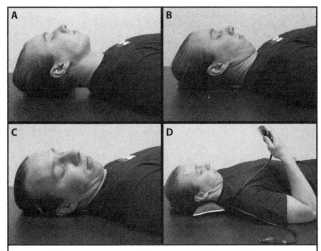

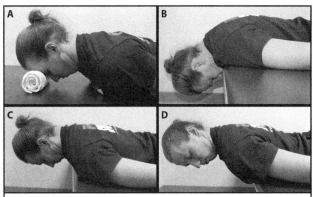

2.03.4 Strengthen: Isotonic; Chin Tuck

<u>Position</u>: Supine

<u>Targets</u>: Strengthening of the deep neck flexors, also called the prevertebrals (longus capitis, longus colli primarily), also activates scalenes and two of the suboccipital muscles (rectus capitis anterior and rectus capitis lateralis)

<u>Instruction</u>: With the arms either at the sides, instruct patient to flatten the curve in neck, bringing the chin inwards towards the neck, making a double chin. Start in the neutral position to utilize both sides of the deep neck flexors (A and B). Adding slight rotation in the advanced stage increases the resistance on one side of the neck and makes the exercise more targeted to one side or the other (C). Use of a blood pressure cuff can help the patient monitor and maintain pressure. Place the cuff under the cervical spine, not the head (D).

<u>Substitutions</u>: Jutting the chin out, lifting the head

<u>Parameters</u>: 1 to 3 sets, 8 to 12 repetitions, 1 to 2 times per day

2.03.5 Strengthen: Isotonic; Chin Tuck Neutral (Beginner) and With Slight Rotation (Advanced), Forehead on Towel Roll (Beginner) and Head off Bed (Advanced)

<u>Position</u>: Prone

<u>Targets</u>: Strengthening of the deep neck flexors, also called the prevertebrals (longus capitis, longus colli primarily), also activates scalenes and two of the suboccipital muscles (rectus capitis anterior and rectus capitis lateralis)

<u>Instruction</u>: With the head either on a towel (beginner) (A) or off the edge of the bed (advanced) (B and C) and the arms either at the sides or hanging off the edge of the bed depending on comfort, instruct patient to flatten the curve in neck, bringing the chin inwards towards the neck making a double chin. Start in the neutral position to utilize both sides of the deep neck flexors. Adding slight rotation in the advanced stage increases the resistance on one side of the neck and makes the exercise more targeted to one side or the other (D).

<u>Substitutions</u>: Slouching, loss of chin tuck, tensing the upper trapezius

<u>Parameters</u>: 1 to 3 sets, 8 to 12 repetitions, 1 time per day or every other day

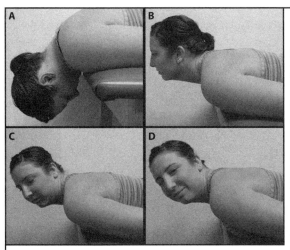

2.03.6 Strengthen: Isotonic; Cervical Extension and Extension With Rotation, Head and Shoulders off Edge of Table (Cervical Extensors)

<u>Position</u>: Prone

<u>Targets</u>: Strengthening cervical extensors (splenius capitis, splenius cervicis, semispinalis capitis, semispinalis cervicis) and erector spinae group (cervical region); this adds a slight sternal lift to activate superior thoracic extensors.

<u>Instruction</u>: With the table end at mid-sternal level, head hanging off the edge of the bed and the arms either at the sides or hanging off the edge of the bed, instruct patient to lift the head up, bringing the top of the head towards the ceiling (A and B). Adding slight rotation (C) and full rotation (D) in the advanced stage increases the resistance on one side of the neck and makes the exercise more targeted to one side or the other.

<u>Substitutions</u>: Tensing the upper trapezius (shrugging shoulders), lifting sternum off of bed

<u>Parameters</u>: 1 to 3 sets, 8 to 12 repetitions, 1 time per day or every other day

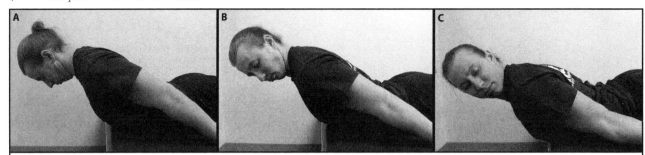

2.03.7 STRENGTHEN: ISOTONIC; LOWER NECK/THORACIC EXTENSION, HEAD LIFT, 5 POSITIONS (CERVICAL EXTENSORS)

POSITION: Prone

TARGETS: Strengthening cervical extensors (splenius capitis, splenius cervicis, semispinalis capitis, semispinalis cervicis) and erector spinae group (cervical and upper thoracic region)

INSTRUCTION: With the table end at mid-sternal level, head hanging off the edge of the bed and arms at the sides, instruct patient to chin tuck first and lift the head and upper sternum while retracting scapula back and down. Chin should stay tucked through the entire movement (A). Positions 2 and 3 are with slight rotation right and left and repeat movement (B). Positions 4 and 5 are with full rotation right and left and repeat movement (C). Allowing a slight lift of the upper sternum encourages upper thoracic extension with the cervical movement.

SUBSTITUTIONS: Tensing the upper trapezius (shrugging shoulders), lower sternum lift and ribs substituting with lower back extensors

PARAMETERS: 1 to 3 sets, 8 to 12 repetitions, 1 time per day or every other day

2.03.8 STRENGTHEN: ISOTONIC; CHIN TUCK CERVICAL FLEXION WITH HEAD LIFT (DEEP NECK FLEXORS)

POSITION: Supine

TARGETS: Strengthening cervical deep neck flexors (longus colli and longus capitis), also activates scalenes, SCM, and two of the suboccipital muscles (rectus capitis anterior and rectus capitis lateralis)

INSTRUCTION: With arms lying along sides, instruct patient to chin tuck first (this initiates craniocervical flexion), followed by lifting the head off the table, clearing the occiput. Chin tuck must be maintained throughout the movement. The patient should hold until fatigue.

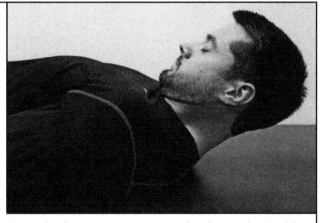

SUBSTITUTIONS: Using only superficial cervical flexors, which results from not maintaining the chin tuck, shoulders should be relaxed. Patients tend to hold the breath, encourage patient to continue to breathe.

PARAMETERS: 1 to 2 sets, 8 to 12 repetitions, 1 time per day or every other day

Where's the Evidence?

Jull, O'Leary, and Falla (2008) identified that patients with neck pain disorders displayed reduced isometric endurance of the deep cervical flexors. In 2012, Falla, O'Leary, Farina, and Jull found that specific training of the deep cervical flexors improved EMG amplitude of these muscles and reduced neck pain. Cervical flexion and craniocervical flexion strengthening exercises have been shown to significantly improve craniocervical flexor muscle performance (O' Leary, Jull, Kim, & Vincenzio, 2007). Falla, Jull, Russell, Vincenzio, and Hodges (2007) also found that people with chronic neck pain demonstrate a reduced ability to maintain an upright posture when distracted. Following intervention with an exercise program targeted at training the craniocervical flexor muscles, subjects with neck pain demonstrated an improved ability to maintain a neutral cervical posture during prolonged sitting.

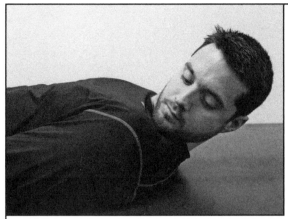

2.03.9 STRENGTHEN: CERVICAL FLEXION WITH ROTATION (STERNOCLEIDOMASTOID)

POSITION: Supine

TARGETS: Strengthening contralateral SCM

INSTRUCTION: With arms in the 90/90 position to decrease substitution with the erector spinae, instruct patient to rotate the head as far as is comfortable. The patient then lifts the head off of the table. Chin should stay slightly tucked through the entire movement to protect the cervical spine. Rotation to one side strengthens the SCM on the contralateral side. Repeat on other side. If the patient has shoulder discomfort or tingling in the hands, arms can be at the sides. Resistance (manual, resistance band or a cuff weight) can be applied as the patient advances.

SUBSTITUTIONS: Tensing the upper trapezius (shrugging shoulders), jutting the chin out, lifting shoulders off table

PARAMETERS: 1 to 3 sets, 8 to 12 repetitions, 1 time per day or every other day

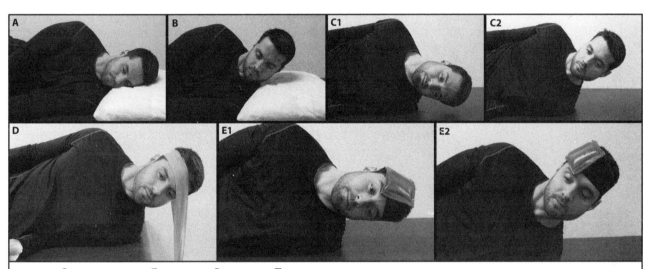

2.03.10 STRENGTHEN: CERVICAL LATERAL FLEXION

POSITION: Side-lying

TARGETS: Strengthening cervical lateral flexors (ipsilateral scalenes, SCM, splenius capitis, longissimus capitis and longissimus cervicis, erector spinae assist)

INSTRUCTION: With arms in a comfortable position, have the patient perform a slight chin tuck to protect the cervical spine and scapular retraction to stabilize scapula from upper trapezius pulling into elevation. Beginners should start with head on a pillow or towel roll in the neutral position (A). Instruct patient to lift head off the table bringing the ear towards the shoulder (B). Advancing the exercise involves removal of the pillow for increase range (C1 and C2). Resistance (manual, resistance band or a cuff weight) can be applied as the patient advances (D through E2).

SUBSTITUTIONS: Tensing the upper trapezius (shrugging shoulders), rolling trunk forward or back to substitute with cervical flexors or extensors, loss of slight chin tuck/jutting chin out

PARAMETERS: 1 to 3 sets, 8 to 12 repetitions, 1 time per day or every other day

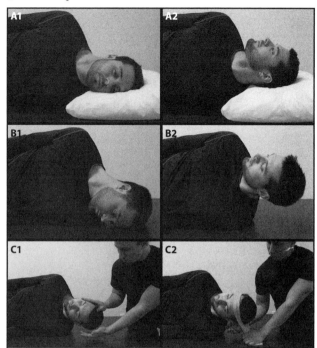

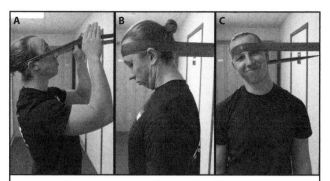

2.03.12 STRENGTHEN: CERVICAL RESISTANCE BAND, 2 PLANES

POSITION: Seated, standing

TARGETS: Strengthening cervical extensors (splenius capitis, splenius cervicis, semispinalis capitis, semispinalis cervicis) and erector spinae group (cervical and upper thoracic region); strengthening cervical deep neck flexors (longus colli and longus capitis), also activates superficial cervical flexors scalenes, SCM, and two of the suboccipital muscles (rectus capitis anterior and rectus capitis lateralis). Strengthening cervical lateral flexors (ipsilateral scalenes, SCM, splenius capitis, longissimus capitis and longissimus cervicis, erector spinae assist).

INSTRUCTION: Resistance band will be at the level of the patient's forehead. The resistance band can be affixed in a doorway, to an anchor, or held by the therapist with resistance band applied around the head at the level of the temples above the ears. Instruct the patient to retract and depress the scapula (pinch shoulder blades together and down like you are trying to put them in your back pockets). The head and neck should be in a neutral position with a slight chin tuck to protect the cervical spine for all of these exercises. For extension, extend the neck to look up toward the ceiling (A). For flexion, have the patient look down towards chest (B). For lateral flexion, bring the ear towards the ipsilateral shoulder. Resistance is applied by the resistance band in the opposite direction (C).

SUBSTITUTIONS: Tensing the upper trapezius (shrugging shoulders), leaning forwards, backwards or sideways with the trunk, jutting the chin out; it is difficult to remove the substitutions if the patient is holding the resistance band with the hands; an external support by anchor or another person is optimal.

PARAMETERS: 1 to 3 sets, 8 to 12 repetitions, 1 time per day or every other day

2.03.11 STRENGTHEN: CERVICAL ROTATION

POSITION: Side-lying

TARGETS: Strengthening cervical rotators (ipsilateral scalenes, splenius capitis, semispinalis capitis, longissimus capitis, contralateral SCM)

INSTRUCTION: With arms in a comfortable position, have the patient perform a slight chin tuck to protect the cervical spine. Beginners should start with head on a pillow or towel roll in the neutral position. Instruct the patient to rotate the chin towards the shoulder (A1 and A2). Advancing the exercise involves removal of the pillow for increase range (B1 and B2). Resistance (manual, resistance band or a cuff weight) can be applied as the patient advances (C1 and C2).

SUBSTITUTIONS: Tensing the upper trapezius (shrugging shoulders), loss of slight chin tuck/jutting chin out, cervical flexion, extension or lateral flexion should not be allowed

PARAMETERS: 1 to 3 sets, 8 to 12 repetitions, 1 time per day or every other day

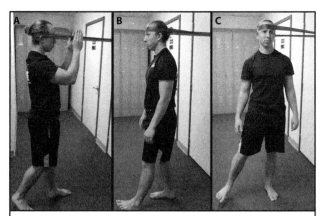

2.03.13 STRENGTHEN: CERVICAL RESISTANCE BAND, WALK-OUTS

POSITION: Standing

TARGETS: Strengthening cervical extensors (splenius capitis, splenius cervicis, semispinalis capitis, semispinalis cervicis) and erector spinae group (cervical and upper thoracic region); strengthening cervical deep neck flexors (longus colli and longus capitis), also activates superficial cervical flexors scalenes, SCM, and two of the suboccipital muscles (rectus capitis anterior and rectus capitis lateralis); strengthening cervical lateral flexors (ipsilateral scalenes, SCM, splenius capitis, longissimus capitis and longissimus cervicis, upper trapezius assist).

INSTRUCTION: Resistance band will be at the level of the patient's forehead. The band can be affixed in a doorway, to an anchor, or held by the therapist with resistance band applied around the head at the level of the temples above the ears. Instruct the patient to retract and depress the scapula (pinch shoulder blades together and down like you are trying to put them in your back pockets). The head and neck should be in a neutral position with a slight chin tuck to protect the cervical spine for all of these exercises. For extension, patient faces anchor with band around the back of the head and walks backwards as neck resists the pull of the band into flexion (A). For flexion, patient faces away from anchor with band around the front of the head and walks forwards as neck resists the pull of the band into extension (B). For lateral flexion, patient's ear faces anchor with band around the side of the head and walks sideways as neck resists the pull of the band into lateral flexion (C).

SUBSTITUTIONS: Tensing the upper trapezius (shrugging shoulders), leaning forwards, backwards or sideways with the trunk, jutting the chin out, loss of slight chin tuck or neutral cervical spine

PARAMETERS: 1 to 3, sets 8 to 12 repetitions, 1 time per day or every other day

REFERENCES

Falla, D., Jull, G., Russell, T., Vicenzino, B., & Hodges, P. (2007). Effect of neck exercise on sitting posture in patients with chronic neck pain. *Physical Therapy, 87*(4), 408-417.

Falla, D., O'Leary, S. P., Farina, D., & Jull, G. (2012). The change in deep cervical flexor activity after training is associated with the degree of pain reduction in patients with chronic neck pain. *Clinical Journal of Pain, 28*(7), 628-634.

Jull, G. A., O'Leary, S. P., & Falla, D. L. (2008). Clinical assessment of the deep cervical flexor muscles: The craniocervical flexion test. *Journal of Manipulative and Physiological Therapeutics, 31*(7), 525-533.

O'Leary, S., Jull, G., Kim, M., & Vicenzino, B. (2007). Specificity in retraining craniocervical flexor muscle performance. *Journal of Orthopedic Sports Physical Therapy, 37*(1), 3-9.

Section 2.04

ADDITIONAL HINTS
CERVICAL

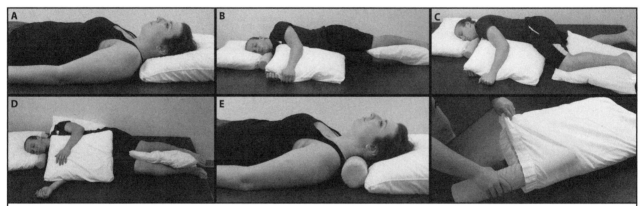

2.04.1 SLEEPING POSITIONS

The way we sleep can have a negative impact on our spinal health. A proper sleep position can positively affect the maintenance of a neutral spine during sleep. Patients may sleep in multiple positions throughout the night, therefore it can be difficult to address sleep postures. General recommendations based on current evidence include using a regular or latex pillow for side-sleeping and a pillow height of 4 inches (10 cm) for supine-sleeping (A). It is also important to encourage the patient to avoid curling up too tightly in side-lying. A pillow between the knees is also recommended for the lower spine and pelvis (B). Rolling the trunk slightly forward or backward in side-lying while hugging a pillow may ease discomfort on the weightbearing shoulder (C and D). Oftentimes, it is recommended to use a small rolled up towel inserted just under the neck in supine or side-lying to support the cervical spine (E). It can also be inserted into the pillowcase to help it stay in place (F). Prone-sleeping is discouraged due to the resultant excessive cervical rotation and extension. Due to differing body types, sizes, and varying cervical disorders, focus should be primarily on maintenance of the neutral spine position and normal cervical lordosis of 31 to 40 degrees with modifications as needed for optimal sleep quality.

Where's the Evidence?

Kim et al. (2015) found that an increase in pillow height caused an increase coronal plane deformity and neck tilt and a decrease in the thoracic inlet angle of the cervical spine. Kim and colleagues concluded the optimal pillow height for maintaining neutral cervical alignment supine-sleeping was 10 cm. Another study found that, for patients with side-sleeping preference, evidence supported the use of a rubber or latex pillow as it performed better than foam regular, foam contour, and polyester pillows in sleep quality, comfort and cervical pain upon waking. Feather pillows were not recommended (Gordon, Grimmer-Somers, & Trott, 2009). This recommendation for side-sleepers to use a latex pillow was also supported in another study comparing latex to polyester, foam regular, foam contour, and feather. Gordon, Grimmer-Somers, and Trott (2010) found that cervical stiffness, headache, and scapular/arm pain were least frequent with use of the latex pillow. There was no difference between foam and foam contour and again, feather pillows performed the worst. Gordon, Grimmer-Somers, and Trott (2011) also found that spinal sloping did not change between regular and contoured pillows. Statistically, cervical pain has been strongly associated with a cervical lordosis of less than 20 degrees (McAviney, Schulz, Bock, Harrison, & Holland, 2005).

REFERENCES

Gordon, S. J., Grimmer-Somers, K., & Trott, P. (2009). Pillow use: The behaviour of cervical pain, sleep quality and pillow comfort in side sleepers. *Manual Therapy, 14*(6), 671-678.

Gordon, S. J., Grimmer-Somers, K. A., & Trott, P. H. (2010). Pillow use: The behavior of cervical stiffness, headache and scapular/arm pain. *Journal of Pain Research, 3*, 137-145.

Gordon, S. J., Grimmer-Somers, K. A., & Trott, P. H. (2011). A randomized, comparative trial: Does pillow type alter cervico-thoracic spinal posture when side lying? *Journal of Multidisciplinary Healthcare*, 321-327.

Kim, H. C., Jun, H. S., Kim, J. H., Ahn, J. H., Chang, I. B., Song, J. H., & Oh, J. K. (2015). The effect of different pillow heights on the parameters of cervicothoracic spine segments. *Korean Journal of Spine, 12*(3), 135-138.

McAviney, J., Schulz, D., Bock, R., Harrison, D. E., & Holland, B. (2005). Determining the relationship between cervical lordosis and neck complaints. *Journal of Manipulative and Physiological Therapeutics, 28*(3), 187-193.

Section 2.05

CERVICAL PROTOCOLS AND TREATMENT IDEAS

2.05.1 NECK PAIN (NON-SPECIFIC) RECOMMENDED EXERCISES

Where's the Evidence?

Although specific studies regarding CROM are currently lacking, a best evidence synthesis performed by the Bone and Joint Decade 2000-2010 task force on neck pain suggests that therapies involving manual therapy and exercise are more effective than alternative strategies for patients with neck pain; this is also true of therapies which include educational interventions addressing self-efficacy. Additionally, for whiplash-associated disorders, evidence shows that educational videos, mobilization, and exercises appear more beneficial than usual care or physical modalities. For other neck pain, the evidence suggests that manual and supervised exercise interventions, low-level laser therapy, and perhaps acupuncture are more effective than no treatment, sham, or alternative interventions; however, none of the active treatments are clearly superior to any other in either the short- or long-term. For both whiplash-associated disorders and other neck pain without radicular symptoms, interventions that focus on regaining function as soon as possible are relatively more effective than interventions that do not have such a focus. Their consensus is based on a synthesis of research from 1980 through 2006 (Hurwitz et al., 2009).

Patients with cervical spine dysfunctions often exhibit UCS in which deep neck flexors, serratus anterior muscle, rhomboids, middle and lower trapezius are weak and inhibited and upper trapezius, levator scapula, suboccipitals, SCM, pectoralis major and pectoralis minor are tight and facilitated. Patients generally exhibit forward head, elevated and protracted shoulders, thoracic kyphosis, and abducted winging scapula (Page, Frank, & Larcher, 2010, p. 176).

Recommended exercises are as follows:

1. CROM
   a. 2.01.2 ROM: Cervical Anterior Semicircles
   b. 2.01.3 ROM: Chin Tuck With Cervical Extension
   c. 2.01.4 ROM: Chin Tuck With Cervical Flexion
   d. 2.01.5 ROM: Chin Tuck With Cervical Rotation
   e. 2.01.6 ROM: Chin Tuck With Cervical Lateral Flexion

2. Chin tuck
   a. 2.01.1 ROM: Chin Tuck
   b. 2.03.4 Strengthen: Isotonic; Chin Tuck
   c. 2.03.5 Strengthen: Isotonic; Chin Tuck Neutral (Beginner) and With Slight Rotation (Advanced), Forehead on Towel Roll (Beginner) and Head off Bed (Advanced)

3. Scapular retraction
   a. 5.03.3 Strengthen: Scapular Retraction and Variations
   b. 5.03.4 Strengthen: Scapular Retraction, Arms by Sides

4. Pectoral stretch
   a. 5.06.8 Stretch: Shoulder Horizontal Adductors, Towel Roll and Swiss Ball
   b. 5.06.5 Stretch: Shoulder Horizontal Adductors, Doorway

5. Upper trapezius stretch
   a. 2.02.3 Stretch: Self-Assisted Cervical Lateral Flexion
6. Levator scapula stretch
   a. 2.02.7 Stretch: Cervical Flexion and Rotation
7. Scalene stretch
   a. 2.02.4 Stretch: Cervical Extension and Rotation
   b. 2.02.5 Stretch: Cervical Rotation and Extension, First Rib Stabilization With Belt/Strap
8. Cervical isometrics
   a. 2.03.1 Strengthen: Isometric; Cervical All Planes Neutral Resist With Hand
   b. 2.03.2 Strengthen: Isometric; Cervical All Planes Multi-Positional Resist With Hand
   c. 2.03.3 Strengthen: Isometric; Cervical Bi-Planar Neutral Resist With Ball on Wall
9. Prone head lift
   a. 2.03.7 Strengthen: Isotonic; Lower Neck/Thoracic Extension, Head Lift, 5 Positions (Cervical Extensors)
10. Supine head lift
    a. 2.03.8 Strengthen: Isotonic; Chin Tuck Cervical Flexion With Head Lift (Deep Neck Flexors)
11. Scapular strengthening: middle and lower trapezius, rhomboid
    a. 5.03.5 Strengthen: Scapular Retraction, "T", "Y", and "I" and Variations
    b. 5.03.8 Strengthen: Scapular Retraction, "W" or "Batwings" **5.03.9**
    c. 5.03.12 Strengthen: Resistance Band, Scapular Row and Variations
    d. 5.07.24 Strengthen: Isotonic; Shoulder, Row (Prone)
    e. 5.07.25 Strengthen: Isotonic; Shoulder, Military Press (Prone)
    f. 5.07.63 Strengthen: Closed Kinetic Chain; Scapular and Shoulder Depression
12. Shoulder external rotators strengthening; assists to correct forward shoulders.
    a. 5.07.22 Strengthen: Isotonic; Shoulder External Rotation
    b. 5.07.23 Strengthen: Isotonic; Shoulder External Rotation 90/90
    c. 5.07.27 Strengthen: Isotonic; Posterior Cuff, 4-Way
    d. 5.07.41 Strengthen: Isotonic; Resistance Band, Shoulder External Rotation and Variations
13. Scapular strengthening; serratus anterior
    a. 5.03.1 Strengthen: Scapular, Push-Up Plus (Beginner)
    b. 5.03.2 Strengthen: Scapular, Ceiling Punch
    c. 5.03.15 Strengthen: Resistance Band, Scapular, Punch
14. Strengthening latissimus dorsi
    a. 5.07.34 Strengthen: Isotonic; Resistance Band and Machine, Shoulder, Lat Pull-Down
    b. 5.07.46 Strengthen: Isotonic; Resistance Band, Shoulder Pull-Over
    c. 5.07.47 Strengthen: Isotonic; Resistance Band, Shoulder Pull-Back
    d. 5.07.54 Strengthen: Exercise Ball, Pull-Over (Latissimus Dorsi)
    e. 5.07.64 Strengthen: Closed Kinetic Chain; Shoulder, Table Top Push-Pull

Other exercises to target these areas may be added as patient advances and based on individual responses to treatment.

2.05.2 WHIPLASH/CERVICAL STRAIN DISCUSSION

Whiplash is generally due to a traumatic event. The mechanism of injury is variable, usually involving a motor vehicle accident but also including causes such as sports injury, child abuse, blows to the head from a falling object, or similar acceleration-deceleration events (Lowe, Norton, Van Horebeek, Bortels, & Kistmatcher, 2015). As this is a traumatic injury, bony structures, ligamentous structures, muscles, neurological structures, and other connective tissue may be affected. Anatomic causes of pain can be any of these structures, with the strain injury resulting in secondary edema, hemorrhage, and inflammation (Lowe et al., 2015). Up to 40% of people continue to report symptoms 15 years after the accident (Binder, 2008).

> ### *Where's the Evidence?*
>
> Neck-specific exercise has been found to be more beneficial than no intervention in individuals with chronic whiplash-associated disorder (Peolsson, Landén Ludvigsson, Tigerfors, & Peterson, 2015). A review of 36 articles suggests early mobilization may lead to improved outcomes (Yadla, Ratliff, & Harrop, 2008). Another systematic review supports this, stating early mobilization may reduce pain in people with acute whiplash injury compared with immobilization or rest with a collar and also supported multimodal treatment (postural training, psychological support, eye fixation exercises, and manual treatment) to be more effective at improving pain at 1 and 6 months in people with whiplash due to a road traffic accident in the previous 2 months (Binder, 2008). Moderate evidence in another systematic review supports the use of postural exercises for decreasing pain and time off work in the treatment of patients with acute whiplash-associated disorder (Drescher et al., 2008). Additionally, a randomized trial of 200 patients reveals early exercise therapy is superior to collar therapy in reducing pain intensity and disability for whiplash injury (Schnabel, Ferrari, Vassiliou, & Kaluza, 2004). Considering all available evidence, exercise and/or mobilization-based therapies currently have the greatest level of evidence in support of their effectiveness for reducing the duration and severity of whiplash-associated neck pain, ROM deficits and disability, at least during the acute and chronic stages of the disorder (Teasell et al., 2010).

ROM exercises, gentle mobilization, muscle re-education, low-load isometrics, postural correction, eye fixation exercises and patient education are the staples of a physical therapy program. Clinical judgment is crucial if symptoms are aggravated and intermittent rest should be implemented if symptoms are severe.

2.05.3 Whiplash/Cervical Strain Recommended Exercises

Recommended exercises are as follows:

1. CROM; *all motions should be done in pain-free range.*
   a. 2.01.2 ROM: Cervical Anterior Semicircles
   b. 2.01.3 ROM: Chin Tuck With Cervical Extension
   c. 2.01.4 ROM: Chin Tuck With Cervical Flexion
   d. 2.01.5 ROM: Chin Tuck With Cervical Rotation
   e. 2.01.6 ROM: Chin Tuck With Cervical Lateral Flexion
2. Chin tuck
   a. 2.01.1 ROM: Chin Tuck
   b. 2.03.4 Strengthen: Isotonic; Chin Tuck
   c. 2.03.5 Strengthen: Isotonic; Chin Tuck Neutral (Beginner) and With Slight Rotation (Advanced), Forehead on Towel Roll (Beginner) and Head off Bed (Advanced)
3. Scapular retraction
   a. 5.03.3 Strengthen: Scapular Retraction and Variations
   b. 5.03.4 Strengthen: Scapular Retraction, Arms by Sides
4. Cervical isometrics; *sub-maximal starting with only < 25% effort.*
   a. 2.03.1 Strengthen: Isometric; Cervical All Planes Neutral Resist With Hand
   b. 2.03.2 Strengthen: Isometric; Cervical All Planes Multi-Positional Resist With Hand
   c. 2.03.3 Strengthen: Isometric; Cervical Bi-Planar Neutral Resist With Ball on Wall
5. Prone head lift; *implement in subacute and chronic stages.*
   a. 2.03.7 Strengthen: Isotonic; Lower Neck/Thoracic Extension, Head Lift, 5 Positions (Cervical Extensors)
6. Supine head lift; *implement in subacute and chronic stages.*
   a. 2.03.8 Strengthen: Isotonic; Chin Tuck Cervical Flexion With Head Lift (Deep Neck Flexors)
7. Oculomotor
   a. 7.01.6 Oculomotor: Saccades
   b. 7.01.7 Oculomotor: Smooth Pursuits
   c. 7.01.8 Gaze Stabilization

Additional postural correction and exercises may be added based on assessed flexibility and weaknesses in the subacute to chronic stages.

2.05.4 Internal Derangement (Disc Bulge) Cervical Discussion and Basic Exercises

The McKenzie method utilizes assessment of the directional preference of the neck, identifying which direction of movement centralizes the pain decreasing the radicular symptoms. Findings of centralization or directional preference at baseline would appear to be useful indicators of management strategies and prognosis. In the McKenzie method, patients are classified first into syndromes, then into sub-syndromes. The McKenzie assessment performed by persons trained in the McKenzie method may allow for reliable classification of patients with cervical and lumbar pain (Clare, Adams, & Maher, 2005). The presence of a directional preference and centralization of symptoms have been associated with improvements in functional outcomes (Edmond et al., 2014). Furthermore, if centralization is not observed by the seventh treatment visit, medical evaluation for physical or nonphysical factors that could be delaying quick resolution of an acute episode is recommended (Werneke, Hart, & Cook, 1999).

Below are some very basic exercises for a *posterior derangement*.

    a. 2.01.1 ROM: Chin Tuck
    b. 2.01.3 ROM: Chin Tuck With Cervical Extension
    c. 2.01.5 ROM: Chin Tuck With Cervical Rotation; hands assist at end range.
    d. 2.01.6 ROM: Chin Tuck With Cervical Lateral Flexion; to painful side.

Where's the Evidence?

May and Aina (2012) performed a systematic review of the literature relating to centralization and directional preference, and specifically report on prevalence, prognostic validity, reliability, loading strategies, and diagnostic implications. Search was conducted June 2011; multiple study designs were considered. Sixty-two studies were included in the review, 54 related to centralization and 8 to directional preference. The prevalence of centralization was 44.4% in 4745 patients with back and neck pain in 29 studies; it was more prevalent in acute (74%) than subacute or chronic (42%) symptoms. The prevalence of directional preference was 70% in 2368 patients with back or neck pain in 5 studies. Twenty-one of 23 studies supported the prognostic validity of centralization, including 3 high quality studies and 4 of moderate quality; whereas 2 moderate quality studies showed evidence that did not support the prognostic validity of centralization. Centralization and directional preference appear to be useful treatment effect modifiers in 7 out of 8 studies.

2.05.5 Cervicogenic Headaches Discussion

Head pain that is referred from the bony structures or soft tissues of the neck is commonly called a cervicogenic headache. It is often a sequela of head or neck injury but may also occur in the absence of trauma (Page, 2011). Patients with a cervicogenic headache will often have altered neck posture or restricted cervical ROM.

Where's the Evidence?

Hall and Robinson (2004) looked at active cervical motion in rotation between the cervicogenic and control groups. Average rotation in flexion was 44 degrees to each side in the asymptomatic group and 28 degrees towards the headache side in the symptomatic group. C1 to C2 was deemed to be the dominant segmental level of headache origin in 24 of 28 subjects. In those 24 subjects, range of rotation during the flexion-rotation test was inversely correlated to headache severity.

The head pain can be triggered or reproduced by active neck movement, passive neck positioning, especially in extension or extension with rotation toward the side of pain, or on applying digital pressure to the involved facet regions or over the ipsilateral greater occipital nerve. Muscular trigger points are usually found in the suboccipital, cervical, and shoulder musculature, and these trigger points can also refer pain to the head when manually or physically stimulated. There are no neurologic findings of cervical radiculopathy, though the patient might report scalp paresthesia or dysesthesia (Page, 2011). It is believed that irritation of the trigeminal nerve refers painful sensations from neck to face and head.

Where's the Evidence?

Biondi's (2005) article reviewing cervicogenic headaches and diagnostic and treatment strategies discusses the trigeminocervical nucleus as a region of the upper cervical spinal cord where sensory nerve fibers in the descending tract of the trigeminal nerve are believed to interact with sensory fibers from the upper cervical roots. He describes a functional convergence of upper cervical and trigeminal sensory pathways allowing the bidirectional referral of painful sensations between the neck and trigeminal sensory receptive fields of the face and head. He also describes a convergence of sensorimotor fibers in the spinal accessory nerve (cranial nerve XI) and upper cervical nerve roots ultimately converging with the descending tract of the trigeminal nerve as a possible source for the referral of cervical pain to the head.

Where's the Evidence?

Several physical therapies, including spinal joint manipulation/mobilization, soft tissue interventions, therapeutic exercises, and needling therapies, are proposed to be effective for the management of headaches. Current evidence has shown that the effectiveness of these interventions will depend on proper clinical reasoning since not all interventions are equally effective for all headache pain conditions. It seems that multimodal approaches including different interventions are more effective for patients with tension type, migraine, and cervicogenic headaches (Fernández-de-Las-Peñas & Cuadrado, 2015). For the prophylactic treatment of cervicogenic headache, there is evidence that neck exercise is effective in the short- and long-term when compared to no treatment (Bronfort et al., 2004). Mechanical neck and back pain identifies the source of pain is in the spine and/or supporting structures. There is moderate evidence that neck strengthening exercises reduce pain, improve function, and global perceived effect for chronic neck disorder with headache in the short- and long-term and a stretching and strengthening program focuses on the cervical or cervical and shoulder/thoracic region, there is moderate evidence of benefit on pain in chronic mechanical neck pain (Kay et al., 2005). Research showed the use of strengthening and endurance exercises for the cervico-scapulothoracic and shoulder may be beneficial in reducing pain and improving function. However, when only stretching exercises were used, no beneficial effects may be expected (Gross et al., 2015).

Where's the Evidence?

Manipulative therapy and exercise can reduce the symptoms of cervicogenic headache and the effects are maintained.

Jull et al. (2002) performed a randomized controlled trial to determine the effectiveness of manipulative therapy and a low-load exercise program for cervicogenic headache when used alone and in combination, as compared with a control group. In this study, 200 participants who met the diagnostic criteria for cervicogenic headache were randomized into four groups: manipulative therapy group, exercise therapy group, combined therapy group, and a control group. The primary outcome was a change in headache frequency. Other outcomes included changes in headache intensity and duration, the Northwick Park Neck Pain Index, medication intake, and patient satisfaction. Physical outcomes included pain on neck movement, upper cervical joint tenderness, a craniocervical flexion muscle test, and a photographic measure of posture. The results indicated at the 12-month follow-up assessment, both manipulative therapy and specific exercise had significantly reduced headache frequency and intensity, and the neck pain and effects were maintained. The combined therapies were not significantly superior to either therapy alone, but 10% more patients gained relief with the combination. Effect sizes were at least moderate and clinically relevant.

The three major criteria for diagnosing cervicogenic headache is head pain brought about by neck movement or awkward sustained neck postures or external pressure over the upper cervical or occipital region on the symptomatic side, restricted ROM, and ipsilateral neck, shoulder or arm pain (Sjaastad, Fredriksen, & Pfaffenrath, 1998).

2.05.6 CERVICOGENIC HEADACHES RECOMMENDED EXERCISES

1. CROM
   a. 2.01.2 ROM: Cervical Anterior Semicircles
   b. 2.01.3 ROM: Chin Tuck With Cervical Extension
   c. 2.01.4 ROM: Chin Tuck With Cervical Flexion
   d. 2.01.5 ROM: Chin Tuck With Cervical Rotation
   e. 2.01.6 ROM: Chin Tuck With Cervical Lateral Flexion
2. Chin tuck
   a. 2.01.1 ROM: Chin Tuck
   b. 2.03.4 Strengthen: Isotonic; Chin Tuck
   c. 2.03.5 Strengthen: Isotonic; Chin Tuck Neutral (Beginner) and With Slight Rotation (Advanced), Forehead on Towel Roll (Beginner) and Head off Bed (Advanced)
3. Cervical extensors stretch
   a. 2.02.1 Stretch: Subocciptal Muscle; stretch arms behind head.
4. Scapular retraction
   a. 5.03.3 Strengthen: Scapular Retraction and Variations
   b. 5.03.4 Strengthen: Scapular Retraction, Arms by Sides
5. Pectoral stretch
   a. 5.06.8 Stretch: Shoulder Horizontal Adductors, Towel Roll and Swiss Ball
   b. 5.06.5 Stretch: Shoulder Horizontal Adductors, Doorway
6. Upper trapezius stretch
   a. 2.02.3 Stretch: Self-Assisted Cervical Lateral Flexion
7. Levator scapula stretch
   a. 2.02.7 Stretch: Cervical Flexion and Rotation
8. Scalene stretch
   a. 2.02.4 Stretch: Cervical Extension and Rotation
   b. 2.02.5 Stretch: Cervical Rotation and Extension, First Rib Stabilization With Belt/Strap
9. Cervical isometrics
   a. 2.03.1 Strengthen: Isometric; Cervical All Planes Neutral Resist With Hand
   b. 2.03.2 Strengthen: Isometric; Cervical All Planes Multi-Positional Resist With Hand
   c. 2.03.3 Strengthen: Isometric; Cervical Bi-Planar Neutral Resist With Ball on Wall
10. Prone head lift
    a. 2.03.7 Strengthen: Isotonic; Lower Neck/ Thoracic Extension, Head Lift, 5 Positions (Cervical Extensors)
11. Supine head lift
    a. 2.03.8 Strengthen: Isotonic; Chin Tuck Cervical Flexion With Head Lift (Deep Neck Flexors)
12. Scapular strengthening; middle trapezius, lower trapezius, rhomboid.
    a. 5.03.5 Strengthen: Scapular Retraction, "T", "Y", and "I" and Variations
    b. 5.03.8 Strengthen: Scapular Retraction, "W" or "Batwings" **5.03.9**
    c. 5.03.12 Strengthen: Resistance Band, Scapular Row and Variations
    d. 5.07.24 Strengthen: Isotonic; Shoulder, Row (Prone)
    e. 5.07.25 Strengthen: Isotonic; Shoulder, Military Press (Prone)
    f. 5.07.63 Strengthen: Closed Kinetic Chain; Scapular and Shoulder Depression
13. Shoulder external rotators strengthening; assists to correct forward shoulders.
    a. 5.07.22 Strengthen: Isotonic; Shoulder External Rotation
    b. 5.07.23 Strengthen: Isotonic; Shoulder External Rotation 90/90
    c. 5.07.27 Strengthen: Isotonic; Posterior Cuff, 4-Way
    d. 5.07.41 Strengthen: Isotonic; Resistance Band, Shoulder External Rotation and Variations
14. Scapular strengthening; serratus anterior
    a. 5.03.1 Strengthen: Scapular, Push-Up Plus (Beginner)
    b. 5.03.2 Strengthen: Scapular, Ceiling Punch
    c. 5.03.15 Strengthen: Resistance Band, Scapular, Punch
15. Strengthening latissimus dorsi
    a. 5.07.34 Strengthen: Isotonic; Resistance Band and Machine, Shoulder, Lat Pull-Down
    b. 5.07.46 Strengthen: Isotonic; Resistance Band, Shoulder Pull-Over
    c. 5.07.47 Strengthen: Isotonic; Resistance Band, Shoulder Pull-Back
    d. 5.07.54 Strengthen: Exercise Ball, Pull-Over (Latissimus Dorsi)
    e. 5.07.64 Strengthen: Closed Kinetic Chain; Shoulder, Table Top Push-Pull

2.05.7 Cervical Postsurgical Fusion, Laminectomy, Discectomy Protocol

Combination of protocols adapted from Center for Spinal Disorders Rehabilitation Department; Cervical Fusion Protocol; IMS Orthopedics, Issada Thong-trangan, MD (Southeast Georgia Health System, 2013).

Post-Operation 1 to 3 Days Up to 4 to 6 Weeks

1. Precautions
   a. Prevent excessive initial mobility or stress on tissues and follow physician recommendations regarding use of cervical collar. Avoid bending head forward if you had a posterior fusion (incision on back of neck). Avoid bending head backward if you had an anterior fusion (incision on front or side of neck).
   b. Sex: Wait 2 weeks. Use the least exerting and most comfortable positions.
   c. Tub baths/shower: If hip graft is present, none for 1 month because of posture and submersing the incision. Shower only in the Philadelphia collar (peach-colored foam rubber).
   d. Household chores: None for 3 to 6 weeks, or as approved by your physician. Progress slowly as you begin. Consult outpatient physical therapist for proper body mechanics.
   e. Yard work: Consult physician before performing yard work. Observe proper body mechanics and lifting limit.
   f. The following observations require a consultation with the referring/consulting physician:
      i. Failure of incision to close or significant redness, swelling, or pain in the area of incision
      ii. Unexpectedly high self-reports of pain in comparison to presurgical state
      iii. Failure to meet progress milestones according to protocol "guidelines" as may be modified by clinical judgment with consideration given to previous presurgical state and typical progression of patients during rehabilitation
      iv. Evidence of acute exacerbation of symptoms: significant increase of pain, sudden increase of radicular symptoms, and/or sudden loss of strength/sensation/reflexes
      v. Development of new unexpected symptoms during the course of rehabilitation
2. Physical therapy includes bed mobility, transfers and education on donning/doffing collar if applicable, gait (with appropriate assistive device if necessary), and discussing increasing walking tolerance. Reinforce sitting, standing, and ADL modifications with neutral spine postures and proper body mechanics.

3. Breathing
   a. 3.03.7 Breathing Techniques: Diaphragmatic and Pursed-Lip Breathing
4. Scapular
   a. 5.03.4 Strengthen: Scapular Retraction, Arms by Sides
   b. 5.03.10 Strengthen: Scapular Elevation, Shrugs
5. LE
   a. 6.11.3 ROM: Ankle/Foot, Long-Sitting and Ankle Pumps, 4-Way, Active
   b. 6.01.8 ROM: Hip Flexion and Extension, Heel Slide, Active
   c. 6.01.14 ROM: Hip Internal Rotation and External Rotation, Active
   d. 6.04.2 Strengthen: Isometric; Hip Extension/ Gluteus Sets
   e. 6.09.1 Strengthen: Isometric; Knee Extension, Quadriceps Set
   f. 6.09.3 Strengthen: Isometric; Knee Flexion, Hamstring Set
   g. 6.09.9 Strengthen: Isotonic; Long-Arc Extension (Quadriceps)
   h. Walking: Walk for short distances at first, twice daily, at a comfortable pace. Choose a safe, paved area. Gradually increase to 1 half mile in the morning and 1 half mile in the evening by 1 to 2 months or start out 5 minutes in 1 direction and 5 minutes back, gradually increase time as tolerated up to 45 minutes total.

Post-Operation 4 to 6 Weeks; Starting Outpatient Physical Therapy

1. Precautions
   a. No bridging, no lifting > 8 lbs
   b. Sit as tolerated, getting up every 30 minutes to adjust posture; avoid slouching
2. CROM; *all motions should be done in pain-free range.*
   a. 2.01.1 ROM: Chin Tuck
   b. 2.01.2 ROM: Cervical Anterior Semicircles
   c. 2.01.3 ROM: Chin Tuck With Cervical Extension
   d. 2.01.4 ROM: Chin Tuck With Cervical Flexion
   e. 2.01.5 ROM: Chin Tuck With Cervical Rotation
3. Cervical isometrics: start at 50%, work up to 75% maximal contraction over 4 weeks
   a. 2.03.1 Strengthen: Isometric; Cervical All Planes Neutral Resist With Hand
   b. 2.03.2 Strengthen: Isometric; Cervical All Planes Multi-Positional Resist With Hand

   c. 2.03.3 Strengthen: Isometric; Cervical Bi-Planar Neutral Resist With Ball on Wall

4. Shoulder AROM
   a. 5.04.28 ROM: Shoulder Flexion, Active
   b. 5.04.29 ROM: Shoulder Abduction, Active
   c. 5.04.33 ROM: Shoulder Extension, Active
   d. 5.04.34 ROM: Shoulder Scaption, Active
5. Thoracic mobility
   a. 3.01.4 ROM: Thoracic Flexion and Extension With and Without Cervical Extension, Cat and Camel
   b. 3.01.5 ROM: Thoracic Rotation, Bow and Arrow Rib Pull Upper, Middle, and Lower
   c. 3.01.7 ROM: Thoracic Extension Over Back of Chair, Head Supported
   d. 3.01.9 ROM: Thoracic Rotation, Active
6. Fingers
   a. 5.16.3 Strengthen: Isometric; Finger Variations
   b. 5.16.4 Strengthen: Isometric; Thumb Variations
7. Overall conditioning
   a. Treadmill walking comfortable pace; *monitor good posture.*
   b. Stationary bike comfortable pace; *monitor good posture.*
   c. 5.04.1 ROM: Shoulder, Warm-Up, Upper Body Ergometer, Active Assistive; *add resistance as tolerated.*
8. Nerve glides; pain-free.
   a. 5.17.1 Nerve Glide: Median Nerve
   b. 5.17.2 Nerve Glide: Radial Nerve
   c. 5.17.3 Nerve Glide: Ulnar Nerve
9. Core stabilization exercises with neutral lumbar spine (no bridging); **4.03.**
10. General upper and lower body strengthening

Post-Operation 2 to 6 Months

1. Precautions: Avoid excessive cervical loading (minimal overhead arm resisted movements), limit lifting to 10 to 15 lbs.
2. Continue with above exercises and emphasize posture.
3. Clear to initiate stretching of cervical spine *if necessary.*
4. Cervical extensors stretch
   a. 2.02.1 Stretch: Suboccipital Muscle
5. Pectoral stretch
   a. 5.06.8 Stretch: Shoulder Horizontal Adductors, Towel Roll and Swiss Ball
   b. 5.06.5 Stretch: Shoulder Horizontal Adductors, Doorway
6. Upper trapezius stretch
   a. 2.02.3 Stretch: Self-Assisted Cervical Lateral Flexion
7. Levator scapula stretch
   a. 2.02.7 Stretch: Cervical Flexion and Rotation
8. Scalene stretch
   a. 2.02.4 Stretch: Cervical Extension and Rotation
   b. 2.02.5 Stretch: Cervical Rotation and Extension, First Rib Stabilization With Belt/Strap
9. Cervical strengthening
   a. 2.03.5 Strengthen: Isotonic; Chin Tuck Neutral (Beginner) and With Slight Rotation (Advanced), Forehead on Towel Roll (Beginner) and Head off Bed (Advanced)
   b. 2.03.7 Strengthen: Isotonic; Lower Neck/Thoracic Extension, Head Lift, 5 Positions (Cervical Extensors)
   c. 2.03.8 Strengthen: Isotonic; Chin Tuck Cervical Flexion With Head Lift (Deep Neck Flexors); scapular stabilization strengthening exercises.
10. Scapular and shoulder strengthening
   a. 5.03.5 Strengthen: Scapular Retraction, "T", "Y", and "I" and Variations
   b. 5.03.8 Strengthen: Scapular Retraction, "W" or "Batwings" **5.03.9**
   c. 5.03.12 Strengthen: Resistance Band, Scapular Row and Variations
   d. 5.07.24 Strengthen: Isotonic; Shoulder, Row (Prone)
   e. 5.07.63 Strengthen: Closed Kinetic Chain; Scapular and Shoulder Depression
11. Shoulder external rotators strengthening; assists to correct forward shoulders.
   a. 5.07.22 Strengthen: Isotonic; Shoulder External Rotation
   b. 5.07.23 Strengthen: Isotonic; Shoulder External Rotation 90/90
   c. 5.07.27 Strengthen: Isotonic; Posterior Cuff, 4-Way
   d. 5.07.41 Strengthen: Isotonic; Resistance Band, Shoulder External Rotation and Variations
12. Scapular strengthening; serratus anterior
   a. 5.03.1 Strengthen: Scapular, Push-Up Plus (Beginner)
   b. 5.03.2 Strengthen: Scapular, Ceiling Punch
   c. 5.03.15 Strengthen: Resistance Band, Scapular, Punch
13. Strengthening latissimus dorsi
   a. 5.07.34 Strengthen: Isotonic; Resistance Band and Machine, Shoulder, Lat Pull-Down
   b. 5.07.46 Strengthen: Isotonic; Resistance Band, Shoulder Pull-Over
   c. 5.07.47 Strengthen: Isotonic; Resistance Band, Shoulder Pull-Back
   d. 5.07.54 Strengthen: Exercise Ball, Pull-Over (Latissimus Dorsi)
14. Work/activity specific training
15. Begin jogging/running if desired

REFERENCES

Binder, A. (2008, Aug 4). Neck pain. *BMJ Clinical Evidence*, pii:1103.

Biondi, D. M. (2005). Cervicogenic headache: A review of diagnostic and treatment strategies. *Journal of the American Osteopathic Association, 105*(4 Suppl 2), 16S-22S.

Bronfort, G., Nilsson, N., Haas, M., Evans, R., Goldsmith, C. H., Assendelft, W. J., & Bouter, L. M. (2004). Non-invasive physical treatments for chronic/recurrent headache. *Cochrane Database of Systematic Reviews*, (3), CD001878.

Clare, H. A., Adams, R., & Maher, C. G. (2005). Reliability of McKenzie classification of patients with cervical or lumbar pain. *Journal of Manipulative and Physiological Therapeutics, 28*(2), 122-127.

Drescher, K., Hardy, S., Maclean, J., Schindler, M., Scott, K., & Harris, S. R. (2008). Efficacy of postural and neck-stabilization exercises for persons with acute whiplash-associated disorders: A systematic review. *Physiotherapy Canada, 60*(3), 215-223.

Edmond, S. L., Cutrone, G., Werneke, M., Ward, J., Grigsby, D., Weinberg, J., . . . Hart, D. L. (2014). Association between centralization and directional preference and functional and pain outcomes in patients with neck pain. *Journal of Orthopedic and Sports Physical Therapy, 44*(2), 68-75.

Fernández-de-Las-Peñas, C., & Cuadrado, M. L. (2016). Physical therapy for headaches. *Cephalgia, 36*(12), 1134-1142.

Gross, A., Kay, T. M., Paquin, J. P., Blanchette, S., Lalonde, P., Christie, T., . . . Cervical Overview Group. (2015). Exercises for mechanical neck disorders. *Cochrane Database of Systematic Reviews, 1*, CD004250

Hall, T., & Robinson, K. (2004). The flexion-rotation test and active cervical mobility—A comparative measurement study in cervicogenic headache. *Manual Therapy, 9*(4), 197-202.

Hurwitz, E. L., Carragee, E. J., van der Velde, G., Carroll, L. J., Nordin, M., Guzman, J., . . . Haldeman, S. (2008). Treatment of neck pain: Noninvasive interventions: Results of the Bone and Joint Decade 2000-2010 Task Force on Neck Pain and Its Associated Disorders. *Spine, 33*(4 Suppl), S123-152.

Jull, G., Trott, P., Potter, H., Zito, G., Niere, K., Shirley, D., . . . Richardson, C. (2002). A randomized controlled trial of exercise and manipulative therapy for cervicogenic headache. *Spine, 27*(17), 1835-1843.

Kay, T. M., Gross, A., Goldsmith, C., Santaguida, P. L., Hoving, J., Bronfort, G.; Cervical Overview Group. (2005). Exercises for mechanical neck disorders. *Cochrane Database of Systematic Reviews*, (3), CD004250.

Lowe, R., Norton, H., Van Horebeek, E., Bortels, S., & Kistmacher, S. (2015). Whiplash associated disorders. *Physiopedia*. Retrieved from http://www.physio-pedia.com/Whiplash_Associated_Disorders

May, S., & Aina, A. (2012). Centralization and directional preference: A systematic review. *Manual Therapy, 17*(6), 497-506.

Page, P. (2011). Cervicogenic headaches: An evidence-led approach to clinical management. *International Journal of Sports Physical Therapy, 6*(3), 254-266.

Page, P., Frank, C. C., & Larcher, R. (2010). *Assessment and treatment of muscle imbalance: The Janda approach*. Champagne, IL: Human Kinetics.

Peolsson, A., Landén Ludvigsson, M., Tigerfors, A. M., & Peterson, G. (2015). Effects of neck-specific exercises compared to waiting list for individuals with chronic whiplash associated disorders: A prospective randomized controlled study. *Archives of Physical Medicine and Rehabilitation, 97*(2), 189-195.

Schnabel, M., Ferrari, R., Vassiliou, T., & Kaluza, G. (2004). Randomised, controlled outcome study of active mobilisation compared with collar therapy for whiplash injury. *Emergency Medicine Journal, 21*(3), 306-310.

Sjaastad, O., Fredriksen, A., & Pfaffenrath, V. (1998). Cervicogenic headache: Diagnostic criteria. *Headache, 38*(6), 442-445.

Southeast Georgia Health System. (2013). Orthopedic protocols: Post-surgical rehabilitation protocol: Cervical laminectomy, discetomy, fusion. Retrieved from http://www.sghs.org/documents/Rehab-Protocols/cervical-fusion-rehabilitation-05-13-2013.pdf

Teasell, R. W., McClure, A., Walton, D., Pretty, J., Salter, K., Meyer, M., . . . Death, B. (2010). A research synthesis of therapeutic interventions for whiplash-associated disorder: Part 1—overview and summary. *Pain Research and Management, 15*(5), 287-294.

Werneke, M., Hart, D. L., & Cook, D. (1999). A descriptive study of the centralization phenomenon. A prospective analysis. *Spine, 24*(7), 676-683.

Yadla, S., Ratliff, J. K., & Harrop, J. S. (2008). Whiplash: Diagnosis, treatment, and associated injuries. *Current Reviews in Musculoskeletal Medicine, 1*(1), 65-68.

Chapter 3
THORACIC EXERCISES

Bryan E. *The Comprehensive Manual of Therapeutic Exercises:*
Orthopedic and General Conditions (pp 55-82).

Section 3.01

THORACIC RANGE OF MOTION

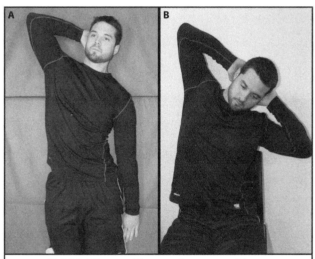

3.01.1 ROM: UPPER TRUNK LATERAL FLEXION, ACTIVE

POSITION: Supine, seated

TARGETS: Mobility of the thoracic spine into side-bending

INSTRUCTION: *Supine*: For side-bending to one side, patient reaches contralateral shoulder overhead into full shoulder abduction. The ipsilateral hand reaches down towards the foot, keeping the hand close to the thigh. Therapist may stabilize the hips as patient reaches towards the foot and overhead on each side, bending the thoracic spine (A). *Seated*: With feet flat on floor, patient clasps hands behind the head and side-bends upper torso bringing elbow towards hip (B).

SUBSTITUTIONS: Leaning forward and side-bending in lumbar spine instead of thoracic

PARAMETERS: Hold long enough to take 1 breath, 3 to 5 repetitions depending on treatment goals, 1 to 3 times per day

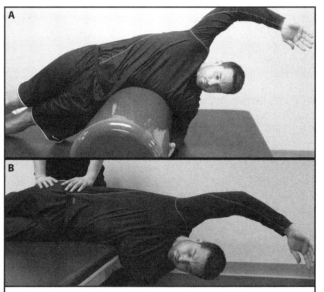

3.01.2 ROM: UPPER TRUNK LATERAL FLEXION, PASSIVE

POSITION: Side-lying

TARGETS: Mobility of the thoracic spine into side-bending

INSTRUCTION: *Towel roll*: Place a large towel roll, bolster or pillow under the upper torso at the level of the scapula and instruct the patient to allow the upper torso to side-bend. Bring the top arm into full shoulder abduction, lying over the top of the head or just behind (A). *Off edge of bed*: Place a towel roll under the upper torso at the level of the scapula as the patient lies with the upper rib cage over the edge of the top of the bed/mat. Instruct the patient to allow the upper torso to side-bend. Patient brings the top arm into full shoulder abduction lying over the top of the head or just behind. Therapist may need to stabilize the hips to allow patient to relax without feeling they may fall off bed (B).

SUBSTITUTIONS: Lifting pelvis off table, rolling forward or backward

PARAMETERS: Hold for 1 to 3 minutes, repeat 1 to 3 times per day

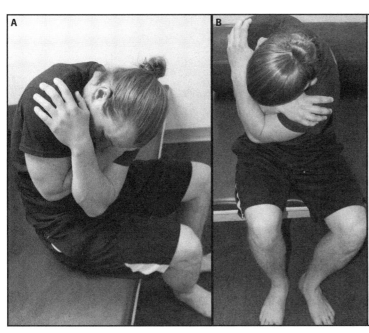

3.01.3 ROM: UPPER TRUNK FLEXION WITH ROTATION, ACTIVE

POSITION: Seated

TARGETS: Mobility of the thoracic spine in flexion/rotation

INSTRUCTION: Seated with feet flat on floor, patient hugs self and flexes forward in the upper torso. Patient then brings one shoulder up towards the ceiling and the other shoulder down towards the floor. Chin stays aligned with sternum (A and B).

SUBSTITUTIONS: Bending at the waist

PARAMETERS: Hold long enough to take 1 breath, 3 to 5 repetitions depending on treatment goals, 1 to 3 times per day

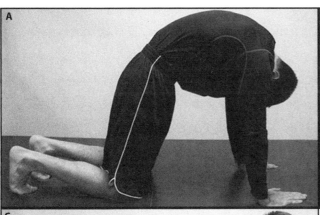

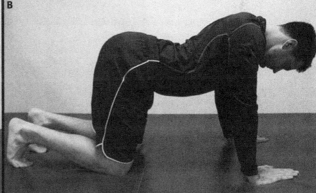

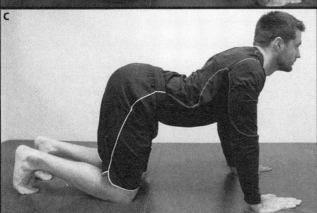

3.01.4 ROM: THORACIC FLEXION AND EXTENSION WITH AND WITHOUT CERVICAL EXTENSION, CAT AND CAMEL

POSITION: Quadruped

TARGETS: Mobility of the thoracic spine into flexion and extension; good exercise for warming-up thoracic spine.

INSTRUCTION: Knees are spaced hip-width apart and hands directly beneath shoulders. *Cat*: Patient tightens abdominal muscles and arches spine upward toward the ceiling. Patient relaxes the head and allows it to droop (A). *Camel*: Patient slowly relaxed back, allowing stomach to fall toward the floor while bringing shoulders together, stretching into a swayback position. Keep the head aligned with the neck, looking at the floor in front (B). Cervical extension may be added to camel by instructing the patient to look up (C). Avoid excessive hyperextension of the neck.

SUBSTITUTIONS: Only moving in the lumbar region, especially with camel; encourage patient to extend and flex in the upper back.

PARAMETERS: Hold each position for at least 10 seconds, 5 to 15 repetitions, 1 to 3 times per day

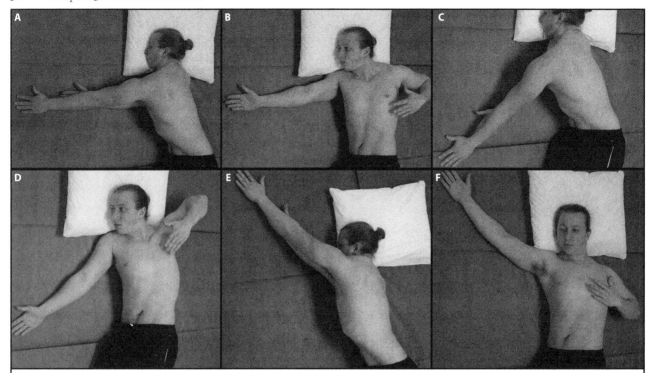

3.01.5 ROM: Thoracic Rotation, Bow and Arrow Rib Pull Upper, Middle, and Lower

<u>Position</u>: Side-lying

<u>Targets</u>: Mobility of the thoracic spine; opening and closing intervertebral and costovertebral facets.

<u>Instruction</u>: Hips and shoulder should start stacked with opposite leg flexed 90 degrees at hip and knee. Place a support under the knee. If the knee is too low, this will create more of a lumbar stretch instead of targeting the thoracic region. Use a cervical spine support to maintain neutral neck. Too much lateral flexion in the neck will enable the tissue to brace. *Middle*: With both shoulders at 90 degrees of flexion and palms facing each other, reach the top hand past the other hand rolling the upper torso forward as if grasping a bow string. The patient pulls the bowstring back, while retracting the scapula and rotating upper torso, almost like trying to touch the top posterior deltoid to the floor. The patient can place the hand on the rib cage to assist with end range. Exhale during the rotation and inhale on the return to starting position (B). *Upper*: With both shoulders at 45 degrees of flexion and palms facing each other, repeat steps for middle ending with the top shoulder at 120 degrees of abduction (C and D). *Lower*: With both shoulders at 120 degrees of flexion and palms facing each other, repeat steps for middle ending with the top shoulder at 45 degrees of abduction and extended (E and F).

<u>Substitutions</u>: Avoid strain in neck or pulling too hard at the end range; this should be a gentle movement; a good benchmark of too much stretch is an inability to breathe through the diaphragm.

<u>Parameters</u>: Hold each position for 2 to 4 breaths allowing soft tissue to relax, 3 to 5 repetitions, 1 to 3 times per day

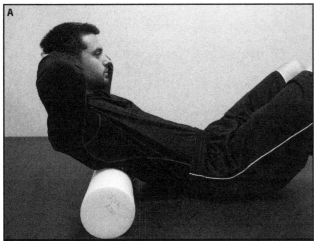

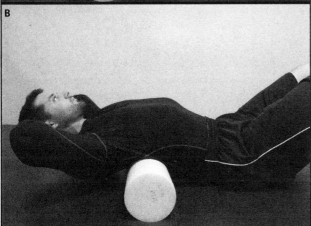

Where's the Evidence?

Jang, Kim, and Kim (2015) studied the effects of thorax correction exercises on flexed posture and chest function in older women with age-related hyperkyphosis. Forty-one elderly women who were divided into a thorax correction exercise group and a control group. Participants in the exercise group completed a specific exercise program that included breathing correction, thorax mobility, thorax stability (strengthening with resistance band), and thorax alignment training performed twice per week, 1 hour each session, for 8 weeks. Outcome measures included the flexed posture (thoracic kyphosis angle, forward head posture) and chest function (vital capacity, forced expiratory volume in a second, and chest expansion length). Participants in the thorax correction exercise group demonstrated significantly greater improvements in thoracic kyphosis angle, forward head, and chest expansion than those in the control group. The study illustrates that exercise interventions may improve flexed posture and chest function in older women with age-related hyperkyphosis.

3.01.6 ROM: Thoracic Extension Over Foam Roll, Head Supported

Position: Hook-lying, supine

Targets: Increase lumbar lordosis (mobility of lumbar spine into extension), facilitate lumbar extensors (erector spinae: iliocostalis, longissimus, spinalis), and iliopsoas (reversal of origin and insertion)

Instruction: Place foam roller under thoracic spine. Patient can keep knees bent in hook-lying or perform supine depending on effectiveness and comfort. Patient clasps hands behind head, pulling elbows as close together as possible. Patient can roll up and down several repetitions prior to extending, but eventually the patient extends the thoracic spine over the foam roller while supporting the head to maintain neutral neck and avoid hyperextension. The patient then rolls back up in a semi crunch and rolls body along the foam roller to the next level to extend. This exercise can be somewhat uncomfortable, as the spine loosens and soft tissue adjusts. Discomfort is considered normal when first initiating the exercise (A and B).

Substitutions: Avoid lifting pelvis

Parameters: Hold each extended position for 1 to 2 breaths, 1 to 3 repetitions each level, 1 to 3 times per day; focus more on levels of discomfort.

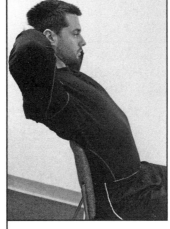

3.01.7 ROM: Thoracic Extension Over Back of Chair, Head Supported

Position: Seated

Targets: Mobility of the upper thoracic spine in the sagittal plane (extension); can mobilize a specific segment or use as a global stretch.

Instruction: Starting in a good seated posture with pelvis in contact with the back of the chair, clasp the hands behind the head. Have the patient slowly extend the thoracic region over the back of the chair while relaxing and breathing into the stretch. Do not overextend to the point of pain. Hands should keep the head supported to avoid neck strain or hyperextension.

Substitutions: Extension of the lumbar spine to compensate for poor thoracic extension, bringing hips away from the back of the chair.

Parameters: Hold 10 to 15 seconds (enough to take 3 to 4 breaths), 5 to 10 repetitions depending on treatment goals, 1 to 2 times per day

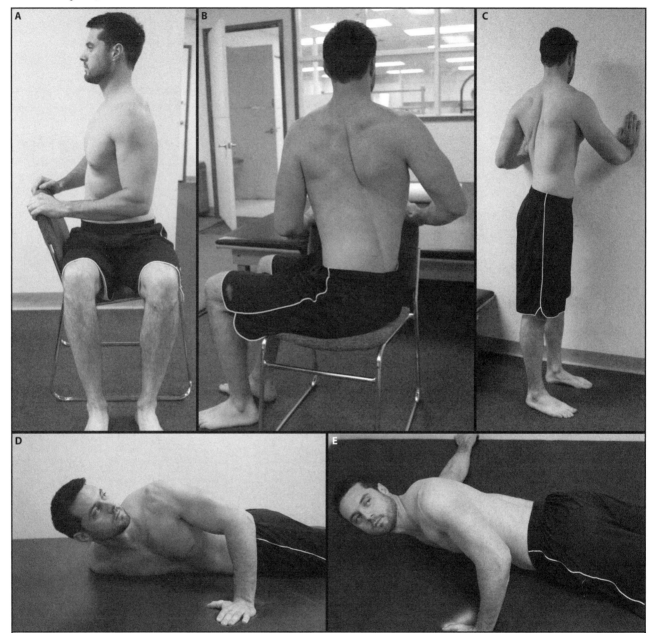

3.01.8 ROM: Thoracic Rotation, Passive

<u>Position</u>: Seated, standing, prone

<u>Targets</u>: Mobility of the upper thoracic spine in the transverse/horizontal plane (rotation)

<u>Instruction</u>: *Seated*: Starting in a good seated posture with pelvis in contact with the back of the chair, patient rotates head and shoulders to one side, grasping the back of the chair with both hands. Feet should be on floor or on blocks. If the chair has an arm rest this can also be used. Take a deep breath in and then rotate further, pulling with the ipsilateral hand and pushing with the contralateral hand. Patient should maintain rotation as they repeat inhale, rotate further and exhale (A and B). *Standing*: With feet, apart and the left side of body about 20 cm from the wall, flex elbows 90 degrees and flex shoulders approximately 45 degrees. Rotate head, shoulders, and spine to the left, so that upper body faces the wall, but keep pelvis fixed. Place palms flat against a wall and use left arms to push further into rotation (C). *Prone*: With feet apart and toes pointing backwards, abduct arms until hands are level with shoulders. Flex one elbow and place hand, palm down, nearer to side. Raise head, ipsilateral shoulder, and elbow off the floor. This will rotate spine to the ipsilaterally. Maintain pelvis on the floor (D and E).

<u>Substitutions</u>: Pelvis rotates, leaning forward or backwards, shoulder shrug, neck strain

<u>Parameters</u>: Hold long enough to take 3 to 4 breaths, 3 to 5 repetitions depending on treatment goals, 1 to 2 times per day

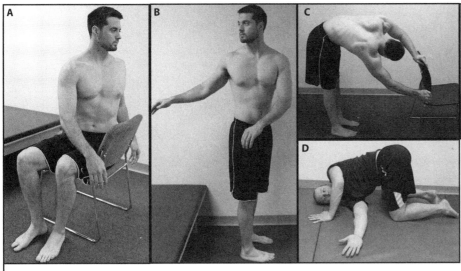

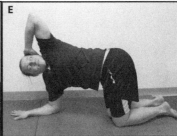

3.01.9 ROM: Thoracic Rotation, Active

Position: Seated, standing, quadruped

Targets: Mobility of the upper thoracic spine in the transverse plane/horizontal (rotation)

Instruction: *Seated*: With back straight and body at right angle to the back of the chair, and the side of thigh resting against the back of the chair, feet should be on floor or on blocks, patient rotates head, neck, shoulders, and spine towards the front of the chair. Place the wrist of the hand nearest to knee against the side of thigh and fully extend forearm at the elbow. Allow other arm to hang freely from the shoulder down at side (A). *Standing*: With feet apart and arms at sides, rotate head, neck, shoulders and spine to the left, but keep pelvis and lower limbs in a fixed position. Shoulders are relaxed and dropped so arms hang freely at sides (B). *Standing flexing at hips*: Standing with feet 30 to 50 cm apart, about 1 m from a chair or table. Patient flexes 90 degrees at the hips and grasp the back of the chair. Patient leans backward, away from the chair and dropping bring one shoulder towards the floor and contralateral shoulder towards ceiling so that upper body faces sideways (C). *Quadruped "Thread the needle"*: Kneeling on hands palms down on the floor in front, patient moves one hand forward and flex the elbow. Slide the other hand along the floor and under body to the opposite side, rotating the spine the same direction. The sliding posterior hand and arm rest on the floor (D). *Quadruped active rotation*: Kneeling with one elbow and forearm on the floor while opposite hand is behind neck, patient rotates elbow and shoulder, twisting torso up towards ceiling. Head should also rotate the same direction, looking up at ceiling (E).

Substitutions: Pelvis rotates, neck out of neutral alignment (keep chin in same line as sternum), shoulder shrug

Parameters: Hold long enough to take 1 to 2 breaths, 3 to 5 repetitions depending on treatment goals, 1 to 2 times per day

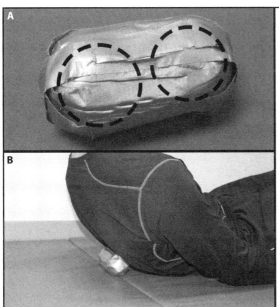

3.01.10 ROM: Thoracic Segmental Extension, Self-Mobilization With Tennis Balls

Position: Hook-lying

Targets: Thoracic spine mobility into extension; can be used for segmental extension and soft tissue work. This is an active shortened duration extension mobilization.

Instruction: Tape two tennis balls together (A). Patient lies on top of balls so that one ball sits just lateral to the thoracic spine on each side. Patient then does a very small forward crunch until feeling the tennis ball pressing into the tissues lateral to the spine and then patient lies back onto the ball. This is generally an uncomfortable exercise at first. Repeat at multiple levels along the thoracic spine by rolling the ball up or down by walking the body up or down along the mat/floor (B). This can also be used for self-soft tissue work on thoracic extensors.

Substitutions: Lifting hips off floor

Parameters: Repeat each level holding 5 to 10 seconds, 3 to 5 repetitions, perform 1 to 2 times per day

Tennis balls underneath the desired thoracic segments

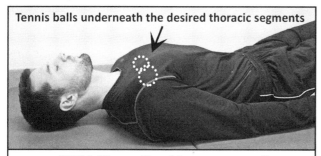

3.01.11 ROM: Upper Rib Mobilization Into Extension With Tennis Balls

Position: Hook-lying

Targets: Thoracic spine mobility into extension; can be used for segmental extension and soft tissue work; this is a prolonged passive extension mobilization.

Instruction: Tape two tennis balls together (**3.01.10-A**). Patient lies on top of balls so that one ball sits just lateral to the thoracic spine on each side at the spinal level of T1. A pillow should be placed under the head to maintain neutral neck alignment. Patient is then instructed to relax weight of upper trunk onto the tennis balls.

Substitutions: Neck extension, inability to relax shoulders

Parameters: Stay in this position 3 to 5 minutes, 1 to 2 repetitions, 1 to 2 times per day

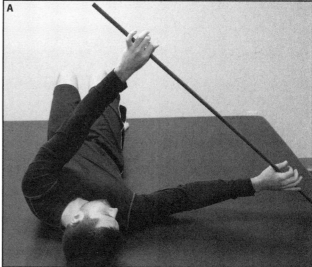

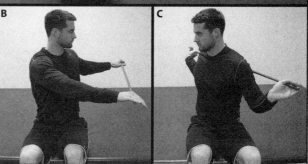

3.01.13 ROM: Spine Elongations, Wall Slide

Position: Standing

Targets: Elongation of the spine

Instruction: Patient stands with toes touching the wall and slides hands up the wall, palms facing forward, gaze is forward. Patient reaches as high as possible, giving a slight tractioning force to the torso. In this position, patient then breathes deeply into the chest, filing the chest while the spine, continues to elongate. Perform for 5 breaths. Relax and repeat.

Substitutions: Shrugging shoulders, lumbar hyperextension

Parameters: 5 to 10 sets with 5 breath holds each repetition, 1 to 2 times per day

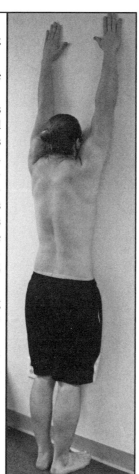

3.01.12 ROM: Thoracic, Broomstick Twist

Position: Supine, seated, standing

Targets: Mobility of the upper thoracic spine in the transverse plane/horizontal plane (rotation); this is a good warm-up before starting other thoracic activities.

Instruction: *Supine*: This is a good place to start with this exercise as it is difficult to keep lumbar spine and hips from rotating in standing. Have patient hold a long stick/wand with shoulders flexed 90 degrees and elbows extended. The patient rotates to one side, bringing one end of the stick towards the floor/mat while the other end moves toward the ceiling. Repeat to other side (A). *Seated or standing*: With feet placed hip-width apart and knees and hips slightly bent, place stick in front (B) or in back (C). Rotate the upper torso towards each side. Exhale on twist and inhale on return.

Substitutions: Avoid rotation of the pelvis and hips, breathe rhythmically

Parameters: 5 to 20 repetitions each direction, 1 to 2 times per day

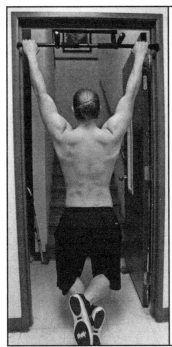

3.01.14 ROM: SPINE ELONGATIONS, BAR HANG

<u>POSITION</u>: Standing

<u>TARGETS</u>: Elongation of the spine

<u>INSTRUCTION</u>: Patient stands underneath a secure bar overhead just above hands reach, gaze is forward. Patient reaches up and grasps bar with a grip as wide as shoulder width or just slightly more. Overhand grip is preferred. Patient brings feet off floor and hangs partial to full body weight as shoulder and scapular muscles keep shoulders from shrugging excessively. Patient hangs as long as they can, usually grip strength limits the amount of time they can hang. While hanging in this position, patient then breathes deeply into the chest, filing the chest while the spine continues to elongate. Perform for 5 breaths. Relax and repeat.

<u>SUBSTITUTIONS</u>: Shrugging shoulders, lumbar hyperextension, swinging or rotational movements; encourage the lower body to hang limp.

<u>PARAMETERS</u>: 5 to 10 sets with up to 5 breath holds each repetition, 1 to 2 times per day

REFERENCE

Jang, H. J., Kim, M. J., & Kim, S. Y. (2015). Effect of thorax correction exercises on flexed posture and chest function in older women with age-related hyperkyphosis. *Journal of Physical Therapy Science, 27*(4), 1161-1164.

Section 3.02

THORACIC STRETCHING

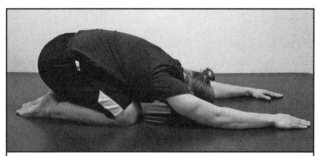

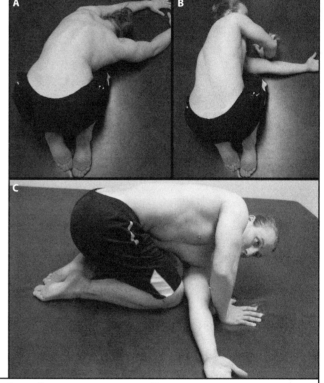

3.02.1 STRETCH: THORACIC FLEXION, "CHILD'S POSE" OR "PRAYER STRETCH"

POSITION: Quadruped

TARGETS: Stretches latissimus dorsi, thoracic and lumbar extensors; good for increasing shoulder flexion.

INSTRUCTION: Have patient sit back on their heels while they extend the arms in front of them, palms down. Press chest into the mat between the knees and rest forehead on the mat.

SUBSTITUTIONS: Hunching upper back, shrugging shoulders

PARAMETERS: Hold for 15 to 30 seconds, 3 to 5 repetitions, 1 to 3 times per day

3.02.2 STRETCH: THORACIC FLEXION, "CHILD'S POSE" OR "PRAYER STRETCH" ADD SIDE-BEND OR ROTATION

POSITION: Quadruped

TARGETS: Stretches latissimus dorsi, thoracic and lumbar extensors; good for increasing shoulder flexion.

INSTRUCTION: *With side-bending*: Have patient sit back on heels while they extend the arms in front of them, palms down. Reach hands towards one side, allowing the ribs to open up on the contralateral side. Patient may grasp side of table to increase stretch (A). *With thoracic rotation*: Patient threads one arm under the other as they rotate from full "child's pose" position (B and C).

SUBSTITUTIONS: Rolling upper trunk forwards or backwards, lower spine and pelvis should remain neutral; hips should be stacked.

PARAMETERS: Hold for 15 to 30 seconds, 3 to 5 repetitions, 1 to 3 times per day

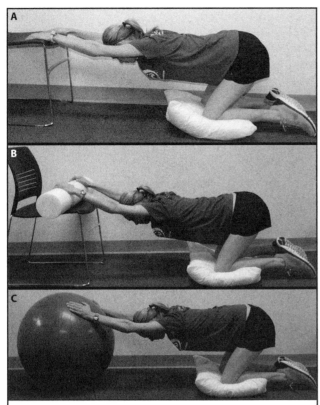

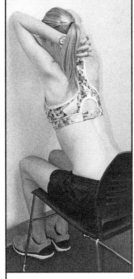

3.02.4 Stretch: Thoracic Extension With Hands Clasped Behind Head, Using Wall

Position: Seated

Targets: Mobility of the thoracic spine into extension

Instruction: Seated in chair, facing the wall, feet planted with toes touching wall, patient clasps hands behind the head while bringing elbows forward. Elbow are then placed on the wall at eye level. Patient then presses chest towards the wall causing an extension stretch to the thoracic spine.

Substitutions: Extension of lower back, hyperextension of the neck

Parameters: Hold for 15 to 30 seconds, 3 to 5 repetitions, 1 to 3 times per day

3.02.3 Stretch: Thoracic With Hands on Bench/Chair/Ball, Using Foam Roll

Position: Quadruped

Targets: Stretches latissimus dorsi while promoting thoracic extension; good for increasing shoulder flexion.

Instruction: Place hands on chair with palms down or thumbs up depending on comfort. Press upper body down towards floor until stretch felt in armpit and thoracic spine (A). A bolster can be used for comfort (B). Patient may also do this with an exercise ball (C).

Substitutions: Shoulder shrug, hips flex beyond 90 degrees (sits back towards heels)

Parameters: Hold for 15 to 30 seconds, 3 to 5 repetitions, 1 to 3 times per day

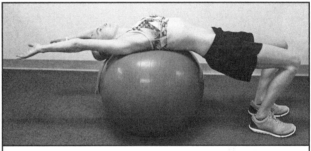

3.02.5 Stretch: Thoracic Extension/Chest Stretch on Exercise Ball

Position: Seated to reverse table top

Targets: Opening chest, stretching pectoral and abdominal muscles

Instruction: Begin seated on the ball and walk feet forward until ball is supporting only the mid-thoracic level. Have the patient relax, sagging the hips down into the ball and arms to the sides. Return to start by walking the feet back up to sitting. Bringing arms overhead will add a latissimus stretch. This is more isolated to the thoracic spine by placing ball in the thoracic region.

Substitutions: Extension of lower back, hyperextension of the neck

Parameters: Hold for 15 to 30 seconds, 3 to 5 repetitions, 1 to 3 times per day

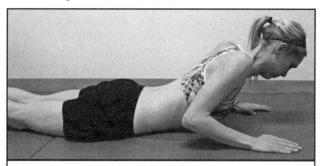

3.02.6 STRETCH: THORACIC EXTENSION, SPHINX POSE

POSITION: Prone

TARGETS: Kyphotic postural correction to improve thoracic extension

INSTRUCTION: Lying face down with feet hip-width distance apart, place elbows directly under the shoulders with palms down in front. Patient then presses up, lifting the upper body off the surface while looking forward (not up). Encourage patient to do this with a long spine, lengthening from the pelvis to the chest. Patient should actively work to pull elbows together for increased stretch. Legs should be kept firm.

SUBSTITUTIONS: Extension of lower back, hyperextension of the neck

PARAMETERS: Hold for 15 to 30 seconds, 3 to 5 repetitions, 1 to 3 times per day

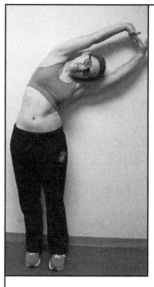

3.02.7 STRETCH: THORACIC AND THORACOLUMBAR SIDE-BEND

POSITION: Seated, standing

TARGETS: Mobility of the thoracic spine into side-bending, stretch obliques and latissimus dorsi

INSTRUCTION: Patient stands or sits with good posture and extends arms overhead to interlace fingers with palms facing outward. Keeping the arms straight, patient deeply inhales then exhales while leaning from the waist to one side without twisting the torso. For increased thoracic stretch, encourage patient to stabilize lower trunk while side-bending primarily in the thoracic region.

SUBSTITUTIONS: Leaning forward, trunk rotation, shoulder tense/shrug; only bending at waist and not thoracic region.

PARAMETERS: Hold for 15 to 30 seconds, 3 to 5 repetitions, 1 to 3 times per day

3.02.8 STRETCH: THORACOLUMBAR ROTATION

POSITION: Long-sitting

TARGETS: Mobility of the thoracic spine into rotation and stretching thoracic rotators

INSTRUCTION: Patient in long-sitting steps one foot across opposite knee and bends bottom leg to tuck foot near opposite hip (can also be held straight depending on comfort). Patient roots down into sit bones while lengthening spine upward. At the tallest point, patient twists toward the top leg and hugs front leg or pins elbow across thigh. Patent then twists from behind the belly button, allowing the twist to spiral up spine until at last the head turns with the chin parallel to the floor.

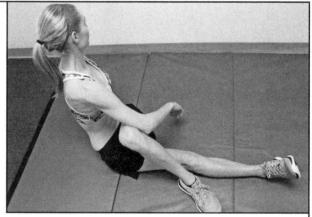

SUBSTITUTIONS: Leaning forward or backward, hips coming off floor, slouching, jutting chin out

PARAMETERS: Hold for 15 to 30 seconds, 3 to 5 repetitions, 1 to 3 times per day

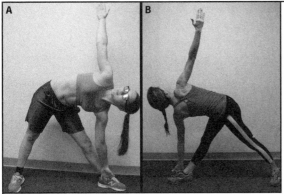

3.02.9 STRETCH: THORACIC ROTATION, EXTENDED TRIANGLE POSE

POSITION: Standing

TARGETS: Mobility of the thoracic spine into rotation, stretching thoracic rotators, chest opening

INSTRUCTION: *For left rotation*: Patient turns left foot in slightly to the right and right foot out to the right 90 degrees, aligning the right heel with the left heel. Instruct patient to firm the thighs and turn right thigh outward so that the center of the right knee cap is in line with the center of the right ankle. Patient exhales and extends torso to the right directly over the plane of the right leg, bending from the hip joint, not the waist, while pressing the outer heel firmly to the floor. Patient then rotates the torso to the left, keeping the two sides equally long and reaches towards the ceiling (and back if able) with the top arm. Encourage the left hip come slightly forward and lengthen the tailbone toward the back heel. Inhale to come up while strongly pressing the back heel into the floor and reaching the top arm toward the ceiling. Eyes follow fingertips. Reverse the feet and repeat to the opposite side (A). Hand placement may also change for an increased stretch the opposite direction (B).

SUBSTITUTIONS: Leaning forward or backwards

PARAMETERS: Hold for 15 to 30 seconds, 3 to 5 repetitions, 1 to 3 times per day

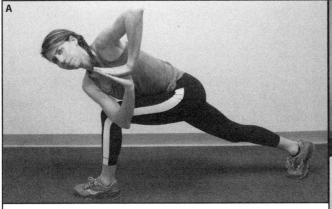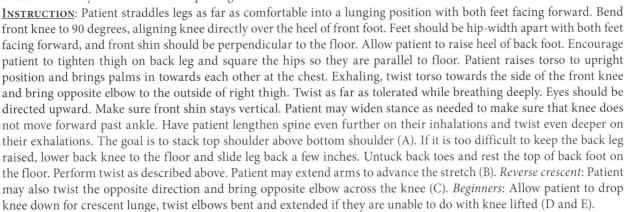

3.02.10 STRETCH: THORACIC, CRESCENT LUNGE TWIST

POSITION: Standing

TARGETS: Mobility of the thoracic spine into rotation, stretching thoracic rotators, chest opening; works muscles of the lower body in addition and requires good balance.

INSTRUCTION: Patient straddles legs as far as comfortable into a lunging position with both feet facing forward. Bend front knee to 90 degrees, aligning knee directly over the heel of front foot. Feet should be hip-width apart with both feet facing forward, and front shin should be perpendicular to the floor. Allow patient to raise heel of back foot. Encourage patient to tighten thigh on back leg and square the hips so they are parallel to floor. Patient raises torso to upright position and brings palms in towards each other at the chest. Exhaling, twist torso towards the side of the front knee and bring opposite elbow to the outside of right thigh. Twist as far as tolerated while breathing deeply. Eyes should be directed upward. Make sure front shin stays vertical. Patient may widen stance as needed to make sure that knee does not move forward past ankle. Have patient lengthen spine even further on their inhalations and twist even deeper on their exhalations. The goal is to stack top shoulder above bottom shoulder (A). If it is too difficult to keep the back leg raised, lower back knee to the floor and slide leg back a few inches. Untuck back toes and rest the top of back foot on the floor. Perform twist as described above. Patient may extend arms to advance the stretch (B). *Reverse crescent*: Patient may also twist the opposite direction and bring opposite elbow across the knee (C). *Beginners*: Allow patient to drop knee down for crescent lunge, twist elbows bent and extended if they are unable to do with knee lifted (D and E).

SUBSTITUTIONS: Twisting through the hips

PARAMETERS: Hold for 15 to 30 seconds, 3 to 5 repetitions, 1 to 3 times per day

3.02.11 STRETCH: THORACIC, GOLFER'S ROTATION AND SIDE-BEND

<u>POSITION</u>: Standing

<u>TARGETS</u>: Mobility of the thoracic spine into side-bending and rotation; good warm-up to golf swings.

<u>INSTRUCTION</u>: *Golfer's side bend*: Patient stands in good posture and places golf club behind the neck sitting on top of the posterior shoulders, holding on both ends with palms facing outward. Patient deeply inhales then exhales while leaning from the waist to one side without twisting the torso (A). *Golfer's twist*: Patient stands in good posture and places golf club behind the neck sitting on top of the posterior shoulders, holding on both ends with palms facing outward. Patient deeply inhales then exhales while rotating shoulders around one side while hips stay facing forward (B).

<u>SUBSTITUTIONS</u>: Leaning forward, trunk rotation, shoulder tense/shrug, only bending at waist and not thoracic region

<u>PARAMETERS</u>: Hold for 5 to 10 seconds, 5 to 10 repetitions, 1 to 3 times per day

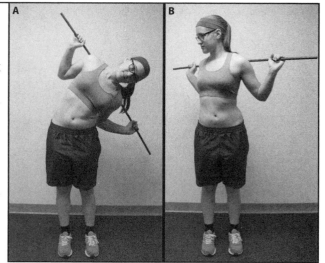

Section 3.03

THORACIC STRENGTHENING

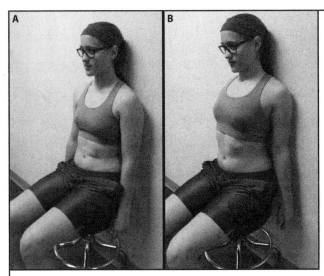

3.03.1 STRENGTHEN: ISOMETRIC; STERNAL LIFT

POSITION: Seated

TARGETS: Kyphotic postural correction to improve thoracic extension, strengthening thoracic extensors and scapular retractors (rhomboids, mid-trapezius) and depressors (lower fibers serratus anterior muscle, lower trapezius, pectoralis minor)

INSTRUCTION: Feet flat on the floor, have patient lift the breastbone (sternum) while drawing the shoulder blades back and down. Patient may perform this with the back against the wall to avoid body sway and give feedback. Encourage the patient to press-up through the chest while retracting and depressing the shoulders and lifting the sternum (A and B).

SUBSTITUTIONS: Slouching, loss of chin tuck, tensing the upper trapezius

PARAMETERS: Hold for 6 to 10 seconds, 1 to 3 sets, 8 to 12 repetitions, 1 time per day or every other day

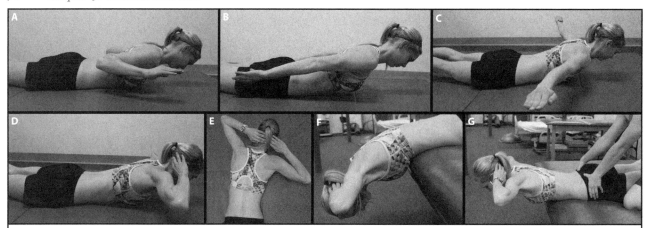

3.03.2 STRENGTHEN: ISOTONIC; STERNAL LIFT, 4-WAY

<u>POSITION</u>: Prone

<u>TARGETS</u>: Kyphotic postural correction to improve thoracic extension, strengthening thoracic extensors and scapular retractors (rhomboids, mid-trapezius) and depressors (lower fibers serratus anterior muscle, lower trapezius, pectoralis minor)

<u>INSTRUCTION</u>: *Hands under shoulders*: Lying face down, patient places hands directly under the shoulders. Patient then lifts sternum off of surface while looking forward at the floor/mat just in front of the head (not up). Encourage patient to do this by contracting muscles in the upper back and not pressing through arms. Beginners may use arms to assist, but progression should be made to eventually do without any UE assist (A). *Hands at sides*: Progression moves to placing the arms by the sides, retracting the scapula and lifting sternum off of the surface. Gaze remains as previously described (B). *"T" position*: Arms are placed with shoulders at 90 degrees of abduction, patient lifts sternum off of table along with arms. Arms should remain at the level of the shoulder joint and not horizontally abduction beyond the torso. This isolates thoracic extensors (C). *Hands behind head*: Clasp hands behind the neck, keeping chin tucked. Patient then lifts sternum off of surface while looking forward at the floor/mat just in front of the head (not up) (D). *With side bend*: Clasp hands behind the neck, keeping chin tucked. Patient then lifts sternum off of surface while looking forward at the floor/ mat just in front of the head (not up). Encourage patient to do this by contracting muscles in the upper back. Patient then side-bends the thoracic region as they bring the elbow towards the ipsilateral hip. Therapist may stabilize the hips as needed (E). *Xiphoid process at edge of mat variation*: Patient may do all of the above exercises with the xiphoid process at the edge of the mat for increased recruitment as they advance (F and G).

<u>PARAMETERS</u>: Hold 2 to 3 seconds, repeat 10 times, 2 to 3 sets, 1 time per day or every other day

Where's the Evidence?

Park, Kang, Kim, An, and Oh (2015) examined the effect of modified prone trunk-extension exercises on selective activity of the thoracic erector spinae in 39 healthy subjects performed four modified prone trunk-extension exercises, involving location of the edge of the table iliac crests vs xiphoid process and the degree of trunk extension horizontal vs hyperextension. EMG signals were collected bilaterally from the longissimus thoracis, iliocostalis thoracis, and iliocostalis lumborum. Activity in the lumbar erector spinae and iliocostalis thoracis muscles was greater when subjects were in the hyper extended position than in the horizontal position. Moreover, activity in the thoracic erector spinae was greater when the table edge was aligned with the iliac crest compared with the xiphoid process. Their findings suggest that prone trunk-extension exercise with the xiphoid process aligned with the table edge and avoiding hyper extension in the lower back increased the selective activation of the thoracic erector spinae muscles.

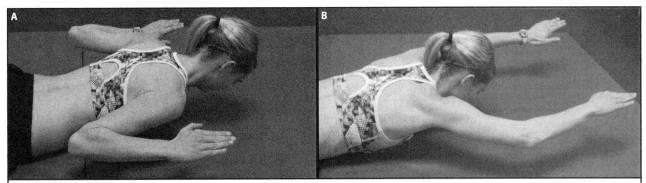

3.03.3 STRENGTHEN: ISOTONIC; STERNAL LIFT WITH SHOULDER MOVEMENTS

<u>POSITION</u>: Prone

<u>TARGETS</u>: Kyphotic postural correction to improve thoracic extension, strengthening thoracic extensors and scapular retractors (rhomboids, mid-trapezius) and depressors (lower fibers, serratus anterior, lower trapezius, pectoralis minor)

<u>INSTRUCTION</u>: Patient starts with arms in the "batwing" position, shoulders abducted 20 degrees, elbow flexed 90 to 100 degrees and palms down, lift arms off table/mat keeping elbows and hands at same height. Patient slightly lifts sternum off mat or table and, holding this position, brings arms into full abduction while extending the elbows. Patient should continue to look at the mat/table/floor during this entire movement and then return to start. Continue with repetitions until fatigue before lowering sternum back down (A and B).

<u>SUBSTITUTIONS</u>: Lifting too far, substituting with lower back, shrugging excessively with the upper trapezius

<u>PARAMETERS</u>: Repeat 10 to 20 times, 1 to 3 sets, 1 time per day or every other day

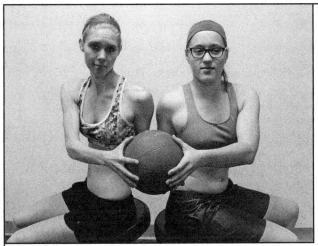

3.03.4 STRENGTHEN: THORACIC, SEATED TWIST WITH MEDICINE BALL/PARTNER

<u>POSITION</u>: Seated

<u>TARGETS</u>: Strengthening thoracic lateral flexors (ipsilateral erector spinae, iliocostalis, longissimus)

<u>INSTRUCTION</u>: Patient and partner straddle a bench seated back-to-back, facing away from each other. A weighted ball is placed in the patient's hands, elbows extended and shoulders flexed 90 degrees. The patient then twists the upper body to pass the ball to the partner who brings the ball around to the other side. The patient must rotate the opposite direction to then grab the ball and repeat rotation towards the other side.

<u>SUBSTITUTIONS</u>: The partners must maintain straight postures to keep in contact with each other. Patient should not lean forward or back. Watch for upper trapezius substitution (shrugging) with holding the ball away from the body.

<u>PARAMETERS</u>: Repeat 10 to 20 times, 1 to 3 sets, 1 time per day or every other day

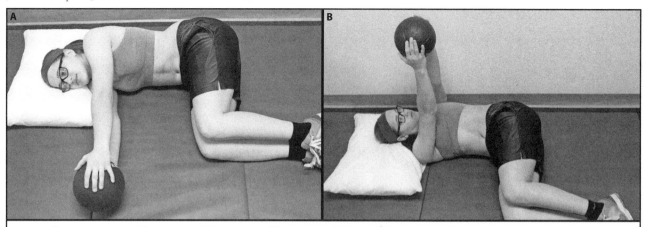

3.03.5 Strengthen: Isotonic; Thoracic Rotation With Weighted Ball

POSITION: Side-lying

TARGETS: Strengthening thoracic rotatores and semispinalis (will also utilize obliques)

INSTRUCTION: Lying on the side, patient bends the top hip and knee to 90 degrees. A support is placed under the top knee to maintain neutral pelvic and lumbar alignment. Place a weighted ball in the patient's hands. The patient should be facing the same direction as the knees with the shoulders flexed 90 degrees, the elbow extended, and the ball in the hands (A). Have the patient then rotate the upper trunk across the body to tap the floor on the opposite side and return to starting. Eyes should follow the ball (B).

SUBSTITUTIONS: Momentum and quick transitions; this should be done slowly, hips should remain stacked and knee on support.

PARAMETERS: 1 to 3 sets, 8 to 12 repetitions, 1 time per day or every other day

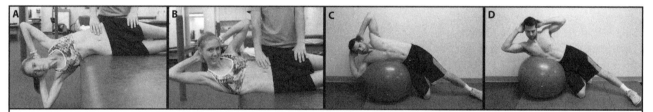

3.03.6 Strengthen: Isotonic; Thoracic Lateral Flexion, Arms Behind Head

POSITION: Side-lying

TARGETS: Strengthening thoracic lateral flexors (ipsilateral erector spinae, iliocostalis, longissimus)

INSTRUCTION: *Table:* Lying on the side with the upper thoracic region off of a table or mat at the level of the nipple line. Pad the end of the table with a towel as needed for comfort. The patient then clasps hands behind the head and allows the upper thoracic to drop toward the floor. Shoulders should remain in the same vertical plane. Patient then raises the upper thoracic up off table, bringing top elbow towards top hip. Stabilization of the legs may assist the patient during this activity (A and B). *Exercise ball:* Place the patient on the exercise ball so that the ball sits at the mid-thoracic region and allow the patient to place feet where they feel the most stable. Top knee should be extended. Placing the ball against a wall allows for greater stability. Patient then repeats the movement as described above (C and D).

SUBSTITUTIONS: Momentum and quick transitions; this should be done slowly, hips should remain stacked and knee on support.

PARAMETERS: 1 to 3 sets, 8 to 12 repetitions, 1 time per day or every other day

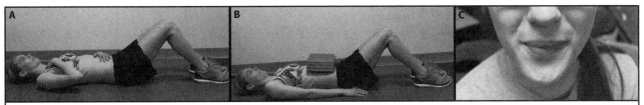

3.03.7 BREATHING TECHNIQUES: DIAPHRAGMATIC AND PURSED-LIP BREATHING

Diaphragmatic breathing, also known as abdominal breathing, belly breathing, or deep breathing, is done by contracting the diaphragm causing a negative vacuum in the thoracic cavity that pulls air into the lungs.

POSITION: Hook-lying

TARGETS: *Diaphragmatic breathing*: Focusing on improving the expansion of the lungs via improving the function of the diaphragm. *Pursed-lip breathing*: Focuses on keeping the lungs inflated for longer period time to improve the gas exchange in the alveoli.

INSTRUCTION: *Diaphragmatic breathing*: Patient places one hand over the chest and one hand over the belly. Patient contracts the pelvic floor muscles to begin, as this will improve the diaphragmatic motion. Patient then deeply inhales through the nose while trying to keep the chest hand still as the belly hand rises, holds 1 second, and exhales through the nose or mouth. Breathing ratio is 1:2 for inhale and exhale; start with 2 seconds: 4 seconds and work up to longer inhale and exhale times (A). To make this a strengthening exercise, place cuff or plate weights over the belly as the patient inhales, lifting the weight with the stomach as a resistive exercise (B). Patient may also use a book or several books at home. *Pursed-lip breathing*: Patient inhales through the nose and exhales through pursed or puckered lips, as if trying to whistle or make a candle flame flicker with a controlled blow). The pursed lips provide resistance to the exhale allowing the air to stay in the lungs longer and prolong lung inflation and air exchange (C).

SUBSTITUTIONS: Accessory breathing pattern; chest rises, shoulders shrug.

PARAMETERS: *For general practice*: 10 breaths, 3 to 4 times per day; *for strengthening*: 1 to 3 sets, 8 to 12 repetitions, 1 time per day or every other day.

Where's the Evidence?

Park and Han (2015) investigated the correlation between the pelvic floor muscles and diaphragmatic motion during breathing. Twenty healthy female students, who listened to an explanation of the study methods and purpose agreed to participate in the experiment. Radiograph equipment was used to examine diaphragmatic motion with contraction of the pelvic floor muscles during breathing, and a spirometer was used to examine lung vital capacity. The results revealed a significant change in the diaphragmatic motion and pulmonary function when the pelvic floor muscles was contracted, concluding diaphragmatic motion and contraction of the pelvic floor muscles correlate with breathing and that breathing is much more effective during contraction of the pelvic floor muscles. Therefore, pelvic floor muscles strengthening exercises should be included in respiratory rehabilitation programs.

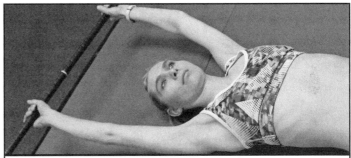

3.03.8 BREATHING TECHNIQUES: DIAPHRAGMATIC BREATHING WITH UPPER EXTREMITY FIXATION

POSITION: Supine

TARGETS: Fixation of the UE allows the inspiratory muscles to pull on the chest wall, reversing origin and insertion and improving chest expansion; diaphragmatic breathing strengthens diaphragm and improves air exchange in the lungs.

INSTRUCTION: Using a fixed bar overhead at 10 inches above the bed, patient lying supine place a small foam or towel rolls 2 to 3 inches in diameter under the mid-thoracic region (do not use if patient has pain or discomfort). Patient reaches overhead to place palms under the bar and grasps bar. Patient, then in a full upper body stretch, practices diaphragmatic breathing as described in **3.07.7**.

SUBSTITUTIONS: Accessory breathing pattern; chest rises, shoulders shrug.

PARAMETERS: *For general practice at home*: 10 breaths, 3 to 4 times per day; *clinically*: 20 to 30 deep breaths in this position, 1 times per day.

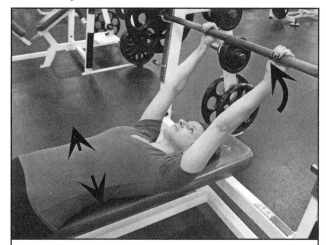

3.03.9 Breathing Techniques: Diaphragmatic Breathing With Upper Extremity Fixation and Isometric Lift

<u>Position</u>: Supine

<u>Targets</u>: Fixation of the UE allows the inspiratory muscles to pull on the chest wall, reversing origin and insertion and improving chest expansion; diaphragmatic breathing strengthens diaphragm and improves air exchange in the lungs. Isometric contraction of the shoulder muscles in this position encourages the pectoralis major to pull at the sternal attachments and increase chest expansion.

<u>Instruction</u>: Using a fixed bar overhead at 10 inches above the bed, patient lying supine place a small foam or towel rolls 2 to 3 inches in diameter under the mid-thoracic region (do not use if patient has pain or discomfort). Patient reaches overhead to place palms under the bar and grasps bar. Patient, then in a full upper body stretch, practices diaphragmatic breathing as described in **3.07.7** and, when the patient inspires, instruct them to attempt to lift the bar (isometrically), holding for 8 seconds then relax. Patient may use a standard weightlifting bar as an alternative with enough weight to resist any movement when isometrically lifting.

<u>Substitutions</u>: Accessory breathing pattern; chest rises, shoulders shrug.

<u>Parameters</u>: 10 breaths/lifts, 3 sets; for improving chest wall expansion optimally, this should be done 3 to 4 times per day.

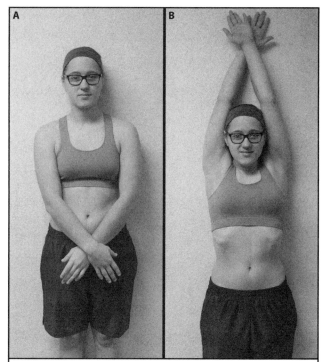

3.03.10 Breathing Techniques: Chest Expansion Breathing With Upper Extremity Movements

<u>Position</u>: Standing

<u>Targets</u>: Increase chest expansion and lung capacity

<u>Instruction</u>: Patient crosses arms at wrists in front of pelvis. Patient inhales deeply as they abduct both shoulders fully, bringing wrists to cross again overhead, focus on expanding the chest/ribs outward. Patient exhales slowly as the arms are lowered back to start (A and B).

<u>Substitutions</u>: Accessory breathing pattern; shoulders shrug, neck muscles should stay relaxed.

<u>Parameters</u>: 10 breaths/lifts, 3 sets; for improving chest wall expansion optimally, this should be done 3 to 4 times per day.

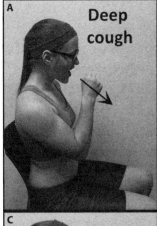
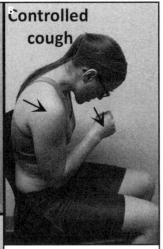

Deep cough

Controlled cough

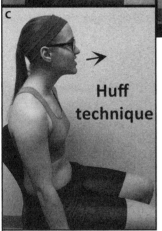

Huff technique

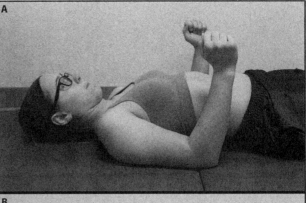

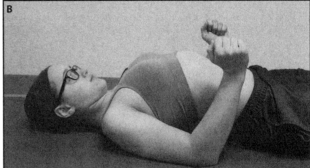

3.03.11 BREATHING TECHNIQUES: DEEP COUGH, CONTROLLED COUGH, AND THE "HUFF" TECHNIQUE

POSITION: Seated

TARGETS: To clear airways with the least amount of thoracic movement; controlled and "huff" techniques are effective for patients who have thoracic or rib pain with coughing.

INSTRUCTION: *Deep cough*: Patient takes a deep breath and holds the breath in for 2 to 3 seconds then uses the abdominals to forcefully expel the air (A). *Controlled cough*: Patient sits on a chair with both feet on the floor. Patient takes a slow, deep breath through the nose and holds for 2 counts, then leans slightly forward coughing 2 short coughs (B). *The "huff" technique*: Patient takes a slow, deep breath through the nose and holds for 2 counts then exhales, opening the mouth to make a "huff" sound in the throat as if fogging up a mirror, huffing 2 to 3 times (C).

SUBSTITUTIONS: Accessory breathing pattern; chest rises, shoulders shrug.

PARAMETERS: Repeat as needed for airway clearance.

3.03.12 STRENGTHEN: BACK-ARCHING SHOULDER PRESS

POSITION: Supine

TARGETS: Kyphotic postural correction to improve thoracic extension, strengthening thoracic extensors and scapular retractors (rhomboids, mid-trapezius) and depressors (lower fibers serratus anterior, lower trapezius, pectoralis minor); also increases chest expansion and lung capacity.

INSTRUCTION: Patient engages the lower abdominals to stabilize the lumbar spine. Patient inhales deeply, expanding the chest/ribs outward and presses elbows down into the mat, lifting the thoracic region off. Patient then exhales slowly while lowering their upper back to the mat (A and B).

SUBSTITUTIONS: Arching lower back excessively; abdominals are engaged to stabilize pelvis; avoid accessory breathing pattern and shoulders shrugging, neck muscles should stay relaxed.

PARAMETERS: 10 breaths/lifts, 3 sets; for improving chest wall expansion optimally, this should be done 3 to 4 times per day.

REFERENCES

Park, H., & Han, D. (2015). The effect of the correlation between the contraction of the pelvic floor muscles and diaphragmatic motion during breathing. *Journal of Physical Therapy Science, 27*(7), 2113-2115.

Park, K. H., Kang, M. H., Kim, T. H., An, D. H., & Oh, J. S. (2015). Selective recruitment of the thoracic erector spinae during prone trunk-extension exercise. *Journal of Back and Musculosketal Rehabilitation, 28*(4), 789-795.

Section 3.04

THORACIC/CHEST PROTOCOLS AND TREATMENT IDEAS

3.04.1 PECTUS EXCAVATUM DISCUSSION

Pectus excavatum also known as "funnel chest" is a congenital (present at birth) abnormality that can be mild or severe. It usually develops during pregnancy. It is caused by excessive growth of the connective tissue that joins the ribs to the breastbone. This causes the sternum to malform inward. The child typically has a depression in the center of the chest over the sternum, and this may appear quite deep. If pectus excavatum is severe, it may affect the heart and lungs, making exercise difficult. Also, the appearance of the chest may cause psychological difficulty for the child. Pectus excavatum may occur as the only abnormality or together with other syndromes (Daller, 2013). Pectus excavatum accounts for >90% of congenital chest wall deformities (Jaroszewski, Notrica, McMahon, Steidley, & Deschamps, 2010). Pectus excavatum occurs in approximately 1 out of 400 to 1000 children and is 3 to 5 times more common in males than females. The deformity usually becomes more severe as the child grows. Some children with pectus excavatum report that they have chest pain and shortness of breath or limited stamina with exercise. Other children have no symptoms. Surgery may not alleviate chest pain (The Regents of the University of California, 2015).

However, in the still-developing adolescent surgery is often considered. Patients with pectus excavatum are often dismissed by physicians as having an inconsequential problem; however, it can be more than a cosmetic deformity. Severe cases can cause cardiopulmonary impairment and physiologic limitations. Evidence continues to present that these physiologic impairments may worsen as the patient ages. Data reports improved cardiopulmonary function after repair and marked improvement in psychosocial function. More recent consensus by both the pediatric and thoracic surgical communities validates surgical repair of the significant pectus excavatum and contradicts arguments that repair is primarily cosmetic (Jaroszewski et al., 2010). Moreover, after corrective surgery, pectus excavatum patients have increased exercise tolerance and a higher oxygen pulse, as a measure of cardiac output, suggesting that surgical repair improves cardiopulmonary function during vigorous exercise (Haller & Loughlin, 2000).

There are two surgical procedures used currently, open and minimally invasive. The open repair, or Ravitch procedure, involves a horizontal incision across the mid-chest. In this repair, the abnormal costal cartilages are removed, preserving the lining of cartilage, thus allowing the sternum to move forward in a more normal position. In certain patients, an osteotomy (a break) in the sternum is done to allow the sternum to be positioned forward. In addition, to keep the sternum elevated in the desired position after the removal of the cartilages and the osteotomy, a temporary metal chest strut (bar) may need to be placed. The minimally invasive repair of pectus excavatum (MIRPE), or Nuss procedure, involves bending a stainless bar to fit the chest wall and inserting, through a small incision under each arm, using the aid of an endoscope to monitor and avoid injury to the heart during insertion. The bar goes over the ribs and under the sternum, to push the sternum forward into the new position. The ends of the bar are secured to the chest wall (The Regents of the University of California, 2015).

A non-surgical option is cup suction which is used to create a vacuum at the chest wall. It utilizes a patient-activated hand pump to reduce pressure up to 15% below atmospheric pressure. In patients with pectus excavatum, application of a vacuum effectively pulled the depressed anterior chest wall forward (Schier, Bahr, & Klobe, 2005). The initial results proved dramatic, although it is not yet known how much time is required for long-term correction. Several studies since have confirmed the vacuum method

holds promise as a valuable adjunct treatment in both surgical and nonsurgical correction of pectus excavatum.

Where's the Evidence?

Haecker (2011) studied 133 patients with pectus excavatum aged 3 to 61 years using the vacuum bell for 1 to a maximum of 36 months. A suction cup is used to create a vacuum at the anterior chest wall. When creating the vacuum, the lift of the sternum is obvious and remains for a different time period. Computed tomographic scans showed that the device lifted the sternum and ribs immediately. In addition, this was confirmed thoracoscopically during the MiRPE procedure. One hundred and five patients showed a permanent lift of the sternum for more than 1 cm after 3 months of daily application. Thirteen patients stopped the application and underwent MIRPE. Relevant side effects were not noted. Haecker recommended the device should be used for a minimum of 30 min (twice a day), and may be used up to a maximum of several hours daily. Furthermore, in 2015 Lopez et al. evaluated the efficacy of cup suction in the correction of pectus excavatum. A total of 73 patients presenting typical pectus excavatum (symmetric in 52 cases and asymmetric in 21 cases) were treated by cup suction. The mean depth of pectus excavatum was 23 mm. At 6 months of treatment, the mean depth of pectus excavatum was 9 mm across all patients except four that left the study. Twenty-three of the remaining 69 patients completed the treatment and exhibited flattening of the sternum. These patients were considered to have an excellent aesthetic result. The mean treatment duration to normal reshape was achieved at 10 months. The remaining patients continue to improve under further active treatment. They concluded treatment using cup suction is a promising, useful alternative in selected cases of symmetric and asymmetric pectus excavatum, providing that the thorax is flexible. The cup suction can also be used for pediatrics and young adults waiting for a treatment, possibly surgery.

Where's the Evidence?

Canavan and Cahalin (2008) in a single case study of a 22-year-old male with moderate to severe pectus excavatum implemented an individualized physical therapy program integrating cardiopulmonary and musculoskeletal interventions and eliminated bilateral shoulder pain and decreased the severity of the excavatum, which was shown through volumetric measurement of the depression from 60 mL to 20 ml (a 60% decrease). They concluded that this treatment, provided to other patients with pectus excavatum, may provide similar result and furthermore suggested that if provided to younger patients with pectus excavatum could be of even greater benefit because of a less mature skeleton.

For patients who have not had surgery, physical therapy has been shown to provide minimal-to-moderate improvements on many characteristics of pectus excavatum.

Physical therapy includes training the inspiratory muscles that help in pulling up the chest wall: anterior and middle scalenes, SCM, pectoralis minor and intercostals. Intercostal muscles help the elevation of the chest wall only when the first ribs are fixed and elevated. None of these muscles can directly add their pull of force on the lower sternum and sunken ribs, which are commonly encountered in pectus excavatum. Their effect of pull seems limited to the upper chest wall. However, if the upper limbs can be anchored by grasping a chair back or table, the sternal origin of the pectoralis major muscles can also assist the elevation process of the chest wall by reversing origin and insertion. This concept provides the direction for the design of the following suggested exercise program. With an increase in strength and muscle tone by training, the chest wall deformity may be diminished or at least maintained. In addition, the increase in intensity of training, especially to the anterior chest wall may help to build up larger muscle bulk and a better cosmetic outlook (Cheung, 2005).

3.04.2 PECTUS EXCAVATUM RECOMMENDED EXERCISES

Precautions should be taken if patient has undergone surgical repair. This protocol is for the non-operative patient; however, these exercises may be implements once cleared by the doctor after substantial healing has occurred.

Recommended exercises
1. Breathing
   a. 3.03.7 Breathing Techniques: Diaphragmatic and Pursed-Lip Breathing

---

Where's the Evidence?

Chanavirut, Khaidjapho, Jaree, and Pongnaratorn (2006) studied short-term yoga training and its effects on chest wall expansion and lung volumes in young healthy adults. Fifty-eight volunteers between the ages of 18 and 25 were studied. The yoga group performed 5 yoga postures: Uttita Kummersana (Cat position), Ardha Matsyendrasana (sitting and twisting the trunk), Vrikshasana (Tree position), Yoga Mudra and Ushtrasana (Camel position) for 20 minutes a day, 1 time a day, and 3 days a week until 6 weeks, whereas the control group had no intervention. At the end of 6 weeks of yoga training, chest wall expansion significantly increased in all 3 levels when compared to their pre-test values and post-test control. The improvement was highest at the upper compared to middle and lower chest levels. The 5 positions of Hatha yoga used in this study had been reported to predominantly effect on prime mover and accessory respiratory muscle such as external and internal intercostal muscle, pectoral, latissimus dorsi, erector spinae, RA, serratus anterior muscle and diaphragm. The authors concluded that short-term yoga exercise improves respiratory breathing capacity by increasing chest wall expansion and forced expiratory lung volumes. Vedala, Mane, and Paul (2014) looked at pulmonary function tests to measure 50 subjects practicing yoga and 50 sedentary subjects in the age group of 20 to 40 years. Pulmonary functions were compared between the yoga practitioners and sedentary group. Yoga exercise significantly increased chest wall expansion as observed by higher values of pulmonary functions compared with sedentary controls. They concluded regular yoga practice increases the vital capacity, timed vital capacity, maximum voluntary ventilation, breath holding time and maximal inspiratory and expiratory pressures.

---

2. Thoracic
   a. 3.02.3 Stretch: Thoracic With Hands on Bench/Chair/Ball, Using Foam Roll **3.03.7**
   b. 3.02.7 Stretch: Thoracic and Thoracolumbar Side-Bend
   c. 5.06.5 Stretch: Shoulder Horizontal Adductors, Doorway
   d. 5.06.6 Stretch: Shoulder Horizontal Adductors, Wall
   e. 3.03.8 Breathing Techniques: Diaphragmatic Breathing With Upper Extremity Fixation
   f. 3.03.9 Breathing Techniques: Diaphragmatic Breathing With Upper Extremity Fixation and Isometric Lift
   g. 3.03.1 Strengthen: Isometric; Sternal Lift
   h. 3.03.2 Strengthen: Isotonic; Sternal Lift, 4-Way
   i. 5.07.41 Strengthen: Isotonic; Resistance Band, Shoulder External Rotation and Variations
   j. 5.07.30 Strengthen: Isotonic; Resistance Band, Shoulder Adduction, 180 degrees, 90 degrees, no anchor.
   k. 5.07.62 Strengthen: Closed Kinetic Chain; Shoulder, Push-Up
   l. 5.17.1 Nerve Glide: Median Nerve
3. Yoga
   a. 3.01.4 ROM: Thoracic Flexion and Extension With and Without Cervical Extension, Cat and Camel
   b. 7.04.2CC Half Lord of the Fishes Pose (Ardha Matsyendrasana)
   c. 7.04.2N Tree Pose (Vrksasana)
   d. Cross-legged sitting and focused diaphragmatic breathing; hands relaxed on knees 5 to 10 minutes.
4. Other considerations
   a. Freestyle swimming
   b. Alternate climbing exercises
   c. Aerobic activities; running, biking, rowing.

5. Other exercises to target these areas may be added as patient advances and based on individual responses to treatment. Exercises should mainly concentrate on realignment of good static and dynamic posture. Consider additional scapulothoracic and shoulder strengthening exercises to progress. Consider some of these in your progression:
   a. Scapular strengthening; middle trapezius, lower trapezius, rhomboid.
      i. 5.03.5 Strengthen: Scapular Retraction, "T", "Y", and "I" and Variations
      ii. 5.03.8 Strengthen: Scapular Retraction, "W" or "Batwings" **5.03.9**
      iii. 5.03.12 Strengthen: Resistance Band, Scapular Row and Variations
      iv. 5.07.24 Strengthen: Isotonic; Shoulder, Row (Prone)
      v. 5.07.25 Strengthen: Isotonic; Shoulder, Military Press (Prone)
      vi. 5.07.63 Strengthen: Closed Kinetic Chain; Scapular and Shoulder Depression
   b. Shoulder external rotators strengthening; assists to correct forward shoulders.
      i. 5.07.22 Strengthen: Isotonic; Shoulder External Rotation
      ii. 5.07.23 Strengthen: Isotonic; Shoulder External Rotation 90/90
      iii. 5.07.27 Strengthen: Isotonic; Posterior Cuff, 4-Way
      iv. 5.07.41 Strengthen: Isotonic; Resistance Band, Shoulder External Rotation and Variations
   c. Scapular strengthening; serratus anterior
      i. 5.03.1 Strengthen: Scapular, Push-Up Plus (Beginner)
      ii. 5.03.2 Strengthen: Scapular, Ceiling Punch
      iii. 5.03.15 Strengthen: Resistance Band, Scapular, Punch

d. Strengthening latissimus dorsi
    i. 5.07.34 Strengthen: Isotonic; Resistance Band and Machine, Shoulder, Lat Pull-Down
    ii. 5.07.46 Strengthen: Isotonic; Resistance Band, Shoulder Pull-Over

iii. 5.07.47 Strengthen: Isotonic; Resistance Band, Shoulder Pull-Back
iv. 5.07.54 Strengthen: Exercise Ball, Pull-Over (Latissimus Dorsi)
v. 5.07.64 Strengthen: Closed Kinetic Chain; Shoulder, Table Top Push-Pull

3.04.3 Thoracic Outlet/Inlet Syndrome Discussion

TOS represents a spectrum of disorders encompassing three related syndromes: compression of the brachial plexus (neurogenic TOS), compression of the subclavian artery or vein (vascular TOS), and the nonspecific or disputed type of TOS (Huang & Zager, 2004). The thoracic outlet, more recently referred to as *thoracic inlet syndrome*, refers to the compression of structures traveling through an anatomical opening at the top of the thoracic cavity. The thoracic inlet is essentially a hole surrounded by a bony ring, through which several vital structures pass. The thoracic inlet is bounded by the first thoracic vertebra (T1) and costovertebral joints posteriorly, the first pair of ribs and costal cartilages laterally, and the superior border of the manubrium anteriorly (Knipe, 2017).

Neurovascular compression may be observed most commonly in the interscalene triangle, but it also has been described in the costoclavicular space and in the subcoracoid space. Patients present with symptoms and signs of arterial insufficiency, venous obstruction, painless wasting of intrinsic hand muscles, paresthesia and pain. A careful and detailed medical history and physical examination are the most important diagnostic tools for proper identification of TOS. EMG, nerve conduction studies, and imaging of the cervical spine and the chest also can provide helpful information regarding diagnosis. Clinical management usually starts with conservative treatment including exercise programs and physical therapy. When these therapies fail, patients are considered for surgery. Two of the most commonly used surgical approaches are the supraclavicular exposure and the transaxillary approach with first rib resection. On occasion, these approaches may be combined or, alternatively, posterior subscapular exposure may be used in selected patients (Huang & Zager, 2004). Causes can be from congenital factors such as cervical rib, fibrous muscular bands, abnormalities of the insertion of the scalene muscles, exostosis of the first rib, cervicodorsal scoliosis, congenital unilateral or bilateral elevated scapula, or location of the subclavian artery and vein in relation to the anterior scalene. TOS can present from acquired conditions such as posture, dropped shoulder condition, heavy mammaries, trauma such as clavicle or rib fractures or neck injuries or repetitive stress injuries i.e., computer use or repetitive UE use. Muscular hypertrophy or shortening

of the scalenes, decreased tone of the middle trapezius, levator scapula and rhomboids or shortening of the middle trapezius, levator scapula, and pectoral muscles may also be linked to TOS (Walker, Keller, Schwarz, Nordin, & Salininger, n.d.).

Physical therapy treatment should address the problems identified during the patient evaluation. Conservative treatment should be utilized unless there is significant vascular compromise, motor loss or as long as the patient is improving. Conservative management of TOS requires accurate evaluation of the peripheral nervous system, posture, and the cervicoscapular muscles. Patients should be instructed in postural correction in sitting, standing and sleeping, stretching exercises (i.e., upper trapezius, levator scapulae, suboccipitals, scalenes, SCM and pectoral muscles), and strengthening exercises of the lower scapular stabilizers beginning in gravity-assisted positions to regain normal movement patterns in the cervicoscapular region. Patient education, compliance to an exercise program, and behavioral modification at home and work are critical to successful conservative management (Novak, 1996).

> ## *Where's the Evidence?*
>
> Hanif et al. (2007) studies 50 consecutive patients with neurogenic TOS, all diagnosed clinically with conformation electrodiagnosis. Patients followed a therapeutic exercises program for 6 months. After 6 months of conservative treatment, 34% of patients showed full recovery, 28% had marked improvement, 32% had partial improvement while 6% patients reported with persistent severe symptoms. Hanif et al. (2006) concluded that a trial of therapeutic exercises provides relief of symptoms of neurogenic TOS in majority of patients.

Surgical treatment typically includes resection of first rib, scalenotomy or clavicular resection, but should be used as a last resort (Powers, 2002). Disputed neurogenic TOS is best managed with a trial of conservative therapy before surgical treatment options are considered. Cases that are resistant to conservative treatment may require surgical intervention. True neurogenic TOS may require surgical intervention to relieve compression of the neural structures in the thoracic outlet. Surgical management is required for cases of vascular TOS because of the potentially serious complications that may arise from venous or arterial compromise. Post-operative rehabilitation is recommended after surgical decompression to address factors that could lead to a reoccurrence of the patient's symptoms (Hooper, Denton, McGalliard, Brismée, & Sizer, 2010).

Where's the Evidence?

Lindgren (1997) evaluated a conservative therapy program that aimed to restore normal function to the upper thoracic aperture in patients with TOS. After therapy, the patients were followed for a mean period of 24.6 months. Therapy was initiated primarily in an inpatient rehabilitation ward over a range of 4 to 24 day stay. One hundred nineteen patients with a positive TOS index participated. At admission, 50% of the patients were employed, 48% were on sick leave or retired, and 2% were unemployed. The patients received instructions on how to restore the normal function of their cervical spine and upper thoracic aperture by means of home exercises. The efficacy of the treatment program was assessed by the frequency of return to work, normalization of the motion of the cervical spine and upper thoracic aperture, and subjective satisfaction with the outcome. At the follow-up examination, 88% of the patients were satisfied with the outcome of their treatment, and the ranges of motion of the cervical spine and upper thoracic aperture had normalized in 8 of 10 patients. Seventy-three percent of the patients returned to work after the therapy, either directly or after retraining, and 88% of the patients carried through the recommendations given at discharge during long-term follow-up. Lindgren (1997) concluded the treatment program provides relief to most patients with symptoms of TOS. However as there was no control group findings may be somewhat inconclusive.

3.04.4 THORACIC OUTLET/INLET RECOMMENDED EXERCISES

This is possibly done in conjunction with mobilization treatments to first rib, SCM joint, acromioclavicular joint, glenohumeral joint, cervical spine and taping. What is listed below in the protocol is the exercise portion only. Precautions should be taken if patient has undergone surgical repair. This protocol is for the non-operative patient; however, these exercises may be implements once cleared by the doctor after substantial healing has occurred.

Recommended exercises:

1. Breathing
   a. 3.03.7 Breathing Techniques: Diaphragmatic and Pursed-Lip Breathing
2. Cervical ROM
   a. 2.01.2 ROM: Cervical Anterior Semicircles
   b. 2.01.3 ROM: Chin Tuck With Cervical Extension
   c. 2.01.4 ROM: Chin Tuck With Cervical Flexion
   d. 2.01.5 ROM: Chin Tuck With Cervical Rotation
   e. 2.01.6 ROM: Chin Tuck With Cervical Lateral Flexion
3. Chin tuck (posture correction: forward head)
   a. 2.01.1 ROM: Chin Tuck
   b. 2.03.4 Strengthen: Isotonic; Chin Tuck
   c. 2.03.5 Strengthen: Isotonic; Chin Tuck Neutral (Beginner) and With Slight Rotation (Advanced), Forehead on Towel Roll (Beginner) and Head off Bed (Advanced)
4. Scapular retraction (posture correction: forward shoulders)
   a. 5.03.3 Strengthen: Scapular Retraction and Variations
   b. 5.03.4 Strengthen: Scapular Retraction, Arms by Sides **5.03.10**
5. Scapular elevation (posture correction: downward shoulders)
   a. 5.03.10 Strengthen: Scapular Elevation, Shrugs
6. Thoracic mobility
   a. 3.01.4 ROM: Thoracic Flexion and Extension With and Without Cervical Extension, Cat and Camel
   b. 3.01.5 ROM: Thoracic Rotation, Bow and Arrow Rib Pull Upper, Middle, and Lower
   c. 3.01.7 ROM: Thoracic Extension Over Back of Chair, Head Supported
   d. 3.01.9 ROM: Thoracic Rotation, Active
7. Pectoral stretch
   a. 5.06.8 Stretch: Shoulder Horizontal Adductors, Towel Roll and Swiss Ball
   b. 5.06.5 Stretch: Shoulder Horizontal Adductors, Doorway
8. Upper trapezius stretch
   a. 2.02.3 Stretch: Self-Assisted Cervical Lateral Flexion

9. Levator Scapula stretch
   a. 2.02.7 Stretch: Cervical Flexion and Rotation
10. Scalene stretch
    a. 2.02.4 Stretch: Cervical Extension and Rotation
    b. 2.02.5 Stretch: Cervical Rotation and Extension, First Rib Stabilization With Belt/Strap
11. Nerve glides; pain-free.
    a. 5.17.1 Nerve Glide: Median Nerve
    b. 5.17.2 Nerve Glide: Radial Nerve
    c. 5.17.3 Nerve Glide: Ulnar Nerve
12. Cervical strengthening
    a. 2.03.7 Strengthen: Isotonic; Lower Neck/Thoracic Extension, Head Lift, 5 Positions (Cervical Extensors)
    b. 2.03.8 Strengthen: Isotonic; Chin Tuck Cervical Flexion With Head Lift (Deep Neck Flexors)
13. Scapular and shoulder strengthening
    a. 5.03.5 Strengthen: Scapular Retraction, "T", "Y", and "I" and Variations
    b. 5.03.8 Strengthen: Scapular Retraction, "W" or "Batwings"
    c. 5.03.12 Strengthen: Resistance Band, Scapular Row and Variations
    d. 5.07.24 Strengthen: Isotonic; Shoulder, Row (Prone)
    e. 5.07.63 Strengthen: Closed Kinetic Chain; Scapular and Shoulder Depression

14. Shoulder external rotators strengthening; assists to correct forward shoulders.
    a. 5.07.22 Strengthen: Isotonic; Shoulder External Rotation
    b. 5.07.23 Strengthen: Isotonic; Shoulder External Rotation 90/90
    c. 5.07.27 Strengthen: Isotonic; Posterior Cuff, 4-Way
    d. 5.07.41 Strengthen: Isotonic; Resistance Band, Shoulder External Rotation and Variations
15. Scapular strengthening; serratus anterior
    a. 5.03.1 Strengthen: Scapular, Push-Up Plus (Beginner)
16. Body mechanics and ergonomics education: regarding postures, positions, and activities that exacerbate the symptoms is of extreme importance to allow the patient to begin modification of work and home activities. The patient should minimize overhead activity, be conscious of head/shoulder postures, avoid sleeping in prone or on the affected side and avoid carrying heavy objects with the affected arm (Powers, 2002).
17. Overall conditioning
    a. Treadmill walking comfortable pace; *monitor good posture.*
    b. Stationary bike comfortable pace; *monitor good posture.*
    c. 5.04.1 ROM: Shoulder, Warm-Up, Upper Body Ergometer, Active Assistive; *add resistance as tolerated.*

3.04.5 BREATHING AND COUGHING TECHNIQUES

Patients may have pain with coughing or difficulties with breathing due to obstructive or resistive airway syndromes. Additionally, coughing can increase thoracic or rib pain. Below are some basic breathing and cough techniques that may assist in guiding these patients.

1. Breathing
   a. 3.03.7 Breathing Techniques: Diaphragmatic and Pursed-Lip Breathing
2. Coughing techniques
   a. 3.03.10 Breathing Techniques: Chest Expansion Breathing With Upper Extremity Movements

REFERENCES

Canavan, P. K., & Cahalin, L. (2008). Integrated physical therapy intervention for a person with pectus excavatum and bilateral shoulder pain: A single-case study. *Archives of Physical Medicine & Rehabilitation, 89*(11), 2195-2204.

Chanavirut, R., Khaidjapho, K., Jaree, P., & Pongnaratorn, P. (2006). Yoga exercise increases chest wall expansion and lung volumes in young healthy Thais. *Thai Journal of Physiological Sciences, 19*(1), 1-7.

Cheung, S. Y. K. (2005). Exercise therapy in the correction of pectus excavatum. *Journal of Pediatric Respiratory and Critical Care, 1*(2), 10-13.

Daller, J. A. (2013). Pectus excavatum. *MedlinePlus.* Retrieved from https://www.nlm.nih.gov/medlineplus/ency/article/003320.htm

Haecker, F. M. (2011). The vacuum bell for conservative treatment of pectus excavatum: The Basle experience. *Pediatric Surgery International, 27*(6), 623-627.

Haller, J. A. Jr, & Loughlin, G. M. (2000). Cardiorespiratory function is significantly improved following corrective surgery for severe pectus excavatum. Proposed treatment guidelines. *Journal of Cardiovascular Surgery, 41*(1), 125-130.

Hanif, S., Tassadaq, N., Rathore, M. F., Rashid, P., Ahmed, N., & Niazi, F. (2007). Role of therapeutic exercises in neurogenic thoracic outlet syndrome. *Journal of Ayub Medical College, 19*(4), 85-88.

Hooper, T. L., Denton, J., McGalliard, M. K., Brismée, J. M., & Sizer, P. S, Jr. (2010). Thoracic outlet syndrome: a controversial clinical condition. Part 2: Non-surgical and surgical management. *Journal of Manual & Manipulative Therapy, 18*(3), 132-138.

Huang, J. H., & Zager, E. L. (2004). Thoracic outlet syndrome. *Neurosurgery, 55*(4), 897-902.

Jaroszewski, D., Notrica, D., McMahon, L., Steidley, D. E., & Deschamps, C. (2010). Current management of pectus excavatum: A review and uposterior deltoidate of therapy and treatment recommendations. *Journal of the American Board of Family Medicine, 23*(2), 230-239.

Knipe, H. (2017). Superior thoracic aperture. Retrieved from https://radiopaedia.org/articles/superior-thoracic-aperture

Lindgren, K. A. (1997). Conservative treatment of thoracic outlet syndrome: A 2-year follow-up. *Archives of Physical Medicine and Rehabilitation, 78*(4), 373-378.

Lopez, M., Patoir, A., Costes, F., Varlet, F., Barthelemy, J. C., & Tiffet, O. (2015). Preliminary study of efficacy of cup suction in the correction of typical pectus excavatum. *Journal of Pediatric Surgery, 51*(1), 183-187.

Novak, C. B. (1996). Conservative management of thoracic outlet syndrome. *Seminar in Thoracic and Cardiovascular Surgery, 8*(2), 201-207.

Powers, W. S. (2002). Evaluation and treatment for thoracic outlet syndrome. *Rehab Insider.* Retrieved from http://rehab-insider.advanceweb.com/evaluation-and-treatment-for-thoracic-outlet-syndrome

Schier, F., Bahr, M., & Klobe, E. (2005). The vacuum chest wall lifter: an innovative, nonsurgical addition to the management of pectus excavatum. *Journal of Pediatric Surgery, 40*(3), 496-500.

The Regents of the University of California. (2015). Pediatric surgery: Pectus excavatum. *University of California San Francisco.* Retrieved from http://pedsurg.ucsf.edu/conditions--procedures/pectus-excavatum.aspx#a3

Vedala, S. R., Mane, A. B., & Paul, C. N. (2014). Pulmonary functions in yogic and sedentary population. *International Journal of Yoga, 7*(2), 155-159.

Walker, C., Keller, J., Schwarz, K., Nordin, J., Slininger, C.; Texas State University Evidence-Based Practice Project. (n.d.). Thoracic outlet syndrome. *Physiopedia.* Retrieved from http://www.physio-pedia.com/Thoracic_Outlet_Syndrome

Chapter 4

LUMBAR EXERCISES

Bryan E. *The Comprehensive Manual of Therapeutic Exercises:*
Orthopedic and General Conditions (pp 83-163).
© 2018 SLACK Incorporated.

Section 4.01

Lumbar Range of Motion

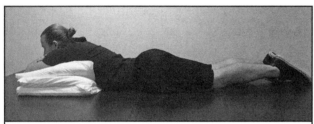

4.01.1 ROM: Lumbar Extension, Pillows Under Chest, Passive

Position: Prone

Targets: Mobility of the lumbar spine into extension

Instruction: Place one to multiple pillows under the patient's chest and allow patient to sink hips into the mat/table. Encourage patient to breathe deeply and relax into the movement of lumbar extension.

Substitutions: Lifting pelvis off table

Parameters: Hold for 3 to 5 minutes, repeat 1 to 3 times per day

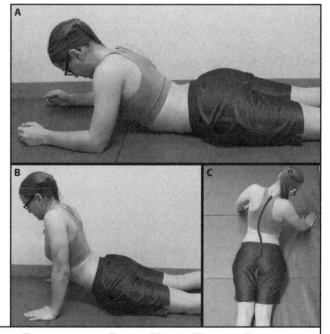

4.01.2 ROM: Lumbar Extension, Prone on Elbows, Progress to Press Up on Hands, Passive

Position: Prone

Targets: Mobility of the lumbar spine into extension

Instruction: *On elbows*: Patient places elbows under shoulders, palms down in front, and presses upper torso upwards while maintaining gaze forward. Encourage patient to sink hips into the mat/table and breathe deeply and relax into the movement of lumbar extension (A). *Press up on hands*: Patient places hands under shoulders, palms down, and presses upper torso upwards while maintaining gaze forward (B). *Lateral preference*: When using for centralization of pain and to target reduction on one side specifically, patient lies in prone with trunk side-bent to desired direction in which centralization occurs. Patient then presses up onto elbows and eventually onto the hands as per tolerance (C).

Substitutions: Lifting pelvis off table

Parameters: *Prone on elbows*: Hold for 3 to 5 minutes, repeat 1 to 3 times per day. *Prone press up on hands*: Hold for 10 seconds, repeat 5 to 15 times, repeat 1 to 3 times per day.

Where's the Evidence?

Beattie, Arnot, Donley, Noda, and Bailey (2010) looked at changes of diffusion of water in the L5 to S1 intervertebral disc between subjects with nonspecific LBP who reported an immediate reduction in pain intensity of 2 or greater on an 11-point (0 to 10) numeric rating scale after a 10-minute session of lumbar joint mobilization, followed by prone press up exercises, compared to those who did not report an immediate reduction in pain intensity of 2 or greater on the pain scale. Subjects underwent T2- and diffusion-weighted lumbar MRI scans before and immediately after receiving a 10-minute session of lumbar pressures in a posterior-to-anterior direction and prone press up exercises. Subjects who reported a decrease in current pain intensity of 2 or greater immediately following treatment were classified as immediate responders, while the remainder were classified as not-immediate responders. Following treatment, immediate responders (n = 10) had a mean increase in the apparent diffusion coefficient in the middle portion of the L5 to S1 intervertebral disc of 4.2% compared to a mean decrease of 1.6% for the not-immediate responders. Beattie et al. (2010) concluded the report of an immediate reduction in pain intensity of 2/10 greater after a treatment of posterior-to-anterior–directed pressures, followed by prone press up exercises, was associated with an increase in diffusion of water in the nuclear region of the L5 to S1 intervertebral disc.

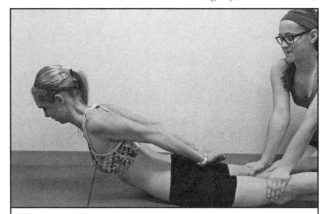

4.01.3 ROM: Lumbar Extension, Active

POSITION: Standing

TARGETS: Mobility of the lumbar spine into extension; good exercise for patients to do after any repeated bending or lifting.

INSTRUCTION: Patient places hands in the back of the pelvis and extends lower back into extension. Feet should be placed hip-width apart and knees slightly bent. Breathe deeply and relax into the movement.

SUBSTITUTIONS: Excessive cervical extension, pressing hips forward and avoiding extension through the lumbar spine, excessive knee bending

PARAMETERS: Hold for 10 seconds, repeat 5 to 15 times, repeat 1 to 3 times per day

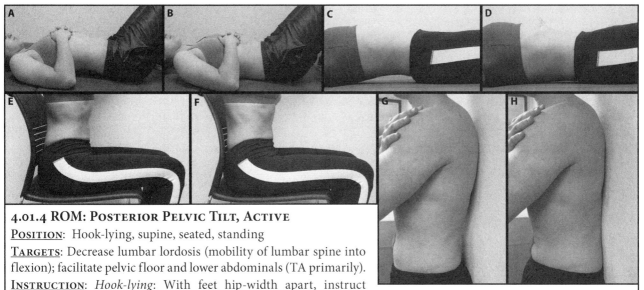

4.01.4 ROM: Posterior Pelvic Tilt, Active

POSITION: Hook-lying, supine, seated, standing

TARGETS: Decrease lumbar lordosis (mobility of lumbar spine into flexion); facilitate pelvic floor and lower abdominals (TA primarily).

INSTRUCTION: *Hook-lying*: With feet hip-width apart, instruct patient to decrease the space between the supporting surface and the lower back by tilting the pelvis posteriorly, drawing the navel in toward the spine. Therapist may place the hand under the lower back to feel the pressure and provide feedback (A and B). *Supine*: This is more difficult than hook-lying and is the next progression for this movement. In this position, repeat the same instructions as for hook-lying (C and D). *Seated and standing*: With feet hip-width apart and planted on the floor, repeat instructions (E through H).

SUBSTITUTIONS: Avoid hunching through the upper torso.

PARAMETERS: Hold for 10 seconds, repeat 5 to 15 times, repeat 1 to 3 times per day

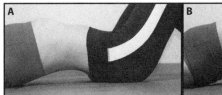
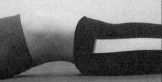
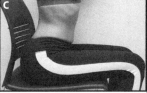
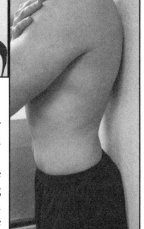

4.01.5 ROM: Anterior Pelvic Tilt, Active

Position: Hook-lying, supine, seated, standing

Targets: Increase lumbar lordosis (mobility of lumbar spine into extension); facilitate lumbar extensors (erector spinae: iliocostalis, longissimus, spinalis) and iliopsoas (reversal of origin and insertion).

Instruction: *Hook-lying*: With feet hip-width apart, instruct patient to increase the space between the supporting surface and the lower back by tilting the pelvis anteriorly, bringing navel up and away from table in an arching motion (A). *Supine*: This is more difficult than hook-lying and is the next progression for this movement. In this position, repeat the same instructions as for hook-lying (B). *Seated and standing*: With feet hip-width apart and planted on the floor, repeat instructions (C and D).

Substitutions: Avoid bringing scapula or pelvis off of table.

Parameters: Hold for 10 seconds, repeat 5 to 15 times, repeat 1 to 3 times per day

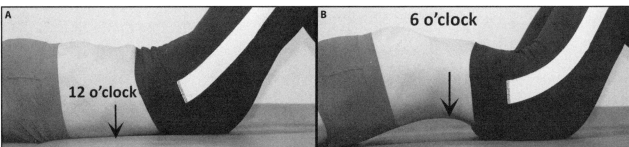
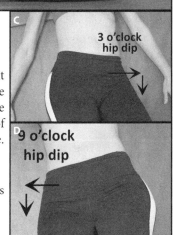

4.01.6 ROM: Pelvic Clocks

Position: Hook-lying

Targets: Mobility of lumbar spine, engages pelvic muscles

Instruction: Lying face up, have the patient imagine a clock on the stomach. Patient performs the following motions. *12 o'clock*: PPT (see previous) (A). *6 o'clock*: APT (see previous) (B). *3 and 9 o'clock*: Have patient imagine people sitting on each side of the pelvis with the pelvis acting as a teeter totter. Have the patient lift up on one side of the pelvis. Knee will push slightly away from the body as the patient elongates one side. Repeat to the other side (C and D).

Substitutions: Do not allow knees to drop in or out.

Parameters: Hold 10 to 15 seconds (enough to take 3 to 4 breaths), repeat 1 to 3 times at each level depending on treatment goals, 1 to 2 times per day

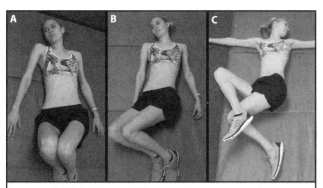

4.01.7 ROM: Lower Trunk Rotation, Active

Position: Hook-lying

Targets: Mobility of the lumbar spine in the transverse plane (rotation)

Instruction: Start with the back flat and feet together flat on mat. Rotate knees fully to the left and then follow by going to the right. Knees should remain together. Movements should be slow. For warm-up, only go part range and then progress to end range rotations (A and B). Therapist may add neck rotation to the opposite to increase rotation. Shoulders should stay in contact with surface. Patient may also cross leading ankle over the opposite knee to add over pressure and stretch component through the lower back and pelvic/hip posterior muscles (C).

Substitutions: Pelvis comes off floor

Parameters: Repeat 10 to 20 times, 1 to 3 times per day

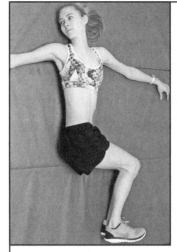

4.01.8 ROM: Lower Trunk Rotation 90/90, in Air and on Exercise Ball, Active

Position: Supine 90/90

Targets: Mobility of the lumbar spine in the transverse plane (rotation); can also be used for strengthening lower trunk rotators (obliques).

Instruction: Start with the back flat and hips and knees at 90 degrees of flexion (90/90). Patient places arms out to the sides and rotates knees fully to the left and then follows by going to the right. Abdominals remain engaged to avoid lumbar extension and knees should remain together. Movements should be slow. For warm-up, only go part range and then progress to end range rotations. Therapist may add neck rotation to the opposite side to increase rotation. Shoulders should stay in contact with surface. *Exercise ball*: Placing legs in 90/90 position on the exercise ball, patient then rotates trunk, bringing exercise ball to each side.

Substitutions: Arching lower back, holding breath

Parameters: Repeat 10 to 20 times, 1 to 3 times per day

4.01.9 ROM: Lower Trunk Lateral Flexion Against Wall, Passive

Position: Standing

Targets: Mobility of the lumbar spine in the coronal plane (side-bending)

Instruction: Start standing sideways to a wall. Patient's feet are close to the wall. Patient presses upper body away with hand while side-bending the trunk away from the wall. The wall press allows the patient to push further into side-bending.

Substitutions: Arching lower back, leaning forward, holding breath

Parameters: Repeat 10 to 20 times, 1 to 3 times per day

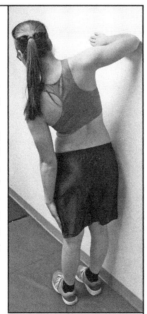

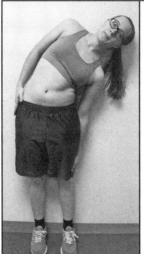

4.01.10 ROM: Lower Trunk Lateral Flexion, Active

Position: Standing

Targets: Mobility of the lumbar spine in the coronal plane (side-bending); can also be used to stretch obliques and quadratus lumborum and open lateral rib cage.

Instruction: Patient stands with side against wall, feet close to wall. Patient pushes away from the wall into side-bending using arm closest to wall and slides opposite hand down the outside of thigh. Patient should keep shoulder in line with body without bending forward or back or rotating trunk to either side. Patient may hold for a stretch here per treatment goals and then slowly return to starting position. Rolling forward will target quadratus lumborum if desired.

Substitutions: Flexion, extension, or rotation of trunk

Parameters: Repeat 5 to 15 times, 1 to 3 times per day; patient may hold 15 to 30 seconds if stretch is intended.

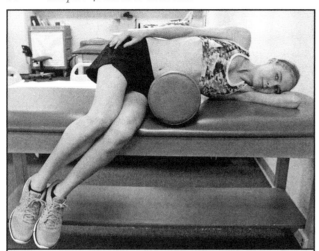

4.01.11 ROM: LOWER TRUNK LATERAL FLEXION WITH TOWEL ROLL AND LEG DROP, PASSIVE

POSITION: Side-lying

TARGETS: Mobility of the lumbar spine in the coronal plane (side-bending)

INSTRUCTION: Patient is in side-lying with the front of the body close to the edge of the table. A bolster, towel roll, or pillow is placed under the lumbar spine. Inferior arm may be placed under the head for comfort or use supporting pillow for head. The top hip and knee are flexed and then allowed to drop slowly off the bed, opening the lumbar spine facets and intervertebral joints on the opposite side. After holding desired length of time, therapist may assist the leg in lowering and returning to decrease discomfort.

SUBSTITUTIONS: Flexion, extension, or rotation of trunk

PARAMETERS: Repeat 2 to 3 times, 1 to 2 times per day; patient may hold up to several minutes depending on treatment goals.

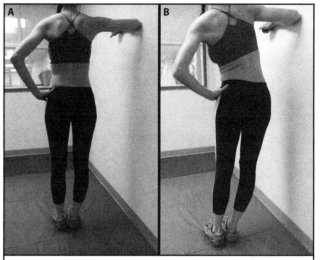

4.01.12 ROM: LATERAL SHIFT, SELF-CORRECTION

POSITION: Standing

TARGETS: Mobility of the lumbar spine in the coronal plane (side-bending); correction of lateral shift.

INSTRUCTION: Patient stands perpendicular to a wall and places both shoulder and elbow against it. Leg closest to the wall steps outward so that feet are approximately 8 to 12 inches from the wall (A). Opposite hand is placed on the iliac crest and presses the pelvis toward the wall. This is done in a pattern of pushing a comfortable distance and then releasing back half of that distance and repeating this "2 steps in, 1 step back" pattern until the pelvis reaches the wall. Once the patient's pelvis reaches the way, this position may be held for several seconds per tolerance (B).

SUBSTITUTIONS: Flexion, extension, or rotation of trunk

PARAMETERS: Repeat 5 to 15 times, 1 to 3 times per day; patient may hold 15 to 30 seconds if stretch is intended.

Where's the Evidence?

Several published case studies in 1998 and 2009 and have shown improvements in patients presenting with an acute lateral shift deformity. In each case, the practitioner used the lateral shift maneuver to manage their patients with acute lumbar lateral shift and obtained favorable results (Fritz, 1998; Laslett, 2009).

REFERENCES

Beattie, P. F., Arnot, C. F., Donley, J. W., Noda, H., & Bailey, L. (2010). The immediate reduction in low back pain intensity following lumbar joint mobilization and prone press-ups is associated with increased diffusion of water in the L5-S1 intervertebral disc. *Journal of Orthopedic Physical Therapy, 40*(5), 256-264.

Fritz, J. M. (1998). Use of a classification approach to the treatment of 3 patients with low back syndrome. *Physical Therapy, 78*(7), 766-777.

Laslett, M. (2009). Manual correction of an acute lumbar lateral shift: Maintenance of correction and rehabilitation: A case report with video. *Journal of Manual and Manipulative Therapy, 17*(2), 78-85.

Section 4.02

LUMBAR STRETCHING

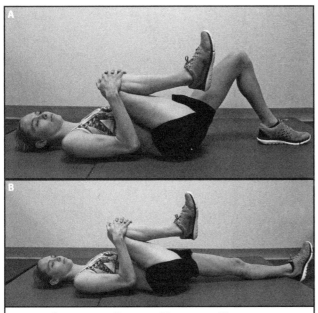

4.02.1 STRETCH: SINGLE KNEE TO CHEST

POSITION: Supine, hook-lying; supine is the most effective way to achieve results but dependent on back pain; hook-lying may be more comfortable for some patients, due to increased stress placed on back during supine.

TARGETS: Stretches proximal end of hamstrings, gluteus maximus, gluteus medius, gluteus minimus, thoracolumbar erector spinae muscles, quadratus lumborum

INSTRUCTION: Bend up one knee and grab with both hands either behind the knee or in front of the bent knee. Relax and keep the opposite leg down and straight (unless hook-lying, then keep foot flat), and then pull bent knee toward chest (A and B).

SUBSTITUTIONS: Lateral trunk flexion; pulling bent knee into abduction.

PARAMETERS: Hold for 15 to 30 seconds, 3 to 5 repetitions, 1 to 3 times per day

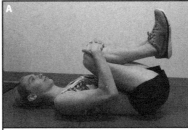
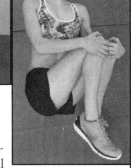

4.02.2 STRETCH: DOUBLE KNEE TO CHEST, 3-WAY

POSITION: Supine or hook-lying

TARGETS: Increase lumbar flexion flexibility; stretch paraspinal muscles of the lumbar spine, gluteus medius, gluteus minimus, gluteus maximus, and quadratus lumborum.

INSTRUCTION: In supine, bring one bent knee to chest and hold knee with ipsilateral hand. Then slowly bring up the other knee to chest and hold knee with ipsilateral hand (A). To target one side further, patient can pull both knees toward left or right shoulder to increase unilateral stretching (B).

SUBSTITUTIONS: Tensing neck and shoulders; knees too far apart becoming a hip stretch rather than lumbar.

PARAMETERS: Hold for 15 to 30 seconds 3 to 5 repetitions, 1 to 3 times per day

Where's the Evidence?

In a study of 40 women with a hyperlordotic lumbar spine, William's flexion exercises led to significant decreases in lumbar angle and back pain, increases in flexibility of hamstring muscles, hip flexor muscles flexibility, lumbar extensor muscles flexibility, and abdominal muscles strength (Fatemi, Javid, & Najafabadi, 2015). William's flexion exercises include PPT, SKTC and DKTC, partial sit-up, hamstring stretch, hip flexor stretch, seated lumbar flexion and squat (Starkey, 2013).

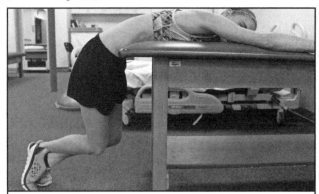

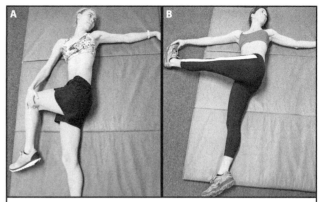

4.02.3 STRETCH: HIP AND LEG HANG OVER EDGE OF BED FOR FLEXION BIAS

POSITION: Prone

TARGETS: Stretches bilateral erector spinae muscles of lumbar spine and quadratus lumborum; mild positional traction of lumbar vertebra.

INSTRUCTION: Lie over the edge of the bed or mat with torso supported and feet resting on the floor. Start out with knees extended and begin to slowly lower by bending knees. Allow hips to roll back and fall down. Hold the end position.

SUBSTITUTIONS: Not relaxing; resting lower torso on the table.

PARAMETERS: Hold for 15 to 60 seconds, 3 to 5 repetitions, 1 to 3 times per day

4.02.4 STRETCH: LOWER TRUNK ROTATION AND TWIST, KNEE FLEXED AND EXTENDED

POSITION: Supine

TARGETS: Lumbar spine rotation and lumbar/hip flexibility; stretch obliques, quadratus lumborum, erector spinae of lumbar and thoracic region, gluteus medius, and gluteus maximus.

INSTRUCTION: With one arm outstretched to the side, bring ipsilateral leg into the 90/90 position. Use opposite hand to grab knee and pull knee toward the floor on the contralateral until a stretch is felt. Patient may look toward stationary hand for added rotation in the cervical region. Shoulders should remain in contact with the surface. Contract core muscles and slowly bring knee toward the other side (A). To advance, repeat entire sequence with the rotating leg in 90 degrees hip flexion and knee fully extended. Patient may modify hand placement to the toes if able or continue to apply overpressure at the knee (B).

SUBSTITUTIONS: Shoulders come off surface, tensing shoulders, neck

PARAMETERS: Hold for 15 to 30 seconds, 3 to 5 repetitions, 1 to 3 times per day

4.02.5 STRETCH: LATERAL TRUNK FLEXION, PRESS-UP

POSITION: Side-lying

TARGETS: Spine mobility into lateral flexion; stretch unilateral external and internal obliques, quadratus lumborum, erector spinae of lumbar and thoracic region.

INSTRUCTION: With hips stacked and extended, press up using bottom elbow and prop the upper body up off of the surface. Pelvis and LEs are to remain on the floor and other arm can be used to maintain side-lying balance. To increase intensity, allow patient to press up through the bottom hand until the elbow is fully extended.

SUBSTITUTIONS: Rolling forward or back, flexion at the hips

PARAMETERS: Hold for 15 to 30 seconds, 3 to 5 repetitions, 1 to 3 times per day

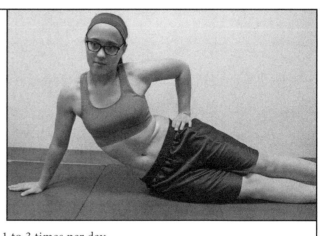

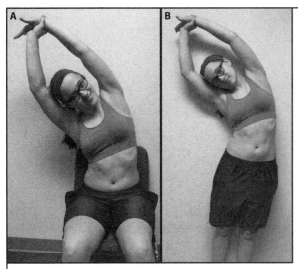

4.02.6 STRETCH: LATERAL TRUNK FLEXION, PULLING FOREARM OVERHEAD

<u>POSITION</u>: Seated, standing

<u>TARGETS</u>: Spine mobility into lateral flexion; stretch unilateral external and internal obliques, quadratus lumborum, erector spinae of lumbar and thoracic region; arm overhead adds latissimus dorsi stretch.

<u>INSTRUCTION</u>: With neutral spine flexion/extension and without the use of the back rest of a chair, patient grabs the forearm of the side to be stretched with the other hand and lifts arms overhead. Have patient lean to the opposite side, pulling the forearm up and away from the side being stretched (A). This can also be done standing as long as pelvis stays neutral and level to avoid hip abduction (B). Encourage patient to depress scapula on side of stretch during overhead pull; this will protect the shoulder joint from excessive impingement.

<u>SUBSTITUTIONS</u>: Leaning forward, trunk rotation, shoulder tense/shrug; only bending at waist and not thoracic region.

<u>PARAMETERS</u>: Hold for 15 to 30 seconds, 3 to 5 repetitions, 1 to 3 times per day

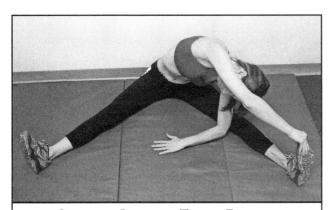

4.02.7 STRETCH: LATERAL TRUNK FLEXION, FLOOR TOE GRAB

<u>POSITION</u>: Seated on a large mat or floor, legs apart

<u>TARGETS</u>: Spine mobility into lateral flexion; advanced stretch unilateral external and internal obliques, quadratus lumborum, erector spinae of lumbar and thoracic region; arm overhead adds latissimus dorsi stretch; patient will need fair hamstring and hip adductor flexibility for this, stretch can be utilized for good combination stretch targeting these areas as well.

<u>INSTRUCTION</u>: Have patient bring right shoulder down toward floor and left shoulder up toward ceiling so that chest is facing the same direction as the inside of the knee. Patient reached overhead with left hand to grab toes on left foot, pulling right shoulder further toward right knee. The right arm lies in lap. Head stays in line with sternum.

<u>SUBSTITUTIONS</u>: Leaning forward with chest facing knee; this will change target to lumbar extensors, shoulder tense/shrug, only bending at waist and not thoracic region.

<u>PARAMETERS</u>: Hold for 15 to 30 seconds, 3 to 5 repetitions, 1 to 3 times per day

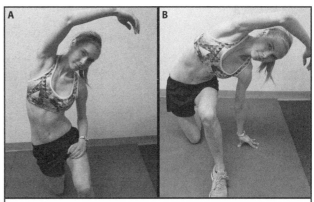

4.02.8 STRETCH: TRUNK SIDE-BEND, ARM OVERHEAD

<u>POSITION</u>: Half-kneeling

<u>TARGETS</u>: Spine mobility into lateral flexion; stretch unilateral external and internal obliques, quadratus lumborum, erector spinae of lumbar and thoracic region; arm overhead adds latissimus dorsi stretch.

<u>INSTRUCTION</u>: In half-kneeling, patient brings posterior leg into further extension by sliding knee back into a slight lunge. Forward lower leg should be perpendicular to the floor and knee should not pass over the foot. In slight lunge, patient reaches up and over with the same arm as the posterior leg. This can also be done standing as long as pelvis stays neutral and level to avoid hip abduction. Encourage patient to depress scapula on side of stretch during overhead pull; this will protect the shoulder joint from excessive impingement. Patient may lay leading hand in lap (A) or place on floor for added support (B).

<u>SUBSTITUTIONS</u>: Leaning forward, trunk rotation, shoulder tense/shrug, only bending at waist and not thoracic region

<u>PARAMETERS</u>: Hold for 15 to 30 seconds, 3 to 5 repetitions, 1 to 3 times per day

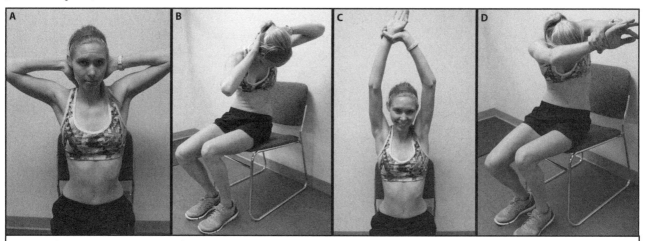

4.02.9 STRETCH: LATERAL TRUNK FLEXION WITH ROTATION

POSITION: Seated, standing

TARGETS: Spine mobility into lateral flexion and ipsilateral rotation; stretch unilateral external and internal obliques, quadratus lumborum, erector spinae of lumbar and thoracic region; flexion/rotation component targets more of the posterior muscles; arm overhead adds latissimus dorsi stretch.

INSTRUCTION: With hands clasped behind the head (A and B) or grasping forearm with arms overhead (C and D) neck neutral, patient leans to the side opposite to end range and then slightly rolls chest around to face toward the ipsilateral hip. Avoiding hip flexion as much as possible and elongating through the posterior and lateral trunk will stretch target area. Tucking chin during stretch will protect the neck. This can also be done standing as long as pelvis stays neutral and level to avoid hip abduction. Encourage patient to depress scapula on side of stretch during overhead pull; this will protect the shoulder joint from excessive impingement.

SUBSTITUTIONS: Leaning forward or backward, hips coming off floor, jutting chin out, pulling on neck

PARAMETERS: Hold for 15 to 30 seconds, 3 to 5 repetitions, 1 to 3 times per day

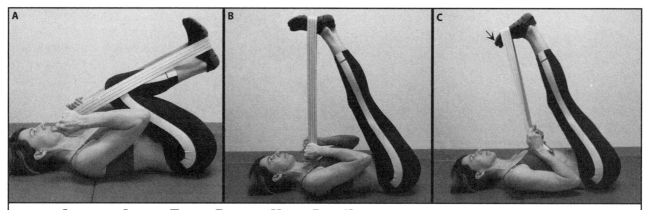

4.02.10 STRETCH: LOWER TRUNK FLEXION USING BELT/STRAP

POSITION: Hook-lying (start)

TARGETS: Lumbar spine mobility into flexion; allows patient to apply assistance and overpressure to increase ROM and stretch the quadratus lumborum and erector spinae of lumbar region; extending knees will add hamstring stretch and give patient greater leverage for pulling; pulling down through toes will add a gastrocnemius stretch.

INSTRUCTION: Loop a belt/strap behind both knees. With both hands on each end of the strap, pull knees to chest until stretch is felt in lumbar region (A). Strap can be moved to foot arches and knees extended to add hamstring stretch (B). Strap can be moved to forefoot/metatarsal heads, and pulling down on toes will add gastrocnemius stretch (C).

SUBSTITUTIONS: Shoulders come off table, overstretch with knees extended and dorsiflexion of ankles can cause significant neural tension; take care with any nerve irritation that you do not overstretch in this position.

PARAMETERS: Hold for 15 to 30 seconds, 3 to 5 repetitions, 1 to 3 times per day

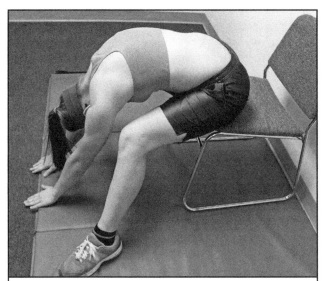

4.02.11 STRETCH: TRUNK FLEXION, KNEES APART, CHAIR

POSITION: Seated

TARGETS: Lumbar spine mobility into flexion; allows patient to apply assistance and overpressure to increase ROM and stretch the quadratus lumborum and erector spinae of lumbar region.

INSTRUCTION: Patient can sit in chair or even on the edge of bed to do the exercise. Patient scoots the buttocks to the front edge of the chair and slowly allows body to bend forward while reaching to the floor. To add overpressure and increase the stretch, patient may grab ankles and gently pull back into more flexion.

SUBSTITUTIONS: Pelvis rises off chair; increase in pain symptoms may indicate this is not an appropriate exercise, especially in the case of an acute lumbar disc herniation.

PARAMETERS: Hold for 15 to 30 seconds, 3 to 5 repetitions, 1 to 3 times per day

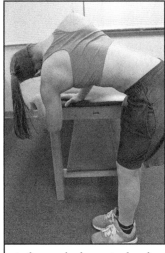

4.02.12 STRETCH: TRUNK FLEXION AND ROTATION

POSITION: Standing near a table on one side

TARGETS: Spine mobility into flexion and rotation; stretch quadratus lumborum, erector spinae, rotatores of lumbar and thoracic region.

INSTRUCTION: Patient bends forward at the trunk, rolling down the vertebra slowly starting at the neck down to lumbar region to finally bending at the hips. Have the patient engage the abdominals to increase the lumbar flexion. Let the patient hang here while deep breathing as spinal muscles relax. Rotation begins as patient rotates one shoulder up toward the ceiling and the other shoulder down toward the floor. Patient may use the arm to push further into rotation for added stretch. Head stays in line with sternum, chin tucked.

SUBSTITUTIONS: Bending solely at the hips, missing the important flexion component through the trunk, excessive neck strain into rotation or jutting chin out, forward roll of shoulder that is pressing further into rotation; avoid excessive shoulder pressure.

PARAMETERS: Hold for 15 to 30 seconds, 3 to 5 repetitions, 1 to 3 times per day

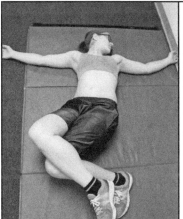

4.02.13 STRETCH: SPINE TWIST, CROSSED KNEES

POSITION: Hook-lying

TARGETS: Mobility of the lumbar spine in the transverse plane (rotation) and stretch obliques, semispinalis, rotatores, multifidus, gluteus medius and minimus

INSTRUCTION: Start with the back flat and feet together flat on mat. Place one ankle to the outside of the opposite knee and lower leg. Use the ankle to push the knee across the body toward the table or mat until a stretch is felt in posterior hip and lower back.

SUBSTITUTIONS: Shoulders come off mat

PARAMETERS: Hold for 15 to 30 seconds, 3 to 5 repetitions, 1 to 3 times per day

4.02.14 STRETCH: SPINE TWIST, LONG-SITTING WITH ONE KNEE BENT

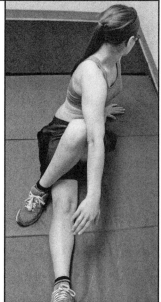

POSITION: Long-sitting, one knee bent

TARGETS: Mobility of the lumbar spine in the transverse plane (rotation) and stretch obliques, semispinalis, rotatores, multifidus, gluteus medius and minimus; may also get rhomboid and posterior deltoid stretch on arm in contact with knee.

INSTRUCTION: In long-sitting with one knee extended, bend the other knee up, placing the ankle on the outside of the opposite knee. Reach across the body with the arm that is on the side of the extended knee and bring the elbow in contact with the outside of the bent knee while placing hand on the extended knee. The other arm is behind the trunk supporting the body. This should be actively pushing down to create length through the spine and minimizing any shoulder shrug. The arm in contact with the knee will then push against the knee, pulling the spine around into rotation, eventually crossing the shoulder past the knee. Patient may also add cervical rotation in the same direction for added spinal rotation through the cervical spine.

SUBSTITUTIONS: Shrugging, leaning backward, jutting chin out

PARAMETERS: Hold for 15 to 30 seconds, 3 to 5 repetitions, 1 to 3 times per day

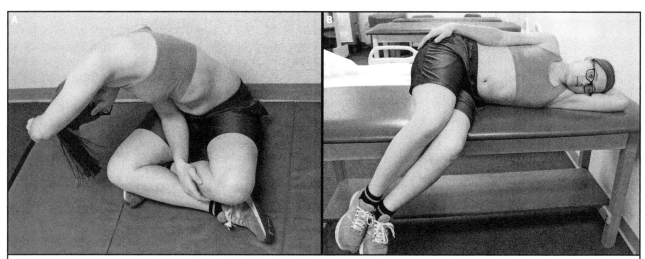

4.02.15 STRETCH: LATERAL TRUNK FLEXION (QUADRATUS LUMBORUM)

POSITION: Seated cross-legged, side-lying

TARGETS: Stretch unilateral quadratus lumborum

INSTRUCTION: *Seated cross-legged*: With arm overhead, neck neutral, patient leans to the side opposite to end range ,allowing leading elbow to offer support on the leg or hand on the floor and then slightly rolls chest around to face toward the ipsilateral hip and bends trunk toward hip. Tucking chin during stretch will protect the neck. Pelvis stays neutral, buttocks on the floor (A). Encourage patient to depress scapula on side of stretch during overhead pull; this will protect the shoulder joint from excessive impingement. *Side-lying*: Lying on contralateral side, bring knees to edge of table or mat and allow lower legs to drop off side of table or mat, allowing pelvis to pull away from rib cage (B).

SUBSTITUTIONS: *Seated cross-legged*: Hips coming off floor, jutting chin out, shrugging shoulder, movement at waist only and not in lumbar region; encourage rounding of the spine. *Side-lying*: No stretch felt indicates to move to seated cross-legged stretch.

PARAMETERS: Hold for 15 to 30 seconds, 3 to 5 repetitions, 1 to 3 times per day

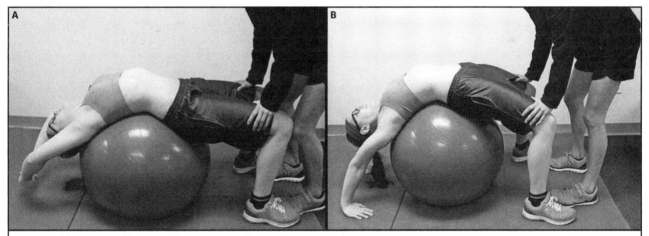

4.02.16 Stretch: Lateral Trunk Flexion Over Exercise Ball

Position: Side-lying on exercise ball

Targets: Stretch unilateral quadratus lumborum and obliques

Instruction: Position patient side-lying over medium exercise ball at the pelvis, ball is against a wall. With arm overhead, neck neutral, patient lies over the ball letting shoulders come toward the floor, reaching with top hand toward floor. Allow bottom knee to flex slightly and stagger feet for stability (A). Patient may lean back slightly to target obliques anteriorly or roll slightly forward to target quadratus lumborum (B).

Substitutions: Feet coming off floor

Parameters: Hold for 15 to 30 seconds, 3 to 5 repetitions, 1 to 3 times per day

4.02.17 Stretch: Trunk Extension Over Exercise Ball

Position: Supine on exercise ball

Targets: Stretch RA

Instruction: Position patient sitting over medium exercise ball with feet flat on the floor and hip-width apart. Patient rolls ball under buttocks and leans back, allowing back to extend over the ball (A). With arm overhead, patient can then reach palms toward the floor into a back-bend position if able (B).

Substitutions: Feet coming off floor

Parameters: Hold for 15 to 30 seconds, 3 to 5 repetitions, 1 to 3 times per day

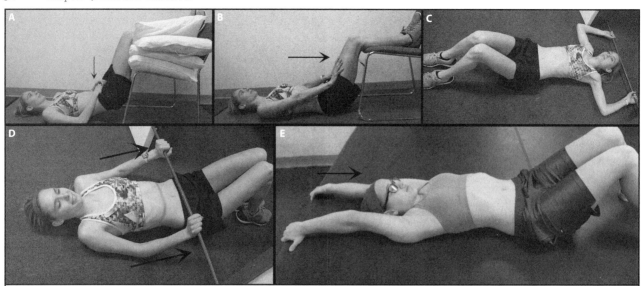

4.02.18 STRETCH: POSITIONAL LUMBAR SELF-TRACTION, 5 TECHNIQUES

<u>POSITION</u>: Supine legs on chair at 90/90 (techniques #1 and #2), hook-lying (techniques #3 through #5)

<u>TARGETS</u>: Traction lumbar spine; good for bulging disc, spinal stenosis, muscle spasms.

<u>INSTRUCTION</u>: *Technique #1*: Position in the 90/90 position with calves supported on chair. Use pillows to increase the height of the chair so that the buttocks are off the floor. Patient then relaxes lumbar spine into flexion while a traction force is enacted by the weight of the hips. This can be held 5 to 10 minutes (A). *Technique #2*: Allowing the hips to lower to the ground, patient applies a force with the hands pushing into the top of the thighs, pushing shoulders away from the hips as traction force is exerted through lumbar spine (B). *Technique #3*: Lie in front of a doorway in hook-lying with bare skin touching the floor to provide friction. Raise both arms overhead and hold a cane or broomstick against the opposite side of the doorway. Gently pull arms against the cane, providing a traction force through the lumbar spine (C). *Technique #4*: Lie in the center of a doorway in hook-lying with bare skin touching the floor to provide friction. Hold a cane or broomstick against the doorway. Gently push against the cane, providing a traction force through the lumbar spine (D). *Technique #5*: On a firm mattress in hook-lying, grasp the head of the bed and pull by flexing the wrists, providing a traction force through the lumbar spine (E).

<u>SUBSTITUTIONS</u>: If there is an increase in radiating pain, stop exercise; may not be appropriate and aggravate condition.

<u>PARAMETERS</u>: *Technique #1*, see above; *techniques #2 through #5*, hold each for 2 minutes and repeat 5 times, perform 1 to 2 times per day as needed for pain relief.

REFERENCES

Fatemi, R., Javid, M., & Najafabadi, E. M. (2015). Effects of William training on lumbosacral muscles function, lumbar curve and pain. *Journal of Back and Musculoskeletal Rehabilitation, 28*(3), 591-597.

Starkey, C. (2013). *Athletic training and sports medicine: An integrated approach* (5th ed.). Burlington, MA: Jones & Bartlett.

Section 4.03

LUMBAR STRENGTHENING

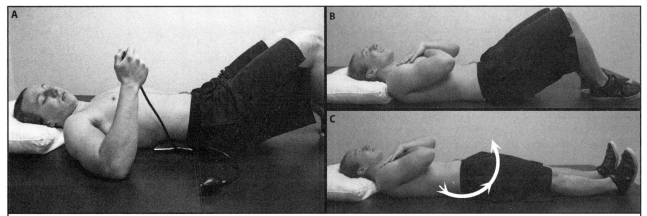

4.03.1 STRENGTHEN: ISOMETRIC; POSTERIOR PELVIC TILT, LUMBAR SPINE, WITH OR WITHOUT BLOOD PRESSURE CUFF FOR BIOFEEDBACK

POSITION: Hook-lying, supine

TARGETS: Decrease lumbar lordosis (mobility of lumbar spine into flexion), facilitate pelvic floor and lower abdominals (TA primarily)

INSTRUCTION: *Hook-lying*: With feet hip-width apart, place blood pressure cuff under the lower back horizontally and inflate to fill the space between, lumbar spine and the supporting surface. Have the patient press the lower back into the surface by tilting pelvis posteriorly, drawing the navel in toward the spine. Note the pressure increase on the sphyngmometer. Patient can then watch the sphyngmometer with each repetition to try to achieve a good posterior tilt as a form of biofeedback (A). This can also be done without the blood pressure cuff (B). *Supine*: This is more difficult than hook-lying and is the next progression for this movement. In this position, repeat the same instructions as for hook-lying (C).

SUBSTITUTIONS: Avoid hunching through the upper torso; patient should exhale with tilt.

PARAMETERS: Hold for 10 seconds, repeat 10 times, perform 2 to 3 sets, repeat 1 times per day or every other day

Where's the Evidence?

Chanthapetch, Kanlayanaphotporn, Gaogasigam, and Chiradejnant (2009) studied the activity of the RA, external abdominal oblique, and transversus abdominis/internal abdominal oblique muscles during abdominal hollowing in 4 positions: hook-lying, prone-lying, quadruped, and wall support standing. Thirty-two healthy participants, average age 21 years, were recruited. During abdominal hollowing in all four starting positions, significant differences were found in the EMG activity of RA, external abdominal oblique, and TA/internal abdominal oblique. The TA/internal abdominal oblique exhibited the highest while the RA exhibited the lowest EMG activity. The results suggest that all four starting positions can facilitate TA/internal abdominal oblique activity with minimal activity from RA and external abdominal oblique.

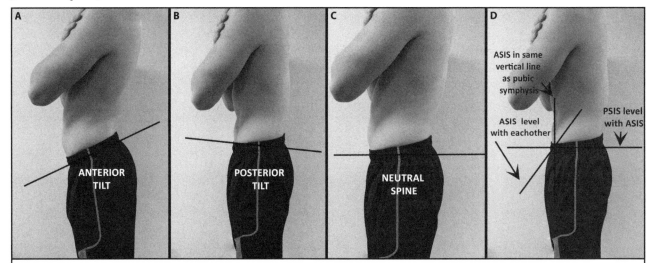

4.03.2 STRENGTHEN: ISOMETRIC; NEUTRAL SPINE, LUMBAR SPINE STABILIZATION

POSITION: Multi-positional

TARGETS: This is the basic lumbar position to maintain with the lumbar stabilization program; this will engage the muscles that stabilize the lumbar spine in a neutral position and targets core lumbar stabilizers; TA, the pelvic floor muscles, the diaphragm and the multifidus.

INSTRUCTION: *How to find the neutral spine*: First the patient must perform a full anterior tilt followed by a posterior tilt. The neutral spine is the position between these two exaggerated anterior and posterior positions (A through C). When the pelvis is in neutral, the bones at the top of the pelvis (back PSIS; front ASIS) are level (D). Patient must learn to utilize the core to initiate movement while in a neutral pelvic alignment to reduce risk of injury and lower back pain and can improve overall general posture. The following 33 exercises are part of the lumbar stabilization program in sequential order. Each exercise begins with finding and stabilizing the neutral lumbar spine before initiating movement. The deep abdominals respond most effectively to a gentle contraction. The patient only needs to create a mild contraction to activate these muscles; much like a light switch, they are either on or off. Once the abdominal muscles are engaged, the patient can confidently use the large muscles for the action phase of the movement. Use of a mirror can be helpful in the beginning of these exercises.

SUBSTITUTIONS: Avoid hunching through the upper torso; patient should breathe normally.

PARAMETERS: Hold 6 to 10 seconds and repeat 10 times, 1 time per day or every other day; progress to lumbar stabilization program once patient has a good understanding.

Where's the Evidence?

Moon et al. (2013) compared the effects of lumbar stabilization exercises and lumbar dynamic strengthening exercises on the maximal isometric strength of the lumbar extensors, pain severity, and functional disability in patients with chronic LBP. Twenty-one patients suffering nonspecific LBP for more than 3 months were included and randomized into lumbar stabilization exercise group or lumbar dynamic strengthening exercise group. Exercises were performed for 1 hour, twice weekly, for 8 weeks. The strength of the lumbar extensors was measured using MedX. The VAS and the Oswestry LBP Disability Questionnaire were used to measure the severity of LBP and functional disability before and after the exercise. Compared with the baseline, LE strength at all angles improved significantly in both groups after 8 weeks. The improvements were significantly greater in the lumbar stabilization exercise group at 0 and 12 degrees of lumbar flexion. VAS decreased significantly after treatment in both groups; however, the Oswestry LBP Disability Questionnaire scores improved significantly only in the stabilization exercise group. Researchers concluded both lumbar stabilization and dynamic strengthening exercise strengthen the lumbar extensors and reduce LBP and that lumbar stabilization exercise is more effective in lumbar extensor strengthening and functional improvement in patients with nonspecific chronic LBP.

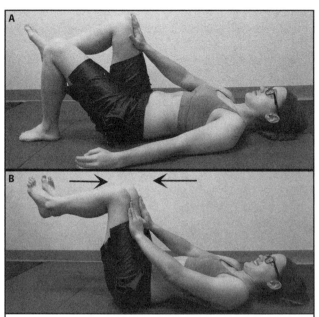

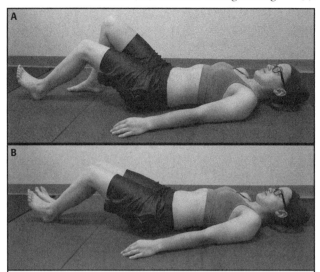

4.03.3 STRENGTHEN: LUMBAR SPINE, UNILATERAL TRUNK FLEXION AND BILATERAL KNEE TO CHEST RESIST WITH HAND

POSITION: Supine 90/90 LE

TARGETS: This will engage the muscles that stabilize the lumbar spine in a neutral position and targets core lumbar stabilizers: TA, the pelvic floor muscles, the diaphragm, and the multifidus while isometrically strengthening RA, obliques, and hip flexors; core muscles are resisting the flexion aspect of the isometric push by maintaining a neutral spine.

INSTRUCTION: With one leg in the 90/90 position and the other in hook-lying with foot flat on surface, patient finds neutral spine and holds while pressing into top of elevated thigh with ipsilateral hand. Repeat to other side (A). Progress to both legs in the 90/90 position. Patient again finds neutral spine and holds while pressing into tops of both elevated thighs with both hands (B).

SUBSTITUTIONS: Loss of neutral spine, holding breath

PARAMETERS: Hold 6 to 10 seconds and repeat 10 times, each up to 3 sets, 1 time per day or every other day

4.03.4 STRENGTHEN: LUMBAR SPINE, ALTERNATING AND BILATERAL HEEL SLIDE

POSITION: Hook-lying

TARGETS: This will engage the muscles that stabilize the lumbar spine in a neutral position and targets core lumbar stabilizers: TA, the pelvic floor muscles, the diaphragm and the multifidus while adding beginning movements of the legs; core muscles are resisting the flexion aspect of the isometric push by maintaining a neutral spine.

INSTRUCTION: With knees and feet hip-width apart and feet planted on surface, patient finds neutral spine and holds while sliding one heel forward, extending the hip and knee. The patient then brings the heel back up to starting position and then repeats to other side (A). Progress to both legs extending at the same time while holding neutral spine (B).

SUBSTITUTIONS: Loss of neutral spine, holding breath

PARAMETERS: 10 times each side up to 3 sets, 1 time per day or every other day

4.03.5 STRENGTHEN: LUMBAR SPINE, ISOMETRIC, TRUNK EXTENSION

POSITION: Seated on stool against a wall

TARGETS: This will engage the muscles that stabilize the lumbar spine in a neutral position and targets core lumbar stabilizers: TA, the pelvic floor muscles, the diaphragm and the multifidus while adding isometric strengthening of erector spinae.

INSTRUCTION: With knees and feet hip-width apart and feet planted on floor, patient finds neutral spine and holds while pressing upper back into the wall as patient attempts to extend the lower back.

SUBSTITUTIONS: Loss of neutral spine, holding breath

PARAMETERS: Hold 6 to 10 seconds and repeat 10 each up to 3 sets, 1 time per day or every other day

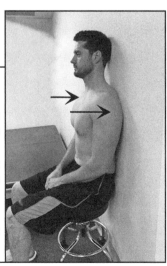

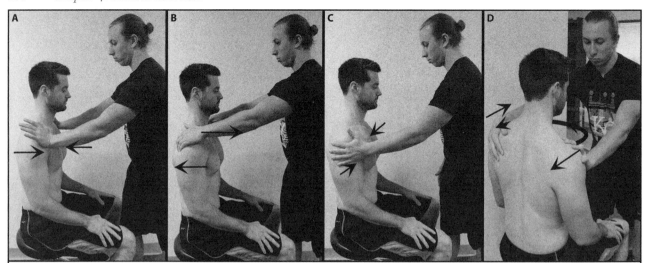

4.03.6 STRENGTHEN: LUMBAR SPINE, PERTURBATIONS

POSITION: Seated on stool

TARGETS: This will engage the muscles that stabilize the lumbar spine in a neutral position and targets core lumbar stabilizers: TA, the pelvic floor muscles, the diaphragm, and the multifidus while adding isometric strengthening of erector spinae, obliques, and RA.

INSTRUCTION: With knees and feet hip-width apart and feet planted on floor, patient finds neutral spine and holds. Therapist applies graded pressure at the shoulder girdle into all planes. Pressures can start slow and unidirectional (flexion/extension) with repeat contractions and then progress to bidirectional (flexion/extension and lateral flexion) lastly adding rotation. Hand placement for flexion/extension will be anterior/posterior shoulder girdle (A and B). Lateral flexion hand placement is at the lateral shoulder aspect (C) and rotation hand placement is with one hand on the anterior shoulder girdle and the other hand at the posterior shoulder girdle on the other side for opposing force to create a torque resistance (D). Patient maintains neutral spine using the deep core muscles and resists the movements in each direction. Progression involves quickening the resistance application and moving to multidirectional. Having the patient close his or her eyes increases proprioceptive training. Diagonal application of resistance can also be applied for further challenge.

SUBSTITUTIONS: Loss of neutral spine, holding breath

PARAMETERS: Start by holding each isometric contraction 6 to 10 seconds and repeat 10 each up to 3 sets, Progress to alternating from one side to the other (alternating isometrics) with the same parameters. Progressing to multidirectional; time measures for each resistance can be shortened and total time of challenges performed for 30 to 60 seconds with rests in between, up to 10 sets, 1 time per day or every other day.

4.03.7 STRENGTHEN: LUMBAR SPINE, BENT-KNEE FALL-OUTS

POSITION: Hook-lying

TARGETS: This will engage the muscles that stabilize the lumbar spine in a neutral position and targets core lumbar stabilizers: TA, the pelvic floor muscles, the diaphragm, and the multifidus while adding beginning movements of the legs.

INSTRUCTION: With knees and feet together, feet planted on floor, patient finds neutral spine and holds. Patient then allows one hip to fall out into abduction and external rotation while maintaining neutral spine. Patient returns to start position and performs on the opposite side (A). Patient may also do this bilaterally with both legs at the same time (B).

SUBSTITUTIONS: Loss of neutral spine, holding breath

PARAMETERS: 10 times each side up to 3 sets, 1 time per day or every other day

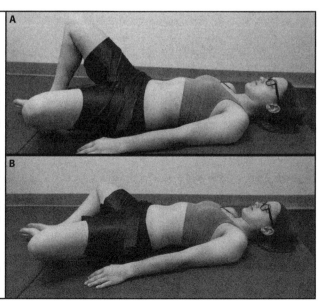

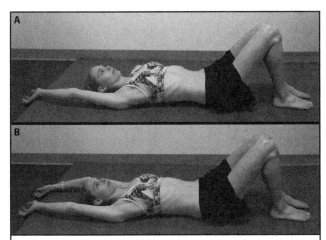

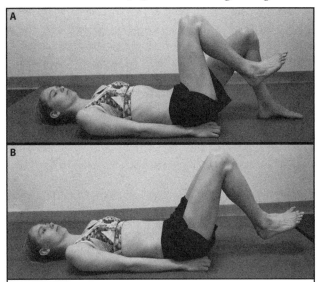

4.03.8 STRENGTHEN: LUMBAR SPINE, ARM LIFT OVERHEAD

POSITION: Hook-lying

TARGETS: This will engage the muscles that stabilize the lumbar spine in a neutral position and targets core lumbar stabilizers: TA, the pelvic floor muscles, the diaphragm, and the multifidus while adding beginning movements of the arms.

INSTRUCTION: With knees and feet hip-width apart and feet planted on floor, patient finds neutral spine and holds. Patient then flexes one shoulder, bringing thumb to mat while maintaining neutral spine. Patient returns to start position and performs on the opposite side (A). To progress, patient will do this bilaterally with both arms at the same time (B). The back will want to arch as patient reaches overhead and deep core muscles will resist this movement.

SUBSTITUTIONS: Loss of neutral spine, holding breath

PARAMETERS: 10 times each side up to 3 sets, 1 time per day or every other day

4.03.9 STRENGTHEN: LUMBAR SPINE, BENT-KNEE LIFT

POSITION: Hook-lying

TARGETS: This will engage the muscles that stabilize the lumbar spine in a neutral position and targets core lumbar stabilizers: TA, the pelvic floor muscles, the diaphragm, and the multifidus while adding beginning movements of the legs.

INSTRUCTION: With knees and feet together, feet planted on floor, patient finds neutral spine and holds. Patient then flexes hip, bringing one foot up and off the surface approximately 6 inches while maintaining neutral spine. Patient returns to start position and performs on the opposite side (A). Further progression involves bringing both legs up together and then lowering one leg at a time (B). The advanced version involves patient flexing both hips, bringing feet up at the same time and then lowering together.

SUBSTITUTIONS: Loss of neutral spine, holding breath

PARAMETERS: 10 times each side up to 3 sets, 1 time per day or every other day

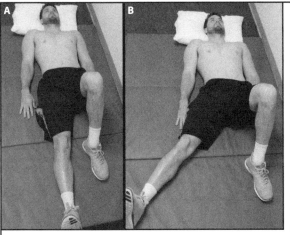

4.03.10 STRENGTHEN: LUMBAR SPINE, HEEL SLIDE ABDUCTION AND ADDUCTION

POSITION: Hook-lying to supine

TARGETS: This will engage the muscles that stabilize the lumbar spine in a neutral position and targets core lumbar stabilizers: TA, the pelvic floor muscles, the diaphragm, and the multifidus while adding beginning movements of the legs.

INSTRUCTION: With knees and feet together, feet planted on floor, patient finds neutral spine and holds. Patient then slowly extends on hip and knee to lying flat on mat, then abducts hip with knee in full extension and adducts to return. Repeat for 1 set and perform on the opposite side (A and B). To progress, patient extends both legs at the same time and then abducts both legs apart and adducts back to center.

SUBSTITUTIONS: Loss of neutral spine, holding breath

PARAMETERS: 10 times each side up to 3 sets, 1 time per day or every other day

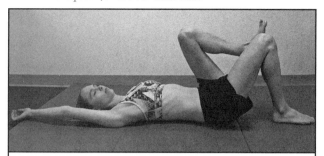

4.03.11 STRENGTHEN: LUMBAR SPINE, OPPOSITE ARM AND BENT-KNEE LIFT

POSITION: Hook-lying

TARGETS: This will engage the muscles that stabilize the lumbar spine in a neutral position and targets core lumbar stabilizers: TA, the pelvic floor muscles, the diaphragm, and the multifidus while adding movements of the arms and legs.

INSTRUCTION: With knees and feet hip-width apart and feet planted on floor or mat, patient finds neutral spine and holds. Patient then flexes one shoulder, bringing thumb to mat and flexed opposite hip bringing one foot up and off the surface approximately 6 inches while maintaining neutral spine. Patient returns to start position and performs on the opposite sides.

SUBSTITUTIONS: Loss of neutral spine, holding breath

PARAMETERS: 10 times each side up to 3 sets, 1 time per day or every other day

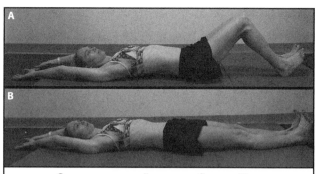

4.03.12 STRENGTHEN: LUMBAR SPINE, BILATERAL ARM LIFT OVERHEAD WITH KNEE EXTENSION

POSITION: Hook-lying

TARGETS: This will engage the muscles that stabilize the lumbar spine in a neutral position and targets core lumbar stabilizers: TA, the pelvic floor muscles, the diaphragm, and the multifidus while adding beginning movements of the arms and legs.

INSTRUCTION: With knees and feet hip-width apart and feet planted on floor or mat, patient finds neutral spine and holds (A). Patient then flexes both shoulders, bringing thumbs to mat while maintaining neutral spine. At the same time, patient slowly extends hip and knee to full extension. Patient returns to start position (B). The back will want to arch at the end range of reaching overhead and deep core muscles will resist this movement.

SUBSTITUTIONS: Loss of neutral spine, holding breath

PARAMETERS: 10 times each side up to 3 sets, 1 time per day or every other day

4.03.13 STRENGTHEN: LUMBAR SPINE, ALTERNATING BENT-KNEE LIFT TO STRAIGHT-LEG LOWER AND HEEL SLIDE TO RETURN

POSITION: Hook-lying

TARGETS: This will engage the muscles that stabilize the lumbar spine in a neutral position and targets core lumbar stabilizers: TA, the pelvic floor muscles, the diaphragm, and the multifidus while adding movements of the legs.

INSTRUCTION: With knees and feet hip-width apart and feet planted on floor or mat, patient finds neutral spine and holds. Patient then flexes one hip, bringing one foot up and off the surface approximately 6 inches. While maintaining neutral spine, patient then fully extends the knee so that bottom of foot is almost facing ceiling. Quadriceps should tighten as knee is held in extension, followed by slowly lowering straight leg to the mat. Patient returns to start position via sliding the heel back to start position. Repeat to other side. An extended knee increases the length of the leg and creates a strong pull into lumbar lordosis which is resisted by the deep core muscles (A through D).

SUBSTITUTIONS: Loss of neutral spine, holding breath

PARAMETERS: 10 times each side up to 3 sets, 1 time per day or every other day

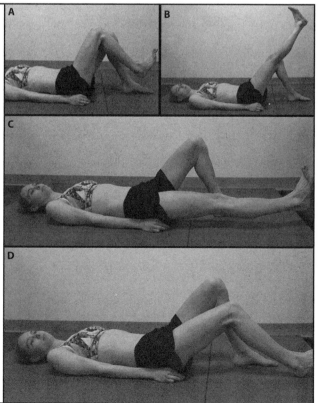

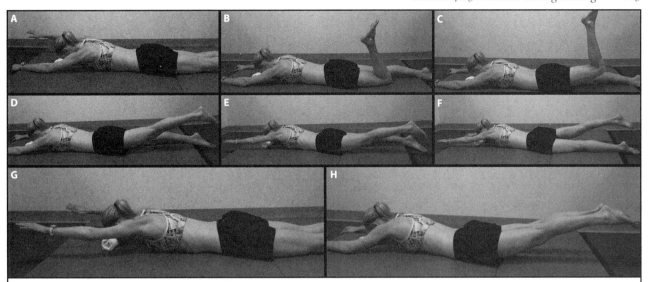

4.03.14 STRENGTHEN: LUMBAR SPINE, ALTERNATING ARM LIFT, LEG LIFT, AND COMBINED

POSITION: Prone

TARGETS: This will engage the muscles that stabilize the lumbar spine in a neutral position and targets core lumbar stabilizers: TA, the pelvic floor muscles, the diaphragm, and the multifidus while adding movements of the arms and legs; erector spinae will be targeting more with prone exercises; with arm movements, lower trapezius and deltoid will also assist; with leg movements, gluteus maximus assists; and for knee extension, a strong contraction of the quadriceps is encouraged.

INSTRUCTION: With arms overhead and legs extended, position patient's forehead on a small roll to maintain neutral neck. A table with a hole for the face will also suffice. *Alternating arms only*: While maintaining neutral spine, patient raises one arm off the table 6 inches with elbow extended (A). *Alternating knee bends*: While maintaining neutral spine, bend one knee to 90 degrees. Repeat to other side (B). *Alternating knee bend and lift*: While maintaining neutral spine, bend one knee to 90 degrees and lift off of the table 6 to 8 inches. Repeat to other side (C). *Alternating legs extended lift*: While maintaining neutral spine, patient raises one leg off the table 6 inches with knee extended. Repeat to other side (D). *Arms and legs same side*: While maintaining neutral spine, patient raises one arm and same side leg off the table 6 inches with elbow and knee extended. Repeat to other side (E). *Arms and legs opposite sides*: While maintaining neutral spine, patient raises one arm and opposite side leg off the table 6 inches with elbow and knee extended. Repeat to opposite sides (F). *Bilateral arms only*: While maintaining neutral spine, patient raises both arms off the table 6 inches with elbows extended (G). *Bilateral legs only*: While maintaining neutral spine, patient raises both legs off the table 6 inches with knees extended (H).

SUBSTITUTIONS: Loss of neutral spine, raising head off table or roll, holding breath

PARAMETERS: Hold 3 to 5 seconds, 10 times each up to 3 sets, 1 time per day or every other day

Where's the Evidence?

Suehiro et al. (2014) examined the effects of lumbopelvic stabilization maneuvers on spine motion and trunk muscle activity during prone hip extension. Fourteen healthy male volunteers (mean age 21) were instructed to perform prone hip extension without any maneuvers (control), with abdominal hollowing, and with abdominal bracing. Surface EMG data were collected from the trunk muscles and the lumbopelvic motion was measured. Lumbar extension and APT degree were significantly lower in the abdominal hollowing and abdominal bracing than in the control condition during prone hip extension. Lumbar extension and APT degree did not differ significantly between the abdominal hollowing and abdominal bracing. Findings suggest that prone hip extension with abdominal hollowing effectively minimizes unwanted lumbopelvic motion, which does not result in global muscle activation.

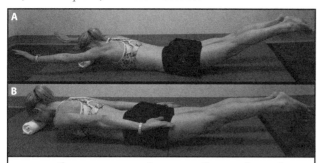

4.03.15 STRENGTHEN: LUMBAR SPINE, LIFT ALL FOURS, "SUPERMAN" AND "ROCKETMAN"

POSITION: Prone

TARGETS: This will engage the muscles that stabilize the lumbar spine in a neutral position and targets core lumbar stabilizers: TA, the pelvic floor muscles, the diaphragm, and the multifidus while adding movements of the arms and legs; erector spinae will be targeting more with prone exercises; with arm movements, lower trapezius and deltoid will also assist; with leg movements, gluteus maximus assists; and for knee extension, a strong contraction of the quadriceps is encouraged.

INSTRUCTION: *"Superman"*: With arms overhead and legs extended, position patient's forehead on a small roll to maintain neutral neck. A table with a hole for the face will also suffice. While maintaining neutral spine, patient raises both arms and legs off the table 6 inches with elbows and knees extended (A). This can also be done with arms by the sides "rocketman" (B).

SUBSTITUTIONS: Loss of neutral spine, raising head off table or roll, holding breath

PARAMETERS: Hold 3 to 5 seconds, to increase endurance holds may be extended, 10 times each up to 3 sets, 1 time per day or every other day

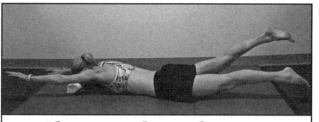

4.03.16 STRENGTHEN: LUMBAR SPINE, "SWIMMING"

POSITION: Prone

TARGETS: This will engage the muscles that stabilize the lumbar spine in a neutral position and targets core lumbar stabilizers: TA, the pelvic floor muscles, the diaphragm, and the multifidus while adding movements of the arms and legs; erector spinae will be targeting more with prone exercises; with arm movements, lower trapezius and deltoid will also assist; with leg movements, gluteus maximus assists; and for knee extension, a strong contraction of the quadriceps is encouraged.

INSTRUCTION: While maintaining neutral spine, patient raises both arms and both legs off the table 6 inches with elbow and knee extended. In a swimming motion that is rapid, the patient raises and lowers opposite arm and leg without allowing extremities to touch table. If arms or legs start to fall to table, a rest break is indicated.

SUBSTITUTIONS: Loss of neutral spine, raising head off table or roll, holding breath

PARAMETERS: Continuous "swimming" 10 to 30 seconds to build endurance 5 to 10 sets, 1 time per day or every other day

4.03.17 STRENGTHEN: LUMBAR SPINE, HEEL LIFT

POSITION: Bridge

TARGETS: This will engage the muscles that stabilize the lumbar spine in a neutral position and targets core lumbar stabilizers: TA, the pelvic floor muscles, the diaphragm, and the multifidus while adding movements of the legs; erector spinae, gluteus maximus, hamstrings, and soleus are targeted.

INSTRUCTION: *Alternating heels*: While maintaining neutral spine in the bridge position, patient raises one heel off the table. Repeat to other side (A). *Bilateral heels*: While maintaining neutral spine in the bridge position, patient raises both heels off the table. Repeat to other side (B).

SUBSTITUTIONS: Loss of neutral spine, loss of neutral hip (maintain extension), pelvis tips to one side; ASIS should remain level, holding breath.

PARAMETERS: Hold 3 to 5 seconds, 10 times each up to 3 sets, 1 time per day or every other day

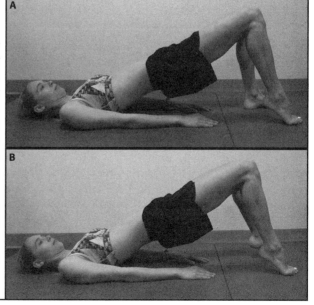

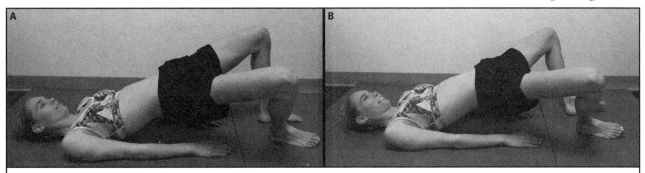

4.03.18 STRENGTHEN: LUMBAR SPINE, HIP ABDUCTION AND ADDUCTION

POSITION: Bridge

TARGETS: This will engage the muscles that stabilize the lumbar spine in a neutral position and targets core lumbar stabilizers: TA, the pelvic floor muscles, the diaphragm, and the multifidus while adding movements of the legs; erector spinae, gluteus maximus, hamstrings, hip rotators, and hip abductors/adductors.

INSTRUCTION: *Alternating hips*: While maintaining neutral spine in the bridge position, patient abducts and externally rotates one hip, opening the knee out. Repeat to other side (A). *Bilateral hips*: While maintaining neutral spine in the bridge position, patient abducts and externally rotates one hip, opening the knee out. Repeat to other side (B).

SUBSTITUTIONS: Loss of neutral spine, loss of neutral extension, pelvis tips to one side; ASIS should remain level, holding breath.

PARAMETERS: Hold 3 to 5 seconds, 10 times each up to 3 sets, 1 time per day or every other day

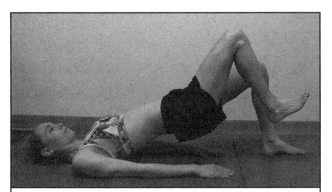

4.03.19 STRENGTHEN: LUMBAR SPINE, BENT-KNEE LIFT, MARCH IN PLACE

POSITION: Bridge

TARGETS: This will engage the muscles that stabilize the lumbar spine in a neutral position and targets core lumbar stabilizers: TA, the pelvic floor muscles, the diaphragm, and the multifidus while adding movements of the legs; erector spinae, gluteus maximus, hamstrings, hip rotators, hip abductors/adductors, and hip flexors.

INSTRUCTION: While maintaining neutral spine in the bridge position, patient flexes hip to bring foot off surface 6 inches. Repeat to other side.

SUBSTITUTIONS: Loss of neutral spine, loss of neutral extension, pelvis tips to one side; ASIS should remain level, holding breath.

PARAMETERS: Hold 3 to 5 seconds, 10 times each up to 3 sets, 1 time per day or every other day

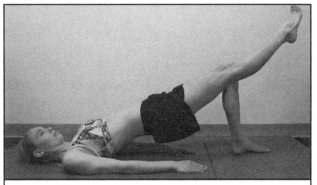

4.03.20 STRENGTHEN: LUMBAR SPINE, ALTERNATING KNEE EXTENSION

POSITION: Bridge

TARGETS: This will engage the muscles that stabilize the lumbar spine in a neutral position and targets core lumbar stabilizers: TA, the pelvic floor muscles, the diaphragm, and the multifidus while adding movements of the legs; erector spinae, gluteus maximus, hamstrings, quadriceps, and general hip stabilizers.

INSTRUCTION: While maintaining neutral spine in the bridge position, patient extends knee while keeping thighs in alignment (level with each other). Repeat to other side.

SUBSTITUTIONS: Loss of neutral spine, loss of neutral extension, pelvis tips to one side; ASIS should remain level, holding breath.

PARAMETERS: Hold 3 to 5 seconds, 10 times each up to 3 sets, 1 time per day or every other day

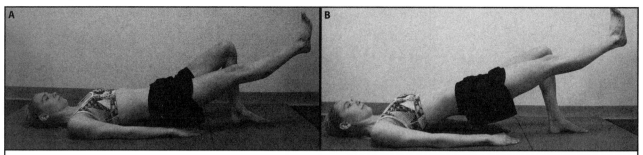

4.03.21 STRENGTHEN: LUMBAR SPINE, UNILATERAL BRIDGE

POSITION: Half-bridge; one knee is extended

TARGETS: This will engage the muscles that stabilize the lumbar spine in a neutral position and targets core lumbar stabilizers: TA, the pelvic floor muscles, the diaphragm and the multifidus while adding movements of the legs; erector spinae, gluteus maximus, hamstrings, and general hip stabilizers.

INSTRUCTION: While maintaining neutral spine in the half-bridge position, in which one knee is fully extended with both thighs at the same level, patient extends hips, keeping thighs lined up at same height. Therapist can choose to finish full set on one side and then repeat to other side or alternate repetitions from side to side (A and B).

SUBSTITUTIONS: Loss of neutral spine, loss of neutral extension, pelvis tips to one side; ASIS should remain level, holding breath.

PARAMETERS: Hold 3 to 5 seconds, 10 times each up to 3 sets, 1 time per day or every other day

4.03.22 STRENGTHEN: LUMBAR SPINE, NEUTRAL SPINE HOLD, QUADRUPED

POSITION: Quadruped

TARGETS: This will engage the muscles that stabilize the lumbar spine in a neutral position and targets core lumbar stabilizers: TA, the pelvic floor muscles, the diaphragm, and the multifidus; active shoulders will engage deltoid, lower trapezius, and serratus anterior; active elbow not allowing hyper extension or locking will target triceps isometrically; and wrist cupping will activate wrist flexors and palmar muscles of the hand.

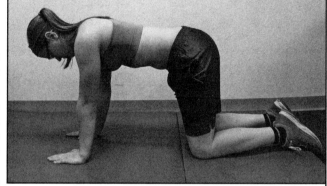

INSTRUCTION: Knees are spaced hip-width apart and hands directly beneath shoulders. Instruct patient to press away from the floor with palms of hands cupping and weight distributed through the fingertips. Shoulders are active and engaged, scapula depressed and retracted slightly. Patient finds neutral spine and holds. Provide verbal and tactile cues to assist patient in maintaining; a mirror to the side can be useful to provide visual feedback. Eyes should gaze between hands.

SUBSTITUTIONS: Sagging abdomen, arching lower back, loss of neutral spine, sagging into shoulders or shrugging, hyperextension of the elbows, poor activation of wrist with no cupping

PARAMETERS: Hold each position for at least 10 to 20 seconds, repeat 5 to 10 times, 1 time per day or every other day

---

Where's the Evidence?

Critchley (2002) investigated the effect of instructing pelvic floor contraction on TA thickness increase during low abdominal hollowing in quadruped. Twenty subjects, male and female, with no LBP in the last 2 years were taught low abdominal hollowing in quadruped. Mean increase in TA thickness during low abdominal hollowing was 49.71%, during low abdominal hollowing with pelvic floor it was 65.81%. Instructing healthy subjects to co-contract pelvic floor results in greater increase in contraction of TA and thus be useful for clinicians training this muscle.

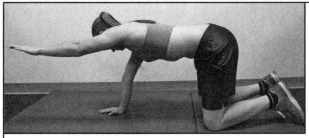

4.03.23 STRENGTHEN: LUMBAR SPINE, ALTERNATING ARM LIFT, QUADRUPED

POSITION: Quadruped

TARGETS: This will engage the muscles that stabilize the lumbar spine in a neutral position and targets core lumbar stabilizers: TA, the pelvic floor muscles, the diaphragm, and the multifidus; active shoulders will engage deltoid, lower trapezius, and serratus anterior; active elbow not allowing hyperextension or locking will target triceps isometrically, and wrist cupping will activate wrist flexors and palmar muscles of the hand; elevating arms will further work deltoid and lower trapezius isotonically.

INSTRUCTION: Knees are spaced hip-width apart and hands directly beneath shoulders. Instruct patient to press away from the floor with palms of hands cupping and weight distributed through the fingertips. Shoulders are active and engaged, scapula depressed and retracted slightly. Patient finds neutral spine and holds. While maintaining shoulders and pelvis level, patient slowly brings one extended arm into shoulder flexion to parallel to the surface.

SUBSTITUTIONS: Sagging abdomen, arching lower back, loss of neutral spine, sagging into shoulders or shrugging, hyperextension of the elbows, poor activation of wrist with no cupping, rolling to one side losing pelvis and shoulder level position

PARAMETERS: Hold 3 to 5 seconds, 10 times each up to 3 sets, 1 time per day or every other day

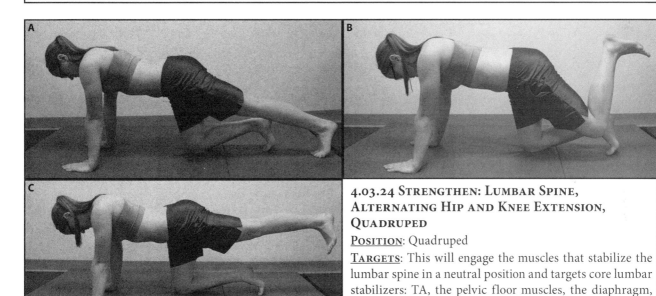

4.03.24 STRENGTHEN: LUMBAR SPINE, ALTERNATING HIP AND KNEE EXTENSION, QUADRUPED

POSITION: Quadruped

TARGETS: This will engage the muscles that stabilize the lumbar spine in a neutral position and targets core lumbar stabilizers: TA, the pelvic floor muscles, the diaphragm, and the multifidus; active shoulders will engage deltoid, lower trapezius, and serratus anterior; active elbow not allowing hyperextension or locking will target triceps isometrically and wrist cupping will activate wrist flexors and palmar muscles of the hand; elevating legs will further work gluteus maximus and quadriceps isotonically.

INSTRUCTION: Knees are spaced hip-width apart and hands directly beneath shoulders. Instruct patient to press away from the floor with palms of hands cupping and weight distributed through the fingertips. Shoulders are active and engaged, scapula depressed and retracted slightly. Patient finds neutral spine and holds. *Leg slide*: Slide one leg back, keeping toes on the floor. Return to start and repeat to other side (A). *Leg lift-bent knee*: While maintaining shoulders and pelvis level, patient slowly extends one hip with knee bent to 90 degrees until lower leg is perpendicular to the surface (B). *Leg reach*: While maintaining shoulders and pelvis level, patient slowly extends one hip and knee until entire leg is parallel to the surface. Instruct patient to imagine patient is pushing against a wall behind patient with heel and tighten quadriceps. Dorsiflexion to neutral can assist with this visualization (C).

SUBSTITUTIONS: Sagging abdomen, arching lower back, loss of neutral spine, sagging into shoulders or shrugging, hyperextension of the elbows, poor activation of wrist with no cupping, rolling to one side losing pelvis and shoulder level position

PARAMETERS: Hold 3 to 5 seconds, 10 times each up to 3 sets, 1 time per day or every other day

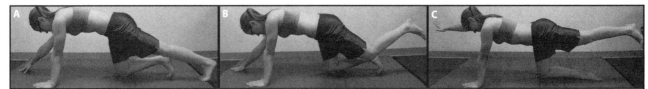

4.03.25 STRENGTHEN: LUMBAR SPINE, OPPOSITE ARM AND LEG LIFT, QUADRUPED

POSITION: Quadruped

TARGETS: This will engage the muscles that stabilize the lumbar spine in a neutral position and targets core lumbar stabilizers: TA, the pelvic floor muscles, the diaphragm, and the multifidus; active shoulders will engage deltoid, lower trapezius, and serratus anterior; active elbow not allowing hyperextension or locking will target triceps isometrically and wrist cupping will activate wrist flexors and palmar muscles of the hand; elevating arms will further work deltoid and lower trapezius isotonically; elevating legs will further work gluteus maximus and quadriceps isotonically.

INSTRUCTION: Knees are spaced hip-width apart and hands directly beneath shoulders. Instruct patient to press away from the floor with palms of hands cupping and weight distributed through the fingertips. Shoulders are active and engaged, scapula depressed and retracted slightly. Patient finds neutral spine and holds. *Arm and leg slide*: While maintaining shoulders and pelvis level, slide one leg back, keeping toes on the floor while bringing opposite arm forward at the same time, keeping fingertips in contact with the floor. Return to start and repeat to opposite side (A). *Arm slide with bent knee lift*: Patient slowly extends one hip while keeping knee flexed 90 degrees until lower leg is perpendicular to the surface, while simultaneously sliding right fingertips forward. Return to start and repeat to opposite sides (B). *Arm and leg reach*: While maintaining shoulders and pelvis level, patient slowly brings one extended arm into shoulder flexion to parallel to the surface, while simultaneously extending the opposite hip and knee to parallel to the surface. Instruct patient to imagine patient is pushing against a wall behind patient with heel, while also reaching forward toward the opposite wall with the hand lengthening the spine. Patient should tighten quadriceps, and dorsiflexion to neutral can assist with this visualization. Repeat to opposite sides (C).

SUBSTITUTIONS: Sagging abdomen, arching lower back, loss of neutral spine, sagging into shoulders or shrugging, hyperextension of the elbows, poor activation of wrist with no cupping, rolling to one side, losing pelvis and shoulder level position

PARAMETERS: Hold 3 to 5 seconds, 10 times each up to 3 sets, 1 time per day or every other day

4.03.26 STRENGTHEN: LUMBAR SPINE, ROCKING

POSITION: Quadruped

TARGETS: This will engage the muscles that stabilize the lumbar spine in a neutral position and target core lumbar stabilizers: TA, the pelvic floor muscles, the diaphragm, and the multifidus; active shoulders will engage deltoid, lower trapezius, and serratus anterior; active elbow not allowing hyperextension or locking will target triceps isometrically and wrist cupping will activate wrist flexors and palmar muscles of the hand; latissimus dorsi will also be strengthening with rocking motion at shoulders.

INSTRUCTION: Knees are spaced hip-width apart and hands directly beneath shoulders. Instruct patient to press away from the floor with palms of hands cupping and weight distributed through the fingertips. Shoulders are active and engaged, scapula depressed and retracted slightly. Patient finds neutral spine and holds. *Forward shift*: Patient shifts weight forward onto arms, holds and returns to start (A). *Backward shift*: Patient

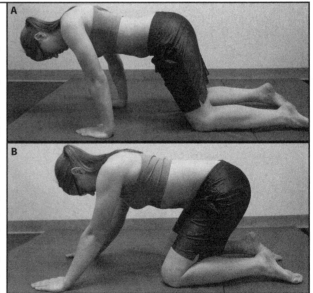

shifts weight backward onto legs, holds and returns to start (B). *Rocking*: Patient forward shifts as described above, holds and then moves straight into backward shift as described above, holds and repeats. Neutral spine should be maintained throughout all of these movement. Gaze is in between hands.

SUBSTITUTIONS: Sagging abdomen, arching lower back, loss of neutral spine, sagging into shoulders or shrugging, hyperextension of the elbows, poor activation of wrist with no cupping, rolling to one side losing pelvis and shoulder level position

PARAMETERS: Hold 3 to 5 seconds, 10 times each up to 3 sets, 1 time per day or every other day

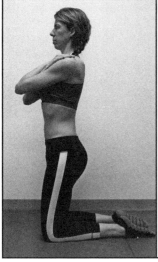

4.03.27 Strengthen: Lumbar Spine, Hold Neutral Spine, Tall-Kneeling

Position: Tall-kneeling

Targets: This will engage the muscles that stabilize the lumbar spine in a neutral position and targets core lumbar stabilizers: TA, the pelvic floor muscles, the diaphragm, and the multifidus.

Instruction: Knees are spaced hip-width apart, feet in plantarflexion resting tops of feet on surface or with toes curled under. Therapist may choose one over the other due to comfort or stability. Hips are in neutral flexion/extension, gluteus maximus is engaged. Instruct patient to elongate the spine, imagining a string pulling from the top of patient's head to the ceiling. Eyes are level and chin slightly tucked so that ears are over the lateral acromion. Scapular depression and retraction are encouraged. Patient finds neutral spine as described in **4.03.2**. Patient uses deep core muscles to hold this position.

Substitutions: Hyperlordosis, hips flex, forward shoulders or jutting chin out

Parameters: Hold 6 to 10 seconds and repeat 10 times, 1 time per day or every other day

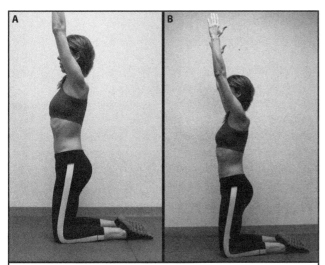

4.03.28 Strengthen: Lumbar Spine, Arm Lift, Tall-Kneeling

Position: Tall-kneeling

Targets: This will engage the muscles that stabilize the lumbar spine in a neutral position and targets core lumbar stabilizers: TA, the pelvic floor muscles, the diaphragm, and the multifidus; arm movements will engage anterior deltoid, long head of biceps, and coracobrachialis.

Instruction: *Unilateral*: Patient uses deep core muscles to hold position described in **4.03.27** and then flexes one shoulder with elbow extended. Thumb should lead the way to clear the acromion. Repeat to other side. A lateral stretch will pull the lumbar spine into extension and should be resisted with the deep core muscles (A). *Bilateral*: For progression, follow previous instructions with flexion of both shoulders at the same time (B).

Substitutions: Hyperlordosis, hips flex, shoulders shrug, chin juts out

Parameters: Hold 3 to 5 seconds, 10 times each up to 3 sets, 1 time per day or every other day

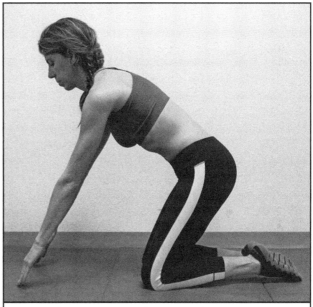

4.03.29 Strengthen: Lumbar Spine, Reach Toward Floor, Tall-Kneeling

Position: Tall-kneeling

Targets: This will engage the muscles that stabilize the lumbar spine in a neutral position and targets core lumbar stabilizers: TA, the pelvic floor muscles, the diaphragm, and the multifidus; gluteus maximus and hamstrings are targeted with hip movement.

Instruction: Patient uses deep core muscles to hold position described in **4.03.27** and then hips flex to reach toward the floor. Patient lightly taps floor with fingertips and returns to start position. Core is engaged the entire exercise and hip movement is isolated; no spinal movement should occur.

Substitutions: Spinal flexion, chin juts out

Parameters: 10 times each up to 3 sets, 1 time per day or every other day

4.03.30 STRENGTHEN: LUMBAR SPINE, REACH TOWARD FLOOR, HALF-KNEELING

POSITION: Half-kneeling

TARGETS: This will engage the muscles that stabilize the lumbar spine in a neutral position and targets core lumbar stabilizers: TA, the pelvic floor muscles, the diaphragm, and the multifidus; gluteus maximus and hamstrings are targeted with hip movement.

INSTRUCTION: Transition from tall-kneeling to place one foot out in front, flat on surface with hip and knee flexed 90 degrees. Knee sits in vertical alignment with ankle. Patient uses deep core muscles to hold position described in **4.03.27** and then hips flex to reach toward the floor to the inside of the bent knee. Patient lightly taps floor with fingertips and returns to start position. Core is engaged the entire exercise and hip movement is isolated; no spinal movement should occur. Once set is finished, perform on the other side.

SUBSTITUTIONS: Spinal flexion, chin juts out

PARAMETERS: 10 times each up to 3 sets, 1 time per day or every other day

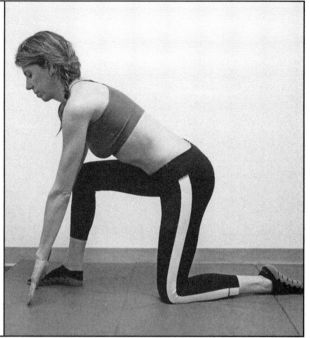

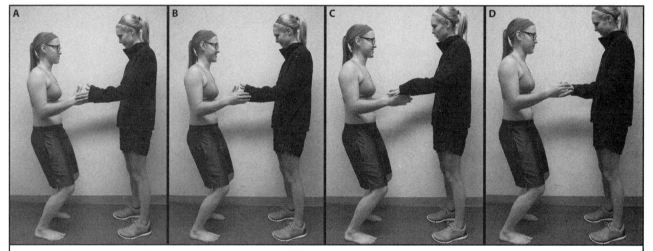

4.03.31 STRENGTHEN: LUMBAR SPINE, QUICK HANDS

POSITION: Mini-squat

TARGETS: This will engage the muscles that stabilize the lumbar spine in a neutral position and targets core lumbar stabilizers: TA, the pelvic floor muscles, the diaphragm, and the multifidus; gluteus maximus, hamstrings and quadriceps, and shoulder internal and external rotators; anterior and posterior deltoid and elbow flexors and extensors are isometrically challenged and targeted with UE resisted movements.

INSTRUCTION: Patient is in standing with feet and knees hip-width apart. Patient slightly flexes at hips and knees with slight dorsiflexion of ankles, trunk is erect and uses deep core muscles to hold position described in **4.03.27**. Shoulders are in neutral with elbows flexed 90 degrees and thumbs pointed up with hands in the fisted position. The therapist then applies resistance to the fists, shoulder internal rotation by pressing outward, external rotation by pressing inward, downward pressure and upward pressure starting slow and rhythmically and progressing to faster movements and with less transition time. Thus, the name "quick hands." The goal is for the patient to maintain the neutral spine alignment by engaging the deep core muscles. An extra challenge may be added by having the patient close his or her eyes to target more proprioceptive training (A through D).

SUBSTITUTIONS: Spinal movement, chin juts out, knees deviate inward or outward, rounding shoulders

PARAMETERS: 10 times each up to 3 sets; may also use a time parameter of 15 to 60 seconds multiplanar with rests in between up to 10 sets, 1 time per day or every other day.

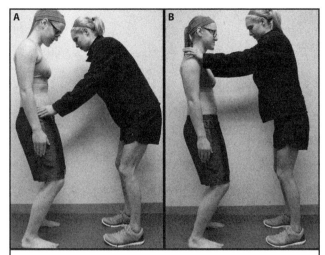

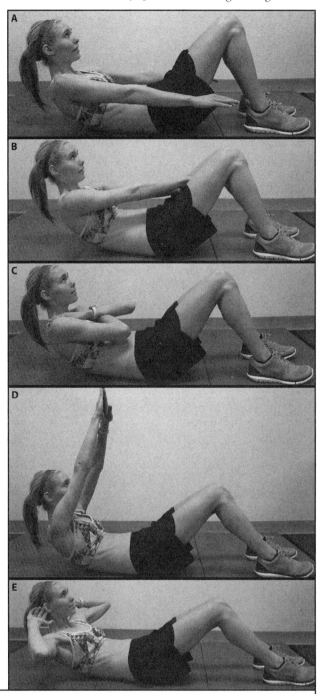

4.03.32 STRENGTHEN: LUMBAR SPINE, BLIND WEIGHT SHIFTS

<u>POSITION</u>: Mini-squat

<u>TARGETS</u>: This will engage the muscles that stabilize the lumbar spine in a neutral position and targets core lumbar stabilizers: TA, the pelvic floor muscles, the diaphragm, and the multifidus; gluteus maximus, hamstrings, and quadriceps are isometrically challenged.

<u>INSTRUCTION</u>: Patient is in standing with feet and knees hip-width apart. Patient slightly flexes at hips and knees with slight dorsiflexion of ankles, trunk is erect and uses deep core muscles to hold position described in **4.03.27**. Hands can be on hips or crossed over chest. Therapist pushes patient at the pelvis or shoulders forward and back, side-to-side, and may even add diagonal challenges as patient resists movements to maintain balance. The goal is for the patient to maintain the neutral spine alignment by engaging the deep core muscles. An extra challenge may be added by having the patient close eyes to target more proprioceptive training. Thus, the term *blind weight shifts* (A and B).

<u>SUBSTITUTIONS</u>: Spinal movement, chin juts out, knees deviate inward or outward, rounding shoulders

<u>PARAMETERS</u>: 10 times each up to 3 sets; may also use a time parameter of 15 to 60 seconds multiplanar with rests in between up to 10 sets, 1 time per day or every other day.

4.03.33 STRENGTHEN: ABDOMINAL, PARTIAL SIT-UP, 5-WAY

<u>POSITION</u>: Supine, hook-lying

<u>TARGETS</u>: This will strengthen the trunk flexors; RA, internal and external obliques, and TA

<u>INSTRUCTION</u>: Patient lies on back in supine or hook-lying with knees and feet hip-width apart depending on comfort. Supine position will remove iliopsoas compensatory strategies and is recommended above hook-lying, but patient comfort may not allow this. Patient will crunch up by rounding spine into a C-curve and bring scapula up off the table while keeping eyes directed toward the ceiling and chin tucked. Hand position from easiest to hardest is hands down by sides (A), hands stacked reaching between knees (B), arms cross over chest (C), hands reaching toward ceiling (D), and fingertips to ears and shoulders externally rotated (E).

<u>SUBSTITUTIONS</u>: Lack of rounding through spine; substituting with hip flexors, fast movement using momentum, holding breath, jutting chin out, pulling on head.

<u>PARAMETERS</u>: 10 times each up to 3 sets, 1 time per day or every other day

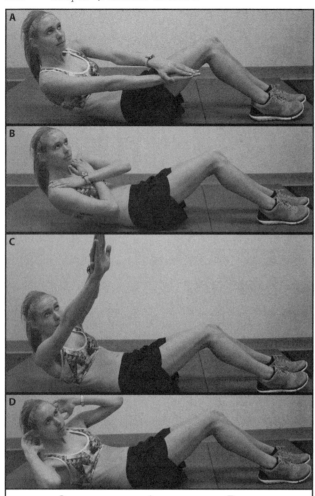

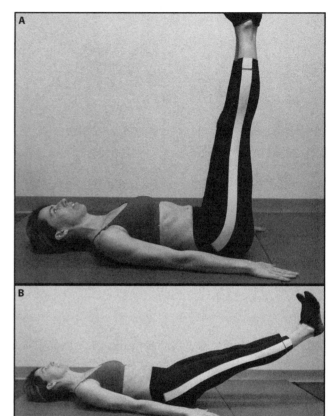

4.03.34 STRENGTHEN: ABDOMINAL, PARTIAL DIAGONAL SIT-UP, 4-WAY

POSITION: Supine, hook-lying

TARGETS: This will strengthen the trunk flexors and rotators primarily internal and external obliques

INSTRUCTION: Patient lies on back in supine or hook-lying with knee and feet hip-width apart depending on comfort. Supine position will remove iliopsoas compensatory strategies and is recommended above hook-lying, but patient comfort may not allow this. Patient will crunch up by rounding spine into a C-curve while simultaneously rotating to one side, bringing sternum in the direction of the ipsilateral knee, bringing scapula up off the table while keeping eyes directed toward the ceiling to that side and chin tucked. Hand position from easiest to hardest is hands stacked reaching to the outside side of the ipsilateral knees (or hip if done supine) (A), arms cross over chest (B), hands reaching toward ceiling on the ipsilateral side (C), and fingertips to ears and shoulders externally rotated (D).

SUBSTITUTIONS: Lack of rounding through spine; substituting with hip flexors, fast movement using momentum, holding breath, jutting chin out, pulling on head, flexing first and rotating at end only or rotating without lifting.

PARAMETERS: 10 times each up to 3 sets, 1 time per day or every other day

4.03.35 STRENGTHEN: ABDOMINAL, POSTERIOR PELVIC TILT, LEG LOWERS

POSITION: Supine

TARGETS: Strengthens RA, TA, and obliques

INSTRUCTION: With knees and feet together, allow knees to bend as patient brings feet up toward ceiling. Instruct patient to straighten knee as much possible. Therapist may hold the legs here while teaching PPT (4.01.4) to ensure the patient has a good tilt before moving to next step. Patient then will contract abdominal muscles to maintain a strong PPT while slowly lowering the heels down toward the bed. Therapist should monitor PPT closely so if patient is unable to maintain, the knees are allowed to bend and patient may rest feet on table in hook-lying. Performing this exercise without maintenance of a strong PPT will place undue stress on the lumbar spine as the iliopsoas attempts to compensate and may cause injury. Once the patient is able to maintain PPT through the entire lowering, progress to patient lifting legs from the table back to perpendicular to floor. Again, PPT must be engaged and before starting lift (A and B).

SUBSTITUTIONS: Loss of strong PPT; holding breath.

PARAMETERS: 10 times up to 3 sets, 1 time per day or every other day

Where's the Evidence?

Shields and Heiss (1997) evaluated the abdominal muscle activity on 15 male subjects during the isometric bent-knee curl and double straight leg lowering exercise to determine if the muscle synergies were specific to a given exercise. The double straight leg lowering exercise resulted in significantly greater activation of the abdominal muscles compared with the curl. Two abdominal muscle synergies emerged during the double straight leg lowering exercise: synergy I exhibited high RA, high external oblique, and low internal oblique muscle activity, whereas synergy II exhibited low RA, high external oblique, and high internal oblique. The results support the use of the double straight leg lowering with the PPT for achieving greater abdominal muscle co-activation in an exercise program.

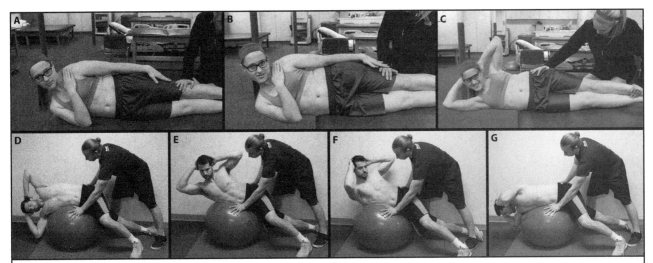

4.03.36 STRENGTHEN: ABDOMINAL, LATERAL TRUNK FLEXION

POSITION: Side-lying

TARGETS: Strengthen unilateral quadratus lumborum, internal and external obliques, and erector spinae

INSTRUCTION: *On table, half-range*: Position patient side-lying on a table with hips and feet stacked. Therapist may stabilize the LEs. The patient's top hand may rest on lateral thigh as bottom hand is placed on top shoulder. Patient raises trunk into lateral flexion, bringing top shoulder up and inferiorly toward hip in a side crunch (A). Progression is to place the hand behind the head with shoulder externally rotated and lead elbow toward lateral pelvis. *Off table full-range*: Position patient over a table in which the rib cage is off the table. Allow the trunk to lower toward floor and then repeat instructions above (B). Progression is to place the hand behind the head with shoulder externally rotated (C). *On exercise ball: (Beginner)* Kneel on left knee with right foot forward, placing the ball against the left thigh and walk the ball up, bringing knee off floor. Hip should now be on the ball. Forward knee is bent with foot flat on floor and back leg has toes on floor. Rest left hand beside on the ball. Set the abdominals and roll left side off of the ball. Roll back down over the ball and repeat. *(Advanced)* With patient side-lying over exercise ball positioned at the pelvis, ball is against a wall. Allow bottom knee to flex slightly and stagger feet for stability. Allow the trunk to lower toward floor and then repeat instructions above. Progression is to place the hand behind the head with shoulder externally rotated (E). Patient may lean back slightly to target obliques anteriorly (F) or roll slightly forward (G) to target quadratus lumborum. Head should stay aligned with sternum and chin tucked.

SUBSTITUTIONS: Feet coming off floor, neck should remain neutral and tucked slightly

PARAMETERS: Hold for 15 to 30 seconds, 3 to 5 repetitions, 1 time per day or every other day

4.03.37 STRENGTHEN: ABDOMINAL, LATERAL TRUNK FLEXION WITH WEIGHT

<u>POSITION</u>: Standing

<u>TARGETS</u>: Strengthen unilateral quadratus lumborum, internal and external obliques, and erector spinae

<u>INSTRUCTION</u>: In a slight mini-squat, with slight flexion of hips and knees and feet hip-width apart and engaging deeper core to address APT or PPT, patient holds weight in hand along the side of the thigh. Patient leans to one side and returns to start while lifting weight (A and B). Repeat full set before switching to other side. Head should stay aligned with sternum and chin tucked.

<u>SUBSTITUTIONS</u>: Hyperextending knees, neck should remain neutral and tucked slightly

<u>PARAMETERS</u>: Hold for 15 to 30 seconds, 3 to 5 repetitions, 1 time per day or every other day

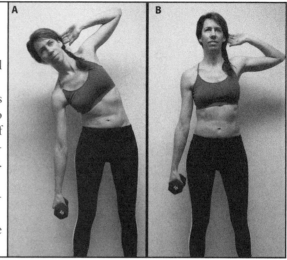

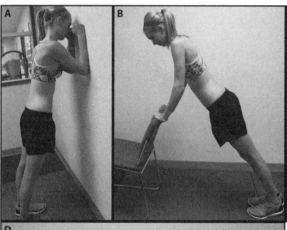

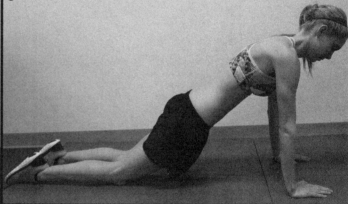

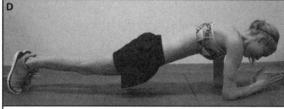

4.03.38 STRENGTHEN: ABDOMINAL, PLANK AND VARIATIONS

<u>POSITION</u>: Standing to start, progress to begin in quadruped, progress to prone

<u>TARGETS</u>: Strengthen primary muscles: erectus spinae, RA, and TA; secondary muscles (synergists/segmental stabilizers): trapezius, rhomboids, RC, the anterior, medial, and posterior deltoid muscles, pectorals, serratus anterior, gluteus maximus, quadriceps, and gastrocnemius

<u>INSTRUCTION</u>: *Standing wall (beginner)*: Patient's feet are hip-width apart, patient places elbows on a wall approximately 4 inches below shoulder height and walks feet back as far as possible without lifting heels. Patient engages core muscles to maintain a neutral spine while pressing forearms into the wall. Patient may lift onto the balls of feet so that heels are hovering off the ground and body is leaning slightly forward. Hold and breathe for up to 1 minute (A). *Standing chair (beginner)*: With the feet hip-width apart, place chair against and facing wall. Patient places hands on chair back and walk feet back as far as possible without lifting heels. Patient engages core muscles to maintain a neutral spine while pressing hands into the back of the chair. Patient may lift onto the balls of feet so that heels are hovering off the ground and body is leaning slightly forward. Hold and breathe for up to 1 minute (B). *Quadruped*: Make sure the patient's hands are directly beneath shoulders and knees directly beneath hips. The tops of feet can either be flat on the floor or with curled toes. Patient engages core muscles to maintain a neutral spine while pressing hands into the floor. Hold and breathe for up to 1 minute (C). *Forearm*: This is what most people consider to be a standard plank. Patient lies face down with legs extended and elbows bent directly under shoulders and hands clasped or in neutral (thumbs up). Feet should be hip-width apart, and elbows should be shoulder-width apart. Patient engages core muscles to maintain a neutral spine while tucking toes and lifting body. Patient should be in a straight line from head to heels. Hold and breathe for up to 1 minute (D). *(continued)*

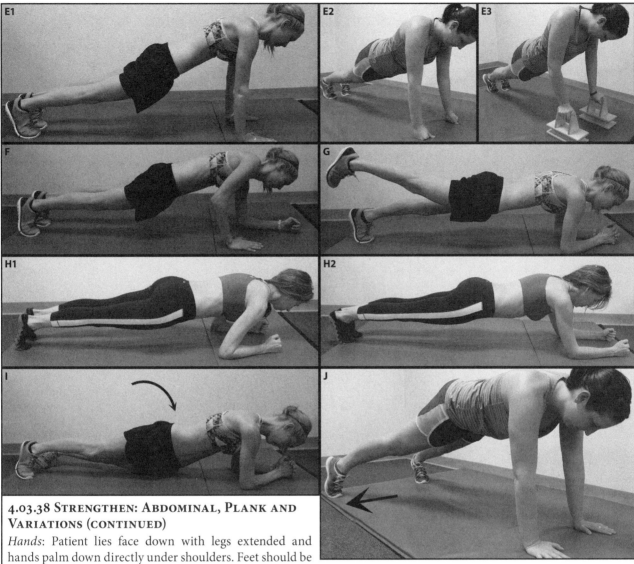

4.03.38 STRENGTHEN: ABDOMINAL, PLANK AND VARIATIONS (CONTINUED)

Hands: Patient lies face down with legs extended and hands palm down directly under shoulders. Feet should be hip-width apart and elbows should be shoulder-width apart. Patient engages core muscles to maintain a neutral spine while tucking toes and lifting body. Patient should be in a straight line from head to heels. Hold and breathe for up to 1 minute (E1). Modification for wrist issues is to bear weight through fisted hand or use push-up blocks (E2 and E3). *Forearms to hands*: Follow instructions for *Hands*, then lower to the right forearm followed by the left forearm so patient is in position described in *Forearm*. Follow with pressing up to right hand and then left returning to start position (F). *Alternating leg lift*: Follow instructions in *Hands*, then lift one leg and return. Repeat on other side. Do not allow lower back to extend or body to roll side-to-side (G). *Rocking*: Follow instructions in *Forearm* or *Hands*. This can be done in either position. Patient shifts weight forward onto arms, holds, and returns to start (H1). Patient then shifts weight backward onto feet, holds, and returns to start (H2). *Cheek dips*: Follow instructions in *Forearm* or *Hands*. This can be done in either position. Patient dips right hip toward floor while maintaining straight spine; do not allow dipping, side-lower back to sag. Return to start and repeat to other side. This is more of a rotational movement as shoulder horizontally adducts and rotation occurs in hips and pelvis (I). *Tap outs*: Follow instructions in *Forearm* or *Hands*. This can be done in either position. Lift one leg slightly off floor and abduct hip to tap the floor. Do not allow dipping, side lower back to sag. Return to start and repeat to other side (J). *(continued)*

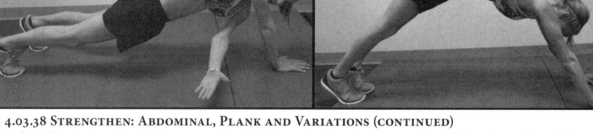

4.03.38 STRENGTHEN: ABDOMINAL, PLANK AND VARIATIONS (CONTINUED)

Jacks: Follow instructions in *Forearm* or *Hands*. This can be done in either position. Patient jumps feet off floor, landing in hip abduction bilaterally like the lower part of a jumping jack and returns to start (K). *Spiderman*: *Knee to same elbow*: Follow instructions in *Forearm* or *Hands*. This can be done in either position. Patient lifts one leg slightly off floor and abducts hip and flexes knee, bringing knee toward ipsilateral elbow. Do not allow dipping, side-lower back to sag. Return to start and repeat to other side (L1). *Knee to opposite elbow*: Patient lifts one leg slightly off floor and adducts hip and flexes knee, bringing knee toward contralateral elbow. Do not allow dipping, side-lower back to sag. Return to start and repeat to other side (L2). *Knee to opposite elbow extend knee*: Patient lifts one leg slightly off floor and adducts hip and flexes knee, bringing knee toward contralateral elbow and then extends the knee. Do not allow dipping, side-lower back to sag. Return to start and repeat to other side (L3). *Thread the needle*: Follow instructions in *Forearm* or *Hands*. This can be done in either position. Patient brings one hand off surface and threads it just inferior to axilla (arm pit) on opposite side. This is more of a rotational movement as shoulder horizontally adducts and rotation occurs in hips and pelvis. Do not allow dipping, side-lower back to sag. Return to start and repeat to other side (M). *Pikes*: Follow instructions in *Forearm* or *Hands*. This can be done in either position. Patient brings hips up toward ceiling by flexing at the hips, spine and knees remain straight. Return to start (N). *(continued)*

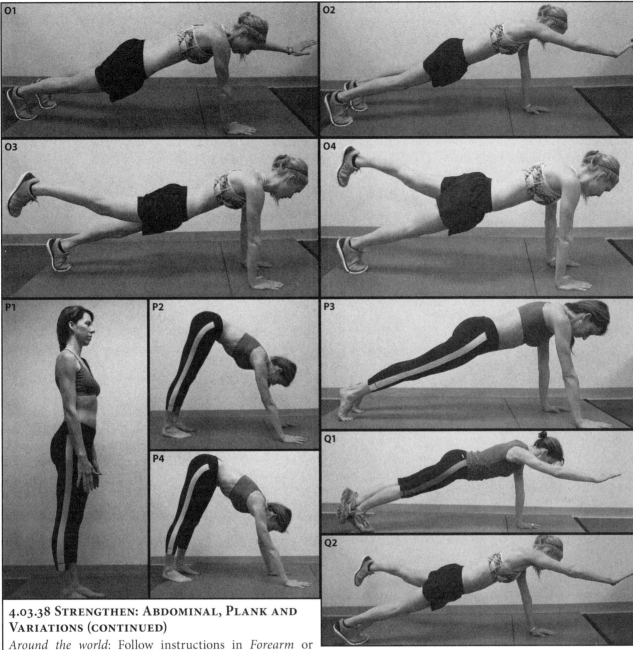

4.03.38 STRENGTHEN: ABDOMINAL, PLANK AND VARIATIONS (CONTINUED)

Around the world: Follow instructions in *Forearm* or *Hands*. This can be done in either position. Patient picks up right hand and reaches forward, replaces on floor, and then follows with left. Patient then lifts left leg and abducts hip and then returns to start, followed by the same movement with the right leg. Cycle continues around going the same direction. Return to start (O1 through O4). *Walkouts*: Patient in standing, bends forward at the hips to reach for the floor. Once hands are on floor, patient walks hands out to full plank on hands and returns to start by piking hips as described in *Pikes* and walks hands back toward feet then extends hips and stands. Neutral spine must be maintained throughout movement. This is a very advanced plank (P1 through P4). *2-point plank*: *Supported*: Follow instructions in *Forearm* or *Hands*, place right foot on top of left ankle and left arm behind the back. Repeat to opposite sides (Q1). *Unsupported*: Follow instructions in *Forearm* or *Hands*, extend right hip and lift foot while flexing opposite shoulder and lifting hand off surface and reaching forward. Repeat to opposite sides (Q2). *(continued)*

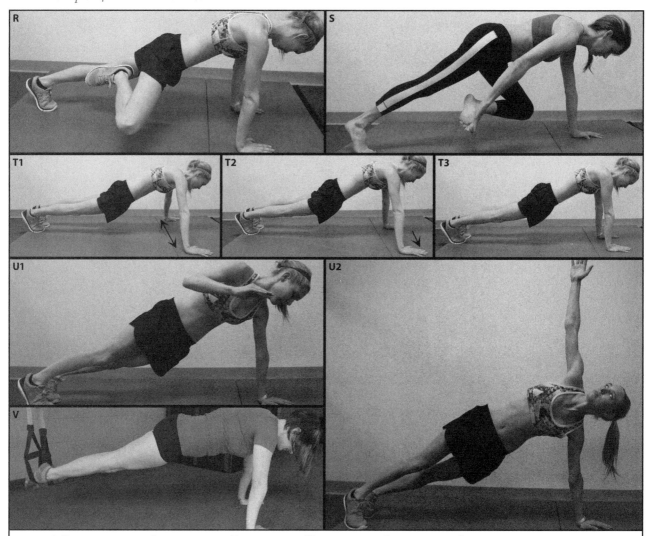

4.03.38 STRENGTHEN: ABDOMINAL, PLANK AND VARIATIONS (CONTINUED)

Tree plank: Follow instructions in *Forearm* or *Hands*, place right foot on inside of left knee. Repeat to opposite sides (R). *Hand to toe*: Follow instructions in *Forearm* or *Hands*, bring right foot off surface and bend knee while externally rotating and abducting hip, opposite hand comes off surface to reach down to touch the opposite foot. Repeat to opposite sides (S). *Out-ins*: Follow instructions in *Forearm* or *Hands*, bring right hand off surface and set out further to the side. Perform same movement on left side. Bring right hand back to start followed by left hand (T1 through T3). *Open rotation*: Follow instructions in *Forearm* or *Hands*, bring one hand off surface and rotate the hand up toward the ceiling while body turns to side plank position and weight shift off ipsilateral foot to lateral aspect of contralateral foot. Return to start. Make sure the humeral head is anchored into glenoid fossa; poor control of the shoulder could result in injury with this movement. Repeat to opposite side (U1 and U2). *Suspension straps*: Position patient's feet in straps so that tops of feet are in contact with strap. Patient then comes up to elbows or hands (advanced) while engaging the core and pelvic floor to maintain a neutral spine. Hold (V).

<u>SUBSTITUTIONS</u>: Neck should remain neutral and tucked slightly, gaze between hands, breathing normally during entire plank. With weightbearing through the hand, cupping/lifting of the palm is important and encourage weight distribution through all fingers. This will engage wrist flexors and decrease wrist stress. The modification for wrist issues is to bear weight through fisted hands or use push-up blocks (E2 and E3). Shoulders are active and engaged, scapula depressed and retracted slightly. Patient maintains neutral spine. Head should stay aligned with sternum and chin tucked.

<u>PARAMETERS</u>: *A-E, Q, R, V*: Hold each position for 10 to 60 seconds, 3 to 5 repetitions; *F-P, S-U*: 10 repetitions, 1 to 3 sets; all exercises: 1 time per day or every other day.

Where's the Evidence?

Atkins (2014) assessed the neuromuscular activation of global core stabilizers when using suspension training techniques, compared to more traditional forms of isometric exercise. Eighteen male youth swimmers performed static bracing of the core using a modified plank position, with and without a Swiss ball, and held for 30 seconds. A mechanically similar plank was then held using suspension straps. Analysis of surface EMG activity revealed that suspension produced higher peak amplitude in the RA than using a prone or Swiss Ball plank. No difference was found between external oblique or erector spinae, concluding that suspension training noticeably improves engagement of anterior core musculature when compared to both lateral and posterior muscles.

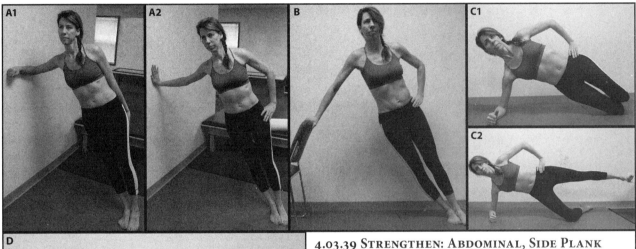

4.03.39 STRENGTHEN: ABDOMINAL, SIDE PLANK AND VARIATIONS

POSITION: Standing to start, progress to side-lying

TARGETS: Strengthen primary muscles: erector spinae, internal and external obliques, RA, and TA; secondary muscle, synergists/segmental stabilizers (trapezius, rhomboids, RC, the anterior, medial, and posterior deltoid muscles, pectorals, serratus anterior, gluteus maximus, quadriceps, and gastrocnemius).

INSTRUCTION: *Standing wall (beginner)*: Facing along the wall with feet together and 8 inches from wall, patient places elbows on a wall approximately 4 inches below shoulder height and walks feet away from the wall. Patient engages core muscles to maintain a neutral spine while pressing forearm into the wall (A1). Feet become stacked as the distance increases. Progress to hand on wall. Hold and breathe for up to 1 minute (A2). *Standing chair (beginner)*: Place chair against and facing wall. Patient facing alongside wall behind the chair then places one hand on chair back and walks feet away from the chair. Patient engages core muscles to maintain a neutral spine while pressing hands into the back of the chair. Feet become stacked as the distance increases. Hold and breathe for up to 1 minute (B). *On elbow and knee (beginner)*: Start in side-lying and bend bottom knee. Prop up on bottom elbow and place top hand on the hip. Engage core and lift torso to straighten the spine (C1). The top knee can be bent or straight (C2). Adding top shoulder horizontal abduction with extended elbow will increase intensity as patient reaches fingertips toward ceiling (C3). Hold and breathe for up to 1 minute. *On elbow and feet*: Start in side-lying with feet stacked. Prop up on bottom elbow and place top hand on the hip. Engage core and lift torso to straighten the spine (D). Adding top shoulder horizontal abduction with extended elbow will increase intensity as patient reaches fingertips toward ceiling. Hold and breathe for up to 1 minute. *(continued)*

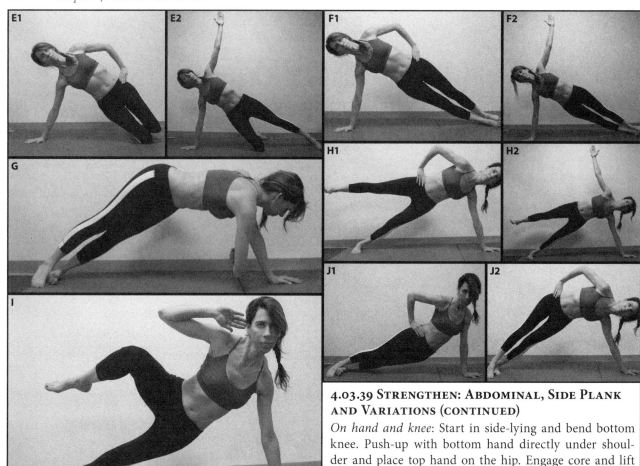

4.03.39 STRENGTHEN: ABDOMINAL, SIDE PLANK AND VARIATIONS (CONTINUED)

On hand and knee: Start in side-lying and bend bottom knee. Push-up with bottom hand directly under shoulder and place top hand on the hip. Engage core and lift torso to straighten the spine (E1). Adding top shoulder horizontal abduction with extended elbow will increase intensity as patient reaches fingertips toward ceiling (E2). Hold and breathe for up to 1 minute. *On hand and feet*: Start in side-lying with feet stacked. Push up with bottom hand directly under shoulder and place top hand on the hip. Engage core and lift torso to straighten the spine (F1). Adding top shoulder horizontal abduction with extended elbow will increase intensity as patient reaches fingertips toward ceiling (F2). Hold and breathe for up to 1 minute. *Curl unders*: Follow instructions *On hand and feet*, adding top shoulder horizontal abduction with extended elbow reaching fingertips toward ceiling. Roll torso toward floor, bringing top hand under rib cage across the body and return to start (G). *With leg lift*: Follow instructions *On hand and feet*, adding top hip abduction with extended knee and toes pointing forward (H1). You can add horizontal abduction of the shoulder with extended elbow to increase intensity. Patient reaches fingertips to ceiling (H2). *Side crunch*: Follow instructions *On hand and feet*, with top hand touching top ear. Bring top elbow toward top knee as patient flexes hip and knee (I). *Hip dip*: Follow instructions *On hand and feet*, with top hand on top hip. Drop bottom pelvis down toward floor and return (J1 and J2). *(continued)*

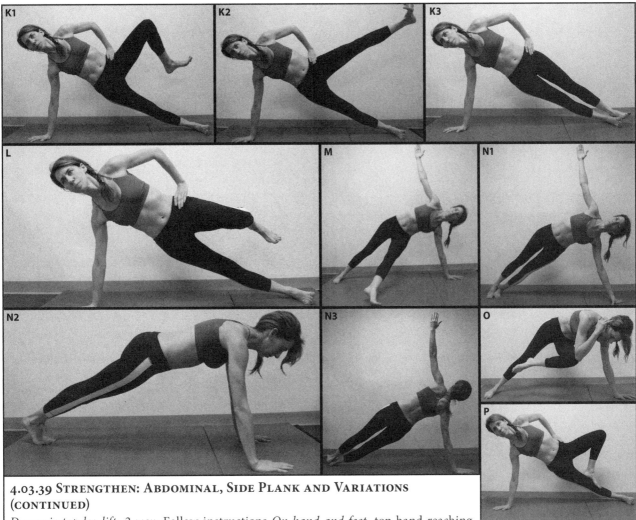

4.03.39 STRENGTHEN: ABDOMINAL, SIDE PLANK AND VARIATIONS (CONTINUED)

Dynamic top leg lift, 2-way: Follow instructions *On hand and feet*, top hand reaching toward ceiling. Bring top hip and knee into flexion and return followed by bringing top hip into abduction and knee flexion and return (K1 through K3). *Marching*: Follow instructions *On hand and feet*, top hand reaching toward ceiling. Bring top hip and knee into flexion and return. Repeat to other side (I). *Dynamic bottom leg flex/extend*: Follow instructions *On hand and feet*, top hand reaching toward ceiling. Bring bottom hip and knee into flexion, tapping floor in front of patient with heel followed by extending the hip and tapping floor behind. Repeat (M). *3-point transition*: Follow instructions in *On hand and feet*. Patient leads with top hand toward floor and torso follows to assume plank position described in *Hands*, then transitions to side plank on other side. Repeat (N1 through N3). *Diagonal crunch*: Follow instructions in *On hand and feet*. Patient leads with top elbow while flexing bottom hip and knee to bring elbow to knee. Repeat (O). *Tree*: Follow instructions in *On hand and feet*. Patient brings bottom of top foot to inside of bottom knee, opening hips and holds (P). *(continued)*

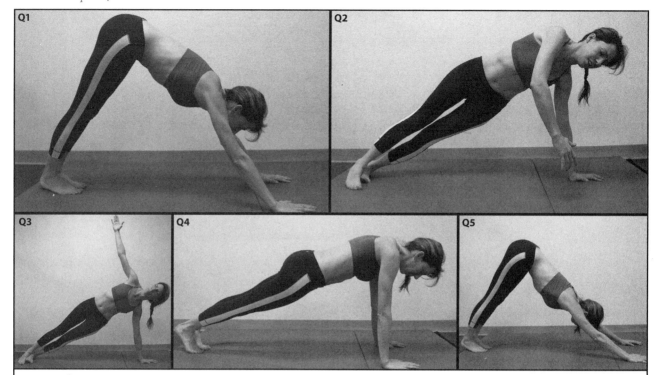

4.03.39 Strengthen: Abdominal, Side Plank and Variations (continued)

Pike split to side plank: Follow instructions in *Hands*. Extend one hip to bring bottom foot up toward ceiling. Transition to side plank by lifting same side hand and rotating trunk onto opposite hand and foot into position described in *on hands and feet* (Q1 through Q5).

<u>Substitutions</u>: Neck should remain neutral and tucked slightly, gaze forward, breathing normally during entire plank. With weightbearing through the hand, cupping/lifting of the palm is important, encourage weight distribution through all fingers. This will engage wrist flexors and decrease wrist stress. The modification for wrist issues is to bear weight through fisted hands or use push-up blocks (E2 and E3). Side planking is especially challenging in the shoulder. To prevent injury, shoulders are active and engaged, scapula depressed and retracted slightly. Patient maintains neutral spine. Head should stay aligned with sternum and chin tucked.

<u>Parameters</u>: *A-F, P*: Hold each position for 10 to 60 seconds, 3 to 5 repetitions; *F-O, Q*: 10 repetitions, 1 to 3 sets; all exercises: 1 time per day or every other day.

Where's the Evidence?

Youdas et al. (2014) used surface EMG to assess muscle activation during a side bridge (side plank) activity. Specifically, they were trying to determine if muscle activation was significant on the non-weightbearing side. They studied 25 subjects looking at RA, external abdominal oblique, lower trapezius, lumbar multifidus, and gluteus medius during 3 repetitions of four side-bridging exercises. They concluded muscle recruitment was greater within muscles of the ipsilateral weightbearing trunk and thigh for all examined muscles except RA during rotational side-bending and lower trapezius during trunk elevated side-bending.

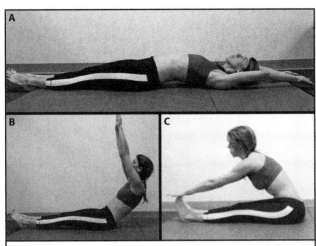

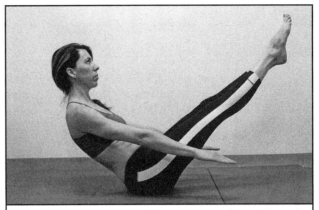

4.03.40 STRENGTHEN: ABDOMINAL, ROLL-UP (ADVANCED)

POSITION: Supine

TARGETS: Decrease lumbar lordosis, facilitate pelvic floor and lower abdominals (TA primarily), strengthen RA, internal and external obliques.

INSTRUCTION: Patient lies flat, inhales while bringing arms overhead while engaging core with a PPT. Patient then slowing brings arms back toward torso while elongating spine and rolling the spine off the floor, following the arms and exhaling as patient rolls up and continuing until reaching the toes or as far forward as possible. Feet are dorsiflexed and buttocks and inner thigh muscles contracted. Patient inhales and then reverses lowering the spine one vertebra at a time (A through C).

SUBSTITUTIONS: Not allowing trunk to curl, but lifting with hip flexors and trunk lagging or is straight, jutting chin out, fast movements of arms to increase momentum assist; movement should be slow and controlled.

PARAMETERS: Repeat 10 times, perform 2 to 3 sets, repeat 1 time per day or every other day

4.03.41 STRENGTHEN: ABDOMINAL, BOAT POSE/ V-SITS (ADVANCED)

POSITION: Long-sitting

TARGETS: Decrease lumbar lordosis, facilitate pelvic floor and lower abdominals and strengthen RA, internal and external obliques.

INSTRUCTION: Patient in long-sitting, inhales and bends knees so feet are flat on the floor. Patient places hands on the side of thighs just below hips, keeping fingers pointed toward the toes, then exhaling and slowly leaning back at the hips lifting legs, with bent knees, a few inches off the floor. Make sure back is straight as the patient draws the shoulder blades together to lift and open the chest. Patient then slowly straightens out legs as far as possible. Patient's hips and trunk should be angled about 45 degrees from the floor. From the side, the body should look like a "V," with the arms still touching the thighs but only lightly, not grasping. If ready, the patient can slowly move the arms alongside the legs with palms facing down until parallel to the floor. Release the pose by dropping the legs and returning to the sitting position.

SUBSTITUTIONS: Jutting chin out, grabbing legs, movement should be slow and controlled

PARAMETERS: Hold each pose 10 to 30 seconds, repeat 5 to 10 times, 1 time per day or every other day

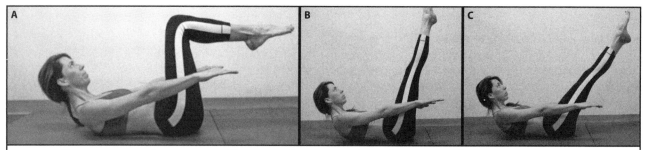

4.03.42 STRENGTHEN: ABDOMINAL, PULSING CRUNCH, 3-WAY (ADVANCED)

POSITION: Supine

TARGETS: Decrease lumbar lordosis, facilitate pelvic floor and lower abdominals (TA primarily), strengthen RA, internal and external obliques.

INSTRUCTION: *Progression #1*: Patient is supine with legs in 90/90 position with arms at the sides palms down. Patient raises head and shoulders off mat, contracting the abdominals and looking up toward the ceiling with the chin slightly tucked. Hands are lifted off the ground and pulsed up and down, keeping fingers just off the floor until resting (A). *Progression #2*: Same instructions as previous with hips at 90 degrees of flexion and knee extended; this requires hamstring flexibility. If patient cannot fully extend the knees, straighten the knees as far as possible (B). *Progression #3*: Same instructions as previous with hips at 45 degrees of flexion and knee extended (C).

SUBSTITUTIONS: Jutting chin out, grabbing legs, movement should be slow and controlled, lifting entire torso; want to see a C-curve in the spine; rounding up toward ceiling at upper torso only.

PARAMETERS: Pulse each for 30 to 100 pulses, repeat 3 to 5 times, 1 time per day or every other day

4.03.43 STRENGTHEN: ABDOMINAL, SCISSOR (ADVANCED)

POSITION: Supine

TARGETS: Strengthens TA and obliques

INSTRUCTION: In supine, instruct patient to perform PPT (**4.01.4**) to ensure a good tilt before moving to next step. Patient then will contract abdominal muscles, lifting shoulders and

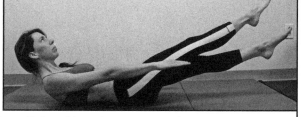

head off surface and looking toward the ceiling, raise legs 4 inches off the table and scissor right foot over left, then left foot over right. Therapist should monitor PPT closely. Performing this exercise without maintenance of a strong PPT will place undue stress on the lumbar spine as the iliopsoas attempts to compensate and may cause injury.

SUBSTITUTIONS: Loss of strong PPT, holding breath

PARAMETERS: 5 to 10 times, 1 to 3 sets, 1 time per day or every other day

4.03.44 STRENGTHEN: ABDOMINAL, SCISSOR LOWER (ADVANCED)

POSITION: Supine

TARGETS: Strengthens TA and obliques

INSTRUCTION: With knees and feet together, allow knees to bend as patient brings feet up toward ceiling. Instruct patient to straighten knee as much as possible. Therapist may hold the legs here while teaching PPT (**4.01.4**) to ensure a good tilt before moving to next step. Patient then will contract abdominal muscles to maintain a strong PPT

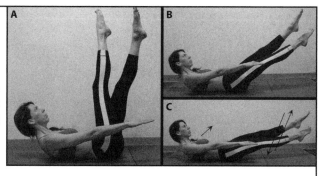

while slowly scissoring the heels down toward the bed, bringing right heel over left ankle and then left ankle over right ankle and repeating until feet meet bed. Therapist should monitor PPT closely, so if patient is unable to maintain the PPT, knees are allowed to bend and patient may rest feet on table in hook-lying. Performing this exercise without maintenance of a strong PPT will place undue stress on the lumbar spine as the iliopsoas attempts to compensate and may cause injury. Once the patient is able to maintain PPT through the entire lowering, allow patient to begin lifting legs and scissoring on the way up as well. Again, PPT must be engaged and held before starting lift (A, B, and C).

SUBSTITUTIONS: Loss of strong PPT, holding breath

PARAMETERS: 5 to 10 times, 1 to 3 sets, 1 time per day or every other day

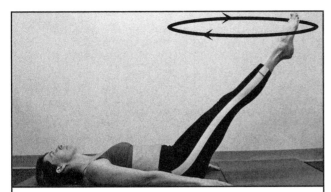

4.03.45 STRENGTHEN: ABDOMINAL, CORKSCREW (ADVANCED)

<u>POSITION</u>: Supine

<u>TARGETS</u>: Strengthens TA and obliques, hip control

<u>INSTRUCTION</u>: Patient is supine with hips flexed 90 degrees, knees extended and arms at their sides, palms down. Instruct patient to straighten knee as much as possible. You may hold the legs here while teaching PPT (**4.01.4**) to ensure a good tilt before moving to next step. Patient then will contract abdominal muscles to maintain a strong PPT while circling the legs clockwise for multiple repetitions, drawing a circle on the ceiling with the toes. Repeat in counter-clockwise direction. Therapist should monitor PPT closely so that if the patient is unable to maintain, the knees are allowed to bend and patient may rest feet on table in hook-lying. Performing this exercise without maintenance of a strong PPT will place undue stress on the lumbar spine as the iliopsoas attempts to compensate and may cause injury. Once the patient is able to maintain PPT through the entire circling, therapist may increase the size of the circle and allow the patient to begin lifting legs and circling on the way up as well.

<u>SUBSTITUTIONS</u>: Loss of strong PPT, holding breath

<u>PARAMETERS</u>: 5 to 10 times, 1 to 3 sets, 1 time per day or every other day

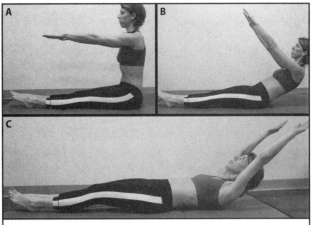

4.03.46 STRENGTHEN: ABDOMINAL, CATAPULT (ADVANCED)

<u>POSITION</u>: Supine with slight bend in knees

<u>TARGETS</u>: Decrease lumbar lordosis, facilitate pelvic floor and lower abdominals (TA primarily), strengthen RA, internal and external obliques.

<u>INSTRUCTION</u>: Patient presses heels into floor and extends arm at shoulder height, palms facing down. With spine straight and upward gaze, inhale deeply then exhale slowly, lowering torso to floor over a 5-count, ending with arms overhead. In one smooth movement, leading with the arms, exhale and explode back to starting position (A, B, and C).

<u>SUBSTITUTIONS</u>: Jutting chin out, grabbing legs, movement should be slow and controlled, lifting entire torso; want to see a C-curve in the spine, rounding up toward ceiling at upper torso only.

<u>PARAMETERS</u>: Pulse each for 30 to 100 pulses, repeat 3 to 5 times, 1 time per day or every other day

4.03.47 STRENGTHEN: ABDOMINAL, OBLIQUE TWIST, MEDICINE BALL TAPS (ADVANCED)

<u>POSITION</u>: Hook-lying

<u>TARGETS</u>: Strengthens TA, obliques, hip control

<u>INSTRUCTION</u>: Allow patient to sit up in hook-lying and then lean back about 30 to 45 degrees from vertical, contracting deep core muscles of the abdomen as a medicine ball is held in hands and on lap. Patient then picks up ball and twists to one side, tapping ball to floor, slowly rotates to opposites side, and repeats (A). Advanced progression is to move into partial boat pose with feet off floor; allow knees to bend and repeat previous instructions (B). Therapist may also stand in front of patient while patient throwing ball to therapist. Therapist returns, throws to each side of the patient and requiring a dynamic twist by the patient (C1 through C4).

<u>SUBSTITUTIONS</u>: Loss of strong PPT, holding breath

<u>PARAMETERS</u>: 5 to 10 times, 1 to 3 sets, 1 time per day or every other day

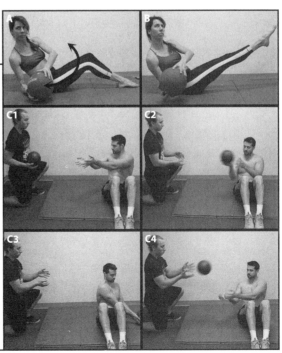

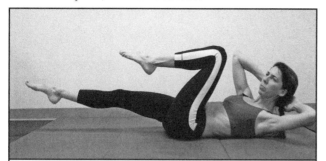

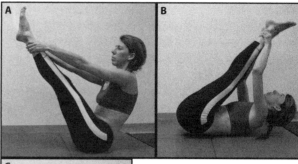

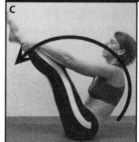

4.03.48 Strengthen: Abdominal, Oblique Twist, Bicycle (Advanced)

<u>Position</u>: Supine

<u>Targets</u>: Strengthens TA, RA, and obliques, hip control

<u>Instruction</u>: Patient is supine 90/90 leg position with legs hip-width distance apart and hands behind head, but not pulling on neck. Patient contracts deep core muscles of the abdomen and raises head and upper body while supporting head with hands while bringing right shoulder toward opposite knee, focusing on twisting in the waist while same-side leg extends to approximately 30 degrees of hip flexion and knee extension. Instruct patient to straighten knee as much as patient can. Repeat on opposite sides.

<u>Substitutions</u>: Loss of strong PPT, holding breath

<u>Parameters</u>: 5 to 10 times, 1 to 3 sets, 1 time per day or every other

4.03.49 Strengthen: Abdominal, Open-Leg Rocker (Advanced)

<u>Position</u>: Long-sitting

<u>Targets</u>: Decrease lumbar lordosis, facilitate pelvic floor and lower abdominals (TA primarily)

<u>Instruction</u>: Patient in long-sitting inhales and bends knees, bringing feet off floor and grabbing ankles with hands. Contract the abdominals and lengthen the legs upward into a "V" shape, hips adducted (A). Inhale, rolling backward from the buttocks all along the spine to the shoulder blades (B). Exhale and return to starting position maintaining balance on the sacrum for 3 to 5 seconds and repeat (C).

<u>Substitutions</u>: Jutting chin out, movement should be slow and controlled

<u>Parameters</u>: Repeat 5 to 10 times, perform 1 to 3 sets, 1 time per day or every other day

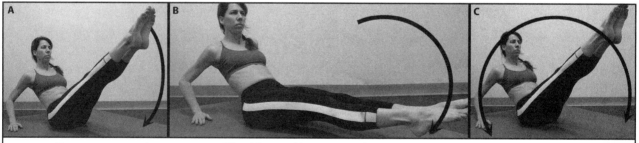

4.03.50 Strengthen: Abdominal, Hip Twist (Advanced)

<u>Position</u>: Long-sitting

<u>Targets</u>: Decrease lumbar lordosis, facilitate and strengthen pelvic floor and abdominals, gain hip control

<u>Instruction</u>: Patient in long-sitting leans back and places hands behind with elbow extended, palms down, thumbs outward, and fingers pointing away from patient. Make sure back is straight as patient draws shoulder blades together to lift and open chest. Patient then slowly brings hips into flexion, about 45 degrees from the floor with knees extended while maintaining a tightened deep core. From the side, patient's body should look like a "V." Patient inhales and circles legs downward and to the right and exhales circling around to the left and returning to start in a circling motion clockwise (A through C). Perform full set before repeating entire sequence counter-clockwise.

<u>Substitutions</u>: Jutting chin out, movement should be slow and controlled

<u>Parameters</u>: Repeat 5 to 10 times, perform 1 to 3 sets, 1 time per day or every other day

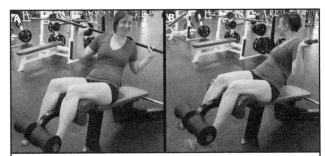

4.03.51 STRENGTHEN: ABDOMINAL, INCLINE BAR TWIST (ADVANCED)

POSITION: Incline bench seated backward

TARGETS: Decrease lumbar lordosis, facilitate and strengthen pelvic floor and abdominals, gain hip control

INSTRUCTION: Patient seated backward on incline bench with ankles locked under roller. Patient leans back to a position of hip flexion at 90 degrees while holding bar behind shoulders. Patient twists from left to right, pausing at end rotation for a 1- to 2-count (A and B). This can also be done on a straight bench by simply leaning forward at the hips, bringing chest toward opposite knee.

SUBSTITUTIONS: Jutting chin out, movement should be slow and controlled

PARAMETERS: Repeat as many repetitions as patient can manage, perform 1 to 3 sets, 1 time per day or every other day

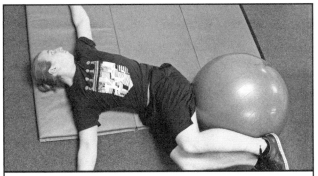

4.03.53 STRENGTHEN: EXERCISE BALL, LOWER TRUNK ROTATION

POSITION: Supine 90/90 legs on ball

TARGETS: Beginner for strengthening lower trunk rotators (obliques), facilitating pelvic floor and TA

INSTRUCTION: Start with the back flat and hips and knees at 90 degrees of flexion (90/90) and calves placed on ball. Patient engages deep core muscles to stabilize neutral spine. Patient places arms out to the sides and rotates knees fully to the left, and then follows by going to the right. Abdominals remain engaged to avoid lumbar extension and knees should remain together. Movements should be slow. Shoulders should stay in contact with surface.

SUBSTITUTIONS: Arching lower back, holding breath

PARAMETERS: Repeat 5 to 10 times, perform 1 to 3 sets, 1 time per day or every other day

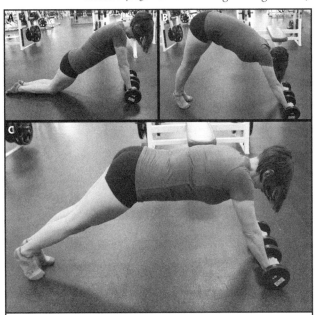

4.03.52 STRENGTHEN: ABDOMINAL, ROLL-UP WITH OLYMPIC BARBELL (ADVANCED)

POSITION: Tall-kneeling, standing

TARGETS: This is a very advanced abdominal exercise that will strengthen pelvic floor, abdominals, and latissimus dorsi primarily; use for the athletic patient only.

INSTRUCTION: Patient begins in tall-kneeling and bends down at hips to place hands on Olympic Barbell 5- to 10-lbs round plate weights on each side (A). Patient tightens core and rolls out to push-up position. Patient should keep a slight arch in the back and then lift hips to roll the barbell toward knee while exhaling. Arms should stay perpendicular to the floor throughout the movement or patient will work out shoulders and back more than the abdominals. For progression, patient begins in standing and bends down at hips to place hands on Olympic Barbell, tightens core, and rolls out to push-up position. Patient should keep a slight arch in the back and then lift hips to roll the barbell toward feet while exhaling. Arms should stay perpendicular to the floor throughout the movement or patient will work out shoulders and back more than the abdominals (B and C).

SUBSTITUTIONS: Jutting chin out, movement should be slow and controlled

PARAMETERS: Repeat 5 to 10 times, perform 1 to 3 sets, 1 time per day or every other day

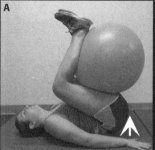
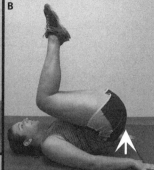
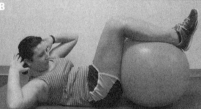

4.03.54 Strengthen: Exercise Ball, Abdominal and Lumbar, Double Knee to Chest/Reverse Crunch

Position: Supine 90/90 legs on ball

Targets: Strengthening RA, iliopsoas and hamstrings, facilitates pelvic floor and TA

Instruction: *Reverse crunch DKTC with ball*: Start with the back flat and hips and knees at 90 degrees of flexion (90/90), arms place by sides, and calves placed on ball. Patient engages deep core muscles to stabilize neutral spine in PPT. Patient squeezes ball between calves and buttocks and then lifts ball, bringing knees to chest. Squeeze abdominals at end range and return to start (A). Shoulders should stay in contact with surface. *Reverse crunch without ball*: Patient lies supine with hips flexed 90 degrees, knees flexed 90 degrees and ankle crossed, patient's hands palms down by the sides. Patient contracts the abdominals and curls lower trunk, lifting knees upward so that lower back and hips are just barely lifted off the floor. Slowly lower until lower back grazes the floor and repeat (B). This can also be done with knees extended for an extra challenge (C).

Substitutions: Arching lower back, holding breath

Parameters: Repeat 5 to 10 times, perform 1 to 3 sets, 1 time per day or every other day

---

Where's the Evidence?

Willett, Hyde, Uhrlaub, Wendel, and Karst (2001) evaluated EMG activity of the upper and lower RA and the external oblique muscles during five commonly performed abdominal strengthening exercises. Twenty-five healthy subjects participated in the study. The reverse curl resulted in the greatest amount of lower rectus activity; the V-sit and reverse curl exercises resulted in the greatest amount of external oblique activity; and the trunk curl, reverse curl, trunk curl with a twist, and V-sit all resulted in similar amounts of upper rectus EMG activity. They concluded abdominal strengthening exercises can differentially activate various abdominal muscle groups, but contradicted some traditionally held assumptions regarding the effects of specific exercises.

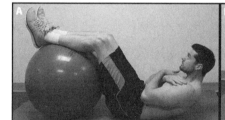
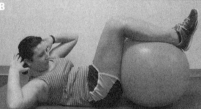
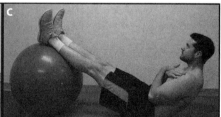

4.03.55 Strengthen: Exercise Ball, Abdominal, Crunch, Legs on Ball

Position: Supine 90/90 legs on ball

Targets: This will strengthen the trunk flexors: RA, internal and external obliques, and TA.

Instruction: Start with the back flat and hips and knees at 90 degrees of flexion (90/90), calves placed on ball. Arms may be placed at various positions, easiest to most difficult: down by sides, stacked reaching between knees, cross over chest, reaching toward ceiling, and fingertips to ears with shoulders externally rotated. Patient will crunch up by rounding spine into a C-curve and bringing scapula up off the table while keeping eyes directed toward the ceiling and chin tucked (A). Diagonal movement may be added to target obliques. Patient rotates to one side while crunching, bringing sternum toward opposite knee (B). This can also be done with knees extended and ankles/lower calves on ball (C).

Substitutions: Lack of rounding through spine; substituting with hip flexors, fast movement using momentum, holding breath, jutting chin out, pulling on head.

Parameters: 10 times each up to 3 sets, 1 time per day or every other day

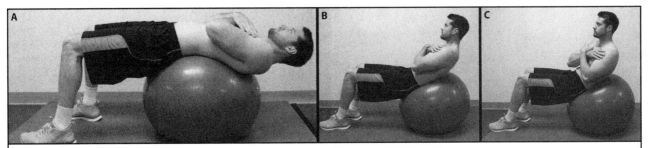

4.03.56 STRENGTHEN: EXERCISE BALL, ABDOMINAL, CRUNCH, TABLE TOP

POSITION: Table top on a ball

TARGETS: This will strengthen the trunk flexors: RA, internal and external obliques, and TA while also isometrically working hip adductors, gluteals, and hamstrings; ball helps to cushion and support the lumbar spine.

INSTRUCTION: Start seated on ball and roll out to table top (also called *reverse bridge*) with ball under lumbar spine. Arms may be placed at various positions, easiest to most difficult: down by sides, stacked reaching between knees, cross over chest, reaching toward ceiling, and fingertips to ears with shoulders externally rotated. Patient will crunch up by rounding spine into a C-curve and maintaining 90 degrees of flexion at the knees (A). Adding a small ball between the knee, and having patient squeeze during exercise can help facilitate hip adductors and keep knees aligned with hips. Keep eyes directed toward the ceiling and chin tucked (B). Diagonal movement may be added to target obliques. Patient rotates to one side while crunching bringing sternum toward opposite knee (C).

SUBSTITUTIONS: Lack of rounding through spine; substituting with hip flexors, fast movement using momentum, holding breath, jutting chin out, pulling on head.

PARAMETERS: 10 times each up to 3 sets, 1 time per day or every other day

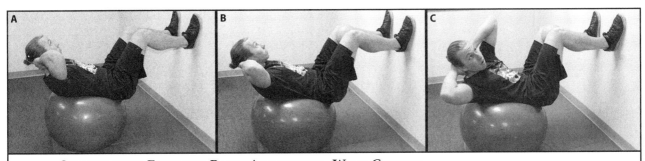

4.03.57 STRENGTHEN: EXERCISE BALL, ABDOMINAL, WALL CRUNCH

POSITION: Supine on ball, feet on wall 90/90

TARGETS: This will strengthen the trunk flexors: RA, internal and external obliques, and TA; ball helps to cushion and support the lumbar spine

INSTRUCTION: Start seated on ball facing a wall approximately 2 feet away. Bringing feet up onto wall, patient rolls out so that ball is positioned under the lumbar spine and legs are in 90/90 position. Arms may be placed at various positions, easiest to most difficult: down by sides, stacked reaching between knees, cross over chest, reaching toward ceiling, and fingertips to ears with shoulders externally rotated. Patient will crunch up by rounding spine into a C-curve and maintaining 90 degrees of flexion at the hips and knees (A). Adding a small ball between the knees and having patient squeeze during exercise can help facilitate hip adductors and keep knees aligned with hips. Keep eyes directed toward the ceiling and chin tucked (B). Diagonal movement may be added to target obliques. Patient rotates to one side while crunching, bringing sternum toward opposite knee (C).

SUBSTITUTIONS: Lack of rounding through spine; substituting with hip flexors, fast movement using momentum, holding breath, jutting chin out, pulling on head.

PARAMETERS: 10 times each up to 3 sets, 1 time per day or every other day

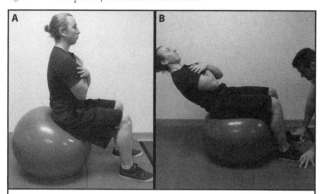

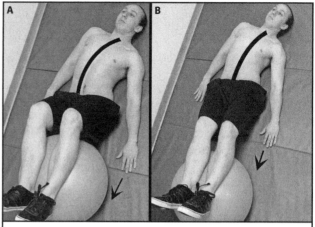

4.03.58 STRENGTHEN: EXERCISE BALL, ABDOMINAL, LEAN-BACKS

POSITION: Seated on ball

TARGETS: Decrease lumbar lordosis, facilitate and strengthen pelvic floor and abdominals

INSTRUCTION: Patient seated backward with feet planted on floor in 90/90 position, legs and arms crossed over chest. Patient leans back while maintaining a rounded spine or C-curve as far as patient can and holds. Return to start by crunching up (A and B).

SUBSTITUTIONS: Jutting chin out, movement should be slow and controlled

PARAMETERS: Hold leaned-back position up to 15 seconds, perform 5 to 10 repetitions, 1 to 3 sets, 1 time per day or every other day

4.03.59 STRENGTHEN: EXERCISE BALL, ABDOMINAL, OBLIQUES, SIDE-REACH

POSITION: Supine legs on ball in 90/90 or knees extended

TARGETS: Strengthens obliques, facilitates pelvic floor and TA

INSTRUCTION: Start with the back flat and hips and knees at 90 degrees of flexion (90/90), arms placed by sides, and calves placed on ball. Patient engages deep core muscles to stabilize neutral spine in PPT. Patient laterally flexes lumbar region to reach hand past ipsilateral hip. Return to start and repeat to other side (A). This can be done with knees extended and ankle on ball (B). Head stays in line with sternum, chin slightly tucked and gaze toward ceiling. Shoulders and entire arm stay in contact with surface.

SUBSTITUTIONS: Arching lower back, holding breath

PARAMETERS: Repeat 5 to 10 times, perform 1 to 3 sets, 1 time per day or every other day

4.03.60 STRENGTHEN: EXERCISE BALL, ABDOMINAL, JACK KNIFE, 4-WAY

POSITION: Prone plank on ball, knees on ball

TARGETS: Strengthens RA, obliques, and latissimus dorsi; facilitates pelvic floor and TA

INSTRUCTION: *Knee flexion*: Start with hands directly below shoulders and extended knees on ball. Crunch abdominals into hip flexion and knee flexion with shins on ball. Shoulders stay flexed 90 degrees (A and B). *Knee flexion: Hip lift*: Crunch abdominals into hip flexion and knee flexion while lifting hips toward ceiling. Shoulders flex further to approximately 110 degrees (C). *Knee extend: Hip lift "pike"*: Crunch abdominals, bringing hips into flexion while keeping knees extended and lifting hips toward ceiling until toes are on ball. Shoulders flex further to approximately 130 degrees (D). *To handstand*: Continue to crunch from *Knees extend: Hip lift "pike"* to a full handstand, shoulders flexed 180 degrees. Patient to push away from the floor, creating shoulder depression to protect the neck and shoulders (E).

SUBSTITUTIONS: Arching lower back, holding breath, head stays in line with sternum, chin slightly tucked and gaze toward floor between hands; cup hands to protect wrists.

PARAMETERS: Repeat 5 to 10 times, perform 1 to 3 sets, 1 time per day or every other day

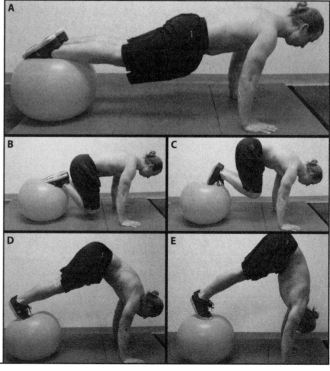

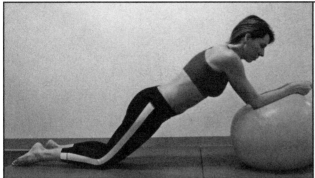

4.03.61 STRENGTHEN: EXERCISE BALL, ABDOMINAL, ROLL-OUT

POSITION: Tall-kneeling

TARGETS: Strengthens RA, obliques, and latissimus dorsi; facilitates pelvic floor and TA

INSTRUCTION: With ball approximately 12 inches in front of knees, patient places clasped hands on ball and braces abdominals. Patient rolls ball away until ball is under forearms, shifting weight into UEs and holding spine neutral.

SUBSTITUTIONS: Arching lower back, holding breath, shrugging shoulders

PARAMETERS: Hold 5 to 15 seconds, repeat 5 to 10 times, perform 1 to 3 sets, 1 time per day or every other day

Where's the Evidence?

Escamilla et al. (2010) found that EMG signals during the roll-out and pike exercises for the RA, external oblique, and internal oblique were significantly greater compared to other exercise ball activities (knee up, skiier, hip extension right, hip extension left, decline push up, and sitting march) and two traditional abdominal exercises (crunch and bent-knee sit-up). latissimus dorsi EMG signals were greatest in the pike, knee up, skiier, hip extension right and left, and decline push up. They determined the roll-out and pike were the most effective exercises in activating upper and lower RA, external and internal obliques, and latissimus dorsi muscles while minimizing lumbar paraspinals and rectus femoris activity.

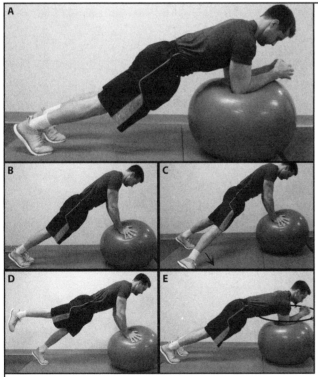

4.03.62 STRENGTHEN: EXERCISE BALL, ABDOMINAL, PLANK AND VARIATIONS, UPPER EXTREMITY

POSITION: Tall-kneeling

TARGETS: Strengthens RA and obliques, facilitates pelvic floor and TA

INSTRUCTION: *Elbows on ball*: With ball approximately 12 inches in front of knees, patient places clasped forearms on ball and rests elbows on ball. Patient braces abdominals and raises knees, while on toes, into a push up position with neutral spine. Hold, return to start, and repeat (A). *Hands on ball*: Start in same position, patient places hands on ball, braces abdominals, and raises knees, while on toes, into a push-up position with neutral spine. Hold, return to start, and repeat (B). *Tap outs*: Lift one leg slightly off floor and abduct hip to tap the floor. Do not allow dipping, lower back to sag. Return to start and repeat to other side (C). *Alternating leg lift*: Lift one leg and return, repeat to other side. Do not allow lower back to extend or body to roll side-to-side (D). *Stir the pot*: Widen foot stance and repeat instructions for *Elbows on ball*, hold lower abdominal region tight and swirl elbows around in a circle clockwise. Perform full set and then repeat counter-clockwise (E).

SUBSTITUTIONS: Arching lower back, sagging hips, holding breath, shrugging shoulders on ball

PARAMETERS: *Elbows on ball* and *hands on balk*: Hold 5 to 30 seconds, repeat 5 to 10 times, perform 1 to 3 sets; *Tap outs, leg lifts,* and *stir the pot*: Repeat 5 to 10 repetitions, perform 1 to 3 sets, 1 time per day or every other day

Where's the Evidence?

Snarr and Esco (2014) investigated EMG activity of the RA, external abdominal oblique, and erector spinae while performing planks with and without multiple instability devices. Twelve healthy men and women volunteered to participate in this study. All participants performed two isometric contractions of five different plank variations, with or without an instability device. Results indicated that planks performed with the instability devices increased EMG activity in the superficial musculature when compared with traditional stable planks. Therefore, a traditional plank performed on an unstable device may be considered an advanced variation and appropriate for use when a greater challenge is warranted.

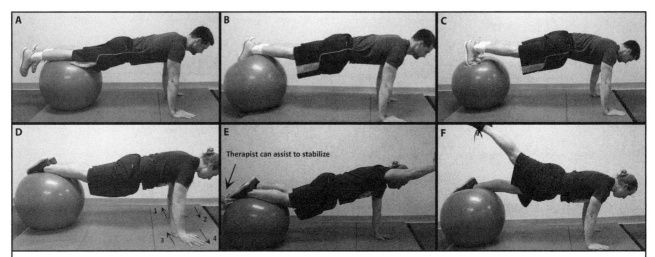

4.03.63 STRENGTHEN: EXERCISE BALL, ABDOMINAL, PLANK AND VARIATIONS, LOWER EXTREMITY

POSITION: Quadruped

TARGETS: Strengthens RA, obliques, and latissimus dorsi; facilitates pelvic floor and TA.

INSTRUCTION: Start with body lying in quadruped over the ball. Knees are extended and feet on floor hip-width apart. Hands are on the floor in front of the patient. *Knees on ball*: Patient braces abdominals and walks hands out, rolling ball to just below the knees. Instruct patient to lengthen legs, pushing heels toward the back of the room. Hands are directly under the shoulders. Continue to hold while pulling abdominals away from the floor. Return to start and repeat (A). *Ankles/feet on ball*: Repeat instructions for *Knees on ball*, except the patient will walk out to ball positioned under the ankles (B) and may even go as far as feet with toes pressing into ball (C). *Tap outs*: Lift one hand slightly off floor and horizontally abduct shoulder to tap the floor. Do not allow dipping, lower back to sag. Return to start and repeat to other side (D). *Alternating shoulder flexion*: Lift one arm into shoulder flexion and return, repeat to other side. Do not allow lower back to extend or body to roll to the side to (E). *Alternating leg lift*: Lift one leg and return, repeat to other side. Do not allow lower back to extend or body to roll to the side to (F).

SUBSTITUTIONS: Arching lower back, sagging hips, holding breath, shrugging shoulders

PARAMETERS: *Knees/ankles on ball plank*: Hold 5 to 30 seconds, repeat 5 to 10 times, perform 1 to 3 sets; *Tap outs, shoulder flexion,* and *leg lift*: Repeat 5 to 10 repetitions, perform 1 to 3 sets, 1 time per day or every other day

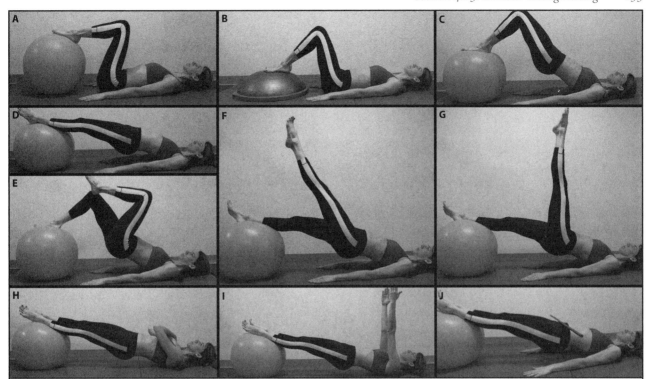

4.03.64 STRENGTHEN: EXERCISE BALL, ABDOMINAL, BRIDGE AND VARIATIONS

POSITION: Supine

TARGETS: Strengthens gluteus maximus, hamstrings, and erector spinae; facilitates pelvic floor and TA.

INSTRUCTION: Start in supine with knees and hips flexed and feet on ball (A), hands are by their sides on the floor. Beginners may start with Bosu ball, which provides gradually transition from stable to unstable surfaces (B). *Feet on ball knees flexed*: Patient braces abdominals and lifts hips up. Continue to hold while maintaining neutral spine and pelvis. Return to start and repeat (C). *Ankles on ball knees extended*: Patient braces abdominals and lifts hips up. Continue to hold while maintaining neutral spine and pelvis. Return to start and repeat (D). *Marching*: This can be done with the *knees flexed* or *knee extended* starting positions. Lift one leg slightly off ball, flexing hip and knee toward ipsilateral shoulder. Do not allow dipping, lower back to sag. Pelvis remains level. Return to start and repeat to other side (E). *Alternating leg lift*: Lift one leg 6 inches off ball, keeping knee fully extended. Pelvis remains level. Return to start and repeat to other side (F). *Alternating leg lift to 90 degrees*: Lift one leg with fully extended knee to heel pointing toward ceiling so that leg is perpendicular to the floor. Pelvis remains level. Return and repeat to other side (G). *Add arms*: With above positions, arms may be added for more intensity. Progression with arms to across chest is a starting progression and then bring shoulder to 90 degrees of flexion, reaching toward ceiling with fingertips and keeping hands shoulder-width apart (H and I). A broomstick may be used sitting just below the ASIS to give the patient increased visual feedback on dropping hips (J).

SUBSTITUTIONS: Arching lower back, sagging hips, holding breath, shrugging shoulders, lifting head

PARAMETERS: *Bridge hold*: Hold 5 to 30 seconds, repeat 5 to 10 times, perform 1 to 3 sets; *Leg movements*: Repeat 5 to 10 repetitions, repeated 1 to 3 sets, 1 time per day or every other day

Where's the Evidence?

Cho and Jeon (2013) examined the effects of an abdominal drawing-in bridge exercise on trunk and abdominal muscles and lumbar stability. Thirty healthy young adults took part in this study. The subjects performed bridge exercises using an abdominal drawing-in method on a stable base and unstable base, and changes in their abdominal muscle thickness on the stable and unstable bases and lumbar stability were evaluated. After the intervention, the stable and unstable bridge exercise groups showed a statistically significant increase in muscle thickness in the transversus abdominis. Additionally, the unstable bridge exercise group showed significantly increased muscle thicknesses of the internal obliques in static and dynamic lumbar stability. The authors concluded that lumbar stability exercise, with the compensation of the lumbar spine minimized, using an abdominal drawing-in method on an unstable support of base is effective in increasing muscle strength and spinal stability.

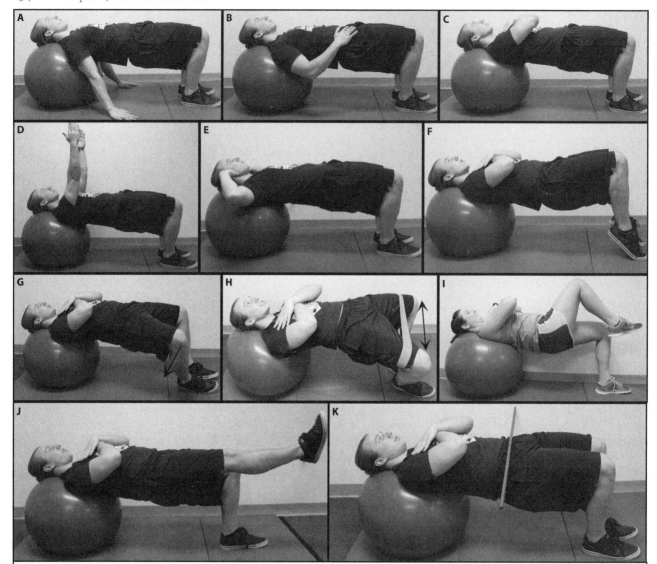

4.03.65 STRENGTHEN: EXERCISE BALL, ABDOMINAL AND LUMBAR, REVERSE BRIDGE AND VARIATIONS

<u>POSITION</u>: Table top on ball

<u>TARGETS</u>: Strengthens gluteus maximus, hamstrings, and erector spinae; facilitates pelvic floor and TA.

<u>INSTRUCTION</u>: Start sitting on ball and roll out to table top (also called reverse bridge) with ball under shoulders and neck. Arms may be placed on the floor to assist with balance (A) and then moved to the hips (B) and then crossed over chest (C) to fingertips reaching toward ceiling (D) to fingertips to ears (E). *Heel raises*: Plantarflex one ankle, lifting heel off ground. Repeat to other side. Progress to bilateral heel raise (F). *Hip abduction/adduction*: Bring knees apart, hold, and bring back together. Repeat to other side (G). Add *resistance band* to further target gluteus medius and minimus with TFL assistance. Loop resistance band around the distal thigh, bring knees apart, hold, and bring back together (H). *Marching*: Lift one foot slightly off floor, flexing hip. Do not allow dipping, lower back to sag. Pelvis remains level. Return to start and repeat to other side (I). *Alternating knee extension*: Lift one foot slightly off floor while extending knee. Keep thighs level with each other. Do not allow dipping, lower back to sag. Pelvis remains level. Return to start and repeat to other side (J). Lift one foot slightly off floor, flexing hip. Do not allow dipping, lower back to sag. Pelvis remains level. Return to start and repeat to other side. A broomstick may be used sitting just below the ASIS to give the patient increased visual feedback on dropping hips (K).

<u>SUBSTITUTIONS</u>: Arching lower back, sagging hips, holding breath, shrugging shoulders, lifting head

<u>PARAMETERS</u>: 10 times each up to 3 sets, 1 time per day or every other day

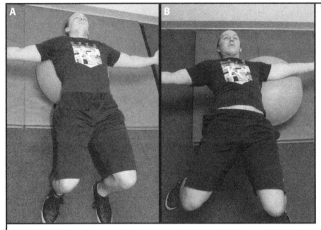

4.03.66 STRENGTHEN: EXERCISE BALL, ABDOMINAL AND LUMBAR, T-BRIDGE FALL-OFF, SIDE-WALKS

POSITION: Seated

TARGETS: Strengthens RA, obliques, gluteus maximus, and hamstrings; facilitates pelvic floor and TA.

INSTRUCTION: Roll out on ball to reverse bridge/table top, seating ball at a level to support the neck and shoulders. Patient creates a strong "table" by tightening from the core and hip extensors. Roll from side-to-side using legs to move the ball to the point where the patient is about to fall off the ball. Close guarding is needed here for safety. Spine should not rotate. Torso and hips remain straight (A and B).

SUBSTITUTIONS: Arching lower back, sagging hips, holding breath, shrugging shoulders, torso rotation

PARAMETERS: Repeat 5 to 10 alternating to each side, repeated 1 to 3 sets, 1 time per day or every other day

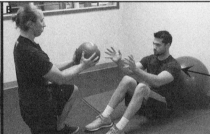

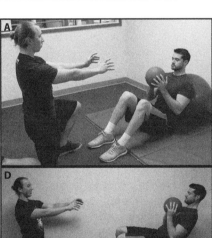

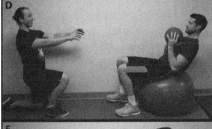

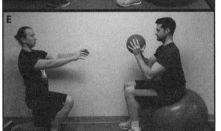

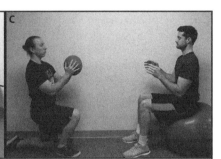

4.03.67 STRENGTHEN: EXERCISE BALL, ABDOMINAL AND LUMBAR, SIT-UPS, BALL THROW

POSITION: Seated

TARGETS: This will strengthen the trunk flexors: RA, internal and external obliques, and TA.

INSTRUCTION: *Beginner:* Start seated on floor with ball behind back and knees in hook-lying position. Patient leans slightly backward followed by crunching up and rounding spine while making a chest pass forward with the medicine ball. Therapist, standing in front, catches ball and returns pass to patient, who brings ball into chest while leaning back to slow the ball down. The exercise ball assists with both motions and is a good place to start this exercise. Repeat entire sequence (A and B). *Advanced:* Start seated on ball and roll out with ball under lumbosacral region, slightly round spine, and medicine ball in hands. Knees should be flexed 90 degrees and feet hip-width apart and flat on floor. Patient leans slightly backward, followed by crunching up and rounding spine while making a chest pass forward with the medicine ball. Therapist, standing in front, catches ball and returns pass to patient, who brings ball into chest while leaning back to slow the ball down. Repeat entire sequence (C through E).

SUBSTITUTIONS: Lack of rounding through spine; substituting with hip flexors, fast movement using momentum, holding breath, jutting chin out.

PARAMETERS: 10 times each up to 3 sets, 1 time per day or every other day

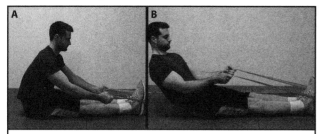

4.03.68 STRENGTHEN: RESISTANCE BAND, LUMBAR EXTENSION

POSITION: Long-sitting

TARGETS: This will strengthen the lumbar erector spinae group

INSTRUCTION: Sitting on floor with knees straight and one end of resistance band looped around the feet, patient grasps the other end of the loop at chest level. With back straight and upright, lean backward away from feet. Do not arch back. Hold and slowly return (A and B).

SUBSTITUTIONS: Lack of rounding through spine; substituting with hip flexors, fast movement using momentum, holding breath, jutting chin out.

PARAMETERS: 10 times each up to 3 sets, 1 time per day or every other day

Where's the Evidence?

Sundstrup, Jakobsen, Andersen, Jay, and Andersen (2012) compared muscle activation as measured by EMG of global core and thigh muscles during abdominal crunches performed on a Swiss ball with elastic resistance or on an isotonic training machine when normalized for training intensity. Forty-two untrained individuals aged 28 to 67 years participated in the study. EMG activity was measured in 13 muscles during 3 repetitions with a 10 RM load during both abdominal crunches on a training ball with elastic resistance and in the same movement utilizing a training machine. When comparing between muscles, normalized EMG was highest in the RA and external obliques. However, crunches on the Swiss ball with elastic resistance showed higher activity of the RA than crunches performed on the machine. By contrast, crunches performed on the Swiss ball induced lower activity of the rectus femoris than crunches in the training machine. The authors concluded crunches on a Swiss ball with added elastic resistance induces high RA activity accompanied by low hip flexor activity, which could be beneficial for individuals with LBP. In opposition, the lower RA activity and higher rectus femoris activity observed in the machine warrant caution for individuals with lumbar pain.

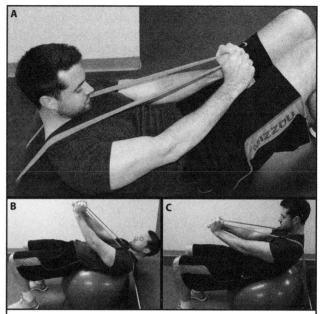

4.03.69 STRENGTHEN: RESISTANCE BAND, ABDOMINAL CRUNCH, FORWARD AND DIAGONAL

POSITION: Hook-lying, seated on exercise ball

TARGETS: This will strengthen the trunk flexors: RA, internal and external obliques (targeted more with diagonal) and TA.

INSTRUCTION: *Forward*: Securely attach the ends of the band to a stationary object near the floor behind patient. Patient extends arms in front and grasps the middle of the loop with hands close together. Keeping elbows straight in front, patient curls trunk upward, lifting shoulder blades from floor. Hold and slowly return. Make sure patient keeps elbows straight and lifts shoulder blades off floor (A). *Diagonal*: Patient holds resistance band in one hand and repeats instructions for forward crunch, bringing chest toward opposite knee. Repeat, alternating to other side. *On exercise ball*: Patient sits on ball then walks feet away while simultaneously going down into a lying position, allowing the ball to stop at the lumbar spine area of the lower back. Feet are 2 feet apart with knees flexed 90 degrees and hands at shoulder level grasping the resistance band. Patient then curls the head, neck, and shoulders up and toward the pelvis region, slowly performing a crunch and then slowly returning to start (B and C).

SUBSTITUTIONS: Lack of rounding through spine; substituting with hip flexors, fast movement using momentum, holding breath, jutting chin out.

PARAMETERS: 10 times each up to 3 sets, 1 time per day or every other day

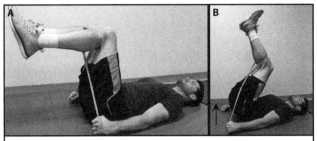

4.03.70 Strengthen: Resistance Band, Abdominal Crunch (Lower Abdominals)

Position: Hook-lying

Targets: This will strengthen the trunk flexors, targeting obliques and TA

Instruction: On back with hips and knees flexed, stretch the band over knees and cross underneath. Secure each end of the band in patient's hands with elbows extended by side. Lift knees upward, lifting hips off the floor. Slowly return (A and B).

Substitutions: Lack of rounding through spine; substituting with hip flexors, fast movement using momentum, holding breath, jutting chin out.

Parameters: 10 times each up to 3 sets, 1 time per day or every other day

4.03.71 Strengthen: Resistance Band, Abdominal and Lumbar, Standing Twist and Derotation

Position: Standing

Targets: This will strengthen the trunk rotators: rotatores and obliques.

Instruction: Securely attach the ends of the band to a stationary object to one side of the patient at elbow height. Patient squats down to flexing at hips and knees about 30 to 45 degrees. Patient grasps the middle of the loop with hands close together and elbows at 90 degrees, shoulders neutral and scapula retracted and depressed. Feet are spaced hip-width apart and there is a slight bend in the knees and hips (mini-squat). Patient walks out until resistance is felt in band. This can be the exercise for beginners as it is an isometric stabilization of the trunk (A). To progress, the patient steps further away, allowing the band to rotate the patient toward the band's anchor. Patient then rotates trunk away from anchor to opposite side while maintaining a forward-facing pelvis. Do not allow twisting through hips or knee and elbows stay tucked into sides. Hold and slowly return (B). A more advanced version involves patient with shoulders at 90 degrees and elbows straight, holding band centered in front of midline of body and not allowing trunk to twist for walk-out isometrics (C). Patient can also then rotate trunk away for isotonic trunk rotation (D).

Substitutions: Twisting through hips and knees, pulling with arms, trunk stays upright, knees stay aligned over second toes, lower abdominal engaged to maintain neutral spine

Parameters: 10 times each up to 3 sets, 1 time per day or every other day

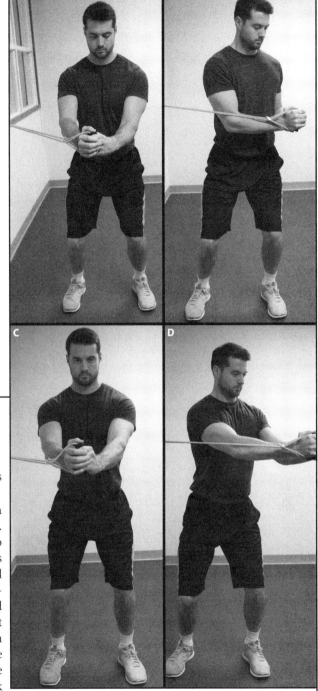

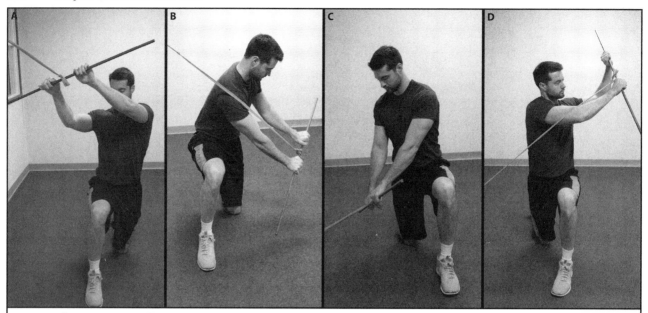

4.03.72 STRENGTHEN: RESISTANCE BAND, TRUNK TWIST, CHOP AND LIFT

<u>POSITION</u>: Standing, half-kneeling, tall-kneeling

<u>TARGETS</u>: Chop will strengthen semispinalis, rotatores, multifidus and obliques, and RA; lift will target semispinalis, rotatores, multifidus, and erector spinae.

<u>INSTRUCTION</u>: *Chop*: Securely attach the ends of the band to a stationary object above the head to one side or in the top of a doorway. Patient grasps the loose end with hands close together and elbows extended above the head and to one side. Walk away from anchor until the patient begins to feel resistance. Feet are spaced hip-width apart and there is a slight bend in knees and hip (mini-squat). Using the trunk movement, the patient pulls the resistance band forward and down toward outside of opposite hip in a motion like chopping wood. Gaze follows hands. Return to start and repeat (A and B). *Lift*: Securely attach the ends of the band to a stationary object below the knee to one side or in the bottom of a doorway. Patient grasps the loose end with hands close together and elbows flexed as patient bends forward at the trunk and rotates toward the anchor side. Walk away from anchor until the patient begins to feel resistance. Feet are spaced hip-width apart and there is a slight bend in knees and hip (mini-squat). Using the trunk movement, the patient pulls the resistance band back and up toward the outside of opposite shoulder in a motion like lifting an axe before chopping wood. Gaze follows hands. Return to start and repeat (C and D).

<u>SUBSTITUTIONS</u>: Twisting through hips and knees, pulling with arms only, shrugging shoulders, jutting chin out

<u>PARAMETERS</u>: 10 times each up to 3 sets, 1 time per day or every other day

Where's the Evidence?

Combining the PNF chop and lift patterns with the half-kneeling and tall-kneeling postures will help bridge the gap between low-level patterns and postures (rolling, crawling, creeping) and high-level, functional patterns and postures (squatting, lunging, stepping, pushing, pulling). The patterns require and promote instantaneous local muscular activity as they tap into early developmental reflex movement and balance reactions. The therapeutic use of both PNF and developmental patterns has been a hallmark of rehabilitation of patients with neurologic dysfunction, but can be equally and effectively applied in the sports and orthopedic rehabilitation setting (Voight, Hoogenboom, & Cook, 2008).

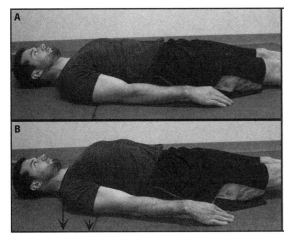

4.03.73 STRENGTHEN: ISOMETRIC, SUPINE LUMBAR EXTENSION

POSITION: Supine

TARGETS: Lumbar extensor strengthening; targets multifidus and erector spinae.

INSTRUCTION: Patient lying supine with legs extended, toes pointed down toward ceiling, hands by sides, presses posterior shoulders into the bed while isometrically contracting the lumbar extensors (A and B).

SUBSTITUTIONS: Therapist may place hand under the lower back to palpate for good contraction and ensure patient is performing correctly.

PARAMETERS: 10 to 20 repetitions up to 3 sets, 1 time per day or every other day (higher repetitions builds endurance)

Where's the Evidence?

Balogun, Olokungbemi, and Kuforiji (1992) compared the effectiveness of spine lumbar extension exercise and prone lumbar extension exercise on spinal mobility and muscular strength. Thirty-four healthy men, average age 23, were randomly assigned to three groups: subjects using spine lumbar extension protocol, subjects using prone lumbar extension protocol, and a control group. The exercise programs were standardized and administered 3 times per week for 6 weeks. The spinal ROM and back extension isometric force of all the subjects was evaluated before training, at the end of the third and sixth weeks of the study, and 9 weeks after the end of the exercise training. Significant progressive increases in spinal ROM and isometric force after the exercise training were noted at the end of the sixth week of training. Improvement in muscular strength was sustained 9 weeks after the end of physical training. The study concluded that both methods were effective at improving ROM and strength of the lumbar spine and further stated the spine lumbar extension method was better for improving the spinal ROM, whereas the prone lumbar extension method was more effective in strengthening of the back.

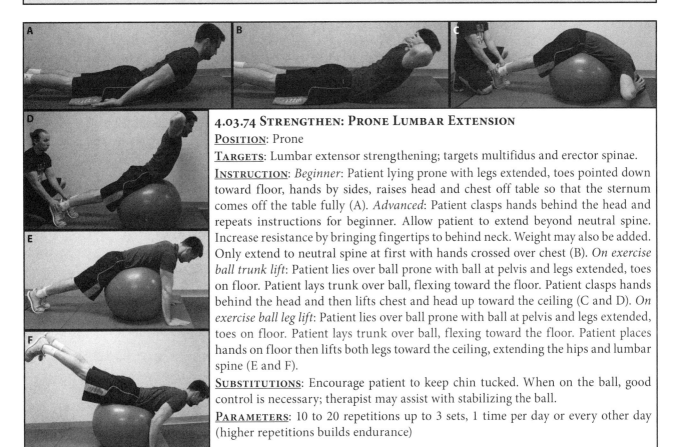

4.03.74 STRENGTHEN: PRONE LUMBAR EXTENSION

POSITION: Prone

TARGETS: Lumbar extensor strengthening; targets multifidus and erector spinae.

INSTRUCTION: *Beginner*: Patient lying prone with legs extended, toes pointed down toward floor, hands by sides, raises head and chest off table so that the sternum comes off the table fully (A). *Advanced*: Patient clasps hands behind the head and repeats instructions for beginner. Allow patient to extend beyond neutral spine. Increase resistance by bringing fingertips to behind neck. Weight may also be added. Only extend to neutral spine at first with hands crossed over chest (B). *On exercise ball trunk lift*: Patient lies over ball prone with ball at pelvis and legs extended, toes on floor. Patient lays trunk over ball, flexing toward the floor. Patient clasps hands behind the head and then lifts chest and head up toward the ceiling (C and D). *On exercise ball leg lift*: Patient lies over ball prone with ball at pelvis and legs extended, toes on floor. Patient lays trunk over ball, flexing toward the floor. Patient places hands on floor then lifts both legs toward the ceiling, extending the hips and lumbar spine (E and F).

SUBSTITUTIONS: Encourage patient to keep chin tucked. When on the ball, good control is necessary; therapist may assist with stabilizing the ball.

PARAMETERS: 10 to 20 repetitions up to 3 sets, 1 time per day or every other day (higher repetitions builds endurance)

Where's the Evidence?

Yaprak (2013) studied the effects of a 10-week dynamic back extension training program on back muscle strength, back muscle endurance, and spinal ROM for healthy young females. Seventy-three young females, average age 19, volunteered for the study and were divided into two groups. The exercise group performed the dynamic back extension exercise 3 days per week for 10 weeks (similar to the advanced prone extension lift). The control group did not participate in any type of exercise. Findings showed that there were significant differences between pre-training and post-training values for back muscle strength and spinal ROM in the exercise group. The control group did not show any significant changes when compared with the pre-training values. The results demonstrate that the 10-week dynamic strength training program was effective for spinal extension ROM and back muscle strength.

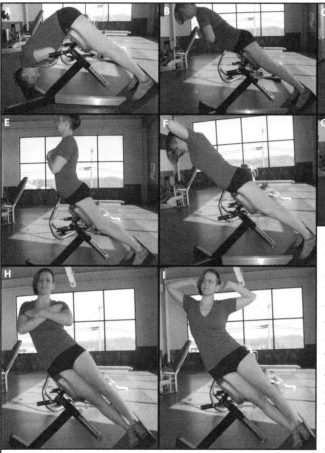

4.03.75 STRENGTHEN: LUMBAR, ROMAN CHAIR AND VARIATIONS

POSITION: Prone

TARGETS: *Extension*: This is an advanced exercise for lumbar and hip extensor strengthening; targets multifidus, erector spinae, gluteus maximus, and hamstrings. *Modification of hip rotation*: Adding slight internal rotation of the hips in positioning will increase the percent of recruitment in the lumbar extensors compared to hip extensors (Mayer, Verna, Manini, Mooney, & Graves, 2002). *Lateral flexion*: Strengthening of lateral flexors: obliques, unilateral erector spinae, quadratus lumborum.

INSTRUCTION: Adjust the bench to a 45-degree angle; patient climbs into device while facing the floor. Lower calves or heels are under a roller pad (or plate as shown), feet flat on foot plate, and pelvic pad just under ASIS. Patient rests pelvis on the pads and allows trunk to relax toward the floor while crossing arms over chest. There are handles to the side to allow patient to use hands to assist for lowering and raising if needed. Patient uses lower back and gluteal muscles to extend the hips and lumbar spine as patient raises the trunk up toward the ceiling. *Beginner*: Only extend to neutral spine at first with hands crossed over chest (A and B). *Hip hinge with dowel*: Adding the use of a long dowel rod to encourage hip hinging can be done by placing the dowel along the posterior spine and encouraging the patient to keep sacrum and thoracic spine in contact with the rod during the trunk lift movement (C and D). *Advanced*: Allow patient to extend beyond neutral spine. Increase resistance by bringing fingertips to behind neck. Weight may also be added in advanced stages. Keep arms at the sides (beginner) or crossed behind the neck (advanced). Neck stays neutral with gaze toward floor in front of device at end range (E and F). *Lateral flexion/side crunch*: Patient positions feet laterally on foot plate so that both legs are under roller and feet are flat. Pelvic roller sits just under lateral iliac crest. Patient allows trunk to side bend to comfort level and follows by bringing trunk up toward ceiling into a side crunch. Arms are crossed over chest for beginner and fingertips behind neck for advanced. Weights may be added to increase intensity (H and I).

SUBSTITUTIONS: Neck hyperextension at end range, lack of hip extension with lumbar extension, bending forward at hips with lateral flexion, pulling on neck

PARAMETERS: 10 times each up to 3 sets, 1 time per day or every other day

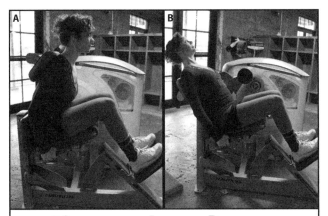

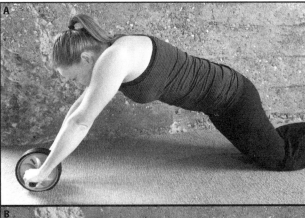

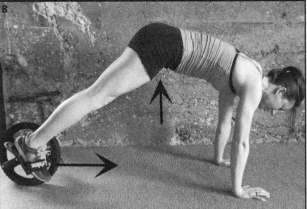

4.03.76 STRENGTHEN: LUMBAR, BACK EXTENSION USING MACHINE

POSITION: Seated

TARGETS: This is an advanced exercise for lumbar and hip extensor strengthening; targets multifidus, erector spinae, gluteus maximus, and hamstrings.

INSTRUCTION: Adjust the bench so it is at a 90-degree angle at the hips with patient. Feet flat on foot plate and back against the back pad at mid-thoracic region. Instruct patient to activate lower abdominals to stabilize the pelvis, followed by pressing the torso backward while keeping the chest lifted (A and B). Pelvic stabilization with this exercise enhances the effectiveness in strengthening the important multifidus muscles and decreases the chance for injury. *Isometric variation*: Lock the weights so that the weights are set at the heaviest. Follow instructions above except when the patient pushes back, patient will be doing an isometric contraction grading the push slowly over 12 seconds to 75% maximal pushing; no movement should occur. Patient holds 6 to 10 seconds and slowly relaxes.

SUBSTITUTIONS: Neck hyperextension at end range, lack of hip extension with lumbar extension, bending forward at hips with lateral flexion, pulling on neck

PARAMETERS: 10 times each up to 3 sets, 1 time per day or every other day

4.03.77 STRENGTHEN: ABDOMINAL, POWER WHEEL

POSITION: Quadruped

TARGETS: Strengthens RA, obliques, and latissimus dorsi; facilitates pelvic floor and TA.

INSTRUCTION: *Roll-up*: *Knees on floor, hands on wheel*: Patient braces abdominals and rolls hands out, rolling wheel as far as possible with good control. Slowly return to start and repeat (A). *Knee-up: Hands on floor, feet on wheel, knees bent*: Patient places bottoms of feet on wheel handles with palms on floor and knees and hips flexed in toward stomach. Bracing the abdominals, the patient extends the hips and knees, rolling wheel as far as patient can with good control. Slowly return to start and repeat. *Pike: Hands on floor, feet on wheel, knees extended*: Patient places bottoms of feet on wheel handles with palms on floor and hips and knees extended. Bracing the abdominals, patient flexes hips, keeping knees straight as patient comes into a "V" position as far as possible with good control. Slowly return to start and repeat (B).

SUBSTITUTIONS: Arching lower back, sagging hips, holding breath, shrugging shoulders

PARAMETERS: Up to 10 repetitions, 3 sets, 1 time per day or every other day

Where's the Evidence?

San Juan et al. (2005) examined the effect of pelvic stabilization on the activity of the lumbar and hip extensor muscles during dynamic back extension exercise. Fifteen volunteers in good general health performed dynamic extension exercise in a seated upright position on a lumbar extension machine with and without pelvic stabilization. During exercise, surface EMG activity of the lumbar multifidus and biceps femoris was recorded. The activity of the multifidus was 51% greater during the stabilized condition, whereas there was no difference in the activity of the biceps femoris between conditions. This study demonstrates that pelvic stabilization enhances lumbar muscle recruitment during dynamic exercise on machines.

Where's the Evidence?

Escamilla et al. (2006) evaluated EMG activity with nontraditional abdominal exercises with devices such as abdominal straps, the Power Wheel (Lifeline), and the Ab Revolutionizer (Thane Direct, Inc) to test the effectiveness of traditional and nontraditional abdominal exercises in activating abdominal and extraneous musculature. Twenty-one men and women who were healthy and between 23 and 43 years of age were recruited. Upper and lower RA, internal oblique, and latissimus dorsimuscle EMG activity were highest for the Power Wheel (pike, knee-up, and roll-out), hanging knee-up with straps, and reverse crunch inclined 30 degrees. External oblique activity was highest for the Power Wheel (pike, knee-up, and roll-out) and hanging knee-up with straps. Rectus femoris muscle EMG activity was highest for the Power Wheel (pike and knee-up), reverse crunch inclined 30 degrees, and bent knee sit-up. Lumbar paraspinal muscle EMG activity was low and similar among exercises. They concluded the Power Wheel (pike, knee-up, and roll-out), hanging knee-up with straps, and reverse crunch inclined 30 degrees not only were the most effective exercises in activating abdominal musculature but also were the most effective in activating extraneous musculature. Caution, the relatively high rectus femoris muscle activity obtained with the Power Wheel may be problematic for some people with low back problems.

REFERENCES

Atkins, S. (2015). Electromyographic response of global abdominal stabilizers in response to stable- and unstable-base isometric exercise. *Journal of Strength and Conditioning Research, 29*(6), 1609-1615.

Balogun, J. A., Olokungbemi, A. A., & Kuforiji, A. R. (1992). Spinal mobility and muscular strength: Effects of supine- and prone-lying back extension exercise training. *Archives of physical medicine and rehabilitation, 73*(8), 745-751.

Chanthapetch, P., Kanlayanaphotporn, R., Gaogasigam, C., & Chiradejnant, A. (2009). Abdominal muscle activity during abdominal hollowing in four starting positions. *Manual Therapy, 14*(6), 642-646.

Cho, M., & Jeon, H. (2013). The effects of bridge exercise on an unstable base of support on lumbar stability and the thickness of the transversus abdominis. *Journal of Physical Therapy Science, 25*(6), 733-736.

Critchley, D. (2002). Instructing pelvic floor contraction facilitates transversus abdominis thickness increase during low-abdominal hollowing. *Physiotherapy Research International, 7*(2), 65-75.

Escamilla, R. F., Babb, E., DeWitt, R., Jew, P., Kelleher, P., Burnham, T., . . ., R. T. (2006). Electromyographic analysis of traditional and nontraditional abdominal exercises: Implications for rehabilitation and training. *Physical Therapy, 86*(5), 656-671.

Escamilla, R. F., Lewis, C., Bell, D., Bramblet, G., Daffron, J., Lambert, S., . . ., Andrews, J. R. (2010). Core muscle activation during Swiss ball and traditional abdominal exercises. *Journal of Orthopedic Sports Physical Therapy, 40*(5), 265-276.

Mayer, J. M., Verna, J. L., Manini, T. M., Mooney, V., & Graves, J. E. (2002). Electromyographic activity of the trunk extensor muscles: effect of varying hip position and lumbar posture during Roman chair exercise. *Archives of Physical Medicine and Rehabilitation, 83*(11), 1543-1546.

Moon, H. J., Choi, K. H., Kim, D. H., Kim, H. J., Cho, Y. K., Lee, K. H., . . ., Choi, Y. J. (2013). Effect of lumbar stabilization and dynamic lumbar strengthening exercises in patients with chronic low back pain. *Annals of Rehabilitation Medicine, 37*(1), 110-117.

San Juan, J. G., Yaggie, J. A., Levy, S. S., Mooney, V., Udermann, B. E., & Mayer, J. M. (2005). Effects of pelvic stabilization on lumbar muscle activity during dynamic exercise. *Journal of Strength & Conditioning Research, 19*(4), 903-907.

Shields, R. K., & Heiss, D. G. (1997). An electromyographic comparison of abdominal muscle synergies during curl and double straight leg lowering exercises with control of the pelvic position. *Spine, 22*(16), 1873-1879.

Snarr, R. L., & Esco, M. R. (2014). Electromyographical comparison of plank variations performed with and without instability devices. *Journal of Strength and Conditioning Research, 28*(11), 3298-3305.

Suehiro, T., Mizutani, M., Watanabe, S., Ishida, H., Kobara, K., & Osaka, H. (2014). Comparison of spine motion and trunk muscle activity between abdominal hollowing and abdominal bracing maneuvers during prone hip extension. *Journal of Bodywork and Movement Therapies, 18*(3), 482-488.

Sundstrup, E., Jakobsen, M. D., Andersen, C. H., Jay, K., & Andersen, L. L. (2012). Swiss ball abdominal crunch with added elastic resistance is an effective alternative to training machines. *International Journal of Sports Physical Therapy, 7*(4), 372-380.

Voight, M. L., Hoogenboom, B. J., & Cook, G. (2008). The chop and lift reconsidered: Integrating neuromuscular principles into orthopedic and sports rehabilitation. *North American Journal of Sports Physical Therapy, 3*(3), 151-159.

Willett, G. M., Hyde, J. E., Uhrlaub, M. B., Wendel, C. L., & Karst, G. M. (2001). Relative activity of abdominal muscles during commonly prescribed strengthening exercises. *Journal of Strength & Conditioning Research, 15*(4), 480-485.

Yaprak, Y. (2013). The effects of back extension training on back muscle strength and spinal range of motion in young females. *Biology of Sport, 30*(3), 201-206.

Youdas, J. W., Boor, M. M., Darfler, A. L., Koenig, M. K., Mills, K. M., & Hollman, J. H. (2014). Surface electromyographic analysis of core trunk and hip muscles during selected rehabilitation exercises in the side-bridge to neutral spine position. *Sports Health, 6*(5), 416-421.

Section 4.04

BED POSITIONING FOR BACK PAIN

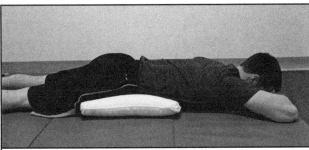

PRONE: Sleeping on the stomach can put undue stress and strain on the lower back as well as the neck. If your patient can only sleep in the prone position, putting a pillow under the stomach may assist to ease back strain.

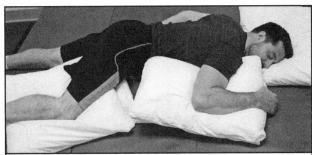

SIDE-LYING QUARTER TURN PRONE: A modification of prone-lying uses several pillows to quarter-turn the body off of one side, pillows under lifted shoulder, pelvis, knee and ankle.

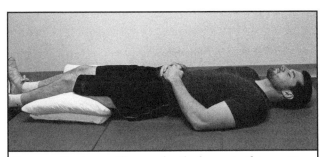

SUPINE: Placing a pillow under the knees in this position will assist the spine in maintaining a natural curve.

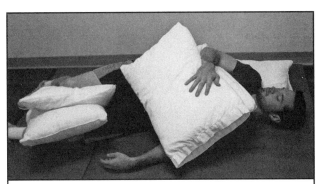

SIDE-LYING QUARTER TURN SUPINE: A modification of prone-lying uses several pillows to quarter-turn the body off of one side, pillows under lifted shoulder, pelvis, knee and ankle.

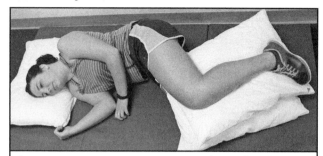

SIDE-LYING BOTH KNEES FLEXED: Place pillow between the knees and ankles to maintain neutral lower spine and pelvis. Patient bends both knees. It is also important to encourage the patient to avoid curling up too tightly in side-lying. Hugging a pillow will also increase comfort.

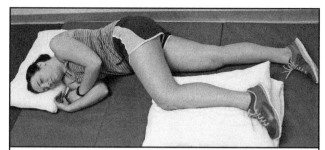

SIDE-LYING TOP KNEE FLEXED: Place pillow between the knees and ankles to maintain neutral lower spine and pelvis while keeping the bottom leg extended and flexing the top leg. Hugging a pillow will also increase comfort.

Where's the Evidence?

A study in 1981 compared four different sleep surfaces in patients with chronic LBP. They compared an orthopedic bed with 720 reinforced coils and a bed board, a softer 500 coil bed, a standard 10-inch thick waterbed, and a hybrid bed of foam and water. In this study, the patients preferred the orthopedic firm bed following with a second preference to the waterbed. The authors recommended that a harder surface be suggested for patients with LBP (Garfin & Pye, 1981). Conversely, a study in 2008 attempted to identify whether different mattresses affected LBP. Patients were divided into three groups: sleeping on waterbed, soft, and firm surfaces for 1 month. Both the waterbed and the soft mattresses seemed superior to the firm mattress (Bergholdt, Fabricius, & Benditimes, 2008). Another study in 2000 compared the use of an airbed vs innerspring mattress and found a highly significant benefit for the airbed design in their short-term comparison. They concluded the airbed appeared to be a useful sleep aid and an adjunct to medical and physical therapies for chronic back pain sufferers (Monsein, Corbin, Culliton, Merz, & Schuck, 2000). Jacobson, Boolani, Dunklee, Shepardson, and Acharya (2010) looked at sleep quality and comfort in a study of participants diagnosed with LBP and stiffness following sleep on individually prescribed mattresses based on dominant sleeping positions. It was concluded that sleep surfaces are related to sleep discomfort and that is indeed possible to reduce pain and discomfort and to increase sleep quality in those with chronic back pain by replacing mattresses based on sleeping position.

REFERENCES

Bergholdt, K., Fabricius, R. N., & Benditimes, T. (2008). Better backs by better beds? *Spine, 33*(7), 703-708.

Garfin, S. R., & Pye, S. A. (1981). Bed design and its effect on chronic low back pain—a limited controlled trial. *Pain, 10*(1), 87-91.

Jacobson, B. H., Boolani, A., Dunklee, G., Shepardson, A., & Acharya, H. (2010). Effect of prescribed sleep surfaces on back pain and sleep quality in patients diagnosed with low back and shoulder pain. *Applied Ergonomics, 42*(1), 91-97.

Monsein, M., Corbin, T. P., Culliton, P. D., Merz, D., & Schuck, E. A. (2000). Short-term outcomes of chronic back pain patients on an airbed vs innerspring mattresses. *Medscape General Medicine, 2*(3), E36.

Section 4.05

SACROILIAC CORRECTION

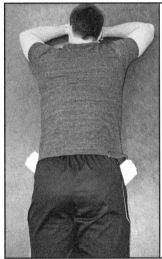

4.05.1 GAPPING TECHNIQUE: SACROILIAC, LYING ON TOWEL ROLLS OR PELVIC BLOCKS

POSITION: Prone

TARGETS: Gap SIJ, pain relief, improve mobility of SIJ; helpful prior to mobilization techniques.

INSTRUCTION: Pelvic blocks act as an extra pair of hands to support areas of the body. In SIJ gapping, the blocks are placed at a 45-degree angle downward, just inferior to the ASIS of the ilium. If pelvic blocks are not available, use rolled-up towels or small bolsters.

SUBSTITUTIONS: Patient should fully relax; a pillow may be placed under stomach for comfort.

PARAMETERS: Allow patient to stay in this position for 5 to 10 minutes; other modalities may be applied at this time to enhance relaxation; this can be done daily.

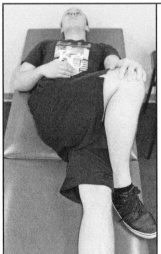

4.05.2 GAPPING TECHNIQUE: SACROILIAC, CROSS LEG

POSITION: Hook-lying

TARGETS: Gap SIJs, pain relief, improve mobility of SIJ; helpful prior to mobilization techniques.

INSTRUCTION: Patient with legs extended brings target-side hip and knee into flexion and grasps knee with opposite hand. Patient then pulls knee across body but keeps pelvis in contact with surface, creating a gapping force through the opposite SIJ.

SUBSTITUTIONS: Patient should fully relax.

PARAMETERS: Allow patient to stay in this position for 15 to 30 seconds and repeat 3 to 5 times; other modalities may be applied at this time to enhance relaxation, 1 to 2 times per day.

4.05.3 SELF-CORRECTION: POSTERIOR INNOMINATE, LEG HANG

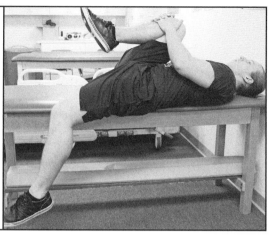

POSITION: Supine

TARGETS: Passive self-correction of a posteriorly rotated innominate using gravity

INSTRUCTION: Patient lies supine with affected side close to edge of bed. Patient then flexes unaffected hip and knee and grasps knee with both hands, pulling toward chest. This locks the unaffected ilia. Patient then scoots toward affected side, letting affected leg drop off side of bed. Patient lets the leg hang and tries to relax.

SUBSTITUTIONS: Patient should fully relax.

PARAMETERS: Allow patient to stay in this position for 1 to 5 minute(s), 1 to 2 times per day or as needed for correction.

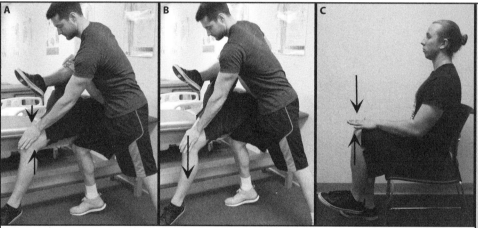

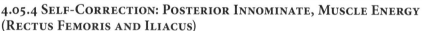

4.05.4 SELF-CORRECTION: POSTERIOR INNOMINATE, MUSCLE ENERGY (RECTUS FEMORIS AND ILIACUS)

POSITION: Supine, seated, standing

TARGETS: Correction of posteriorly rotated innominate using muscle energy, reversing origin, insertion of rectus femoris

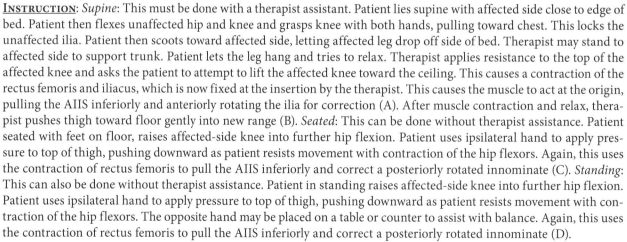

INSTRUCTION: *Supine:* This must be done with a therapist assistant. Patient lies supine with affected side close to edge of bed. Patient then flexes unaffected hip and knee and grasps knee with both hands, pulling toward chest. This locks the unaffected ilia. Patient then scoots toward affected side, letting affected leg drop off side of bed. Therapist may stand to affected side to support trunk. Patient lets the leg hang and tries to relax. Therapist applies resistance to the top of the affected knee and asks the patient to attempt to lift the affected knee toward the ceiling. This causes a contraction of the rectus femoris and iliacus, which is now fixed at the insertion by the therapist. This causes the muscle to act at the origin, pulling the AIIS inferiorly and anteriorly rotating the ilia for correction (A). After muscle contraction and relax, therapist pushes thigh toward floor gently into new range (B). *Seated:* This can be done without therapist assistance. Patient seated with feet on floor, raises affected-side knee into further hip flexion. Patient uses ipsilateral hand to apply pressure to top of thigh, pushing downward as patient resists movement with contraction of the hip flexors. Again, this uses the contraction of rectus femoris to pull the AIIS inferiorly and correct a posteriorly rotated innominate (C). *Standing:* This can also be done without therapist assistance. Patient in standing raises affected-side knee into further hip flexion. Patient uses ipsilateral hand to apply pressure to top of thigh, pushing downward as patient resists movement with contraction of the hip flexors. The opposite hand may be placed on a table or counter to assist with balance. Again, this uses the contraction of rectus femoris to pull the AIIS inferiorly and correct a posteriorly rotated innominate (D).

SUBSTITUTIONS: Too much abduction at the hip can cause substitution with the hip adductors; avoid hyperextension of the lumbar spine.

PARAMETERS: *Supine:* Patient contracts isometrically for 10 seconds, relaxes for 10 seconds into new range, and repeats 3 to 5 times. Recheck for alignment after set. If the correction is only partial, repeat steps, maximum 3 sets. *Seated and standing:* Patient holds isometric contraction 10 seconds, maintains position for 5 seconds, and repeats 3 to 5 times, 1 to 2 times per day as need for correction.

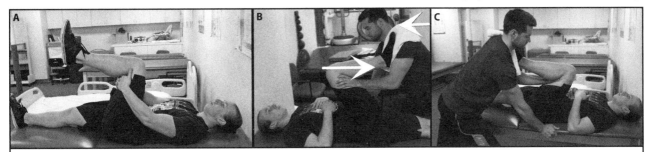

4.05.5 SELF-CORRECTION: ANTERIOR INNOMINATE, MUSCLE ENERGY (HAMSTRING AND GLUTEUS MAXIMUS)

POSITION: Supine

TARGETS: Correction of anteriorly rotated innominate using muscle energy, reversing origin, insertion of hamstring and gluteus maximus

INSTRUCTION: Patient lies supine and flexes affected hip and knee and grasps knee with both hands, pulling toward chest, pulling the affected innominate into a posteriorly rotated position. Patient applies resistance to proximal tibia while trying to extend the hip. Unaffected leg should be maintained against the supporting surface. This causes a contraction of the hamstring and gluteus maximus, which is now fixed at the insertion by the therapist. This causes the muscle to act at the origin, pulling the posterior iliac crest (gluteus maximus) and ischial tuberosity (hamstring), rotating the ilia posteriorly for correction (A). After muscle contraction and relax, therapist pushes thigh toward floor gently into new range. *Therapist assist*: This can be done with therapist assistance. Therapist props patient's leg on the table on the affected side facing the patient. Patient's calf is placed on the therapist's shoulder girdle using a towel for cushioning. Therapist places one hand on unaffected thigh to stabilize leg and instruct patient to push toward the therapist, attempting to extend hip (B). Therapist may use other hand hooked under table to assist resisting this motion (C).

SUBSTITUTIONS: Too much abduction at the hip can cause substitution with the hip adductors; focus needs to be on hip extension and not knee extension, particularly with the therapist assistance.

PARAMETERS: Contract isometrically for 10 seconds, relax for 10 seconds into new range, and repeat 3 to 5 times. Recheck for alignment after set. If correction only partial, repeat steps, maximum 3 sets, 1 to 2 times per day as need for correction.

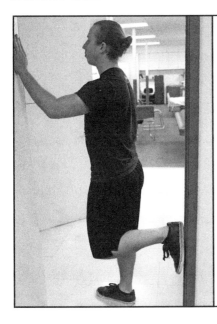

4.05.6 SELF-CORRECTION: ANTERIOR INNOMINATE, MUSCLE ENERGY (HAMSTRING AND GLUTEUS MAXIMUS), DOORWAY

POSITION: Standing in doorway

TARGETS: Correction of anteriorly rotated innominate using muscle energy, reversing origin, insertion of hamstring and gluteus maximus

INSTRUCTION: Patient stands in a doorway. The affected-side hip and knee are flexed with foot flat against the door frame. Patient places affected hand on opposite door frame. Patient then attempts to extend the hip isometrically while the door frame resists. This causes a contraction of the hamstring and gluteus maximus, which is now fixed at the insertion by the door frame. This causes the muscle to act at the origin, pulling the posterior iliac crest (gluteus maximus) and ischial tuberosity (hamstring) rotating the ilia posteriorly for correction.

SUBSTITUTIONS: Unaffected leg and foot come away from the wall or frame or patient leans forward

PARAMETERS: Contract isometrically for 10 seconds, relax for 10 seconds, and repeat 3 to 5 times. Recheck for alignment after set. If correction only partial, repeat steps, maximum 3 sets, 1 to 2 times per day as need for correction.

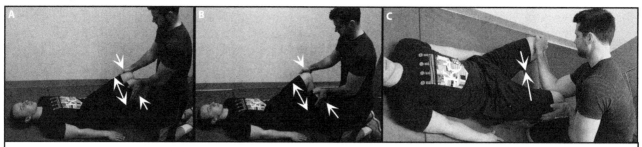

4.05.7 SELF-CORRECTION: PUBIC REPOSITIONING, HIP ABDUCTION AND ADDUCTION, "SHOTGUN TECHNIQUE"

<u>POSITION</u>: Hook-lying

<u>TARGETS</u>: Contracts hip abductors followed by adductors to correct pubic misalignments

<u>INSTRUCTION</u>: Therapist stands to the side of the patient. Patient in hook-lying with feet hip-width apart, therapist places fist between knee and asks patient to squeeze knees together for 10 seconds. Therapist then moves hands to outside of knee furthest away while body is on the outside of the other knee. Ask patient to push knees apart while therapist resists movement. Knees are opened up partially, repeat. Knees are opened even further, repeat. Knees are opened even further, repeat. This done three times, once at each position. Therapist then places a hand inside the furthest knee with wrist extended and elbow placed on inside of closest knee. Patient then squeeze knees together again. Occasionally, a pop may be elicited and is a normal sound associated with pubic correction. Recheck alignment (A, through C).

<u>SUBSTITUTIONS</u>: Lifting head or torso off bed

<u>PARAMETERS</u>: Contracts isometrically for 10 seconds, relax for 10 seconds, and repeat 3 to 5 times. Recheck for alignment after set. If correction only partial, repeat steps, maximum 3 sets, 1 to 2 times per day as need for correction.

Section 4.06

LUMBAR AND SACROILIAC PROTOCOLS AND TREATMENT IDEAS

4.06.1 LUMBAR AND SACROILIAC STABILIZATION DISCUSSION

A lumbar stabilization program is designed to teach a patient strengthening and flexibility exercises to maintain the normal curves of the lower spine. Facilitation of the TA and the lumbar multifidus are key to this approach. MRI results demonstrated that during a drawing-in action, the TA contracts bilaterally to form a musculofascial band that appears to tighten (like a corset) and most likely improves the stabilization of the lumbopelvic region (Hides et al., 2006). Additionally, motor control of the multifidus has been shown to be an underlying factor in chronic LBP via imaging studies (Massé-Alarie, Beaulieu, Preuss, & Schneider, 2015).

The key to determining whether a patient will respond favorably to lumbar stabilization lies in proper evaluation,

Where's the Evidence?

Exercise using abdominal bracing with LE movements has demonstrated improvements in thickness of the internal oblique and TA muscles (Lee, Kim, & Lee, 2014). The multifidus and longissimus thoracis has been shown to be most active via EMG measurement during prone lumbar extension to end range with resistance applied, identified to produce an average of 92% of MVC. Prone lumbar extension to neutral, resisted lumbar extension while sitting, and prone extension with the UEs and LEs lifted produced an average of 77% MVC and bridging exercises, the side-bridge exercise, and UE and LE raises in either the prone or quadruped positions produced an average of less than 50% MVC (Esktrom, Osborn, & Hauer, 2008). Lee also found that lumbar extension exercise with pelvic stabilization may be more effective for multifidus and iliocostalis lumborum muscle activity compared to that without pelvic stabilization (Lee, 2015).

looking at several important variables such as age, straight-leg raise, prone instability test, aberrant motions, lumbar hypermobility, and fear-avoidance beliefs. It appears that the response to a stabilization exercise program in patients with LBP can be predicted from variables collected from the clinical examination (Hicks, Fritz, Delitto, & McGill, 2005).

The SIJ is another structure that can be a source of dysfunction with and without lumbar pain. Generally, the source of SIJ pain can be from an inflammatory condition

Where's the Evidence?

Hayden, van Tulder, Malmivaara, and Koes evaluated evidence in 2005 looking at the effectiveness of exercise therapy in adult nonspecific acute, subacute, and chronic LBP vs no treatment and other conservative treatments. They found 61 randomized controlled trials (6390 participants) that met their inclusion criteria and found effectiveness in chronic populations relative to comparisons at all follow-up periods. There was also evidence of effectiveness of graded-activity exercise program in subacute LBP in occupational settings and evidence of equal effectiveness relative to comparisons in acute populations. They concluded that exercise therapy appeared to be slightly effective at decreasing pain and improving function in adults with chronic LBP, particularly in health care populations. In subacute LBP, there was some evidence that a graded activity program improved absenteeism outcomes and in acute LBP, exercise therapy was as effective as either no treatment or other conservative treatments. Macedo, Maher, Latimer, and McAuley (2009) in a later systematic review randomized controlled trials evaluating the effectiveness of motor control exercises for persistent LBP. Fourteen trials were included. Seven trials compared motor control exercise with minimal intervention or evaluated it as a supplement to another treatment. Four trials compared motor control exercise with manual therapy. Five trials compared motor control exercise with another form of exercise. One trial compared motor control exercise with lumbar fusion surgery. The pooling revealed that motor control exercise was better than minimal intervention in reducing pain at short-term, intermediate and long-term follow-up, and motor control exercise was better than manual therapy for pain, disability, and quality-of-life outcomes at intermediate follow-up and better than other forms of exercise in reducing disability at short-term follow-up. They concluded motor control exercise was superior to minimal intervention and confers benefit when added to another therapy for pain at all time points and for disability at long-term follow-up. Motor control exercise is not more effective than manual therapy or other forms of exercise. Additionally, there was insufficient evidence to derive that motor control exercises were superior to manual therapy or other exercise treatments. Another large study in Australia by Costa et al. (2009) looked at 154 patients with LBP lasting greater than 12 weeks. Twelve sessions of motor control exercises designed to improve function of specific muscles of the low back region and the control of posture and movement or placebo in the control group consisting of detuned ultrasound therapy and detuned short-wave therapy were conducted over 8 weeks. The exercise intervention improved activity and patients' global impression of recovery but did not significantly reduce pain at 2 months. They concluded motor control exercise produced short-term improvements in global impression of recovery and activity, but not necessarily on pain, for people with chronic LBP. Most of the effects observed in the short-term were maintained at the 6- and 12-month follow-ups. Brumitt, Matheson, and Meira performed a systematic review in 2013 of randomized controlled trials that assessed the effects of a motor control exercise approach, a general exercise approach or both for patients with LBP that were published in scientific peer-reviewed journals. Fifteen studies were identified (8 motor control exercise approach without general exercise comparison and 7 general exercise approach with or without motor control exercise approach comparison). Current evidence suggested that exercise interventions may be effective at reducing pain or disability in patients with LBP. They concluded that stabilization exercises for patients with LBP may help to decrease pain and disability.

within the joint, either causing or associated with the pain or instability through ligamentous laxity or tearing of the joint capsule (Laslett, 2008). Proper assessment and treatment of malignments in the sacrum and ilium should be successfully addressed before beginning a stabilization program in an effort to only reinforce correct positioning.

The lumbar stabilization and SIJ protocol is designed to guide an exercise program with primary focus on gaining static and dynamic control of the lumbar spine with trunk and extremity movements.

> ### *Where's the Evidence?*
>
> Mooney, Pozos, Vleeming, Gulick, and Swenski (2001) looked at the relationship of the latissimus dorsi and the gluteus maximus in patients with SIJ pain. EMG studies were performed in 15 healthy individuals as the baseline for evaluation of 5 symptomatic patients with SIJ dysfunction. Abnormal hyperactivity of the gluteus muscle on the involved side and increased activity of the latissimus on the contralateral side was contrasted with the normal function of the healthy individuals. All patients in the rotary strengthening exercise program improved in strength and return of myoelectric activity to more normal patterns. Richardson et al. (2002) looked at abdominal muscle patterns and their effects were compared in relation to SIJ laxity. One pattern was contraction of the transversus abdominis, independently of the other abdominals; the other was a bracing action that used all of the lateral abdominal muscles. Thirteen healthy individuals who could perform the test patterns were included. SIJ laxity values were recorded by means of Doppler imaging with participants in the prone position during the two abdominal muscle patterns. Simultaneous EMG recordings and ultrasound imaging were used to verify the two muscle patterns. The range of SIJ laxity values observed in this study was comparable with levels found in earlier studies of healthy individuals. These values decreased significantly in all individuals during both muscle patterns; however, the independent transversus abdominis contraction decreased SIJ to a significantly greater degree than the general abdominal exercise pattern. They concluded contraction of the transversus abdominis significantly decreases the laxity of the SIJ. This decrease in laxity is larger than that caused by a bracing action using all the lateral abdominal muscles.

4.06.2 LUMBAR AND SACROILIAC STABILIZATION RECOMMENDED EXERCISES

Other exercises to target these areas may be added as patient advances and based on individual responses to treatment. General ROM and stretches affecting the lumbar region may also be added but are not listed here. Refer to **4.01**, **4.02** and **4.03** for ideas.

1. Lumbar stabilization (also affects SIJ)
   a. 4.03.1 Strengthen: Isometric; Posterior Pelvic Tilt, Lumbar Spine, With or Without Blood Pressure Cuff for Biofeedback
   b. 4.03.2 Strengthen: Isometric; Neutral Spine, Lumbar Spine Stabilization
   c. 4.03.4 Strengthen: Lumbar Spine, Alternating and Bilateral Heel Slide
   d. 4.03.5 Strengthen: Lumbar Spine, Isometric, Trunk Extension
   e. 4.03.6 Strengthen: Lumbar Spine, Perturbations
   f. 4.03.7 Strengthen: Lumbar Spine, Bent-Knee Fall-Outs
   g. 4.03.8 Strengthen: Lumbar Spine, Arm Lift Overhead
   h. 4.03.9 Strengthen: Lumbar Spine, Bent-Knee Lift
   i. 4.03.10 Strengthen: Lumbar Spine, Heel Slide Abduction and Adduction
   j. 4.03.11 Strengthen: Lumbar Spine, Opposite Arm and Bent-Knee Lift
   k. 4.03.12 Strengthen: Lumbar Spine, Bilateral Arm Lift Overhead With Knee Extension
   l. 4.03.13 Strengthen: Lumbar Spine, Alternating Bent-Knee Lift to Straight-Leg Lower and Heel Slide to Return
   m. 4.03.14 Strengthen: Lumbar Spine, Alternating Arm Lift, Leg Lift, and Combined
   n. 4.03.15 Strengthen: Lumbar Spine, Lift All Fours, "Superman" and "Rocketman"
   o. 4.03.16 Strengthen: Lumbar Spine, "Swimming"
   p. 4.03.17 Strengthen: Lumbar Spine, Heel Lift
   q. 4.03.18 Strengthen: Lumbar Spine, Hip Abduction and Adduction
   r. 4.03.19 Strengthen: Lumbar Spine, Bent-Knee Lift, March in Place
   s. 4.03.20 Strengthen: Lumbar Spine, Alternating Knee Extension
   t. 4.03.21 Strengthen: Lumbar Spine, Unilateral Bridge
   u. 4.03.22 Strengthen: Lumbar Spine, Neutral Spine Hold, Quadruped
   v. 4.03.23 Strengthen: Lumbar Spine, Alternating Arm Lift, Quadruped
   w. 4.03.24 Strengthen: Lumbar Spine, Alternating Hip and Knee Extension, Quadruped
   x. 4.03.25 Strengthen: Lumbar Spine, Opposite Arm and Leg Lift, Quadruped
   y. 4.03.26 Strengthen: Lumbar Spine, Rocking
   z. 4.03.27 Strengthen: Lumbar Spine, Hold Neutral Spine, Tall-Kneeling
   aa. 4.03.28 Strengthen: Lumbar Spine, Arm Lift, Tall-Kneeling
   ab. 4.03.29 Strengthen: Lumbar Spine, Reach Toward Floor, Tall-Kneeling
   ac. 4.03.30 Strengthen: Lumbar Spine, Reach Toward Floor, Half-Kneeling
   ad. 4.03.31 Strengthen: Lumbar Spine, Quick Hands
   ae. 4.03.32 Strengthen: Lumbar Spine, Blind Weight Shifts

2. Sacroiliac-specific stabilization ideas
    a. 6.04.3 Strengthen: Isometric; Hip Abduction (hook-lying with belt version)
    b. 6.04.4 Strengthen: Isometric; Hip Adduction
    c. 6.04.5 Strengthen: Isometric; Hip Internal Rotation
    d. 6.04.6 Strengthen: Isometric; Hip External Rotation
    e. 6.04.14 Strengthen: Isotonic; Hip Extension, Bridge and Variations
    f. 4.03.33 Strengthen: Abdominal, Partial Sit-Up, 5-Way
    g. 4.03.34 Strengthen: Abdominal, Partial Diagonal Sit-Up, 4-Way
    h. 4.03.35 Strengthen: Abdominal, Posterior Pelvic Tilt, Leg Lowers
    i. 4.03.41 Strengthen: Abdominal, Boat Pose/V-Sits (Advanced)
    j. 4.03.40 Strengthen: Abdominal, Roll-Up (Advanced)
    k. 4.03.38 Strengthen: Abdominal, Plank and Variations
    l. 4.03.39 Strengthen: Abdominal, Side Plank and Variations
    m. 4.03.60 Strengthen: Exercise Ball, Abdominal, Jack Knife, 4-Way
    n. 4.03.61 Strengthen: Exercise Ball, Abdominal, Roll-Out
    o. 4.03.42 Strengthen: Abdominal, Pulsing Crunch, 3-Way (Advanced)
    p. 4.03.73 Strengthen: Isometric; Supine Lumbar Extension

4.06.3 LUMBAR LAMINECTOMY/DISCECTOMY/FUSION

Adapted from protocols from Southeast Georgia Health System (Southeast Georgia Health System, 2013).

Other exercises to target these areas may be added as patient advances and based on individual responses to treatment.

Post-Operation 1 to 3 Days Up to 4 to 6 Weeks

1. Precautions
    a. Prevent excessive initial mobility or stress on tissues and follow physician recommendations regarding use of back brace. Sometimes, hard braces, or thoracolumbosacral orthosis, are issued to patients. These must be worn at all times except when lying down.
    b. Lifting: 5 lbs for the first 4 weeks; dependent on physician restriction.
    c. Driving: No driving for 2 weeks
    d. Sex: Wait 2 weeks; use the least exerting and most comfortable positions.
    e. Sitting: 20-minute intervals for first 4 weeks, slowly increase to 30- to 40-minute intervals after 4 weeks.
    f. Tub baths: None for 1 month because of posture and submersing the incision, then only for short durations. Avoid use of extremely hot water; *skin should not turn red.*
    g. Household chores: None for 4 to 6 weeks, or as approved by your physician; progress slowly at beginning; consult outpatient physical therapist for proper body mechanics.
    h. Yard work: Wait at least 2 to 3 months; consult physician before performing yard work; observe proper body mechanics and lifting limit.
    i. The following observations require a consultation with the referring or consulting physician:
        i. Failure of incision to close or significant redness, swelling, or pain in the area of incision
        ii. Unexpectedly high self-reports of pain in comparison to presurgical state
        iii. Failure to meet progress milestones according to protocol guidelines as may be modified by clinical judgment with consideration given to previous presurgical state and typical progression of patients during rehabilitation
        iv. Evidence of acute exacerbation of symptoms: significant increase of pain, sudden increase of radicular symptoms, and/or sudden loss of strength, sensation and reflexes
        v. Development of new unexpected symptoms during the course of rehabilitation
2. Physical therapy includes bed mobility, transfers, and education on donning/doffing collar if applicable; gait, with appropriate assistive device if necessary; and discussion of increasing walking tolerance. Reinforce sitting, standing, and ADL modifications with neutral spine postures and proper body mechanics.
3. Breathing
    a. 3.03.7 Breathing Techniques: Diaphragmatic and Pursed-Lip Breathing
4. LE (recommended to do every hour)
    a. 6.09.3 Strengthen: Isometric; Knee Flexion, Hamstring Set

b. 6.01.8 ROM: Hip Flexion and Extension, Heel Slide, Active

c. 6.01.14 ROM: Hip Internal Rotation and External Rotation, Active

d. 6.04.2 Strengthen: Isometric; Hip Extension/ Gluteus Sets

e. 6.08.1 Stretch: Quadriceps

f. 6.08.3 Stretch: Hamstrings

g. 6.04.26 Functional: Hip, Wall Squat

h. Walking: Walk for short distances at first, twice daily, at a comfortable pace. Choose a safe, paved area. Gradually increase to one-half mile in the morning and one-half mile in the evening by 1 to 2 months or start out 5 minutes in one direction and 5 minutes back. Gradually increase time as tolerated up to 45 minutes total.

Post-Operation 4 to 6 Weeks to 2 Months

1. Stretching
    a. 6.03.2 Stretch: Hip Flexor, Kneeling Lunge
    b. 6.03.3 Stretch: Hip Flexor, Standing Lunge
    c. 6.07.1 Self-Joint Mobilization: Knee Flexion
    d. 6.08.3 Stretch: Hamstrings
    e. 6.11.5 ROM: Ankle/Foot, Mini-Ball on Wall
    f. 6.11.8 ROM: Ankle/Foot, Alphabet, Active
    g. 4.02.1 Stretch: Single Knee to Chest
    h. 4.02.2 Stretch: Double Knee to Chest, 3-Way
    i. 4.02.4 Stretch: Lower Trunk Rotation and Twist, Knee Flexed and Extended
    j. 6.03.22 Stretch: Piriformis, Figure 4 and Variations
    k. 4.01.2 ROM: Lumbar Extension, Prone on Elbows, Progress to Press Up on Hands, Passive *as tolerated.*

2. Lumbar stabilization (also affects SIJ)
    a. 4.03.1 Strengthen: Isometric; Posterior Pelvic Tilt, Lumbar Spine, With or Without Blood Pressure Cuff for Biofeedback
    b. 4.03.2 Strengthen: Isometric; Neutral Spine, Lumbar Spine Stabilization
    c. 4.03.4 Strengthen: Lumbar Spine, Alternating and Bilateral Heel Slide
    d. 4.03.5 Strengthen: Lumbar Spine, Isometric, Trunk Extension
    e. 4.03.6 Strengthen: Lumbar Spine, Perturbations
    f. 4.03.7 Strengthen: Lumbar Spine, Bent-Knee Fall-Outs
    g. 4.03.8 Strengthen: Lumbar Spine, Arm Lift Overhead
    h. 4.03.9 Strengthen: Lumbar Spine, Bent-Knee Lift
    i. 4.03.10 Strengthen: Lumbar Spine, Heel Slide Abduction and Adduction
    j. 4.03.11 Strengthen: Lumbar Spine, Opposite Arm and Bent-Knee Lift
    k. 4.03.12 Strengthen: Lumbar Spine, Bilateral Arm Lift Overhead With Knee Extension
    l. 4.03.13 Strengthen: Lumbar Spine, Alternating Bent-Knee Lift to Straight-Leg Lower and Heel Slide to Return
    m. 4.03.14 Strengthen: Lumbar Spine, Alternating Arm Lift, Leg Lift, and Combined
    n. 4.03.15 Strengthen: Lumbar Spine, Lift All Fours, "Superman" and "Rocketman"
    o. 4.03.16 Strengthen: Lumbar Spine, "Swimming"
    p. 4.03.17 Strengthen: Lumbar Spine, Heel Lift
    q. 4.03.18 Strengthen: Lumbar Spine, Hip Abduction and Adduction
    r. 4.03.19 Strengthen: Lumbar Spine, Bent-Knee Lift, March in Place
    s. 4.03.20 Strengthen: Lumbar Spine, Alternating Knee Extension
    t. 4.03.21 Strengthen: Lumbar Spine, Unilateral Bridge
    u. 4.03.22 Strengthen: Lumbar Spine, Neutral Spine Hold, Quadruped
    v. 4.03.23 Strengthen: Lumbar Spine, Alternating Arm Lift, Quadruped
    w. 4.03.24 Strengthen: Lumbar Spine, Alternating Hip and Knee Extension, Quadruped
    x. 4.03.25 Strengthen: Lumbar Spine, Opposite Arm and Leg Lift, Quadruped
    y. 4.03.26 Strengthen: Lumbar Spine, Rocking
    z. 4.03.27 Strengthen: Lumbar Spine, Hold Neutral Spine, Tall-Kneeling
    aa. 4.03.28 Strengthen: Lumbar Spine, Arm Lift, Tall-Kneeling
    ab. 4.03.29 Strengthen: Lumbar Spine, Reach Toward Floor, Tall-Kneeling
    ac. 4.03.30 Strengthen: Lumbar Spine, Reach Toward Floor, Half-Kneeling
    ad. 4.03.31 Strengthen: Lumbar Spine, Quick Hands
    ae. 4.03.32 Strengthen: Lumbar Spine, Blind Weight Shifts

3. Pool therapy as indicated
4. Treadmill walking progression program
5. May begin lifting and bending using proper mechanics 10 to 20 lbs; clear with physician.
6. General extremity strengthening

Post-Operation 2 to 6 Months

1. Functional training exercises for sports or work-specific activities; clear with physician.
2. Running progression program; clear with physician.
3. Resume all activities at 6 months post-operation; clear with physician.

4.06.4 LUMBAR SPONDYLOLISTHESIS DISCUSSION

Spondylolisthesis is a pathological condition characterized by the slipping of a vertebral body, compared with the underlying one, following structural and degenerative changes of the spine (Ferrari, Vanti, & O'Reilly, 2012). This can be an anterior slippage (anterolisthesis) or posterior slippage (retrolisthesis) often due to a fracture of the pars interarticularis of the lumbar vertebra. In addition, ligamentous structures, including the iliolumbar ligament (between L5 and the sacrum) are stronger than those between L4 and L5, by which the vertebral slip commonly develops in L4 (Cormond, Mesmaeker, Lowe, Myracle, & Thomas, 2016). Improvement was found in bracing, bracing and exercises emphasizing lumbar extension, ROM and strengthening exercises focusing on lumbar flexion, and strengthening specific abdominal and lumbar muscles (Garet, Reiman, Mathers, & Sylvain, 2013). It is suggested that if a conservative treatment program is elected, back flexion or isometric back strengthening exercises should be considered.

Where's the Evidence?

Sinaki, Lutness, Ilstrup, Chu, and Gramse (1989) studied 48 patients with symptomatic back pain secondary to spondylolisthesis who were treated conservatively and were followed for 3 years after initial examination to compare the outcomes of two exercise programs. The patients were divided into two groups: those doing flexion and those doing extension back-strengthening exercises. All patients received instructions on posture, lifting techniques, and the use of heat for relief of symptoms. After 3 months, only 27% of patients who were instructed in flexion exercises had moderate or severe pain and only 32% were unable to work or had limited their work. Of the patients who were instructed in extension exercises, 67% had moderate or severe pain and 61% were unable to work or had limited their work. At 3-year follow-up, only 19% of the flexion group had moderate or severe pain and 24% were unable to work or had limited their work. The overall recovery rate after 3 months was 58% for the flexion group and 6% for the extension group. At 3 years, these figures improved to 62% for the flexion group and dropped to 0% for the extension group. Based on their findings, they suggested that if a conservative treatment program is elected, back flexion or isometric back-strengthening exercises should be considered.

4.06.5 LUMBAR SPONDYLOLISTHESIS RECOMMENDED EXERCISES

Other exercises to target these areas may be added as patient advances and based on individual responses to treatment.

1. Breathing
    a. 3.03.7 Breathing Techniques: Diaphragmatic and Pursed-Lip Breathing
2. An excellent exercise is stationary bicycling because it promotes spine flexion (Cormond et al., 2016)
3. Stretching
    a. 6.03.2 Stretch: Hip Flexor, Kneeling Lunge; *avoid LE.*
    b. 6.03.3 Stretch: Hip Flexor, Standing Lunge; *avoid LE.*
    c. 6.08.1 Stretch: Quadriceps
    d. 6.08.3 Stretch: Hamstrings
    e. 6.13.5 Stretch: Gastrocnemius Using Strap
    f. 6.13.8 Stretch: Calf on Ramp
    g. 4.02.1 Stretch: Single Knee to Chest
    h. 4.02.2 Stretch: Double Knee to Chest, 3-Way
    i. 3.02.11 Stretch: Thoracic, Golfer's Rotation and Side-Bend
    j. Stretch: Trunk Flexion Knees Apart Chair
    k. 7.04.2C "Rag Doll" or Standing Forward Bend (Uttanasana)
    l. 4.02.4 Stretch: Lower Trunk Rotation and Twist, Knee Flexed and Extended
    m. 6.03.22 Stretch: Piriformis, Figure 4 and Variations
4. Lumbar stabilization (also affects SIJ)
    a. 4.01.4 ROM: Posterior Pelvic Tilt, Active
    b. 4.03.1 Strengthen: Isometric; Posterior Pelvic Tilt, Lumbar Spine, With or Without Blood Pressure Cuff for Biofeedback
    c. 4.03.2 Strengthen: Isometric; Neutral Spine, Lumbar Spine Stabilization
    d. 4.03.4 Strengthen: Lumbar Spine, Alternating and Bilateral Heel Slide
    e. 4.03.5 Strengthen: Lumbar Spine, Isometric, Trunk Extension
    f. 4.03.6 Strengthen: Lumbar Spine, Perturbations
    g. 4.03.7 Strengthen: Lumbar Spine, Bent-Knee Fall-Outs
    h. 4.03.8 Strengthen: Lumbar Spine, Arm Lift Overhead
    i. 4.03.9 Strengthen: Lumbar Spine, Bent-Knee Lift
    j. 4.03.10 Strengthen: Lumbar Spine, Heel Slide Abduction and Adduction

k. 4.03.11 Strengthen: Lumbar Spine, Opposite Arm and Bent-Knee Lift

l. 4.03.12 Strengthen: Lumbar Spine, Bilateral Arm Lift Overhead With Knee Extension

m. 4.03.13 Strengthen: Lumbar Spine, Alternating Bent-Knee Lift to Straight-Leg Lower and Heel Slide to Return

n. 4.03.14 Strengthen: Lumbar Spine, Alternating Arm Lift, Leg Lift, and Combined

o. 4.03.15 Strengthen: Lumbar Spine, Lift All Fours, "Superman" and "Rocketman"

p. 4.03.16 Strengthen: Lumbar Spine, "Swimming"

q. 4.03.17 Strengthen: Lumbar Spine, Heel Lift

r. 4.03.18 Strengthen: Lumbar Spine, Hip Abduction and Adduction

s. 4.03.19 Strengthen: Lumbar Spine, Bent-Knee Lift, March in Place

t. 4.03.20 Strengthen: Lumbar Spine, Alternating Knee Extension

u. 4.03.21 Strengthen: Lumbar Spine, Unilateral Bridge

v. 4.03.22 Strengthen: Lumbar Spine, Neutral Spine Hold, Quadruped

w. 4.03.23 Strengthen: Lumbar Spine, Alternating Arm Lift, Quadruped

x. 4.03.24 Strengthen: Lumbar Spine, Alternating Hip and Knee Extension, Quadruped

y. 4.03.25 Strengthen: Lumbar Spine, Opposite Arm and Leg Lift, Quadruped

z. 4.03.26 Strengthen: Lumbar Spine, Rocking

aa. 4.03.27 Strengthen: Lumbar Spine, Hold Neutral Spine, Tall-Kneeling

ab. 4.03.28 Strengthen: Lumbar Spine, Arm Lift, Tall-Kneeling

ac. 4.03.29 Strengthen: Lumbar Spine, Reach Toward Floor, Tall-Kneeling

ad. 4.03.30 Strengthen: Lumbar Spine, Reach Toward Floor, Half-Kneeling

ae. 4.03.31 Strengthen: Lumbar Spine, Quick Hands

af. 4.03.32 Strengthen: Lumbar Spine, Blind Weight Shifts

5. Suggested additional advanced core strengthening. These target extension, strengthening without extending beyond neutral and flexor strengthening.

a. 4.03.68 Strengthen: Resistance Band, Lumbar Extension

b. 4.03.76 Strengthen: Lumbar, Back Extension Using Machine

c. 4.03.33 Strengthen: Abdominal, Partial Sit-Up, 5-Way

d. 4.03.34 Strengthen: Abdominal, Partial Diagonal Sit-Up, 4-Way

e. 4.03.35 Strengthen: Abdominal, Posterior Pelvic Tilt, Leg Lowers

f. 4.03.41 Strengthen: Abdominal, Boat Pose/V-Sits (Advanced)

g. 4.03.40 Strengthen: Abdominal, Roll-Up (Advanced)

h. 4.03.38 Strengthen: Abdominal, Plank and Variations

i. 4.03.39 Strengthen: Abdominal, Side Plank and Variations

j. 4.03.60 Strengthen: Exercise Ball, Abdominal, Jack Knife, 4-Way

k. 4.03.61 Strengthen: Exercise Ball, Abdominal, Roll-Out

l. 4.03.42 Strengthen: Abdominal, Pulsing Crunch, 3-Way (Advanced)

m. 4.03.75 Strengthen: Lumbar, Roman Chair and Variations, Beginner and Hip Hinge With Dowel; do not extend beyond neutral spine.

4.06.6 McKenzie Extension (for Centralization of Radiating Pain With Extension) Discussion

The McKenzie method is a classification system and a classification-based treatment for patients with LBP. Another term for the McKenzie method is mechanical diagnosis and therapy. The McKenzie method was developed in 1981 by Robin McKenzie, a physical therapist from New Zealand. The evaluation uses repeated movements and sustained positions with the aim to elicit a pattern of pain responses called *centralization*. The symptoms of the lower limbs and lower back are classified into three subgroups: derangement syndrome, dysfunction syndrome, and postural syndrome. The choice of exercises in the McKenzie method is based upon the direction (flexion, extension, or lateral shift) of the spine. The aims of the therapy are reducing pain, centralization of symptoms (symptoms migrating into the middle line of the body), and the complete recovery of pain. All exercises for the lumbar spine are repeated a number of times to end range on spinal symptoms in one direction. Doing only one repetition may cause pain; however, when repeated several times, the pain should decrease. A single direction of repeated movements or sustained postures leads to sequential and lasting abolition of all distal referred symptoms and subsequent abolition of any remaining spinal pain (Tourwe, Pagare, Buton, Thomas, & Vrije Universiteit Brussel's Evidence-based Practice Project, n.d.).

Where's the Evidence?

In patients with LBP for more than 6 weeks presenting with centralization or peripheralization of symptoms, McKenzie method was found to be slightly more effective than manipulation when used adjunctive to information and advice (Petersen et al., 2011). Furthermore, lumbar extension has been shown to reduce stresses in the posterior annulus in discs that exhibited the lowest compressive stresses in the neutral posture in vivo (Adams, May, Freeman, Morrison, & Dolan, 2000). Mbada et al. (2014) looked at 84 patients who received treatment 3 times per week for 8 weeks. Participants were assigned to the McKenzie protocol group, McKenzie protocol plus static back endurance exercise group or McKenzie protocol plus dynamic endurance exercise group using permuted randomization. Adding endurance exercises such as prone chest lift with arms at sides, prone chest lift with hands behind head, prone chest lift with arms fully flexed, prone alternating arm and leg lift, and prone chest lift with arms at 90/90, positively affected health-related quality-of-life of patients with long-term LBP decreases with severity of pain. The McKenzie protocol had significant therapeutic effect on health-related quality-of-life in patients with long-term LBP; however, the addition of dynamic back extensors endurance exercise to the McKenzie protocol led to even more improvement. Based on this, it is recommended that static or dynamic endurance exercise (**4.03**) be combined with McKenzie protocol in patients with long-term LBP.

The McKenzie method is intended to be used by clinicians that have been trained in the McKenzie method. A general interpretation of the basic extension exercises used in one specific McKenzie treatment is provided here for you, but it is encouraged that it be provided and or guided by a certified McKenzie provider.

4.06.7 McKenzie Extension (for Centralization of Radiating Pain With Extension) Protocol

1. Extension progression prone-lying
   a. Patient starts prone-lying with pillows under abdomen and progresses to less pillows and eventually none. This may take one treatment to several treatments. Do not progress to the next exercise until tolerance with no pillows is achieved.
   b. 4.01.1 ROM: Lumbar Extension, Pillows Under Chest, Passive
2. Extension progression prone on elbows
   a. Patient progresses to gently pressing up onto elbows in prone. This may take one treatment to several treatments. Patient may gently progress to on elbows position with a series of placing pillows under the chest and increasing pillows until height or prone on elbows is reached. Do not progress to prone press up until tolerance is achieved. Lateral preference may be added to prone on elbows and prone press up as desired.
   b. 4.01.2 ROM: Lumbar Extension, Prone on Elbows, Progress to Press Up on Hands, Passive
3. Extension progression prone press up; includes lateral preference press-up.
   a. Do not progress to prone press up until tolerance is achieved in prone on elbows. Lateral preference may be added to prone on elbows and prone press up as desired for increased centralization if unilateral directional preference determined.

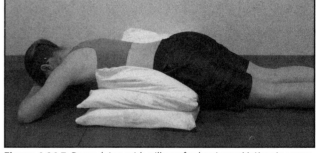

Figure 4.06.7. Prone-lying with pillows for beginner McKenzie extension.

   b. 4.01.2 ROM: Lumbar Extension, Prone on Elbows, Progress to Press Up on Hands, Passive
4. Extension progression prone press up; includes lateral preference press-up.
   a. Do not progress to standing extension until after implementing steps 1 to 3
   b. 4.01.3 ROM: Lumbar Extension, Active (hold for 20 seconds)
5. Adding endurance exercises, such as prone chest lift with arms at sides, prone chest lift with hands behind head, prone chest lift with arms fully flexed, prone alternating arm and leg lift, and prone chest lift with arms at 90/90 has been recommended by research studies (Mbada et al., 2014).

4.06.8 WILLIAMS' FLEXION BASIC EXERCISES

Williams' lumbar flexion exercises are a set or system of related physical exercises intended to enhance lumbar flexion, avoid lumbar extension, and strengthen the abdominal and gluteal musculature in an effort to manage LBP nonsurgically. The system was first devised in 1937 by Dr. Paul C. Williams (1900-1978). Williams' flexion exercises have been a cornerstone in the management of LBP for many years for treating a wide variety of back problems, regardless of diagnosis or chief complaint. Williams' flexion protocol is helpful when flexion is desirable, such as with conditions of anterolisthesis of the lumbar spine to spinal stenosis.

1. Williams' flexion basic program
   a. 4.01.4 ROM: Posterior Pelvic Tilt, Active
   b. 4.02.1 Stretch: Single Knee to Chest
   c. 4.02.2 Stretch: Double Knee to Chest, 3-Way
   d. 4.03.33 Strengthen: Abdominal, Partial Sit-Up, 5-Way
   e. 6.08.3 Stretch: Hamstrings
   f. 6.03.2 Stretch: Hip Flexor, Kneeling Lunge; *avoid lumbar extension.*
   g. 6.03.3 Stretch: Hip Flexor, Standing Lunge; *avoid lumbar extension.*
   h. 6.04.26 Functional: Hip, Wall Squat

4.06.9 SPINAL STENOSIS DISCUSSION

Spinal stenosis is a condition in which the spinal canal narrows and the nerve roots and spinal cord become compressed. Because not all patients with spinal narrowing develop symptoms, the term *spinal stenosis* actually refers to the symptoms of pain and not to the narrowing itself (Lu, Simon, Ritchie, Brachotte, & Van Haver, n.d.). Conservative management centers around a flexion-based exercise program.

> ## Where's the Evidence?
>
> Delitto et al.'s (2015) study of 169 participants with spinal stenosis compared 74 patients who underwent surgery with 73 patients who received only physical therapy treatment. At 24-month follow-up, mean improvement in physical function for the surgery and physical therapy groups was 22.4 and 19.2, respectively, using the Short Form-36 Health Survey. Sensitivity analyses using causal-effects methods to account for the high proportion of crossovers from physical therapy to surgery showed no significant differences in physical function between groups. They concluded surgical decompression yielded similar effects to a physical therapy regimen among patients with lumbar spinal stenosis who were surgical candidates. The study was limited as there was no control group to contrast whether either intervention had a favorable outcome compared to no intervention.

4.06.10 SPINAL STENOSIS RECOMMENDED EXERCISES

1. Breathing
   a. 3.03.7 Breathing Techniques: Diaphragmatic and Pursed-Lip Breathing
2. Stretching
   a. 6.03.2 Stretch: Hip Flexor, Kneeling Lunge; *avoid LE.*
   b. 6.03.3 Stretch: Hip Flexor, Standing Lunge; *avoid LE.*
   c. 6.08.1 Stretch: Quadriceps
   d. 6.08.3 Stretch: Hamstrings
   e. 6.13.5 Stretch: Gastrocnemius Using Strap
   f. 6.13.8 Stretch: Calf on Ramp
   g. 4.02.1 Stretch: Single Knee to Chest
   h. 4.02.2 Stretch: Double Knee to Chest, 3-Way
   i. 3.02.11 Stretch: Thoracic, Golfer's Rotation and Side-Bend
   j. 7.04.2C "Rag Doll" or Standing Forward Bend (Uttanasana)
   k. 4.02.4 Stretch: Lower Trunk Rotation and Twist, Knee Flexed and Extended
   l. 6.03.22 Stretch: Piriformis, Figure 4 and Variations
3. Nerve glides
   a. 6.15.2 Nerve Glide: Femoral Nerve, Flossing and Variations
   b. 6.15.1 Nerve Glide: Sciatic Nerve, Flossing and Variations

4. Lumbar stabilization (also affects SIJ)
    a. 4.01.4 ROM: Posterior Pelvic Tilt, Active
    b. 4.03.1 Strengthen: Isometric; Posterior Pelvic Tilt, Lumbar Spine, With or Without Blood Pressure Cuff for Biofeedback
    c. 4.03.2 Strengthen: Isometric; Neutral Spine, Lumbar Spine Stabilization; use for lumbar stabilization program **4.03.3-33**.
    d. 4.03.4 Strengthen: Lumbar Spine, Alternating and Bilateral Heel Slide
    e. 4.03.5 Strengthen: Lumbar Spine, Isometric, Trunk Extension
    f. 4.03.6 Strengthen: Lumbar Spine, Perturbations
    g. 4.03.7 Strengthen: Lumbar Spine, Bent-Knee Fall-Outs
    h. 4.03.8 Strengthen: Lumbar Spine, Arm Lift Overhead
    i. 4.03.9 Strengthen: Lumbar Spine, Bent-Knee Lift
    j. 4.03.10 Strengthen: Lumbar Spine, Heel Slide Abduction and Adduction
    k. 4.03.11 Strengthen: Lumbar Spine, Opposite Arm and Bent-Knee Lift
    l. 4.03.12 Strengthen: Lumbar Spine, Bilateral Arm Lift Overhead With Knee Extension
    m. 4.03.13 Strengthen: Lumbar Spine, Alternating Bent-Knee Lift to Straight-Leg Lower and Heel Slide to Return
    n. 4.03.14 Strengthen: Lumbar Spine, Alternating Arm Lift, Leg Lift, and Combined
    o. 4.03.15 Strengthen: Lumbar Spine, Lift All Fours, "Superman" and "Rocketman"
    p. 4.03.16 Strengthen: Lumbar Spine, "Swimming"
    q. 4.03.17 Strengthen: Lumbar Spine, Heel Lift
    r. 4.03.18 Strengthen: Lumbar Spine, Hip Abduction and Adduction
    s. 4.03.19 Strengthen: Lumbar Spine, Bent-Knee Lift, March in Place
    t. 4.03.20 Strengthen: Lumbar Spine, Alternating Knee Extension
    u. 4.03.21 Strengthen: Lumbar Spine, Unilateral Bridge
    v. 4.03.22 Strengthen: Lumbar Spine, Neutral Spine Hold, Quadruped
    w. 4.03.23 Strengthen: Lumbar Spine, Alternating Arm Lift, Quadruped
    x. 4.03.24 Strengthen: Lumbar Spine, Alternating Hip and Knee Extension, Quadruped
    y. 4.03.25 Strengthen: Lumbar Spine, Opposite Arm and Leg Lift, Quadruped
    z. 4.03.26 Strengthen: Lumbar Spine, Rocking
    aa. 4.03.27 Strengthen: Lumbar Spine, Hold Neutral Spine, Tall-Kneeling
    ab. 4.03.28 Strengthen: Lumbar Spine, Arm Lift, Tall-Kneeling
    ac. 4.03.29 Strengthen: Lumbar Spine, Reach Toward Floor, Tall-Kneeling
    ad. 4.03.30 Strengthen: Lumbar Spine, Reach Toward Floor, Half-Kneeling
    ae. 4.03.31 Strengthen: Lumbar Spine, Quick Hands
    af. 4.03.32 Strengthen: Lumbar Spine, Blind Weight Shifts
5. Suggested additional advanced core strengthening. These target extension, strengthening without extending beyond neutral and flexor strengthening
    a. 6.04.26 Functional: Hip, Wall Squat
    b. 4.03.68 Strengthen: Resistance Band, Lumbar Extension
    c. 4.03.76 Strengthen: Lumbar, Back Extension Using Machine
    d. 4.03.33 Strengthen: Abdominal, Partial Sit-Up, 5-Way
    e. 4.03.34 Strengthen: Abdominal, Partial Diagonal Sit-Up, 4-Way
6. Treadmill walking and bicycling progression program
7. General UE and LE strengthening

4.06.11 SCOLIOSIS DISCUSSION

When a person's spine twists and develops an "S"-shaped, side-to-side curve, it is a condition known as *scoliosis*. A scoliosis curve can occur in a variety of areas throughout the spine. The abnormal curve can occur in the thoracic spine, the lumbar spine, or both areas at the same time. The curves can range in size from as minor as 10 degrees to severe cases of more than 100 degrees. The measurement of the degrees of curvature from the normal is a measure of how severe the scoliosis is. Usually, curves of less than 40 degrees will be treated without surgery. The most common types of scoliosis are first discovered and treated in childhood or adolescence.

The most common type is idiopathic adolescent scoliosis, occurring in teenagers just at the growth spurt of puberty. When scoliosis occurs, or is discovered after puberty, the condition is called *adult scoliosis* to distinguish it from the curves caused during growth. There are several types of adult scoliosis: *idiopathic* which is the most common and can include *degenerative* scoliosis that typically develops after age 50 years; *congenital* meaning present at birth; *paralytic* means that muscles do not work around the spine, throwing it out of balance, often caused by spinal paralysis; *myopathic* meaning muscles do not work properly, resulting from a muscular or neuromuscular disease, such as muscular dystrophy or cerebral palsy; and *secondary* which develops in adulthood and can be caused by another spinal condition that affects the vertebrae, such as leg length discrepancy, degeneration, osteoporosis, or osteomalacia, or even spinal surgery (DePuy Acromed, 2003).

Surgical management consists of either decompression, correction, stabilization, and fusion procedures or a combination of all of these. Surgical procedure is usually complex and has to deal with a whole array of specific problems, like the age and general medical condition of the patient, the length of the fusion, the condition of the adjacent segments, the condition of the lumbosacral junction, osteoporosis and possibly previous scoliosis surgery, and usually with a long history of chronic back pain and muscle imbalance, which may be very difficult to be influenced (Aebi, 2005). A growing body of evidence from independent sources is consistent with the hypothesis that exercise-based approaches can be used effectively to reverse the signs and symptoms of spinal deformity and to prevent progression in children and adults (Hawes, 2003).

Where's the Evidence?

Negrini et al.'s (2008) systematic review found 18 studies that all confirmed the efficacy of exercises in reducing the progression rate mainly in early puberty, improving the Cobb angles around the end of growth and reducing brace prescription.

Supervised physical therapy may be more effective than one-time treatment in reducing pain and improving function in patients with adolescent idiopathic scoliosis and LBP. Zapata et al. (2015) compared 8 weeks of weekly supervised spinal stabilization exercises with one-time treatment in participants with LBP and AIIS. Seventeen participants in the supervised group received weekly physical therapy, and 17 participants in the unsupervised group received a one-time treatment followed by home exercises. Significant between-group differences were found in the Numeric Pain Rating Scale and the Patient-Specific Functional Scale scores after 8 weeks, indicating the supervised group had significantly more pain reduction and functional improvements than the unsupervised group. However, no between-group differences were found in back muscle endurance, the revised Oswestry Back Pain Disability Questionnaire scores, or the Global Rating of Change scores.

Additionally, Schroth exercises have been shown to improve lung vital capacity, strength, and postural improvements in outpatient adolescents (Otman, Kose, & Yakut, 2005). The Schroth Method is a conservative exercise approach designed to elongate the trunk, correct imbalances of the spine, and develop the inner muscles of the rib cage in order to change the shape of the upper trunk and improve spinal abnormalities. Training and certification courses in the Schroth Method are available as well as a handbook with over 100 scoliosis exercises, written by Christa Lehnert-Schroth, the daughter of Katharina Schroth, who founded the Schroth Method, and may be useful for therapists treating scoliosis. The central concept of Schroth is overcorrection of the laterally shifted section beyond midline to help reduce the deformity. Special equipment such as wall bars are instrumental in this approach.

The Schroth method follows a 3-step process:
1. First, make proper pelvic correction.
2. Do spinal elongation and then rotational angular breathing techniques to move spine and ribs into best possible posture.
3. Tense the trunk muscles isometrically in order to strengthen weak muscles to preserve corrected posture (Schroth Method, 2015).

Where's the Evidence?

Schreiber et al. (2015) assessed 50 patients with small adolescent idiopathic scoliosis, aged 10 to 18 years, with curves 10 to 45 degrees. They were randomized to receive standard of care or supervised Schroth exercises plus standard of care for 6 months. Schroth exercises were taught over 5 sessions in the first 2 weeks, after which a daily home program was adjusted during weekly supervised sessions. Outcomes were measured using outcomes included in the Biering-Sorensen test, Scoliosis Research Society, and Spinal Appearance Questionnaires scores. After 3 months, the Biering-Sorensen in the Schroth group improved by 32.3 seconds, and in the control by 4.8 seconds. From 3 to 6 months, the self-image improved in the Schroth group by 0.13 and deteriorated in the control by 0.17. A difference between groups for the change in the Scoliosis Research Society pain score was observed from 3 to 6 months, where pain decreased significantly more than the control group. Researchers noted that age, self-efficacy, brace wear, Schroth classification, and height had significant main effects on some outcomes. Overall, they concluded supervised Schroth exercises provided added benefit to the standard of care by improving Scoliosis Research Society pain, self-image scores, and the Biering-Sorensen. Yang, Lee, & Lee (2015) performed a case study with consecutive application of stretching, Schroth, and strengthening exercises in a 26-year-old woman with idiopathic scoliosis, Cobb's angle of 20.51 degrees, and back pain. The exercise program consisted of 3 sessions: 10 minutes of stretching exercises, 20 minutes of Schroth exercises, and 10 minutes of strengthening exercises, 3 times per week, for 8 weeks. After treatment was completed, thoracic Cobb's angle decreased from 20.51 degrees to 16.35 degrees, and the rib hump decreased from 15 degrees to 9 degrees, concluding the application of stretching, Schroth, and strengthening exercises may help reduce Cobb's angle and the rib hump in adults with idiopathic scoliosis.

4.06.12 Scoliosis Recommended Exercises

The key to implementing a program for scoliosis is proper identification of the curve(s) before beginning a program. Clinicians must tailor the program specifically to the patient's curve(s) to have positive outcomes.

Following is a basic protocol to improve pulmonary function and chest expansion, spine lengthening, self-mobilization for curve correction, and exercises to promote muscle balance.

1. Breathing techniques
   a. 3.03.7 Breathing Techniques: Diaphragmatic and Pursed-Lip Breathing
   b. 3.03.9 Breathing Techniques: Diaphragmatic Breathing With Upper Extremity Fixation and Isometric Lift
   c. 3.03.8 Breathing Techniques: Diaphragmatic Breathing With Upper Extremity Fixation
2. Curve correction: Encourage deep breathing during these stretches to expand rib cage on concave side.
   a. Performed lying on the convex side of the thoracic C-curve:
      i. 3.01.2 ROM: Upper Trunk Lateral Flexion, Passive
   b. Performed toward the convex side of the thoracic C-curve:
      i. 3.01.1 ROM: Upper Trunk Lateral Flexion, Active
      ii. 3.02.2 Stretch: Thoracic Flexion, "Child's Pose" or "Prayer Stretch," Add Side-Bend or Rotation
      iii. 3.03.2 Strengthen: Isotonic; Sternal Lift, 4-Way
      iv. 3.03.6 Strengthen: Isotonic; Thoracic Lateral Flexion, Arms Behind Head
3. Spine elongation: Symmetry exercises
   a. 3.01.14 ROM: Spine Elongations, Bar Hang
   b. 3.01.13 ROM: Spine Elongations, Wall Slide
4. Breathing; diaphragmatic and chest expansion.
   a. 3.03.8 Breathing Techniques: Diaphragmatic Breathing With Upper Extremity Fixation
   b. 3.03.10 Breathing Techniques: Chest Expansion Breathing With Upper Extremity Movements
   c. 3.03.9 Breathing Techniques: Diaphragmatic Breathing With Upper Extremity Fixation and Isometric Lift
5. Spine ROM: Symmetry exercises
   a. 3.01.4 ROM: Thoracic Flexion and Extension With and Without Cervical Extension, Cat and Camel
   b. 3.01.6 ROM: Thoracic Extension Over Foam Roll, Head Supported
   c. 3.01.7 ROM: Thoracic Extension Over Back of Chair, Head Supported
6. Spine strengthening: Symmetry exercises
   a. 3.03.1 Strengthen: Isometric; Sternal Lift
   b. 3.03.2 Strengthen: Isotonic; Sternal Lift, 4-Way
   c. 3.03.3 Strengthen: Isotonic; Sternal Lift With Shoulder Movements
   d. 3.03.12 Strengthen: Back-Arching Shoulder Press
   e. 4.03.15 Strengthen: Lumbar Spine, Lift All Fours, "Superman" and "Rocketman"
7. Other considerations
   a. Forward head correction:
      i. 2.01.1 ROM: Chin Tuck
      ii. 2.03.4 Strengthen: Isotonic; Chin Tuck
      iii. 2.03.5 Strengthen: Isotonic; Chin Tuck Neutral (Beginner) and With Slight Rotation (Advanced), Forehead on Towel Roll (Beginner) and Head off Bed (Advanced)
      iv. 2.03.8 Strengthen: Isotonic; Chin Tuck Cervical Flexion With Head Lift (Deep Neck Flexors)
      v. Stretching upper trapezius, scalenes, levator scapula, pectoralis major and minor, quadriceps, hamstrings, hip adductors
      vi. Core strengthening: curls ups, planks, bridge, lumbar stabilization, scapular stabilization, upper and lower body strengthening
      vii. Overall conditioning to improve cardiovascular function: swimming, cycling, rowing

---

Where's the Evidence?

Diab (2012) investigated the effectiveness of forward head correction on 3-dimensional posture parameters and functional level in 76 adolescent idiopathic scoliotic patients with Cobb angle ranged from 10 to 30 degrees and craniovertebral angle less than 50 degrees. All patients received traditional treatment in the form of stretching and strengthening exercises. In addition, patients in the study group received a forward head posture corrective exercise program. After 10 weeks and at 3-month follow-up, there was a significant difference between the study and control groups with respect to the following parameters: craniovertebral angle, trunk inclination, lordosis, kyphosis, trunk imbalance, lateral deviation, pelvic torsion, and surface rotation. At 3-month follow-up, there were still significant differences in all of the previous variables. In contrast, while there was no significant difference with respect to Functional Rating Index at 10 weeks, the 3-month follow-up showed a significant difference. Diab (2012) concluded a forward head corrective exercise program combined with conventional rehabilitation improved 3-dimensional scoliotic posture and functional status in patients with adolescent idiopathic scoliosis.

4.06.13 PREGNANCY DISCUSSION

LBP during pregnancy is not uncommon, occurring in up to 2 of 3 pregnancies. Additional pelvic pain is experienced in 1 of 5 pregnant women (Pennick & Liddel, 2013). Most cases are either anterior or posterior LBP. Weight pre-pregnancy, as well as weight gain during pregnancy, has been correlated to increased LBP during pregnancy (Mogren & Pohjanen, 2005). In addition to changes in weight and posture due to pregnancy, the hormone relaxin, which is normally released during pregnancy to assist in the stretching of the pubic symphysis to prepare for child birth, causes ligamentous laxity elsewhere and can lead to instability of the spine and SIJs leading to back pain; however, serum relaxin levels have not been correlated to pelvic pain incidence (Aldabe, Ribeiro, Milosavljevic, & Dawn Bussey, 2012; Björklund, Bergström, Nordström, & Ulmsten, 2000).

Where's the Evidence?

According to Pennick and Liddle (2013), moderate-quality evidence suggested that acupuncture or exercise, tailored to the stage of pregnancy, significantly reduced evening pelvic pain or lumbopelvic pain more than usual care alone, and acupuncture was significantly more effective than exercise for reducing evening pelvic pain. Low-quality evidence suggested that exercise significantly reduced pain and disability from LBP. Physical therapy, osteopathic manipulation, acupuncture, a multi-modal intervention, or the addition of a rigid pelvic belt to exercise seemed to relieve pelvic or back pain more than usual care alone. However, Gutke, Betten, Degerskär, Pousette, and Olsén (2015), in a more recent systematic review, found strong evidence for positive effects of acupuncture and pelvic belts on or LBP during pregnancy and low evidence for exercise in general and for specific stabilizing exercises. The evidence was also very limited for efficacy of water gymnastics, progressive muscle relaxation, a specific pelvic tilt exercise, osteopathic manual therapy, craniosacral therapy, electrotherapy, and yoga.

4.06.14 PREGNANCY RECOMMENDED EXERCISES

The protocol described is to illustrate some very basic and safe exercises for pregnant patients. Proper assessment is encouraged to identify the specific cause of the back pain in developing the best treatment.

1. Sleeping postures
   a. 4.04 Bed Positioning
      i. Side-lying quarter turn prone
      ii. Side-lying quarter turn supine
      iii. Side-lying both knees flexed
      iv. Side-lying top knee flexed
2. Stretching
   a. 6.03.3 Stretch: Hip Flexor, Standing Lunge; *avoid lumbar extension.*
   b. 6.08.1 Stretch: Quadriceps
   c. 6.08.3 Stretch: Hamstrings
   d. 6.13.5 Stretch: Gastrocnemius Using Strap
   e. 6.13.8 Stretch: Calf on Ramp
   f. 4.02.1 Stretch: Single Knee to Chest
   g. 4.02.2 Stretch: Double Knee to Chest, 3-Way; spread knees wide to allow room for stomach as needed.
   h. 3.02.11 Stretch: Thoracic, Golfer's Rotation and Side-Bend
   i. 6.03.22 Stretch: Piriformis, Figure 4 and Variations
   j. 3.01.4 ROM: Thoracic Flexion and Extension With and Without Cervical Extension, Cat and Camel
   k. 3.02.2 Stretch: Thoracic Flexion, "Child's Pose" or "Prayer Stretch," Add Side-Bend or Rotation
3. Lumbar Stabilization (also affects SIJ)
   a. 4.03.1 Strengthen: Isometric; Posterior Pelvic Tilt, Lumbar Spine, With or Without Blood Pressure Cuff for Biofeedback
   b. 4.03.2 Strengthen: Isometric; Neutral Spine, Lumbar Spine Stabilization
   c. 4.03.4 Strengthen: Lumbar Spine, Alternating and Bilateral Heel Slide
   d. 4.03.7 Strengthen: Lumbar Spine, Bent-Knee Fall-Outs
   e. 4.03.8 Strengthen: Lumbar Spine, Arm Lift Overhead
   f. 4.03.9 Strengthen: Lumbar Spine, Bent-Knee Lift
   g. 4.03.10 Strengthen: Lumbar Spine, Heel Slide Abduction and Adduction
   h. 4.03.11 Strengthen: Lumbar Spine, Opposite Arm and Bent-Knee Lift

    i. 4.03.12 Strengthen: Lumbar Spine, Bilateral Arm Lift Overhead With Knee Extension

    j. 4.03.14 Strengthen: Lumbar Spine, Alternating Arm Lift, Leg Lift, and Combined

4. SIJ specific stabilization ideas

    a. 6.04.3 Strengthen: Isometric; Hip Abduction (hook-lying with belt version)

    b. 6.04.4 Strengthen: Isometric; Hip Adduction

    c. 6.04.5 Strengthen: Isometric; Hip Internal Rotation

    d. 6.04.6 Strengthen: Isometric; Hip External Rotation

    e. 6.04.14 Strengthen: Isotonic; Hip Extension, Bridge and Variations

5. More advanced abdominal ideas; perform only beginner versions of sit-up, leg lowers and planks.

    a. 4.03.33 Strengthen: Abdominal, Partial Sit-Up, 5-Way

    b. 4.03.34 Strengthen: Abdominal, Partial Diagonal Sit-Up, 4-Way

    c. 4.03.35 Strengthen: Abdominal, Posterior Pelvic Tilt, Leg Lowers

    d. 4.03.38 Strengthen: Abdominal, Plank and Variations

    e. 4.03.39 Strengthen: Abdominal, Side Plank and Variations

    f. 4.03.61 Strengthen: Exercise Ball, Abdominal, Roll-Out

6. Other ideas for overall conditioning while minimizing stress to the lower back and pelvis.

    a. Walking, swimming, gentle water aerobics, tai chi, recumbent bicycle

REFERENCES

Adams, M. A., May, S., Freeman, B. J., Morrison, H. P., & Dolan, P. (2000). Effects of backward bending on lumbar intervertebral discs. Relevance to physical therapy treatments for low back pain. *Spine, 25*(4), 431-437.

Aebi, M. (2005). The adult scoliosis. *European Spine Journal, 14*(10), 925-948.

Aldabe, D., Ribeiro, D. C., Milosavljevic, S., & Dawn Bussey, M. (2012). Pregnancy-related pelvic girdle pain and its relationship with relaxin levels during pregnancy: A systematic review. *European Spine Journal, 21*(9), 1769-1776.

Björklund, K., Bergström, S., Nordström, M. L., & Ulmsten, U. (2000). Symphyseal distention in relation to serum relaxin levels and pelvic pain in pregnancy. *Acta Obstetricia Gynecologica Scandinavica, 79*(4), 269-275.

Brumitt, J., Matheson, J. W., & Meira, E. P. (2013). Core stabilization exercise prescription, part 2: A systematic review of motor control and general (global) exercise rehabilitation approaches for patients with low back pain. *Sports Health, 5*(6), 510-513.

Cormond, M., De Mesmaeker, M., Lowe, R., Myracle, M., & Thomas, E. (2016). Spondylolisthesis. *Physiopedia.* Retrieved from http://www.physio-pedia.com/Spondylolisthesis#cite_note-Garet-3

Costa, L. O., Maher, C. G., Latimer, J., Hodges, P. W., Herbert, R. D., Refshauge, K. M., . . . Jennings, M. D. (2009). Motor control exercise for chronic low back pain: A randomized placebo-controlled trial. *Physical Therapy, 89*(12), 1275-1286.

Delitto, A., Piva, S. R., Moore, C. G., Fritz, J. M., Wisniewski, S. R., Josbeno, D. A., . . . Welch, W. C. (2015). Surgery versus nonsurgical treatment of lumbar spinal stenosis: A randomized trial. *Annals of Internal Medicine, 162*(7), 465-473.

DePuy Acromed. (2003). Adult scoliosis. *University of Maryland Medical Center.* Retrieved from http://umm.edu/programs/spine/health/guides/adult-scoliosis

Diab, A. A. (2012). The role of forward head correction in management of adolescent idiopathic scoliotic patients: A randomized controlled trial. *Clinical Rehabilitation, 26*(12), 1123-1132.

Ekstrom, R. A., Osborn, R. W., & Hauer, P. L. (2008). Surface electromyographic analysis of the low back muscles during rehabilitation exercises. *Journal of Orthopedic Sports Physical Therapy, 38*(12), 736-745.

Ferrari, S., Vanti, C., & O'Reilly, C. (2012). Clinical presentation and physiotherapy treatment of 4 patients with low back pain and isthmic spondylolisthesis. *Journal of Chiropractic Medicine, 11*(2), 94-103.

Garet, M., Reiman, M. P., Mathers, J., & Sylvain, J. (2013). Nonoperative treatment in lumbar spondylolysis and spondylolisthesis: A systematic review. *Sports Health, 5*(3), 225-232.

Gutke, A., Betten, C., Degerskär, K., Pousette, S., & Olsén, M. F. (2015). Treatments for pregnancy-related lumbopelvic pain: A systematic review of physiotherapy modalities. *Acta Obstetricia Gynecologica Scandinavica, 94*(11), 1156-1167.

Hawes, M. C. (2003). The use of exercises in the treatment of scoliosis: An evidence-based critical review of the literature. *Pediatric Rehabilitation, 6*(3-4), 171-182.

Hayden, J. A., van Tulder, M. W., Malmivaara, A., & Koes, B. W. (2005). Exercise therapy for treatment of non-specific low back pain. *Cochrane Database of Systematic Reviews,* (3), CD000335.

Hicks, G. E., Fritz, J. M., Delitto, A., & McGill, S. M. (2005). Preliminary development of a clinical prediction rule for determining which patients with low back pain will respond to a stabilization exercise program. *Archives of Physical Medicine & Rehabilitation, 86*(9), 1753-1762.

Hides, J., Wilson, S., Stanton, W., McMahon, S., Keto, H., McMahon, K., . . . Richardson, C. (2006). An MRI investigation into the function of the transversus abdominis muscle during "drawing-in" of the abdominal wall. *Spine, 31*(6), 175-178.

Laslett, M. (2008). Evidence-based diagnosis and treatment of the painful sacroiliac joint. *Journal of Manual & Manipulative Therapy, 16*(3), 142-152.

Lee, H. S. (2015). Enhanced muscle activity during lumbar extension exercise with pelvic stabilization. *Journal of Exercise Rehabilitation, 11*(6), 372-377.

Lee, S. H., Kim, T. H., & Lee, B. H. (2014). The effect of abdominal bracing in combination with low extremity movements on changes in thickness of abdominal muscles and lumbar strength for low back pain. *Journal of Physical Therapy Science, 26*(1), 157-160.

Lu, M., Simon, L., Ritchie, L., Brachotte, F., & Van Haver, E. (n.d.). Lumbar spinal stenosis. *Physiopedia.* Retrieved from http://www.physio-pedia.com/Spinal_Stenosis

Macedo, L. G., Maher, C. G., Latimer, J., & McAuley, J. H. (2009). Motor control exercise for persistent, nonspecific low back pain: A systematic review. *Physical Therapy, 89*(1), 9-25.

Massé-Alarie, H., Beaulieu, L. D., Preuss, R., & Schneider, C. (2015). Corticomotor control of lumbar multifidus muscles is impaired in chronic low back pain: Concurrent evidence from ultrasound imaging and double-pulse transcranial magnetic stimulation. *Experimental Brain Research, 234*(4), 1033-1045.

Mbada, E. M., Ayanniyi, O., Ogunlade, S. O., Orimolade, E. A., Oladiran, A. B., & Ogundele, A. O. (2014). Influence of McKenzie protocol and two modes of endurance exercises on health-related quality of life of patients with long-term mechanical low-back pain. *Pan African Medical Journal, 17*(Suppl 1), 5.

Mogren, I. M., Pohjanen, A. I. (2005). Low back pain and pelvic pain during pregnancy: Prevalence and risk factors. *Spine, 30*(8), 983-991.

Mooney, V., Pozos, R., Vleeming, A., Gulick, J., & Swenski, D. (2001). Exercise treatment for sacroiliac pain. *Orthopedics, 24*(1), 29-32.

Negrini, S., Fusco, C., Minozzi, S., Atanasio, S., Zaina, F., & Romano, M. (2008). Exercises reduce the progression rate of adolescent idiopathic scoliosis: Results of a comprehensive systematic review of the literature. *Disability & Rehabilitation, 30*(10), 772-785.

Otman, S., Kose, N., & Yakut, Y. (2005). The efficacy of Schroth's 3-dimensional exercise therapy in the treatment of adolescent idiopathic scoliosis in Turkey. *Saudi Medical Journal, 26*(9), 1429-1435.

Pennick, V., & Liddle, S. D. (2013). Interventions for preventing and treating pelvic and back pain in pregnancy. *Cochrane Database of Systematic Reviews,* (8), CD001139.

Petersen, T., Larsen, K., Nordsteen, J., Olsen, S., Fournier, G., & Jacobsen, S. (2011). The McKenzie method compared with manipulation when used adjunctive to information and advice in low back pain patients presenting with centralization or peripheralization: A randomized controlled trial. *Spine, 36*(24), 1999-2010.

Richardson, C. A., Snijders, C. J., Hides, J. A., Damen, L., Pas, M. S., & Storm, J. (2002). The relation between the transversus abdominis muscles, sacroiliac joint mechanics, and low back pain. *Spine, 27*(4), 399-405.

Schreiber, S., Parent, E. C., Moez, E. K., Hedden, D. M., Hill, D., Moreau, M. J., . . . Southon, S. C. (2015). The effect of Schroth exercises added to the standard of care on the quality of life and muscle endurance in adolescents with idiopathic scoliosis-an assessor and statistician blinded randomized controlled trial: "SOSORT 2015 Award Winner". *Scoliosis, 10,* 24.

Schroth Method. (2015). Schroth exercises for scoliosis. Retrieved from http://www.schrothmethod.com/scoliosis-exercises

Sinaki, M., Lutness, M. P., Ilstrup, D. M., Chu, C. P., & Gramse, R. R. (1989). Lumbar spondylolisthesis: Retrospective comparison and three-year follow-up of two conservative treatment programs. *Archives of Physical Medicine & Rehabilitation, 70*(8), 594-598.

Southeast Georgia Health System. (2013). Post-surgical rehabilitation protocol: Lumbar laminectomy/diskectomy/rusion. Retrieved from http://www.sghs.org/fullpanel/uploads/files/lumbar-fusion-protocol-05-13-2013.pdf

Tourwe, J., Pagare, V., Buxton, S., Thomas, E.; Vrije Universiteit Brussel's Evidence-Based Practice project. (n.d.). McKenzie method. *Physiopedia.* Retrieved from http://www.physio-pedia.com/McKenzie_Method

Yang, J. M., Lee, J. H., & Lee, D. H. (2015). Effects of consecutive application of stretching, Schroth, and strengthening exercises on Cobb's angle and the rib hump in an adult with idiopathic scoliosis. *Journal of Physical Therapy Science, 27*(8), 2667-2669.

Zapata, K. A., Wang-Price, S. S., Sucato, D. J., Thompson, M., Trudelle-Jackson, E., & Lovelace-Chandler, V. (2015). Spinal stabilization exercise effectiveness for low back pain in adolescent idiopathic scoliosis: A randomized trial. *Pediatric Physical Therapy, 27*(4), 396-402.

Chapter 5

UPPER EXTREMITY EXERCISES

Bryan E. *The Comprehensive Manual of Therapeutic Exercises:*
Orthopedic and General Conditions (pp 165-358).
© 2018 SLACK Incorporated.

Section 5.01

SCAPULAR RANGE OF MOTION

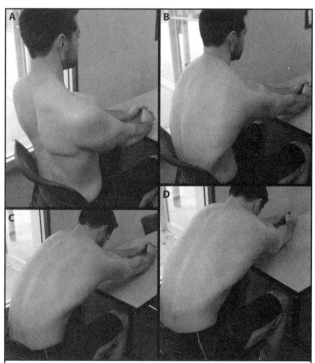

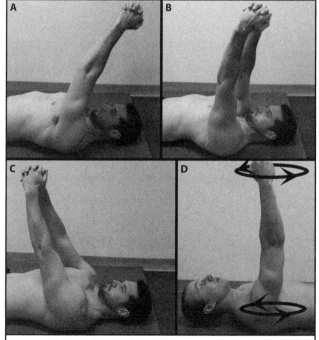

5.01.1 ROM: SCAPULAR PROTRACTION AND UPWARD ROTATION, RETRACTION AND DOWNWARD ROTATION

POSITION: Seated

TARGETS: Mobility of the scapula into protraction and upward rotation, retraction, and downward rotation

INSTRUCTION: Seated with feet flat on floor facing a table, patient places clasped hands on table (A). Patient fully retracts scapula, pinching together, then protracts the scapula, actively reaching forward, sliding hands forward on table (B). Patient then leans forward to increase upward rotation (C). This can also be done diagonally toward each side to target opposite scapula (D).

SUBSTITUTIONS: Shrugging shoulders

PARAMETERS: Hold long enough to take 1 breath, repeat 10 to 15 times depending on treatment goals, 1 to 3 times per day

5.01.2 ROM: SCAPULAR "AROUND THE WORLD"

POSITION: Supine

TARGETS: Mobility of the scapula and gaining control of scapular movements by facilitating contraction of scapular stabilizing muscles (rhomboids, upper trapezius, middle trapezius, lower trapezius, and serratus anterior)

INSTRUCTION: Patient reaches toward the ceiling, clasping hands together, then makes large circular movements as if drawing circles on the ceiling with scapular movements into protraction, depression, retraction, and elevation clockwise for one set and then counter-clockwise. This can be assisted with the other hand (A through C) performed with one arm only (D).

SUBSTITUTIONS: Using the shoulder to move hands in a circle; this motion comes from the scapulothoracic joint, not the shoulder.

PARAMETERS: 10 to 20 times each direction, 1 set, 1 to 3 times per day

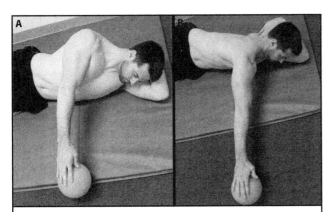

5.01.3 ROM: Scapular Protraction and Retraction Using Ball, Active

Position: Side-lying

Targets: Mobility of the scapula into protraction and retraction, gaining control of scapular movements by facilitating contraction of scapular stabilizing muscles (rhomboids, middle and lower trapezius, serratus anterior)

Instruction: Place an 8- to 10-inch ball under the top palm, shoulder flexed 90 degrees and elbow extended. Patient rolls ball forward, activating the serratus anterior and protracting the scapula, then rolls ball back toward patient by activating the scapular retractors and pinching the scapula in toward the spine (A and B).

Substitutions: Using the shoulder to move the ball; this motion comes from the scapulothoracic joint and not the shoulder.

Parameters: 10 to 20 times each direction, 1 set, 1 to 3 times per day

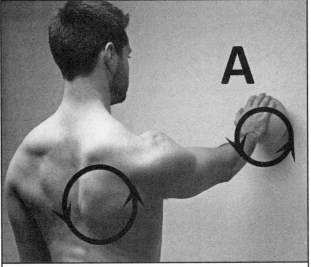

5.01.4 ROM: Scapular Circles and Alphabet Ball on Wall

Position: Standing

Targets: Mobility of the scapula, gaining control of scapular movements by facilitating contraction of scapular stabilizing muscles (rhomboids, upper trapezius, middle trapezius, lower trapezius, and serratus anterior) to improve proprioception.

Instruction: Patient faces a wall. Place a small ball under the palm of hand at shoulder level. Patient steps away from the wall until elbow is extended and the shoulder is at 90 degrees of flexion. Patient initiates small circles with the scapula to rolls ball in small circles. Perform one full set clockwise before repeating counterclockwise. Patient can also "write" imaginary letters of the alphabet with the middle of the palm as another alternative to increase proprioception.

Substitutions: Using the shoulder to move the ball in a circle; this motion comes from the scapulothoracic joint and not the shoulder.

Parameters: 10 to 20 times each direction, 1 set, 1 to 3 times per day

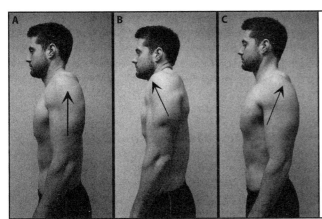

5.01.5 ROM: Scapular Elevation

Position: Standing, seated

Targets: Mobility of the scapula into elevation

Instruction: *Shrug*: Patient shrugs shoulders up toward ears, lowers and repeats (A). To add variation, ask patient to shrug up and forward or up and back to target different regions of the upper trapezius (B and C).

Substitutions: Jutting chin forward

Parameters: 10 to 20 times, 1 to 3 times per day

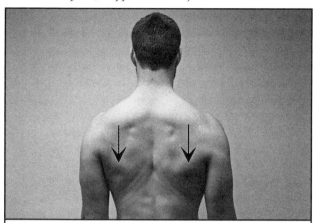

5.01.6 ROM: Scapular Depression

Position: Standing, seated

Targets: Mobility of the scapula into depression

Instruction: Patient actively depresses shoulders, pulling them further away from the ears while slightly retracting scapula, relaxes and repeats.

Substitutions: Jutting chin forward

Parameters: 10 to 20 times, 1 to 3 times per day

Where's the Evidence?

Smith et al. (2006) studied EMG activity in the immobilized shoulder girdle musculature during scapulothoracic exercises. Smith and colleagues monitored supraspinatus, infraspinatus, upper subscapularis, deltoids, trapezii, biceps and serratus anterior electrodes during scapular clock, elevation, depression, protraction, and retraction exercises completed during a single testing session in random order. Biceps activity was uniformly low, < 20% MVC, whereas upper subscapularis activity was uniformly high, 40% to 63% MVC. Both scapular depression and protraction elicited low activity, < 20% MVC in the supraspinatus, infraspinatus, anterior deltoid, and biceps brachii muscles, while generally producing high activity, > 20% MVC in the trapezii and serratus anterior. Scapular depression produced the largest serratus anterior activity, 47% MVC. They concluded that during periods of shoulder immobilization, (1) scapular depression and protraction exercises could potentially be safely performed after RC repair to facilitate scapulothoracic rehabilitation, (2) all exercises studied could potentially be safe after superior labral anteroposterior shoulder repair, and (3) all exercises studied should be avoided after subscapularis repair.

Reference

Smith, J., Dahm, D. L., Kufman, K. R., Boon, A. J., Laskowski, E. R., Kotajarvi, B. R., & Jacofsky, D. J., (2006). Electromyographic activity in the immobilized shoulder girdle musculature during scapulothoracic exercises. *Archives of Physical Medicine and Rehabilitation, 87*(7) 923-927.

Section 5.02

SCAPULAR STRETCHING

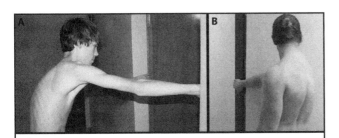

5.02.1 STRETCH: SCAPULAR, DOOR PULL

POSITION: Standing

TARGETS: Mobility of the scapula into protraction, stretching of rhomboid and middle trapezius

INSTRUCTION: Standing in front of a doorway, patient turn palms outward with thumbs down and grasps door frame on each side. Patient then steps back and leans posteriorly until stretch is felt between scapulae (A). This can also be done unilaterally for a more intense stretch by grasping with only one hand and stepping back, allowing body to rotate slightly toward the outstretched hand, and leaning posteriorly (B).

SUBSTITUTIONS: Shrugging shoulders

PARAMETERS: Hold for 15 to 30 seconds, 3 to 5 repetitions, 1 to 3 times per day

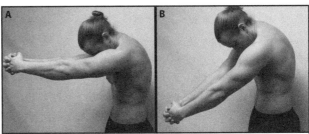

5.02.2 STRETCH: SCAPULAR PROTRACTION, HAND GRASP

POSITION: Seated, standing

TARGETS: Mobility of the scapula into protraction while stretching rhomboid and middle trapezius, downward orientation will also stretch the upper trapezius.

INSTRUCTION: Patient clasps hands in front, shoulders at 90 degrees and elbows extended. Patient protracts scapula as far as possible, reaching hands out further, chin stays tucked (A). Dropping the arms to 45 degrees of shoulder flexion will target the upper trapezius (B).

SUBSTITUTIONS: Shrugging shoulders

PARAMETERS: Hold for 15 to 30 seconds, 3 to 5 repetitions, 1 to 3 times per day

Section 5.03

SCAPULAR STRENGTHENING

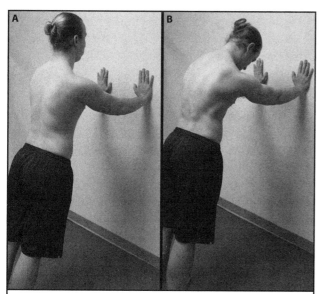

5.03.1 STRENGTHEN: SCAPULAR, PUSH-UP PLUS (BEGINNER)

POSITION: Standing

TARGETS: Strengthen serratus anterior; this is a beginner exercise with no weightbearing through the UE.

INSTRUCTION: Patient positions palms on wall at shoulder height, feet 6 to 12 inches from wall. Patient pushes away from the wall into scapular protraction, rounding upper back slightly. Patient then leans toward wall, allowing elbows to bend, until reaching the upper torso. Press away from the wall, like a push-up, and continue until scapulae are fully protracted and elbows are extended (A and B).

SUBSTITUTIONS: Shrugging shoulders, excessive thoracic flexion

PARAMETERS: 10 repetitions each side, up to 3 sets, 1 time per day or every other day

Where's the Evidence?

During maximum humeral elevation, the scapula normally upwardly rotates 45 to 55 degrees, posterior tilts 20 to 40 degrees, and externally rotates 15 to 35 degrees. The scapular muscles are important during humeral elevation because they cause these motions, especially the serratus anterior, which contributes to scapular upward rotation, posterior tilt, and external rotation. The serratus anterior also helps stabilize the medial border and inferior angle of the scapular, preventing scapular internal rotation (winging), and anterior tilt. If normal scapular movements are disrupted by abnormal scapular muscle firing patterns, weakness, fatigue, or injury, the shoulder complex functions less efficiently and risk of injury increases. Scapula position and humeral rotation can affect injury risk during humeral elevation. Compared with scapular protraction, scapular retraction has been shown to both increase subacromial space width and enhance supraspinatus force production during humeral elevation. Moreover, scapular internal rotation and scapular anterior tilt, both decrease subacromial space width and increase impingement risk (Escamilla, Yamashiro, Paulos, & Andrews, 2009).

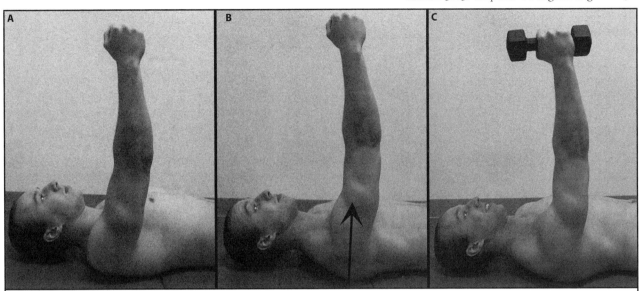

5.03.2 STRENGTHEN: SCAPULAR, CEILING PUNCH

<u>POSITION</u>: Supine

<u>TARGETS</u>: Strengthen serratus anterior

<u>INSTRUCTION</u>: Patient brings shoulder into 90 degrees of flexion with fisted hand, thumb pointing toward the head, protracts scapula then reaches fist closer toward ceiling (A). Patient may use both arms and a cane (B) or add weight for increased intensity (C).

<u>SUBSTITUTIONS</u>: Shrugging shoulders, rotating thoracic spine; this movement can be accomplished with upper trapezius shrug and should be monitored closely. Tapping the serratus will help facilitate the patient's understanding of from where the movement comes.

<u>PARAMETERS</u>: 10 repetitions per side, up to 3 sets, 1 time day or every other day

---

Where's the Evidence?

Decker, Hintermeister, Faber, and Hawkins (1999) studied EMG activity and applied resistance associated with 8 scapulohumeral exercises performed below shoulder height. The following exercises were studied: shoulder extension, forward punch, serratus anterior punch, dynamic hug, scaption (with external rotation), press-up, push-up plus, and knee push-up plus. EMG data were collected from the middle serratus anterior, upper trapezius and middle trapezius, and anterior and posterior deltoid. Resistance was provided by body weight, elastic cord, or dumbbells. The serratus anterior punch, scaption, dynamic hug, knee push-up plus, and push-up plus exercises consistently elicited serratus anterior muscle activity > 20% MVC. The exercises that maintained an upwardly rotated scapula while accentuating scapular protraction, such as the push-up plus and dynamic hug, elicited the greatest EMG activity from the serratus anterior muscle.

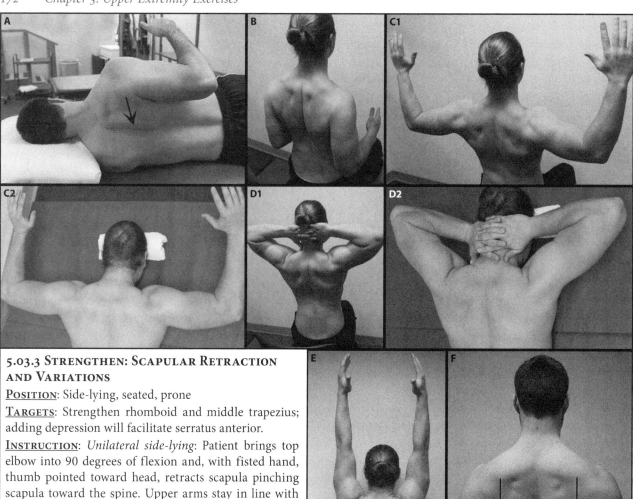

5.03.3 STRENGTHEN: SCAPULAR RETRACTION AND VARIATIONS

POSITION: Side-lying, seated, prone

TARGETS: Strengthen rhomboid and middle trapezius; adding depression will facilitate serratus anterior.

INSTRUCTION: *Unilateral side-lying*: Patient brings top elbow into 90 degrees of flexion and, with fisted hand, thumb pointed toward head, retracts scapula pinching scapula toward the spine. Upper arms stay in line with torso. Do not allow patient to extend shoulder past neutral. Relax and repeat (A). *Bilateral seated*: Patient bends elbows to 90 degrees of flexion and, with fisted hand, thumb pointed toward head, retracts scapula pinching scapula toward the spine. Upper arms stay in line with torso. Do not allow patient to extend shoulder past neutral. Relax and repeat (B). *90/90 with external rotation*: Patient bends elbows to 90 degrees of flexion, flexes shoulder to 90 degrees and externally rotates shoulder, thumb pointed toward head patient retracts scapula, pinching scapula toward the spine. Upper arms stay in line with torso. Do not allow patient to extend shoulder past neutral. Relax and repeat (C1). This can also be done prone to add gravity resistance. Place towel roll under forehead to neutralize neck position (C2). *Hands clasped behind head*: Repeat instructions for *90/90 with external rotation*, but have the patient clasp the hands behind the head (D1). This can also be done prone to add gravity resistance. Place towel roll under forehead to neutralize neck position (D2). *Retraction arms overhead*: Patient stands with arms extended overhead and performs scapular retraction, holds squeeze 2 to 3 seconds (E). *Add depression*: For any of the above exercises, the therapist can cue patient to add depression of the scapula with retraction by asking patient to "tuck shoulder blades into the back pockets" (F).

SUBSTITUTIONS: Shrugging shoulders, thoracic extension rather than retraction, extending shoulder past neutral

PARAMETERS: Hold pinch 3 to 5 seconds, 10 repetitions, up to 3 sets, 1 time per day or every other day

Where's the Evidence?

Smith et al. (2006) studied EMG activity in the shoulder girdle musculature during scapulothoracic exercises performed in a shoulder immobilizer in asymptomatic men. Electrodes recorded EMG activity from each muscle during scapular clock—elevation, depression, protraction, and retraction—exercises completed during a single testing session in random order. Biceps activity was uniformly low, whereas upper subscapularis activity was uniformly high. Both scapular depression and protraction elicited low activity in the supraspinatus, infraspinatus, anterior deltoid, and biceps brachii. muscles, while generally producing greater activity in the trapezii and serratus. Scapular depression produced the largest serratus anterior activity. These data are the first to describe the EMG activity during scapulothoracic exercises while in a shoulder immobilizer. Based on electrophysiological data in normal volunteers, the findings suggest that during periods of shoulder immobilization, (1) scapular depression and protraction exercises could potentially be safely performed after RC repair to facilitate scapulothoracic rehabilitation, (2) all exercises studied could potentially be safe after superior labral anteroposterior shoulder repair, and (3) all exercises studied should be avoided after subscapularis repair.

Castelein, Cools, Parlevliet, and Cagnie (2015) compared muscle activity using both surface and fine-wire electrodes of the medial scapular muscles during different shoulder joint positions while performing shrug and retraction exercises. They found the "retraction overhead" was the most effective exercise in activating the medial scapular muscles (rhomboid major, middle and lower trapezius).

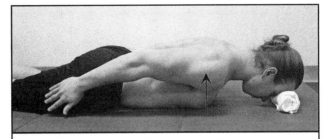

5.03.4 STRENGTHEN: SCAPULAR RETRACTION, ARMS BY SIDES

POSITION: Prone

TARGETS: Strengthen rhomboid, middle trapezius, and posterior RC

INSTRUCTION: *Straight*: Place towel roll under forehead to neutralize neck position. With arms down by the sides, palms facing inward and thumbs down, patient retracts scapula, pinching scapula toward spine with a slight lift in the arms, rolling shoulders back. The arms stay in line with torso. Do not allow patient to extend shoulder past neutral. Relax and repeat. *Behind back*: Patient can also externally rotate shoulders further, bringing hands behind the lower back so that thumb has rotated around to point at ceiling. These can be done unilaterally or bilaterally. Weight may be added for increased resistance.

SUBSTITUTIONS: Shrugging shoulders, thoracic extension rather than retraction, excessive translation of humeral head anteriorly, lifting head; cue patient to bring shoulders "back and down."

PARAMETERS: Hold pinch 3 to 5 seconds, 10 repetitions, up to 3 sets, 1 time per day or every other day

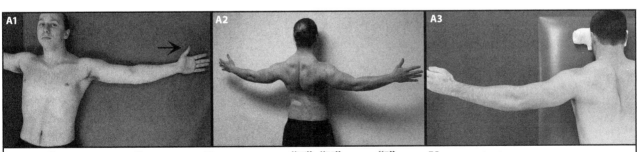

5.03.5 STRENGTHEN: SCAPULAR RETRACTION, "T", "Y", AND "I" AND VARIATIONS

POSITION: Prone, supine

TARGETS: "Y": Strengthen lower trapezius, "T": Strengthen posterior deltoid, rhomboid, and middle trapezius, "I": Strengthen anterior deltoid and lower trapezius, and "W": Strengthen posterior deltoid and lower trapezius

INSTRUCTION: *"T" palm up beginner isometric*: In supine, patient places shoulder in 120 degrees of abduction palm up. Patient retracts scapula, pressing arm into mat (A1). *"T" palm forward facing wall*: Standing facing wall, patient places shoulder in 120 degrees of abduction, palms forward. Patient retracts scapula lifting arm away from wall (A2). *"T" palm down advanced prone*: Place towel roll under forehead to neutralize neck position. With shoulder at 90 degrees of abduction, palms facing down, patient retracts scapula, pinching scapula toward the spine with a slight lift in the arms, rolling shoulders back. The arms stay in line with the torso. Do not allow patient to horizontally abduct excessively which forces humeral head anteriorly. Relax and repeat (A3). *(continued)*

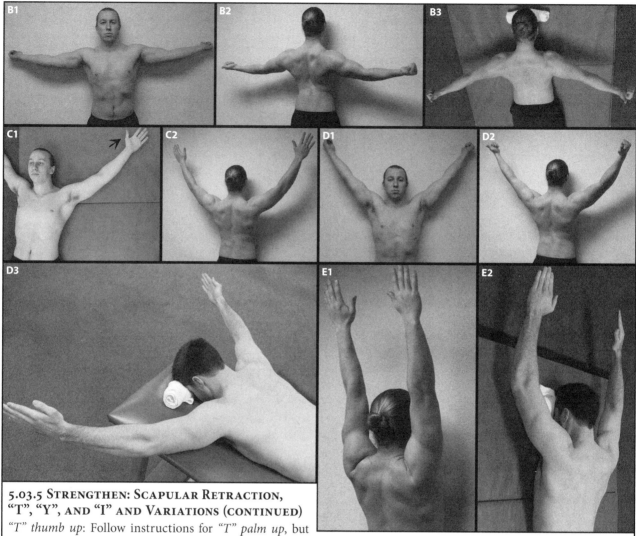

5.03.5 STRENGTHEN: SCAPULAR RETRACTION, "T", "Y", AND "I" AND VARIATIONS (CONTINUED)

"T" thumb up: Follow instructions for *"T" palm up*, but change hand position to thumbs up (thumbs point posteriorly) (B1 through B3).

"Y" palm up isometric beginner: As this exercise is challenging, it may be a good idea for the patient to start in a gravity-assisted position of supine. With shoulder at 120 degrees of abduction, palms facing forward, patient retracts scapula, pinching scapula toward the spine while pushing arms into table or wall (C1). *"Y" Standing facing wall palm forward*: Patient stands against and facing a wall, palms on wall. Patient brings arms off wall by retracting scapula back and down (C2). *"Y" prone palm down advanced*: Place towel roll under forehead to neutralize neck position. With shoulder at 120 degrees of abduction palms facing down, patient retracts scapula, pinching scapula toward the spine with a slight lift in the arms, rolling shoulders back. The arms stay in line with the torso. Do not allow patient to horizontally abduct excessively, which forces humeral head anteriorly. Relax and repeat (not shown). *"Y" thumb up*: Follow instructions for *"Y" palm up*, but change hand position to thumbs up (thumbs point posteriorly) (D1 through D3). *"I" Palm forward isometric beginner*: As this exercise is challenging, it may be a good idea for patient to start in a gravity-assisted position of supine. With shoulder at 170 to 180 degrees of abduction, palms facing forward, patient retracts scapula, pinching scapula toward the spine while pushing arms into table or wall (not shown). *"I" Standing facing wall, palm forward*: Patient stands against and facing a wall, palms on wall. Patient brings arms off wall by retracting scapula back and down (E1). *"I" prone palm down advanced*: Place towel roll under forehead to neutralize neck position. With shoulder at 120 degrees of abduction, palms facing down, patient retracts scapula, pinching scapula toward the spine with a slight lift in the arms, rolling shoulders back. The arms stay in line with the torso. Do not allow patient to horizontally abduct excessively, which forces humeral head anteriorly. Relax and repeat (E2). *(continued)*

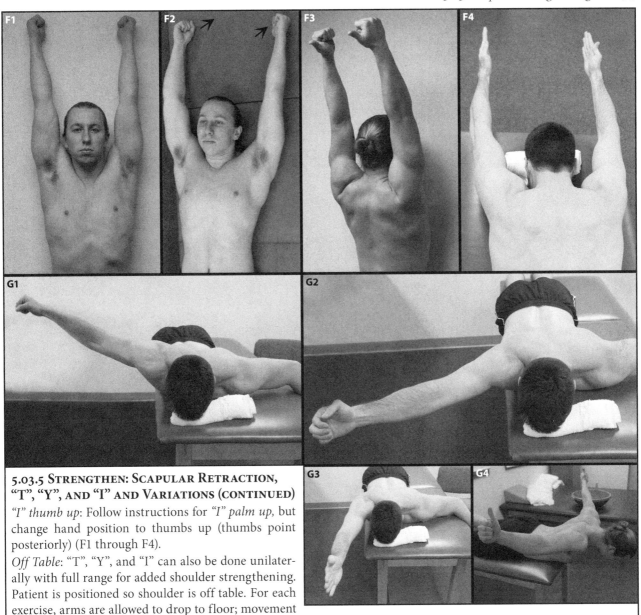

5.03.5 STRENGTHEN: SCAPULAR RETRACTION, "T", "Y", AND "I" AND VARIATIONS (CONTINUED)

"I" thumb up: Follow instructions for *"I" palm up*, but change hand position to thumbs up (thumbs point posteriorly) (F1 through F4).

Off Table: "T", "Y", and "I" can also be done unilaterally with full range for added shoulder strengthening. Patient is positioned so shoulder is off table. For each exercise, arms are allowed to drop to floor; movement follows same instructions while bringing arms up toward ceiling (G1 through G3). To do this bilaterally, bring edge of mat to mid-sternal level, dropping both arms off the front of the table (G4).

SUBSTITUTIONS: Shrugging shoulders excessively; "T" can be done with no upper trapezius, but "Y" and "I" will have some normal recruitment of the upper trapezius; thoracic extension rather than retraction, excessive translation of humeral head anteriorly, lifting head.

PARAMETERS: Hold pinch 3 to 5 seconds, 10 repetitions, up to 3 sets, 1 time per day or every other day

5.03.6 STRENGTHEN: SCAPULAR RETRACTION, ARM OFF TABLE

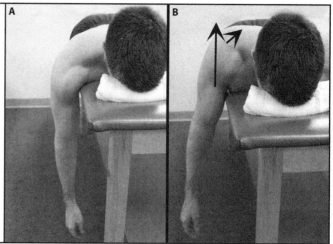

POSITION: Prone

TARGETS: Strengthen rhomboid and middle trapezius

INSTRUCTION: Place towel roll under forehead to neutralize neck position. With arm and shoulder hanging off the side of the bed, allow arm to drop toward the floor, protracting scapula. Patient retracts scapula, pinching scapula toward the spine, with a slight lift in the arm, rolling shoulder back, elbow stays extended. Relax and repeat (A and B).

SUBSTITUTIONS: Shrugging shoulders, thoracic rotation rather than retraction, lifting head

PARAMETERS: Hold pinch 3 to 5 seconds, 10 repetitions, up to 3 sets, 1 time per day or every other day

5.03.7 STRENGTHEN: SCAPULAR RETRACTION AND DEPRESSION WITH WALL SQUAT

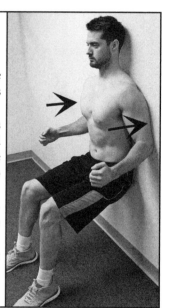

POSITION: 90/90 LE wall squat (or less than 90 at hips depending on LE strength)

TARGETS: Strengthen rhomboid, middle and lower trapezius, while encouraging deep core stabilizers of the trunk to activate; in LE, quadriceps, hamstrings and gluteus maximus are targeted.

INSTRUCTION: Feet are hip-width apart. Patient leans against wall with the back and walks feet out to 90/90 LE position. Patient bends elbows to 90 degrees of flexion with fisted hand and thumb pointing toward the ceiling, retracting scapula, pinching scapula toward the spine while simultaneously depressing scapula. Ask patient to "tuck shoulder blades into the back pockets." Head, shoulders, and buttocks stay against the wall. Relax and repeat.

SUBSTITUTIONS: Shrugging shoulders, thoracic extension rather than retraction, extending shoulder past neutral, torso comes off wall, engaging deep core muscles required to maintain neutral lumbar spine.

PARAMETERS: Hold pinch 3 to 5 seconds, 10 repetitions, up to 3 sets, 1 time per day or every other day

5.03.8 STRENGTHEN: SCAPULAR RETRACTION, "W" OR "BATWINGS"

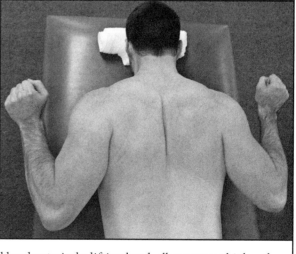

POSITION: Prone

TARGETS: Strengthens rhomboid; these can be done unilaterally or bilaterally.

INSTRUCTION: Place towel roll under forehead to neutralize neck position. With shoulder at 30 degrees of abduction, elbow fully flexed, palms facing down, patient retracts scapula, pinching scapula toward the spine with a slight lift in the arms, rolling shoulders back. The wrist and elbow stay in the same horizontal plane. Do not allow patient to extend shoulder excessively which forces humeral head anteriorly. Relax and repeat. These can all be done unilaterally or bilaterally, and weight may be added for increased resistance.

SUBSTITUTIONS: Shrugging shoulders excessively, thoracic extension rather than retraction, excessive translation of humeral head anteriorly, lifting head; elbow comes higher than wrist, which should be in same horizontal plane.

PARAMETERS: Hold pinch 3 to 5 seconds, 10 repetitions, up to 3 sets, 1 time per day or every other day

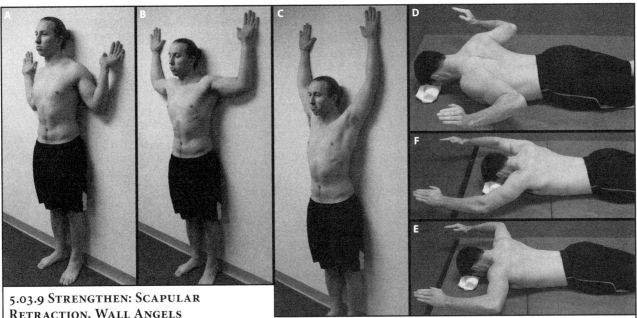

5.03.9 STRENGTHEN: SCAPULAR RETRACTION, WALL ANGELS

<u>POSITION</u>: Standing, prone

<u>TARGETS</u>: Strengthen lower trapezius, primarily due to isolating downward rotation of scapula

<u>INSTRUCTION</u>: *Wall*: Begin facing away from wall and position feet, 3 to 4 inches away from wall, knees and hips slightly flexed. Buttocks and shoulders are against the wall. Patient starts with placing arms at 70 degrees of shoulder abduction and full external rotation with flexed elbows, tops of wrists against the wall. Patient raises the arms above head, keeping shoulders, elbows and wrists in contact with the wall at all times. Lower and repeat (A through C). *Prone advanced*: Place towel roll under forehead to neutralize neck position. In the same position as described above for the arms, patient repeats movements. Elbow, wrist, shoulder, and torso stay in same horizontal plane (D through F).

<u>SUBSTITUTIONS</u>: Shrugging shoulders excessively, arms coming off wall at wrist or elbow; if this occurs, have patient only go as far as possible without lifting arms and repeat in that range.

<u>PARAMETERS</u>: 10 repetitions, up to 3 sets, 1 time per day or every other day

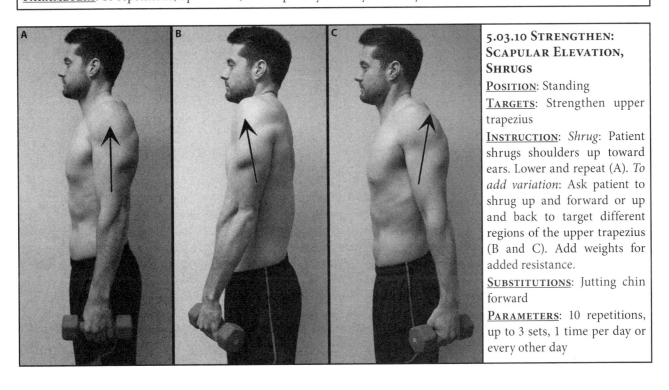

5.03.10 STRENGTHEN: SCAPULAR ELEVATION, SHRUGS

<u>POSITION</u>: Standing

<u>TARGETS</u>: Strengthen upper trapezius

<u>INSTRUCTION</u>: *Shrug*: Patient shrugs shoulders up toward ears. Lower and repeat (A). *To add variation*: Ask patient to shrug up and forward or up and back to target different regions of the upper trapezius (B and C). Add weights for added resistance.

<u>SUBSTITUTIONS</u>: Jutting chin forward

<u>PARAMETERS</u>: 10 repetitions, up to 3 sets, 1 time per day or every other day

5.03.11 STRENGTHEN: RESISTANCE BAND, ISOLATED SCAPULAR RETRACTION

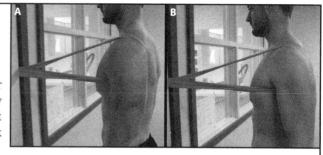

POSITION: Seated

TARGETS: Strengthen rhomboid and middle trapezius

INSTRUCTION: With resistance band anchored at shoulder height, loop band around the shoulder. Scoot chair away from anchor to where resistance is felt at shoulder. Patient retracts scapula, pinching scapula toward the spine. Relax and repeat (A and B).

SUBSTITUTIONS: Shrugging shoulders

PARAMETERS: Hold pinch 3 to 5 seconds, 10 repetitions, up to 3 sets, 1 time per day or every other day

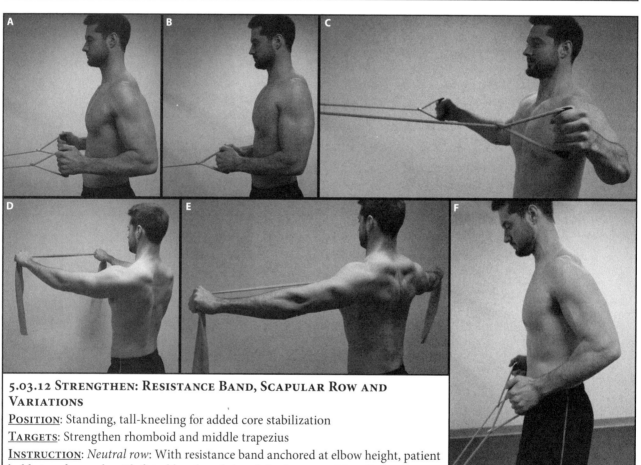

5.03.12 STRENGTHEN: RESISTANCE BAND, SCAPULAR ROW AND VARIATIONS

POSITION: Standing, tall-kneeling for added core stabilization

TARGETS: Strengthen rhomboid and middle trapezius

INSTRUCTION: *Neutral row*: With resistance band anchored at elbow height, patient holds two free ends with fisted hand, and thumb in the up position. Patient moves away from anchor, allowing arms to come forward, until resistance is felt at arm forward position. Patient has shoulders in neutral rotation and pulls resistance band back while flexing elbows to 90 degrees and retracting scapula. Do not let shoulders come back into hyperextension, but target retraction by adding squeeze once arms reach torso (A). *Narrow grip row*: Patient holds bands with a narrow grip and pulls resistance band back, hand to navel, while flexing elbow to 90 degrees and retracting scapula. Do not let shoulders come back into hyperextension, but target retraction by adding squeeze once arms reach torso (B). *Wide row horizontal abduction*: Move resistance band to anchor at shoulder height. Patient holds bands with a narrow grip and pulls resistance band back, horizontally abducting, with elbows extended and retracting scapula. Do not let shoulders come back into horizontal abduction past the torso, and avoid humeral head translation anteriorly. Target retraction by adding squeeze once the arms reach torso (C). This can also be done holding resistance band without an anchor and repeating instructions (D and E). *Pull-up row*: Secure band at floor level with two free ends. Patient pulls the hands up toward the chin with thumbs up, allowing elbows to bend, retracting scapula (F).

SUBSTITUTIONS: Shrugging shoulders, humeral head forward translation with hyper extension/horizontal abduction past torso

PARAMETERS: Hold pinch 3 to 5 seconds, 10 repetitions up to 3 sets, 1 time per day or every other day

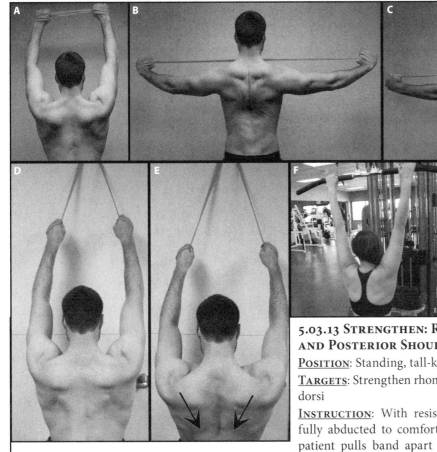

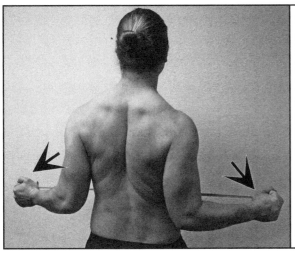

5.03.13 STRENGTHEN: RESISTANCE BAND, SCAPULAR AND POSTERIOR SHOULDER, OVERHEAD PULL-DOWN

POSITION: Standing, tall-kneeling (for added core stabilization)

TARGETS: Strengthen rhomboid, middle trapezius, and latissimus dorsi

INSTRUCTION: With resistance band held overhead, shoulders fully abducted to comfort level and elbows slightly flexed, (A) patient pulls band apart while adducting the shoulders down toward the body to shoulder height. This can be done in front of the head (B) or behind (C). Target retraction by adding squeeze at end range. *Scapular depression and retraction only*: To target only scapular movement, resistance band is anchored overhead in front of patient. Patient is sitting close to the wall, facing away. Band is held overhead with tension on band, patient's shoulders fully abducted to comfort level, elbows slightly flexed. Patient then only retracts and depressed scapula against the resistance (D and E).

Scapular depression and retraction only, lateral pull-down machine: To target only scapular movement with heavier resistance/weights, patient holds latissimus pull-down bar overhead, shoulders fully abducted to comfort level, elbows slightly flexed. Bar should be directly overhead. Patient then only retracts and depresses scapula against the resistance (F and G).

SUBSTITUTIONS: Shrugging shoulders, chin should stay tucked; do not allow jutting out of chin especially with going behind the head.

PARAMETERS: Hold pinch 3 to 5 seconds, 10 repetitions up to 3 sets, 1 time per day or every other day

5.03.14 STRENGTHEN: RESISTANCE BAND, SCAPULAR AND ROTATOR CUFF, RETRACTION AND EXTERNAL ROTATION

POSITION: Standing

TARGETS: Strengthen rhomboid, middle trapezius, and latissimus dorsi

INSTRUCTION: With resistance band held in front of navel, about 6 inches from the body, elbows flexed 90 degrees, patient pulls band apart while externally rotating the shoulders, bringing arms out to the sides. Target retraction by adding a squeeze at end range.

SUBSTITUTIONS: Shrugging shoulders, chin should stay tucked, upper arms stay by the sides

PARAMETERS: Hold pinch 3 to 5 seconds, 10 repetitions, up to 3 sets, 1 time per day or every other day

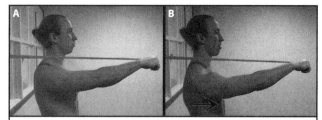

5.03.15 STRENGTHEN: RESISTANCE BAND, SCAPULAR, PUNCH

<u>POSITION</u>: Supine

<u>TARGETS</u>: Strengthen serratus anterior

<u>INSTRUCTION</u>: With resistance band anchored at shoulder height, patient holds end of band facing away from anchor and brings shoulder into 90 degrees of flexion with fisted hand and thumb pointed toward the ceiling. Patient protracts scapula and reaches hand closer forward (A and B).

<u>SUBSTITUTIONS</u>: Shrugging shoulders, rotating thoracic spine; this movement can be accomplished with upper trapezius shrug and should be monitored closely, tapping the serratus anterior will help to facilitate the patient's understanding of from where the movement comes from.

<u>PARAMETERS</u>: 10 repetitions on each side, up to 3 sets, 1 time per day or every other day

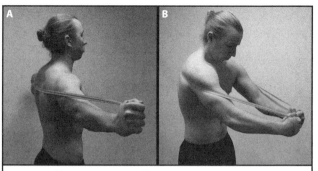

5.03.16 STRENGTHEN: RESISTANCE BAND, SCAPULAR, DYNAMIC HUG

<u>POSITION</u>: Supine

<u>TARGETS</u>: Strengthen serratus anterior

<u>INSTRUCTION</u>: With resistance band looped around posterior shoulders, patient holds the ends of the resistance band in each hand. Patient starts with hands in front of shoulders and horizontally adducts, as if giving a hug, while resistance band resists; emphasize scapular protraction at end range (A and B).

<u>SUBSTITUTIONS</u>: Shrugging shoulders, rotating thoracic spine; this movement can be accomplished with upper trapezius shrug and should be monitored closely, tapping the serratus anterior will help to facilitate the patient's understanding of where the movement comes from.

<u>PARAMETERS</u>: 10 repetitions on each side, up to 3 sets, 1 time per day or every other day

5.03.17 STRENGTHEN: RESISTANCE BAND, SERRATUS WALL SLIDES

<u>POSITION</u>: Standing

<u>TARGETS</u>: Strengthen serratus anterior

<u>INSTRUCTION</u>: Patient begins facing wall and position feet so that, with elbows flexed 90 degrees, forearms rest on wall. Loop resistance band around wrists. Patient protracts the scapula and slides forearms up the wall keeping tension on the band. Return to start and repeat (A and B).

<u>SUBSTITUTIONS</u>: Shrugging shoulders excessively, forearms coming off wall at wrist or elbow; if this occurs, have patient only go as far as possible without lifting arms, and repeat in that range.

<u>PARAMETERS</u>: 10 repetitions, up to 3 sets, 1 time per day or every other day

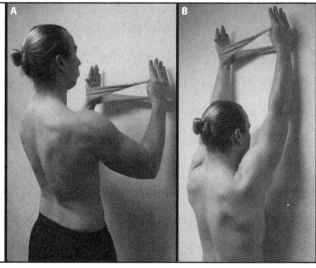

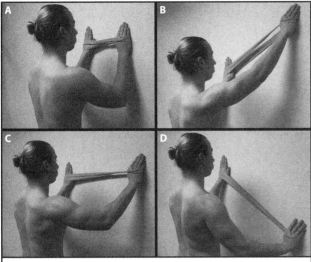

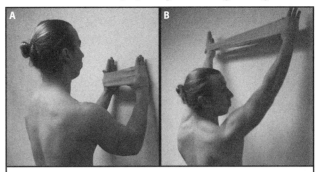

5.03.19 STRENGTHEN: RESISTANCE BAND, SCAPULAR "Vs"

POSITION: Standing

TARGETS: Strengthen serratus anterior, middle and lower trapezius, rhomboids

INSTRUCTION: Patient begins facing wall and positions feet so that, with elbows flexed 100 degrees and shoulders 45 degrees, pinky side of hands rest on wall. Loop resistance band around hands. Patient pulls hands apart and brings arms upward, making a "V" pattern overhead, slowly brings arms down and repeats. Patient uses scapular muscles to accomplish the movements along with shoulder (A and B).

SUBSTITUTIONS: Shrugging shoulders excessively, forearms coming off wall at wrist or elbow; if this occurs, have patient only go as far as possible without lifting arms, and repeat in that range

5.03.18 STRENGTHEN: RESISTANCE BAND, SCAPULAR CLOCKS

POSITION: Standing

TARGETS: Strengthen serratus anterior, middle and lower trapezius, rhomboids

INSTRUCTION: Patient begins facing wall and positions feet so that, with elbows flexed 70 degrees and shoulders 90 degrees, palms rest on wall. Loop resistance band around wrists. Patient pictures a clock in front. Keeping one hand planted, patient uses other hand to tap each number on the clock—1, 3, 5 for right arm or 11, 9, 7 for left hand. Patient uses scapular muscles to accomplish the movements along with shoulder (A through D).

SUBSTITUTIONS: Shrugging shoulders excessively, forearms coming off wall at wrist or elbow; if this occurs, have patient only go as far as possible without lifting arms, and repeat in that range.

PARAMETERS: 10 repetitions, up to 3 sets, 1 time per day or every other day

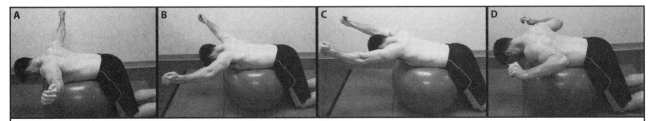

5.03.20 STRENGTHEN: SCAPULAR RETRACTION: "T", "Y", "I", AND "W" ON BALL

POSITION: Prone on exercise ball

TARGETS: "Y": Strengthen lower trapezius "T": Strengthen posterior deltoid, rhomboid, and middle trapezius, "I": Strengthen anterior deltoid and lower trapezius, "Y": Strengthen posterior deltoid and lower trapezius, "W": Strengthening rhomboids

INSTRUCTION: Patient lies face down on the ball with arms stretched forward (just the torso will be on the ball), keeping toes down and knees slightly bent while knees are slightly lifted off the floor. Patient tightens abdominal muscles, lifts arms into a "T", "Y", "I", or "W" position, and retracts scapula at the end of the range. **5.03.5** and **5.03.8** for descriptions of each movement (A through D). Adding the exercise ball creates an unstable surface and is more challenging.

SUBSTITUTIONS: Shrugging shoulders excessively; "T" and "W" can be done without upper trapezius, but "Y" and "I" will have some normal recruitment of the upper trapezius; thoracic extension rather than retraction, excessive translation of humeral head anteriorly, lifting head.

PARAMETERS: Hold pinch 3 to 5 seconds, 10 repetitions, up to 3 sets, 1 time per day or every other day

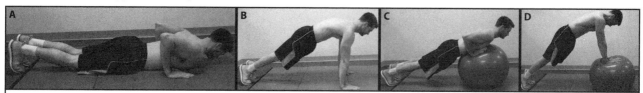

5.03.21 STRENGTHEN: SCAPULAR, PUSH-UP PLUS (ADVANCED)

POSITION: Quadruped

TARGETS: Strengthen serratus anterior

INSTRUCTION: *Advanced stable*: Hands and toes on floor, knees lifted in a push-up position, and elbows extended to neutral, patient presses up away from floor and protracts scapula, rounding the upper thoracic spine (A and B). *Unstable advanced*: Hands on exercise ball, fingers point outward for greater control of ball, toes on floor, knees lifted in a push-up position, elbows extended to neutral, patient presses up away from exercise ball and protracts scapula, rounding the upper thoracic spine (C and D). Gaze is between the hands and chin is slightly tucked.

SUBSTITUTIONS: Shrugging shoulders, this movement can be accomplished with upper trapezius shrug and should be monitored closely; tapping the serratus anterior will help to facilitate the patient's understanding of from where the movement comes from, avoid hyperextension at the elbows and jutting chin out or looking up.

PARAMETERS: 10 repetitions, up to 3 sets, 1 time per day or every other day

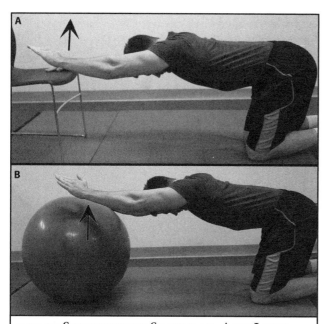

5.03.22 STRENGTHEN: SCAPULAR, ARM LIFTS

POSITION: Quadruped

TARGETS: Strengthen lower trapezius and anterior deltoid

INSTRUCTION: Patient is positioned in quadruped with palms down on a chair (A) or exercise ball (B). Shoulders are in full flexion with elbows extended. Patient retracts and depresses scapula, lifting hands off table while maintaining a neutral spine and tightened deep core. Gaze remains toward the floor with slight chin tuck. Alternate from right to left.

SUBSTITUTIONS: Trunk rotation, sagging abdomen, jutting chin out or looking up

PARAMETERS: 10 repetitions, up to 3 sets, 1 time per day or every other day

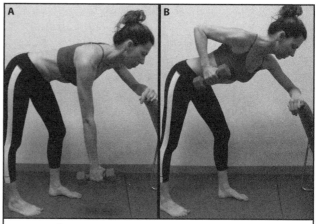

5.03.23 STRENGTHEN: SCAPULAR, BENT ROW

POSITION: Standing

TARGETS: Strengthen rhomboids and middle trapezius

INSTRUCTION: Patient is positioned in standing, bent forward with chair in front and unaffected arm supporting. Patient holds weight and allows affected arm to dangle down, protracting scapula. Patient then retracts scapula and lifts weight, bringing arm up. Focus is on scapular retraction, not shoulder extension (A and B).

SUBSTITUTIONS: Trunk rotation, sagging abdomen, jutting chin out or looking up, torso should stay parallel to floor

PARAMETERS: 10 repetitions, up to 3 sets, 1 time per day or every other day

REFERENCES

Castelein, B., Cools, A., Parlevliet, T., & Cagnie, B. (2015, Sep). Modifying the shoulder joint position during shrugging and retraction exercises alters the activation of the medial scapular muscles. *Manual Therapy, 21,* 250-255.

Decker, M. J., Hintermeister, R. A., Faber, K. J., & Hawkins, R. J. (1999). serratus anterior muscle activity during selected rehabilitation exercises. *American Journal of Sports Medicine, 27*(6), 784-791.

Escamilla, R. F., Yamashiro, K., Paulos, L., & Andrews, J. R. (2009). Shoulder muscle activity and function in common shoulder rehabilitation exercises. *Sports Medicine, 39*(8), 663-685.

Smith, J., Dahm, D. L., Kaufman, K. R., Boon, A. J., Laskowski, E. R., Kotajarvi, B. R., & Jacofsky, D. J. (2006). Electromyographic activity in the immobilized shoulder girdle musculature during scapulo-thoracic exercises. *Archives of Physical Medicine and Rehabilitation, 87*(7), 923-927.

Section 5.04

SHOULDER RANGE OF MOTION

5.04.1 ROM: SHOULDER, WARM-UP, UPPER BODY ERGOMETER, ACTIVE ASSISTIVE

A UBE is a piece of exercise equipment similar to a bicycle that is pedaled with the arms. Settings can be adjusted on the UBE to control resistance and change the amount of work the upper body performing. Typical UBE machines have an adjustable seat and many allow use of the machine while standing.

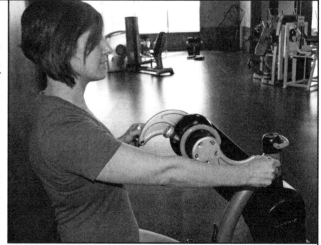

POSITION: Seated

TARGETS: Warm-up of the shoulder and shoulder girdle

INSTRUCTION: Patient seated with feet flat on floor facing the ergometer, adjust settings so that the axis of the crank is slightly below shoulder height and, at the furthest point of reach, shoulder is at slightly below 90 degrees of flexion without any scapular protraction, elbow is flexed only 5 to 10 degrees. This will allow the patient to keep the humeral head seated in the joint. If reach is too far, repeated arm movements may cause inflammation in the subacromial region. Therapist will set the amount of resistance on the ergometer; less resistance is better for warm-up, but if strengthening is desired, increase the resistance. Patient may cycle forward and backward for 30 seconds each or longer intervals. Instruct patient when pulling back to use the scapular retractors to facilitate scapular stability with arm movements.

SUBSTITUTIONS: Shrugging shoulders, torso rotation, forward head, slouching

PARAMETERS: Cycle 5 to 10 minutes, at least 30 second intervals from backward to forward; if using for cardiovascular endurance or cross-training, up to 30 minutes.

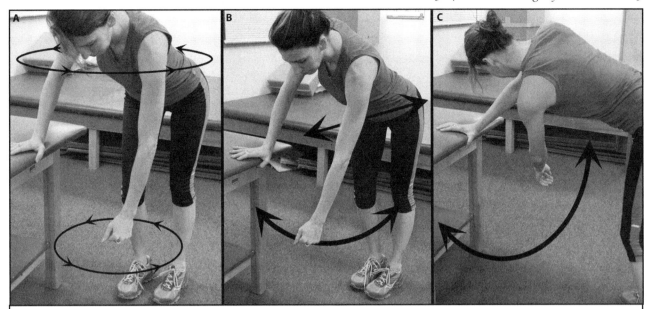

5.04.2 ROM: Shoulder, Pendulum, Passive

Position: Standing

Targets: Warm-up of the shoulder and shoulder girdle causes a slight traction of the glenohumeral joint and oscillatory movement to enhance blood flow and synovial fluid lubrication of joint surfaces; *Postsurgical RC repair*: Limit diameter of movements to 20 inches (50 centimeters).

Instruction: *Circles*: Patient leans over, unaffected arm supporting on a table or chair, affected arm relaxing, hanging straight down, hips and knees are slightly flexed. Patient starts to move the hips and trunk via hip and knee flexion and extension in a circular motion clockwise while momentum slowly begins to swing the relaxed arm. Repeat full set, then repeat counter-clockwise (A). *Flexion/extension*: Patient bends and straightens hips and knees, rocking forward and backward on the unaffected arm, allow the affected arm to swing into flexion and return (B). *Horizontal abduction/ adduction*: Rocking body side to side, allow arm to swing away from body laterally and return to across the body. These are not large movements, but stay within a pain-free range (C).

Substitutions: Use of shoulder muscles to accomplish movement; this is done passively using momentum to create the movements in the shoulder, full relaxation of the shoulder allows joint to distract slightly, which improves the lubrication process. Often patients perform the standard pendulum incorrectly by actively moving the surgical arm to swing it, rather than the appropriate passive swing of the arm through body and hip sway. If this happens, try **5.04.3** as an alternative.

Parameters: 1 minute of each movement, 1 to 3 times per day

Where's the Evidence?

Long et al. (2010) evaluated EMG signal amplitude in the supraspinatus, infraspinatus, and deltoid muscles during pendulum exercises and light activities in a group of healthy subjects. Muscle activity was recorded in 13 subjects performing pendulum exercises incorrectly and correctly in both large (51-cm) and small (20-cm) diameters while typing, drinking, and brushing their teeth. Incorrect and correct large pendulums elicited more than 15% MVC in the supraspinatus and infraspinatus. The supraspinatus EMG signal amplitude was greater during large, incorrectly performed pendulums than during those performed correctly. Both correct and incorrect large pendulums resulted in statistically higher muscle activity in the supraspinatus than the small pendulums. The authors concluded that larger pendulums may require more force than is desirable early in rehabilitation after RC repair.

5.04.3 ROM: Shoulder, Cradle Rocks, Passive

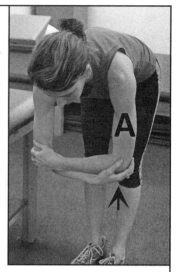

POSITION: Standing

TARGETS: Warm-up of the shoulder and shoulder girdle causes a slight traction of the glenohumeral joint and oscillatory movement to enhance blood flow and synovial fluid lubrication of joint surfaces; this exercise can be done post-surgery and may replace the standard pendulum as it allows the patient to control the surgical arm with the non-surgical arm, protecting the surgical repair from unnecessary stress that the standard pendulum can cause if performed incorrectly.

INSTRUCTION: Bending forward at the hips, patient cradles the affected arm, like holding a baby, using the unaffected arm. The affected hand may grasp the upper arm of the unaffected arm for security. The unaffected arm is intended to provide all the movement of the affected arm. The patient then gently rocks the arm forward and backward, side-to-side, and in clockwise and counter-clockwise circles as is done with the standard **5.04.2**.

SUBSTITUTIONS: Use of shoulder muscles to accomplish movement; this is done passively using unaffected arm to create the movements in the affected shoulder. Full relaxation of the shoulder allows joint to distract slightly, which improves the lubrication process.

PARAMETERS: 1 minute of each movement, 1 to 3 times per day

5.04.4 ROM: Shoulder, Saws, Active Assistive

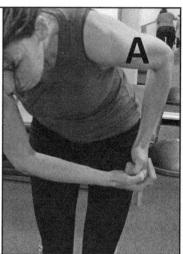

POSITION: Standing

TARGETS: Warm-up of the shoulder and shoulder girdle

INSTRUCTION: Bending forward at the hips, patient leans forward, allowing affected arm to hang. Patient places cupped hand of the unaffected arm under the affected arm's fist and uses unaffected arm to bring the affected fist up toward the chest in a sawing motion and returns to start. Unaffected arm does all (passive) or most (active assistive) of the work.

SUBSTITUTIONS: Use of affected shoulder muscles to accomplish movement; this is done passively using unaffected arm to create the movements in the affected shoulder.

PARAMETERS: 1 minute, 1 to 3 times per day

5.04.5 ROM: Shoulder Girdle Circles, Active Assistive

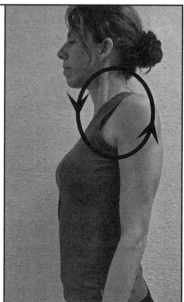

POSITION: Standing

TARGETS: Mobility of the scapula and gaining control of scapular movements by facilitating contraction of scapular stabilizing muscles (rhomboids, upper trapezius, middle trapezius, and lower trapezius, serratus anterior) while creating passive movement in the glenohumeral joint

INSTRUCTION: Patient initiates small circles in the sagittal plane with the scapula rolling forward, up, back, and down while the arms hangs loose at the shoulder joint.

SUBSTITUTIONS: Active use of shoulder; shoulder remains relaxed while shoulder girdle and scapulothoracic create the movements

PARAMETERS: 10 to 20 repetitions each direction, 1 set, 1 to 3 times per day

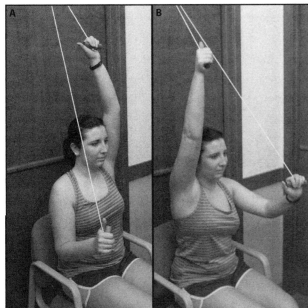

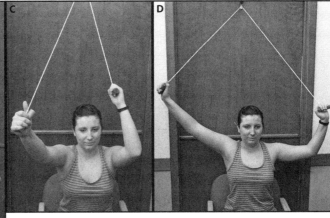

5.04.6 ROM: Pulleys; Shoulder Flexion, Scaption, and Abduction, Passive

Position: Seated, standing

Targets: Mobility of the glenohumeral joint using unaffected arm to assist in movements

Instruction: Anchor the pulleys overhead in a doorway; patient can be seated with the back of the chair against a doorway or standing. Bring one handle to affected hand, allowing it to remain relaxed in the lap while unaffected hand reaches up to grasp the other handle. With thumbs pointed up toward ceiling, patient pulls down with unaffected arm, bringing affected shoulder into flexion. Instruct patient to keep affected shoulder relaxed only using hand to hold handle. This should be a passive exercise for the shoulder elbow can be bent or straight (A through D). Repeat for entire set. Patient can also pull into scaption (C) and abduction (D) in the same manner. Make sure that patient slowly lowers using unaffected arm.

Substitutions: Active use of target shoulder; shoulder remains relaxed while unaffected arm creates the movements, encourage patient to sit up tall with shoulders back.

Parameters: 10 to 20 repetitions holding 1 to 3 seconds at end range each direction, 1 set, 1 to 3 times per day

Where's the Evidence?

Uhl, Muir, and Lawson (2010) used EMG studies to assess muscle activation during passive, active assistive and active shoulder exercises. Passive exercises generated the lowest mean EMG activity, < 10% MVC for all muscles studied (supraspinatus, infraspinatus, anterior deltoid, upper trapezius, lower trapezius, and serratus anterior). The standing active shoulder elevation exercises generated the greatest mean EMG activity, 40% MVC. Overall the active assistive exercises generated a small, < 10%, increase in muscle activity compared with the passive exercises for the supraspinatus and infraspinatus muscles. Data in normal volunteers suggest that many exercises used during the early phase of rehabilitation to regain active elevation do not exceed 20% MVC. Progression from passive to active assisted can potentially be performed without significantly increasing muscular activation levels exercises. Upright active exercises demonstrated a significant increase in muscular activities, supporting that these exercises should be prescribed later in a rehabilitation program.

5.04.7 ROM: PULLEYS; SHOULDER INTERNAL ROTATION, PASSIVE

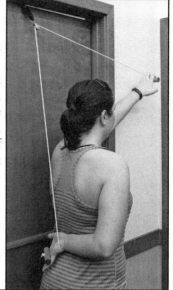

POSITION: Seated, standing

TARGETS: Mobility of the glenohumeral joint using unaffected arm to assist in movements

INSTRUCTION: Anchor the pulleys overhead in a doorway. Patient can be seated with the back of the chair against a doorway or standing. Bring one handle to affected hand, allowing it to remain relaxed in the lap while unaffected hand reaches up to grasp the other handle. Patient places affected arm behind the ipsilateral buttock with thumb up, bringing the rope with. Patient pulls down with the unaffected arm on the other end of the pulley, sliding the affected hand up along the patient's posterior torso. Instruct patient to keep affected shoulder relaxed, only using hand to hold handle. This should be a passive exercise for the shoulder. Make sure that patient slowly lowers using unaffected arm.

SUBSTITUTIONS: Active use of target shoulder; shoulder remains relaxed while unaffected arm creates the movements, encourage scapular retraction and good posture to minimize anterior humeral translation.

PARAMETERS: 10 to 20 repetitions, holding 1 to 3 seconds at end range, 1 set, 1 to 3 times per day

5.04.8 ROM: PULLEYS; SHOULDER EXTERNAL ROTATION, PASSIVE

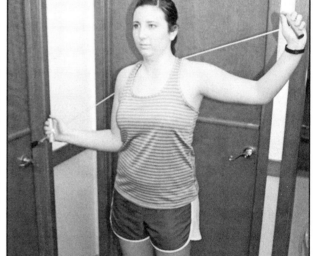

POSITION: Seated, standing

TARGETS: Mobility of the glenohumeral joint using unaffected arm to assist in movements

INSTRUCTION: Anchor the pulleys near the middle hinge in a doorway. Patient can be seated 2 to 3 feet away from the doorway, sideways. Place towel roll between elbows, flexed 90 degrees at patient's side, and have patient squeeze to hold in place throughout entire sequence. Bring one handle to affected hand, allowing it to remain relaxed in the lap while unaffected hand reaches up to grasp the other handle. Patient pulls down with the unaffected arm, pulling the opposite shoulder into external rotation as hand moves away from the side. Instruct patient to keep affected shoulder relaxed, only using to hand to hold handle. This should be a passive exercise for the shoulder.

SUBSTITUTIONS: Active use of target shoulder; shoulder remains relaxed while unaffected arm creates the movements, encourage scapular retraction and good posture to minimize anterior humeral translation.

PARAMETERS: 10 to 20 repetitions, holding 1 to 3 seconds at end range, 1 set, 1 to 3 times per day

5.04.9 ROM: WAND/CANE; SHOULDER CIRCLES, ACTIVE ASSISTIVE

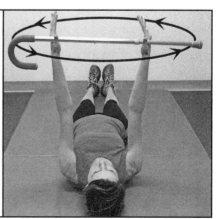

POSITION: Supine

TARGETS: Mobility of the glenohumeral joint using unaffected arm to assist in movements

INSTRUCTION: Patient holds the wand with both hands outstretched. Encourage patient to seat the humeral head in the glenoid fossa by retracting and depressing scapula. Patient then makes small circles clockwise for a full set with both arms using the unaffected arm to assist the affected side. Repeat counter-clockwise. A good cue to use is "draw circles on the ceiling."

SUBSTITUTIONS: Encourage scapular retraction and good posture to minimize anterior humeral translation and subacromial irritation

PARAMETERS: 10 to 20 repetitions each direction, 1 set, 1 to 3 times per day

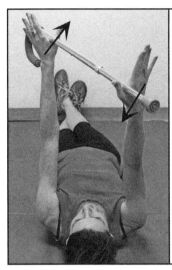

5.04.10 ROM: Wand/Cane; Shoulder Twists, Active Assistive

Position: Supine

Targets: Mobility of the glenohumeral joint using unaffected arm to assist in movements

Instruction: Patient holds the wand with both hands outstretched. Encourage patient to seat the humeral head in the glenoid fossa by retracting and depressing scapula. Patient then twists right hand inferiorly while bringing opposite arm superiorly followed by repeating in opposite directions.

Substitutions: Encourage scapular retraction and good posture to minimize anterior humeral translation and subacromial irritation

Parameters: 10 to 20 repetitions, holding 1 to 3 seconds at end range, 1 set, 1 to 3 times per day

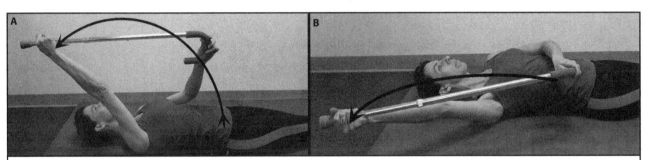

5.04.11 ROM: Wand/Cane; Shoulder Flexion and Scaption, Active Assistive

Position: Supine, seated, standing

Targets: Mobility of the glenohumeral joint using unaffected arm to assist in flexion

Instruction: *Flexion*: Patient holds the wand with both hands, arms by side, affected palm up and unaffected palm down. Encourage patient to seat the humeral head in the glenoid fossa by retracting and depressing scapula. Patient pushes the affected arm into shoulder flexion by pushing up toward the head with the unaffected arm. Affected elbow remains extended (A). *Scaption*: With shoulder 30 degrees forward from abducted position, patient performs the same maneuver as described for flexion, except into the scapular plane (B).

Substitutions: Encourage scapular retraction to minimize subacromial irritation

Parameters: 10 to 20 repetitions holding 1 to 3 seconds at end range, 1 set, 1 to 3 times per day

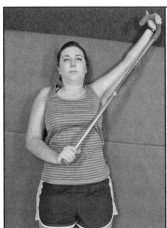

5.04.12 ROM: Wand/Cane; Shoulder Abduction, Active Assistive

Position: Supine, seated, standing

Targets: Mobility of the glenohumeral joint using unaffected arm to assist in abduction

Instruction: Patient holds the wand with both hands, arms by side, affected palm up and unaffected palm down. Encourage patient to seat the humeral head in the glenoid fossa by retracting and depressing scapula. Patient pushes the affected arm into shoulder abduction by crossing over the body with the unaffected arm. Affected elbow remains extended.

Substitutions: Encourage scapular retraction to minimize subacromial irritation

Parameters: 10 to 20 repetitions, holding 1 to 3 seconds at end range, 1 set, 1 to 3 times per day

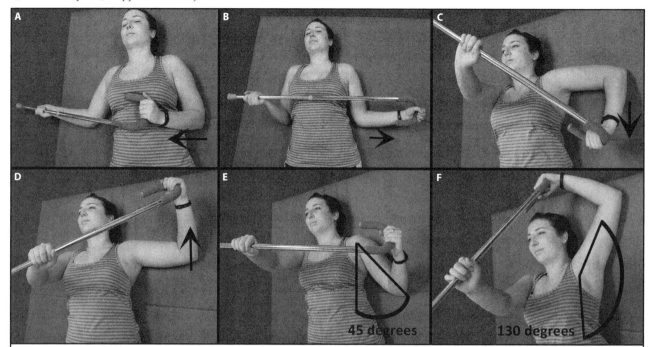

5.04.13 ROM: WAND/CANE; SHOULDER INTERNAL ROTATION, EXTERNAL ROTATION, AND COMBINED, ACTIVE ASSISTIVE

<u>POSITION</u>: Supine, seated

<u>TARGETS</u>: Mobility of the glenohumeral joint using unaffected arm to assist in internal and external rotation

<u>INSTRUCTION</u>: Patient holds the wand with both hands, elbows flexed to 90 degrees. Encourage patient to seat the humeral head in the glenoid fossa by retracting and depressing scapula. *Neutral abduction, internal rotation*: Patient pulls the affected arm into shoulder internal rotation crossing over the body. Affected elbow remains tucked into the patient's side (A). *Neutral abduction, external rotation*: Patient pushes the affected arm into shoulder external rotation crossing unaffected arm over the body. Affected elbow remains tucked into the patient's side (B). *Combined*: Therapist may combine these two movements into one exercise depending on treatment goals. *90/90 internal rotation*: With shoulders abducted 90 degrees, elbows flexed 90 degrees, patient holds wand in both hands and pushes wand inferiorly with unaffected side into internal rotation of the affected shoulder (C). *90/90 external rotation*: With shoulders abducted 90 degrees, and elbows flexed 90 degrees, patient holds wand in both hands and pushes wand inferiorly with unaffected side into external rotation of the affected shoulder (D). Therapist can do this at any angle of abduction in the shoulder depending on treatment goals (i.e. 45 degrees or 120 degrees shoulder abduction) (E and F).

<u>SUBSTITUTIONS</u>: Encourage scapular retraction to minimize subacromial irritation

<u>PARAMETERS</u>: 10 to 20 repetitions, holding 1 to 3 seconds at end range, 1 set, 1 to 3 times per day

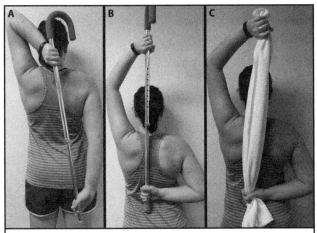

5.04.14 ROM: WAND/CANE/STRAP; SHOULDER INTERNAL ROTATION BEHIND BACK, ACTIVE ASSISTIVE

POSITION: Standing

TARGETS: Mobility of the glenohumeral joint using unaffected arm to assist in movements to increase internal rotation

INSTRUCTION: Patient holds the wand behind the back with unaffected hand overhead, palm facing forward, and affected hand at buttock, palm facing outward. Encourage patient to seat the humeral head in the glenoid fossa by retracting and depressing scapula. Patient pulls the affected arm into shoulder internal rotation as the affected hands slides superiorly along the posterior trunk. Hold and lower slowly (A and B). This can also be done with a towel, strap or sheet (C).

SUBSTITUTIONS: Encourage scapular retraction to minimize subacromial irritation

PARAMETERS: 10 to 20 repetitions, holding 1 to 3 seconds at end range, 1 set, 1 to 3 times per day

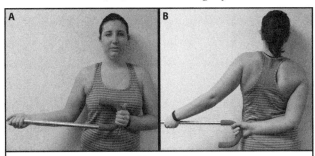

5.04.15 ROM: WAND/CANE; SHOULDER INTERNAL ROTATION, PULLS ACROSS FRONT AND BACK, ACTIVE ASSISTIVE

POSITION: Standing

TARGETS: Mobility of the glenohumeral joint using unaffected arm to assist in movements to increase internal rotation; the pull across also assists in increasing shoulder adduction.

INSTRUCTION: *Pull across front*: Patient holds the wand in front, elbows bent 90 degrees. Encourage patient to seat the humeral head in the glenoid fossa by retracting and depressing scapula. Patient pulls affected hand across the front of the body into internal rotation and adduction (A). *Pull across back*: Patient holds the wand behind the back with both hands facing outward. Encourage patient to seat the humeral head in the glenoid fossa by retracting and depressing scapula. Patient pulls affected hand across the lower back into internal rotation and adduction (B).

SUBSTITUTIONS: Encourage scapular retraction to minimize subacromial irritation

PARAMETERS: 10 to 20 repetitions, holding 1 to 3 seconds at end range, 1 set, 1 to 3 times per day

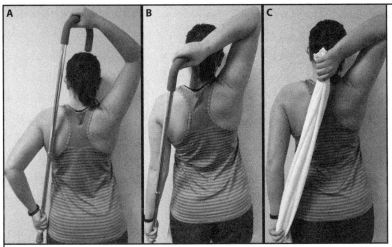

5.04.16 ROM: WAND/CANE/STRAP; SHOULDER EXTERNAL ROTATION BEHIND HEAD, ACTIVE ASSISTIVE

POSITION: Standing

TARGETS: Mobility of the glenohumeral joint using unaffected arm to assist in movements to increase external rotation

INSTRUCTION: Patient holds the wand behind the back with unaffected hand, palm facing out and holding behind the lower back. Patient grasps top of wand just above the head, palm facing forward. Encourage patient to seat the humeral head in the glenoid fossa by retracting and depressing scapula. Patient pulls down on the wand with the affected arm over the head moving behind the head and neck to upper back, which is the functional movement of external rotation. Hold and return slowly (A and B). This can also be done with a towel, strap or sheet (C).

SUBSTITUTIONS: Encourage scapular retraction to minimize subacromial irritation

PARAMETERS: 10 to 20 repetitions, holding 1 to 3 seconds at end range, 1 set, 1 to 3 times per day

5.04.17 ROM: WAND/CANE; SHOULDER EXTENSION, ACTIVE ASSISTIVE

<u>POSITION</u>: Prone, standing

<u>TARGETS</u>: Mobility of the glenohumeral joint using unaffected arm to assist in extension

<u>INSTRUCTION</u>: *Prone*: Lying face down with towel under forehead, patient holds the wand with both

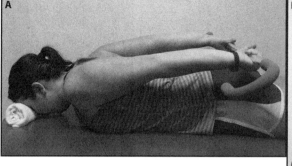
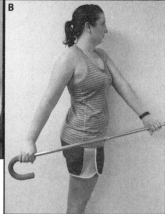

hands, elbows are extended and palms facing each other. Encourage patient to seat the humeral head in the glenoid fossa by retracting and depressing scapula. Patient then lifts the wand toward the ceiling using unaffected arm to assist affected arm (A). *Standing*: Patient pushes the affected arm into shoulder extension crossing unaffected arm over the body. Affected elbow can be flexed or extended (B).

<u>SUBSTITUTIONS</u>: Encourage scapular retraction to minimize subacromial irritation

<u>PARAMETERS</u>: 10 to 20 repetitions, holding 1 to 3 seconds at end range, 1 set, 1 to 3 times per day

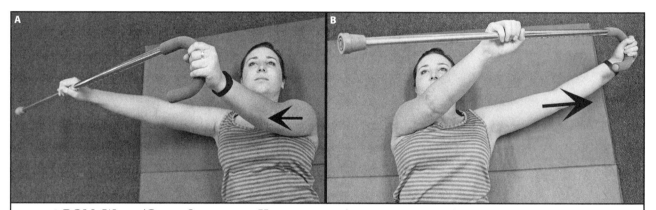

5.04.18 ROM: WAND/CANE; SHOULDER, HORIZONTAL ABDUCTION AND ADDUCTION, ACTIVE ASSISTIVE

<u>POSITION</u>: Supine, seated

<u>TARGETS</u>: Mobility of the glenohumeral joint using unaffected arm to assist in horizontal abduction/adduction

<u>INSTRUCTION</u>: Patient holds the wand with both hands outstretched, affected palm up and unaffected palm down. Encourage patient to seat the humeral head in the glenoid fossa by retracting and depressing scapula. Patient pushes the affected arm into shoulder horizontal abduction by crossing over the body with the unaffected arm, affected elbow remains extended. Patient then pulls affected arm across the body into horizontal adduction, allowing affected elbow to bend (A and B).

<u>SUBSTITUTIONS</u>: Encourage scapular retraction to minimize subacromial irritation

<u>PARAMETERS</u>: 10 to 20 repetitions, holding 1 to 3 seconds at end range, 1 set, 1 to 3 times per day

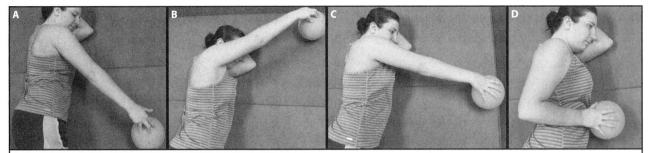

5.04.19 ROM: Shoulder Flexion and Saws, Ball Rolls, Active Assistive

Position: Side-lying

Targets: Mobility of the glenohumeral joint using ball or roller board to eliminate gravity resistance and promote active flexion throughout maximum ROM

Instruction: *Flexion*: Patient is lying on the unaffected side. Affected palm is placed on 8- to 10-inch ball or roller board with elbow extended. Patient begins to flex the shoulder using fingers, walking along the ball as it rolls under the palm throughout the motion, return to start (A and B). Finger walking is not needed with a roller board. *Saws*: Patient, again with palm on ball, and moves arms out in front and back to body in a sawing motion (C and D).

Substitutions: Encourage scapular retraction to minimize subacromial irritation, avoid arching back, chin jutting out, gaze remains forward

Parameters: 10 to 20 repetitions, holding 1 to 3 seconds at end range, 1 set, 1 to 3 times per day

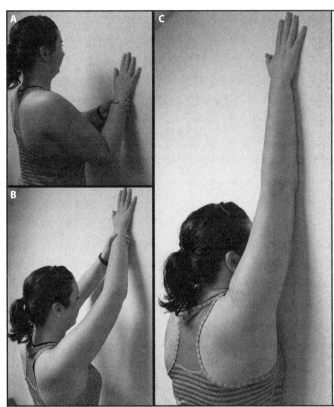

5.04.20 ROM: Shoulder Flexion, Wall Slide, Active Assistive

Position: Standing

Targets: Mobility of the glenohumeral joint using unaffected arm to assist in flexion

Instruction: Standing 4 inches from wall, facing the wall, patient holds affected wrist with unaffected hand and places affected palm on wall in front. Encourage patient to seat the humeral head in the glenoid fossa by retracting and depressing scapula. Patient slides affected hand up the wall into shoulder flexion while extending elbow at end range and assisting with the unaffected hand (A and B). If arms go overhead, patient may step closer or into the wall for a greater stretch into flexion near end range (C).

Substitutions: Encourage scapular retraction to minimize subacromial irritation, avoid arching back, chin jutting out, gaze remains toward wall in front.

Parameters: 10 to 20 repetitions, holding 1 to 3 seconds at end range, 1 set, 1 to 3 times per day

5.04.21 ROM: Shoulder Flexion and Abduction, Towel Slide, Active Assistive

Position: Standing

Targets: Mobility of the glenohumeral joint using wall to support partial weight of arm during arm elevation into flexion and abduction

Instruction: *Flexion*: Standing 4 inches from wall, facing the wall, patient places affected palm on wall in front with small towel under palm. Encourage patient to seat the humeral head in the glenoid fossa by retracting and depressing scapula. Patient slides affected hand up the wall into shoulder flexion while extending elbow at end range (A and B). This may also be done bilaterally (C). *Abduction*: Standing 18 inches from wall, facing sideways, patient places affected palm on wall to the side with small towel under palm. Encourage patient to seat the humeral head in the glenoid fossa by retracting and depressing scapula. Patient slides affected hand up the wall into shoulder abduction while extending elbow at end range. If arms go overhead, patient may step closer or into the wall for a greater stretch into flexion near end range (D).

Substitutions: Encourage scapular retraction to minimize subacromial irritation, avoid arching back or chin jutting out gaze remains forward

Parameters: 10 to 20 repetitions, holding 1 to 3 seconds at end range, 1 set, 1 to 3 times per day

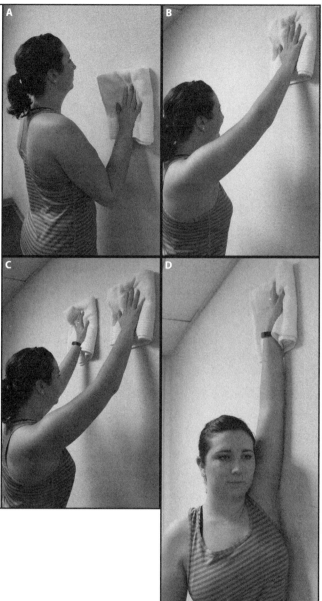

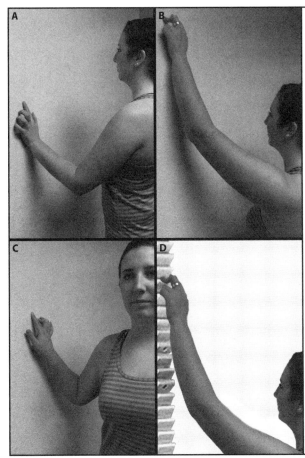

5.04.22 ROM: SHOULDER FLEXION AND ABDUCTION, WALL WALKS, ACTIVE ASSISTIVE

POSITION: Standing

TARGETS: Mobility of the glenohumeral joint using fingers and wall to support partial weight of arm during arm elevation into flexion and abduction

INSTRUCTION: *Flexion*: Standing 4 inches from wall for flexion, facing the wall, patient places affected palm on wall in front. Encourage patient to seat the humeral head in the glenoid fossa by retracting and depressing scapula. Patient walks the fingertips of affected hand up the wall into shoulder flexion while extending elbow at end range (A and B). *Abduction*: Standing 18 inches from wall for flexion, facing sideways, patient places affected palm on wall to the side. Encourage patient to seat the humeral head in the glenoid fossa by retracting and depressing scapula. Patient walks the fingertips of affected hand up the wall into shoulder abduction while extending elbow at end range (C). If arms go overhead, patient may step closer or into the wall for a greater stretch into flexion near end range. A finger ladder is a useful tool for this exercise (D).

SUBSTITUTIONS: Encourage scapular retraction to minimize subacromial irritation, avoid arching back or chin jutting out, gaze remains forward

PARAMETERS: 10 to 20 repetitions, holding 1 to 3 seconds at end range, 1 set, 1 to 3 times per day

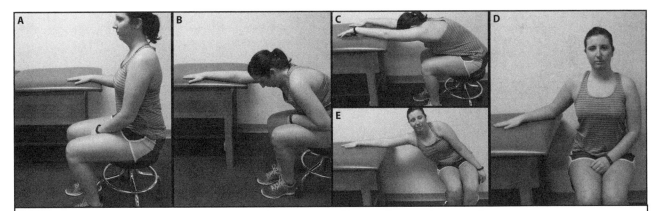

5.04.23 ROM: SHOULDER FLEXION AND ABDUCTION, TABLE SLIDE, ACTIVE ASSISTIVE

POSITION: Seated on rolling stool

TARGETS: Mobility of the glenohumeral joint using table; can be considered passive if done using trunk movement only.

INSTRUCTION: *Flexion*: Seated facing a table, patient slides the affected hand forward on the table while head and chest advance toward the table, hips roll posteriorly. Patient is not actively using shoulder for this motion (A and B). This may also be done bilaterally (C). *Abduction*: Seated sideways by table, patient slides the affected hand out toward the side on the table while the head and chest advance toward the table, hips roll to the opposite side. Patient is not actively using shoulder for this motion (D and E).

SUBSTITUTIONS: Encourage scapular retraction to minimize subacromial irritation, avoid arching back or chin jutting out, gaze remains forward

PARAMETERS: 10 to 20 repetitions, holding 1 to 3 seconds at end range, 1 set, 1 to 3 times per day

Where's the Evidence?

Jung, Kim, Rhee, and Lee (2016) looked at EMG activity of the RC muscles during several different types of passive shoulder and active elbow exercises in 15 healthy subjects. Passive forward flexion of the shoulder was performed using a table, pulley, and cane, and external rotation was performed using a cane and a wall. The active elbow flexion-extension exercise was also performed while holding the upper arm with the contralateral hand. During passive forward flexion, the supraspinatus and infraspinatus muscles exhibited lower activity when using a table compared with a cane and a pulley. Flexion of < 90 degrees decreased supraspinatus activation compared with 170 degrees. During external rotation of the shoulder ,while using the cane and wall, there was no difference in the activity of any muscles. EMG activity during the active elbow exercise was lower in the supraspinatus while holding the upper arm. The authors concluded table sliding exercise may reduce stress on the RC during passive forward flexion more than the other exercises do. Decreasing the ROM to < 90 degrees in forward flexion activated the supraspinatus less. Moreover, movement of the elbow can be performed holding the upper arm to activate the RC to a lesser extent.

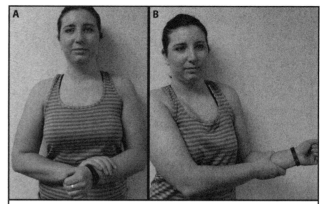

5.04.24 ROM: SHOULDER INTERNAL ROTATION AND EXTERNAL ROTATION USING OTHER HAND, ACTIVE ASSISTIVE

POSITION: Seated

TARGETS: Mobility of the glenohumeral joint using unaffected arm to assist in internal and external rotation; this exercise can be done anywhere, with no equipment and is useful for a home program.

INSTRUCTION: Patient sits with elbows flexed to 90 degrees. Encourage patient to seat the humeral head in the glenoid fossa by retracting and depressing scapula. Patient pulls the affected wrist across the body toward the navel to internally rotate the shoulder. Affected elbow remains tucked into the patient's side (A). Patient pushes the affected wrist outward into shoulder external rotation crossing unaffected arm over the body. Affected elbow remains tucked into the patient's side (B).

SUBSTITUTIONS: Encourage scapular retraction to minimize subacromial irritation

PARAMETERS: 10 to 20 repetitions, holding 1 to 3 seconds at end range, 1 set, 1 to 3 times per day

5.04.25 ROM: SHOULDER INTERNAL ROTATION USING GRAVITY, ACTIVE ASSISTIVE

POSITION: Prone

TARGETS: Mobility of the glenohumeral joint using gravity assist for internal rotation

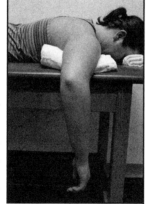

INSTRUCTION: Patient brings shoulder out to 90 degrees and elbow flexed to 90 degrees. Encourage patient to seat the humeral head in the glenoid fossa by retracting and depressing scapula. Patient then slides to let forearm drop off table into internal rotation, allowing gravity to assist.

SUBSTITUTIONS: Encourage scapular retraction to minimize subacromial irritation

PARAMETERS: 1 to 5 minutes, 1 set, 1 to 3 times per day

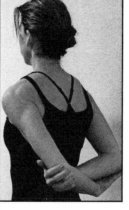

5.04.26 ROM: SHOULDER EXTENSION, ACTIVE ASSISTIVE

POSITION: Standing

TARGETS: Mobility of the glenohumeral joint using unaffected arm to assist in movements to increase extension

INSTRUCTION: Patient grasps elbows behind the back and lifts elbows away from the body. Encourage patient to seat the humeral head in the glenoid fossa by retracting and depressing scapula. Patient holds and lowers slowly.

SUBSTITUTIONS: Encourage scapular retraction to minimize subacromial irritation; do not allow patient to lean forward or round upper back

PARAMETERS: 10 to 20 repetitions, holding 1 to 3 seconds at end range, 1 set, 1 to 3 times per day

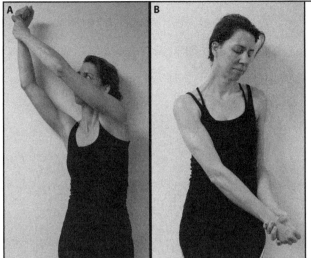

5.04.27 ROM: Shoulder, Chop And Lift, Active Assistive

Position: Standing

Targets: Self-assisted functional movement of flexion, abduction, and external rotation followed by extension, adduction, and internal rotation with associated trunk movements. The chop and lift patterns are applications of the UE diagonals that involve the use of bilateral UEs. One UE is performing the diagonal one pattern, while the other UE is performing the diagonal two pattern, either or both moving into flexion (the lift) or extension (the chop) while using rotational (spiral) and diagonal or combination movements that cross the midline. The chop and lift patterns are combined movements of paired extremities which are asymmetrical (Voight, Hoogenboom, & Cook, 2008).

Instruction: Feet are spaced hip-width apart, a slight bend in knees and hip. Patient grasps affected side at the wrist with unaffected hand and pulls to start position across the waist toward the opposite hip with unaffected palm facing the hip. *Lift*: Patient then lifts the affected arm into shoulder flexion, abduction, and external rotation while following hands with gaze. Allow the upper trunk to twist toward the movement while patient engages deep core to stabilize lower spine (A). Lifted arm is moving in D2 pattern while arm doing the lifting underneath is moving D1 pattern. *Chop*: Patient reaches across body to grasp affected wrist and brings the affected arm across the body into flexion, adduction, and internal rotation, hand coming toward opposite ear while following hands with gaze. Chop happens when coming back down as if chopping wood. Supporting hand moves in D1 pattern and supported arm moves in D2 pattern (B).

Substitutions: Excessive twisting through hips and knees, shrugging shoulders, jutting chin out

Parameters: 10 to 20 repetitions, holding 1 to 3 seconds at end range, 1 set, 1 to 3 times per day

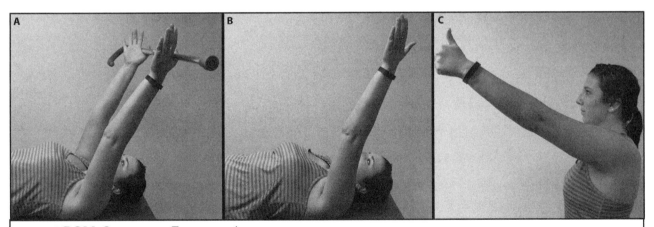

5.04.28 ROM: Shoulder Flexion, Active

Position: Supine, seated, standing

Targets: Mobility of the glenohumeral joint into flexion, activation of shoulder flexors (anterior deltoid, coracobrachialis, long head of biceps, upper fibers pectoralis major) 0 to 60 degrees with minor assist from teres major and subscapularis

Instruction: *With wand/cane bilateral supine*: Patient holds the wand with both hands by sides, palms facing each other, wand sits resting in web space between thumb and index finger. Encourage patient to seat the humeral head in the glenoid fossa by retracting and depressing scapula. Patient brings wand overhead by flexing the shoulders. Elbows remain extended (A). *Without wand/cane supine*: Patient performs shoulder flexion, thumbs lead the way, either bilaterally or unilaterally (B). This is also shown in standing (C).

Substitutions: Encourage scapular retraction to minimize subacromial irritation, avoid arching back, and chin jutting out

Parameters: 10 to 20 repetitions, holding 1 to 3 seconds at end range, 1 set, 1 to 3 times per day

5.04.29 ROM: SHOULDER ABDUCTION, ACTIVE

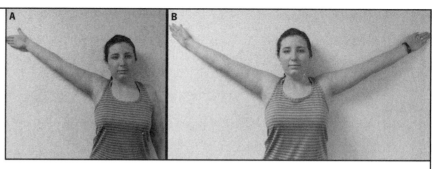

POSITION: Supine, seated, standing

TARGETS: Mobility of the glenohumeral joint into abduction, activation of shoulder abductors (middle deltoid, supraspinatus 0 to 30 degrees, long head of biceps, upper fibers pectoralis major 0 to 60 degrees) with minor assist from teres major and subscapularis

INSTRUCTION: Encourage patient to seat the humeral head in the glenoid fossa by retracting and depressing scapula. Patient performs shoulder abduction, leading with thumb while elbow remains extended; this can be done unilaterally or bilaterally (A and B).

SUBSTITUTIONS: Encourage scapular retraction to minimize subacromial irritation, avoid arching back, and chin jutting out

PARAMETERS: 10 to 20 repetitions holding 1 to 3 seconds at end range, 1 set, 1 to 3 times per day

5.04.30 ROM: SHOULDER ABDUCTION, PARTIAL GRAVITY ASSIST, ACTIVE

POSITION: Side-lying

TARGETS: Mobility of the glenohumeral joint into abduction, activation of shoulder abductors (middle deltoid, supraspinatus 0 to 30 degrees, long head of biceps, upper fibers pectoralis major 0 to 60 degrees) with minor assist from teres major and subscapularis

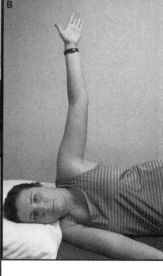

INSTRUCTION: Encourage patient to seat the humeral head in the glenoid fossa by retracting and depressing scapula. Patient performs shoulder abduction, leading with thumb while elbow remains extended. Movement is against gravity for the first 90 degrees but then has gravity assisting and can be useful in early stages of active abduction (A and B). Beyond 90 degrees, the movement becomes gravity assisted (C).

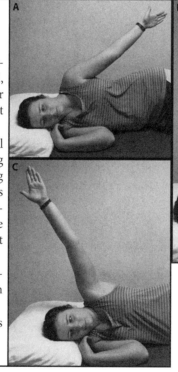

SUBSTITUTIONS: Encourage scapular retraction to minimize subacromial irritation, avoid arching back, and chin jutting out

PARAMETERS: 10 to 20 repetitions, holding 1 to 3 seconds at end range, 1 set, 1 to 3 times per day

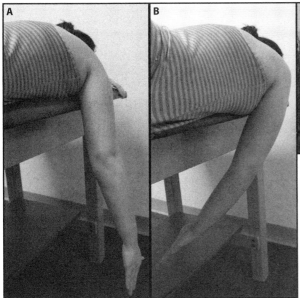
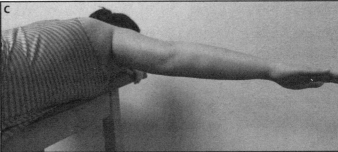

5.04.31 ROM: SHOULDER HORIZONTAL ABDUCTION AND ADDUCTION, ACTIVE

POSITION: Prone

TARGETS: Mobility of the glenohumeral joint into horizontal abduction and horizontal adduction; activation of horizontal abductors (posterior deltoid, infraspinatus, teres minor, latissimus dorsi) and horizontal adductors (pectoralis major and anterior deltoid).

INSTRUCTION: Patient slides to edge of table, allowing affected arm to hang, and slides out to mid-sternum to allow for adduction without hitting table. Patient rests forehead on opposite forearm or towel roll. Patient then lifts arm directly out to the side to horizontally abduct, then returns to horizontally adduct. Encourage patient to seat the humeral head in the glenoid fossa by retracting and depressing scapula throughout the movement (A through C).

SUBSTITUTIONS: Shrugging shoulders excessively, excessive translation of humeral head anteriorly, lifting head

PARAMETERS: 10 to 20 repetitions, holding 1 to 3 seconds at end range, 1 set, 1 to 3 times per day

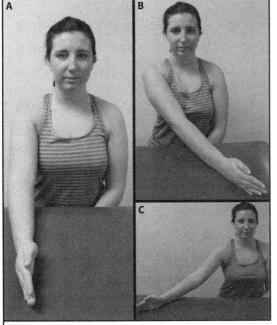

5.04.32 ROM: SHOULDER HORIZONTAL ABDUCTION AND ADDUCTION WITH TABLE SUPPORT, ACTIVE

POSITION: Seated in front of table at shoulder height

TARGETS: Mobility of the glenohumeral joint into horizontal abduction and horizontal adduction; activation of horizontal abductors (posterior deltoid, infraspinatus, teres minor, latissimus dorsi) and horizontal adductors (pectoralis major and anterior deltoid).

INSTRUCTION: With arm resting on table directly in front of patient, body turned slightly outward, elbow extended and thumb or palm up to help clear the humeral head under the acromion, patient slides arm out to the side into horizontal abduction as far as possible, returns to start, and then moves to crossing midline into horizontal adduction. Repeat in one continuous movement holding only at end ranges. Patient then lifts arm directly out to the side, horizontally abducting, then returns to horizontally adduct. Encourage patient to seat the humeral head in the glenoid fossa by retracting and depressing scapula throughout the movement (A through C).

SUBSTITUTIONS: Shrugging shoulders excessively, excessive translation of humeral head anteriorly, lifting head, rolling shoulder forward when at end range of horizontal adduction; cue scapular retraction for control, twisting trunk.

PARAMETERS: 10 to 20 repetitions, holding 1 to 3 seconds at end range, 1 set, 1 to 3 times per day

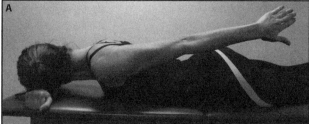

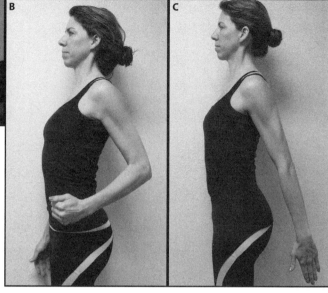

5.04.33 ROM: Shoulder Extension, Active

Position: Prone, standing

Targets: Mobility of the glenohumeral joint using unaffected arm to assist in extension, activation of posterior deltoid, latissimus dorsi, subscapularis, teres major

Instruction: *Prone*: Lying face down with towel under forehead, patient slides to edge of table allowing affected arm to hang, palm facing inward. Encourage patient to seat the humeral head in the glenoid fossa by retracting and depressing scapula. Patient then lifts the arm toward the buttocks and upwards toward ceiling (A). *Standing*: Brings the arm back into shoulder extension; this can be done with a flexed elbow thumbs up or extended elbow (B and C).

Substitutions: Shrugging shoulders excessively, excessive translation of humeral head anteriorly, lifting head.

Parameters: 10 to 20 repetitions, holding 1 to 3 seconds at end range, 1 set, 1 to 3 times per day

5.04.34 ROM: Shoulder Scaption, Active

Position: Standing

Targets: Mobility of the glenohumeral joint into scaption, activation of shoulder flexors in scapular plane (supraspinatus 0 to 30 degrees, anterior and middle deltoid, coracobrachialis, long head of biceps, upper fibers pectoralis major 0 to 60 degrees) with minor assist from teres major and subscapularis

Instruction: Patient performs shoulder scaption; movement in between flexion and abduction approximately 30 degrees forward from the frontal plane, thumbs lead the way; elbows remain extended either bilaterally or unilaterally.

Substitutions: Encourage scapular retraction to minimize subacromial irritation, avoid arching back, chin jutting out, shrugging

Parameters: 10 to 20 repetitions, holding 1 to 3 seconds at end range, 1 set, 1 to 3 times per day

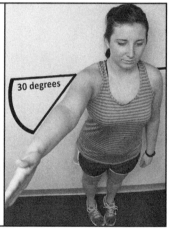

5.04.35 ROM: Shoulder Scaption Figure 8s, Active

Position: Standing

Targets: Activation of shoulder flexors in scapular plane: supraspinatus 0 to 30 degrees, anterior and middle deltoid, coracobrachialis, long head of biceps, upper fibers pectoralis major0 to 60 degrees with minor assist from teres major and subscapularis, encouraging control of the glenohumeral joint

Instruction: Patient performs shoulder scaption, movement in between flexion and abduction approximately 30 degrees forward from the frontal plane, thumbs lead the way, elbows remain extended either bilaterally or unilaterally. With arm elevated to 45 degrees of scaption, patient performs small figure 8 movements with arm while retracting and stabilizing the scapula (A). Repeat at 110 degrees of scaption (B).

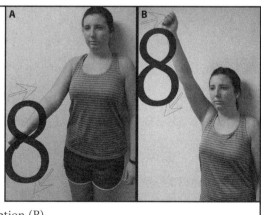

Substitutions: Encourage scapular retraction to minimize subacromial irritation, avoid arching back, chin jutting out, shrugging

Parameters: 10 to 20 repetitions, holding 1 to 3 seconds at end range, 1 set, 1 to 3 times per day

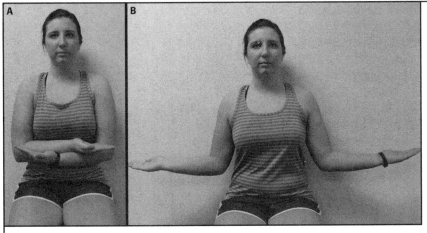

5.04.36 ROM: SHOULDER INTERNAL ROTATION AND EXTERNAL ROTATION, ACTIVE

POSITION: Seated

TARGETS: Mobility of the glenohumeral joint in internal and external rotation; this exercise can be done anywhere with no equipment and is useful for a home program.

INSTRUCTION: Patient sits with elbows flexed to 90 degrees with palms facing up. Encourage patient to seat the humeral head in the glenoid fossa by retracting and depressing scapula. Patient brings pinky toward the navel to internally rotate the shoulder. Affected elbow remains tucked into the patient's side (A). Patient brings thumb outward into shoulder external rotation retracting scapula at end range. Affected elbow remains tucked into the patient's side (B). This can be done bilaterally with increased activation of scapular retractors at end range of external rotation, also called "no money."

SUBSTITUTIONS: Encourage scapular retraction to minimize subacromial irritation

PARAMETERS: 10 to 20 repetitions, holding 1 to 3 seconds at end range, 1 set, 1 to 3 times per day

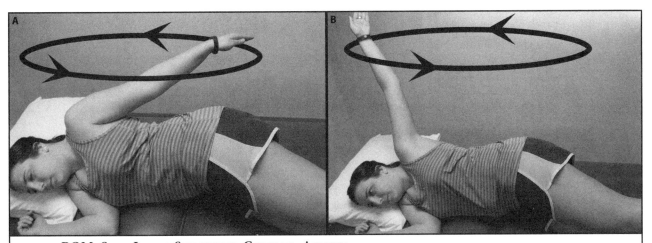

5.04.37 ROM: SIDE-LYING SHOULDER CIRCLES, ACTIVE

POSITION: Side-lying

TARGETS: Mobility of the glenohumeral joint in sagittal plane with gravity assist to seat humeral head in glenoid fossa; this exercise can be done anywhere with no equipment and is useful for a home program.

INSTRUCTION: Patient lies on unaffected side and seats the humeral head of the affected shoulder in the glenoid fossa using scapular retraction and RC. Patient then makes large circles with the arm, maintaining this stable position of the glenohumeral and scapulothoracic joint. Trunk should not move (A and B).

SUBSTITUTIONS: Encourage scapular retraction to minimize subacromial irritation

PARAMETERS: 10 to 20 repetitions, holding 1 to 3 seconds at end ranges, 1 set, 1 to 3 times per day

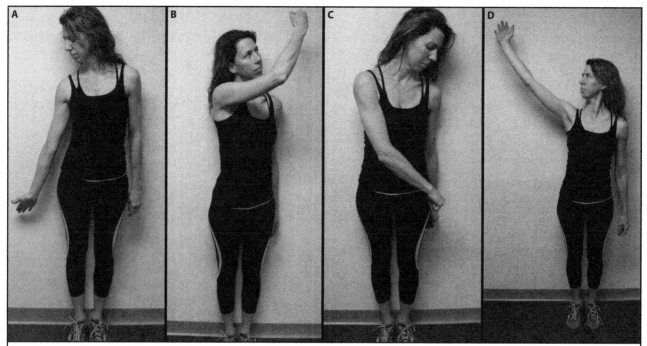

5.04.38 ROM: SHOULDER, PNF D1 AND D2, ACTIVE

<u>POSITION</u>: Standing

<u>TARGETS</u>: Mobility of the glenohumeral joint and activation of functional movements in the shoulder.

<u>INSTRUCTION</u>: Patient performs movements through combined pattern, working the shoulder in all three movement planes. D1 and D2 patterns may start in either the flexed or extended position. Patient should follow the hand movement with the eyes and head.

D1 extension: "Tissue Toss": Starting in a position of scapular retraction, shoulder extension, abduction and internal rotation, forearm is pronated, wrist is ulnarly deviated, fingers are extended (A), patient brings arm across the body and moves to *D1 flexion: "Throwing salt over opposite shoulder"*: Shoulder ends in flexion, adduction, external rotation with forearm supinated, wrist radially deviated and flingers flexed (B).

D2 extension: "Unsheath the sword": Starting in a position of shoulder extension, abduction and internal rotation across the body, forearm is pronated, wrist is ulnarly deviated, fingers are flexed (C), patient brings arm across the body and moves to *D2 flexion: "Tada!"*: Ending with scapula retracted, shoulder flexed, abducted, externally rotated, forearm pronated, wrist in ulnar deviation and fingers extended (D).

<u>SUBSTITUTIONS</u>: Encourage scapular retraction to minimize subacromial irritation, avoid arching back, chin jutting out, shrugging

<u>PARAMETERS</u>: 10 to 20 repetitions, holding 1 to 3 seconds at end range, 1 set, 1 to 3 times per day

REFERENCES

Jung, M. C., Kim, S. J., Rhee, J. J., & Lee, D. H. (2016). Electromyographic activities of the subscapularis, supraspinatus and infraspinatus muscles during passive shoulder and active elbow exercises. *Knee Surgery, Sports Traumatology and Arthroscopy, 24*(7), 2238-2243.

Long, J. L., Ruberte Thiele, R. A., Skendzel, J. G., Jeon, J., Hughes, R. E., Miller, B. S., & Carpenter, J. E. (2010). Activation of the shoulder musculature during pendulum exercises and light activities. *Journal of Orthopedic and Sports Physical Therapy, 40*(4), 230-237.

Uhl, T. L., Muir ,T. A., & Lawson, L. (2010). Electromyographical assessment of passive, active assistive, and active shoulder rehabilitation exercises. *pectoralis majorand R: The Journal of Injury, Function and Rehabilitation, 2*(2), 132-141.

Voight, M. L., Hoogenboom, B. J., & Cook, G. (2008). The chop and lift reconsidered: Integrating neuromuscular principles into orthopedic and sports rehabilitation. *North American Journal of Sports Physical Therapy, 3*(3), 151-159.

Section 5.05

Shoulder Joint Self-Mobilization/Stretching

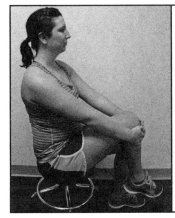

5.05.1 SELF-JOINT MOBILIZATION/STRETCH: SHOULDER, KNEE HOLD, DISTRACTION

POSITION: Seated

TARGETS: Mobility of the glenohumeral joint anterior and inferior capsule stretch

INSTRUCTION: Patient flexes hip and knee off chair and grasps hands together around anterior knee. Patient relaxes leg slowly, allowing gravity pull of the leg to distract the glenohumeral joint in an anterior and inferior direction.

SUBSTITUTIONS: Encourage scapular retraction during distraction

PARAMETERS: Hold 15 to 30 seconds, 3 to 5 repetitions, 1 to 3 times per day

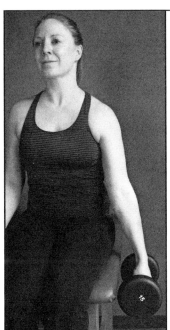

5.05.2 SELF-JOINT MOBILIZATION/STRETCH: SHOULDER, DISTRACTION WITH WEIGHT

POSITION: Seated

TARGETS: Mobility of the glenohumeral joint and inferior capsule stretch

INSTRUCTION: Place a towel roll under the axilla to distract glenohumeral joint and, while holding weight, patient relaxes shoulder slowly, allowing gravity pull to traction the glenohumeral joint in an inferior direction.

SUBSTITUTIONS: Encourage scapular retraction during distraction

PARAMETERS: Hold 15 to 30 seconds up to 5 minutes; repeat 1 to 5 times, 1 to 3 times per day (if doing for longer period of time, only 1 repetition is necessary).

5.05.3 SELF-JOINT MOBILIZATION/STRETCH: SHOULDER DISTRACTION WITH CHAIR PULL

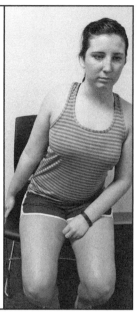

POSITION: Seated

TARGETS: Mobility of the glenohumeral joint inferior capsule stretch

INSTRUCTION: Patient grasps side of chair seat and leans body away to distract glenohumeral joint in an inferior direction.

SUBSTITUTIONS: Encourage scapular retraction during distraction.

PARAMETERS: Hold 15 to 30 seconds, 3 to 5 repetitions, 1 to 3 times per day

5.05.4 SELF-JOINT MOBILIZATION/STRETCH: SHOULDER, ARM HANG, ANTERIOR GLIDE WITH WEIGHT

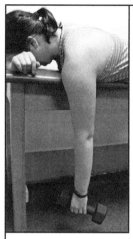

POSITION: Prone

TARGETS: Mobility of the glenohumeral joint anterior capsule stretch

INSTRUCTION: Patient scoots sideways to allow shoulder and arm to drop off table. While holding weight, patient relaxes shoulder slowly, allowing gravity pull to distract the glenohumeral joint in an anterior direction.

SUBSTITUTIONS: Shoulder shrugs

PARAMETERS: Hold 15 to 30 seconds up to 5 minutes; repeat 1 to 5 times, 1 to 3 times per day (if doing for longer period of time, only 1 repetition is necessary).

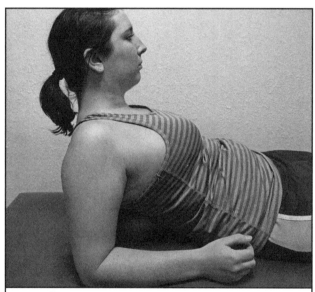

5.05.5 SELF-JOINT MOBILIZATION/STRETCH: ANTERIOR CAPSULE STRETCH, SUPINE ON ELBOWS

POSITION: Supine

TARGETS: Mobility of the glenohumeral joint anterior capsule stretch

INSTRUCTION: Patient props up on elbows, with elbows directly under the shoulders. Patient allows upper back to sag toward the table as humeral head is pushed into the anterior capsule for a stretch.

SUBSTITUTIONS: Shoulder shrug; keep scapula actively retracted.

PARAMETERS: Hold 15 to 30 seconds up to 5 minutes; repeat 1 to 5 times, 1 to 3 times per day (if doing for longer period of time, only 1 repetition is necessary).

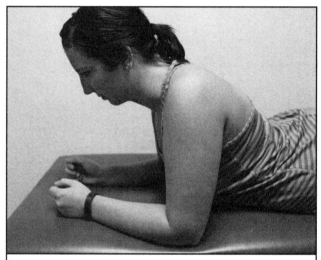

5.05.6 SELF-JOINT MOBILIZATION/STRETCH: POSTERIOR CAPSULE STRETCH, PRONE ON ELBOWS

POSITION: Prone

TARGETS: Mobility of the glenohumeral joint posterior capsule stretch

INSTRUCTION: Patient props up on elbows, with elbows directly under the shoulders. Patient allows upper back to sag toward the table as humeral head is pushed into the posterior capsule for a stretch.

SUBSTITUTIONS: Shoulder shrug; keep scapula actively retracted.

PARAMETERS: Hold 15 to 30 seconds up to 5 minutes; repeat 1 to 5 times, 1 to 3 times per day (if doing for longer period of time, only 1 repetition is necessary).

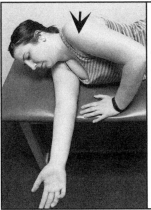

5.05.7 SELF-JOINT MOBILIZATION/STRETCH: POSTERIOR CAPSULE STRETCH, SIDE-LYING CROSSOVER

POSITION: Side-lying

TARGETS: Mobility of the glenohumeral joint posterior capsule stretch

INSTRUCTION: Patient places affected shoulder underneath the body at 90 degrees of flexion and slowly rolls the body over, bringing top shoulder toward the affected arm's elbow until stretch is felt in posterior shoulder. The therapist may apply pressure on the scapula toward the rib cage to increase the stretch.

SUBSTITUTIONS: Shoulder shrug; keep scapula actively retracted to avoid subacromial compression.

PARAMETERS: 15 to 30 seconds at end range, 3 to 5 repetitions, 1 set, 1 to 3 times per day (if doing for longer period of time, only 1 repetition is necessary)

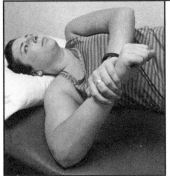

5.05.8 SELF-JOINT MOBILIZATION/STRETCH: SHOULDER INTERNAL ROTATION, "SLEEPER STRETCH", 90/90

POSITION: Side-lying (on affected side; quarter turned toward supine)

TARGETS: Mobility of the glenohumeral joint; increases ROM into internal rotation, stretches posterior glenohumeral capsule.

INSTRUCTION: Using a firm surface, patient lies on target side with quarter turn of body toward supine so pressure not directly on shoulder. Patient is not to lie flat on scapula with rounded shoulder, but mostly on rib cage and outside border of scapula. Patient can roll forward to get scapula off surface, then roll back. Make sure body is not straight up and down but rolled back about 45 degrees. Keep head neutral with pillows. Bottom arm is in 90/90 position. Encourage patient to seat the humeral head in the glenoid fossa by retracting and depressing scapula. Patient uses other arm to press palm of hand arm toward the table for a mild stretch felt in posterior shoulder. Pain in the subacromial region indicates insufficient scapular retraction and depression or positioning errors and should be addressed.

SUBSTITUTIONS: Encourage scapular retraction to minimize subacromial irritation, avoid arching back or chin jutting out; gaze remains forward, avoid any anterior shoulder discomfort as this movement, if pushed too hard, can create impingement.

PARAMETERS: 15 to 30 seconds at end range, 3 to 5 repetitions, 1 set, 1 to 3 times per day

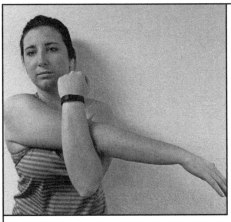

5.05.9 SELF-JOINT MOBILIZATION/STRETCH: POSTERIOR CAPSULE STRETCH, CROSSOVER

POSITION: Seated, standing (on affected side)

TARGETS: Mobility of the glenohumeral joint posterior capsule stretch; also stretches posterior deltoid.

INSTRUCTION: Patient grasps elbow with opposite hand, retracts scapulae- and pulls arm across the front of the body into adduction, or horizontal adduction if tolerated until a stretch is felt in the back of shoulder.

SUBSTITUTIONS: Encourage scapular retraction to minimize subacromial irritation, avoid arching back or chin jutting out; gaze remains forward, avoid any anterior shoulder discomfort as this movement, if pulled too hard, an create impingement.

PARAMETERS: 15 to 30 seconds at end range, 3 to 5 repetitions, 1 set, 1 to 3 times per day

Where's the Evidence?

McClure and Flowers (1992) demonstrated that the cross-arm stretch was more effective than the sleeper stretch for the posterior shoulder. Manske, Meschke, Porter, Smith, and Reiman (2010) found the cross-arm stretch with joint mobilization and the cross-arm stretch alone can significantly increase shoulder internal rotation following 4 weeks of intervention in a group of asymptomatic college-age students.

5.05.10 SELF-JOINT MOBILIZATION/STRETCH: ANTEROINFERIOR CAPSULE

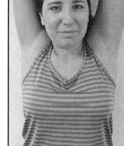

POSITION: Standing

TARGETS: Mobility of the glenohumeral joint using unaffected arm to assist in movements to increase external rotation with anteroinferior capsule stretch

INSTRUCTION: Patient brings hand over the head and behind the neck andupper back. With unaffected hand, apply pressure to the affected elbow into shoulder abduction behind the head. Hold and return slowly.

SUBSTITUTIONS: Encourage scapular retraction to minimize subacromial irritation

PARAMETERS: 15 to 30 seconds at end range, 3 to 5 repetitions, 1 set, 1 to 3 times per day

5.05.11 SELF-JOINT MOBILIZATION/STRETCH: ANTERIOR MIDDLE CAPSULE

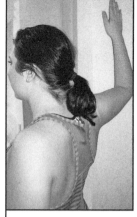

POSITION: Standing

TARGETS: Mobility of the glenohumeral joint to increase external rotation with anterior middle capsule stretch

INSTRUCTION: Patient stands in a doorway with a staggered stance and trunk straight, scapula retracted and depressed slightly, and scaptions the shoulder to 90 degrees and flexes the elbow to 90 degrees, placing the hand and forearm on the door jamb. Patient slowly twists the body away from the affected arm until stretch is felt in the anterior glenohumeral joint. Hold and return slowly.

SUBSTITUTIONS: Encourage scapular retraction and depression to minimize subacromial irritation

PARAMETERS: 15 to 30 seconds at end range, 3 to 5 repetitions, 1 set, 1 to 3 times per day

5.05.12 SELF-JOINT MOBILIZATION/STRETCH: ANTEROSUPERIOR CAPSULE

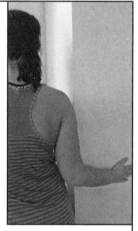

POSITION: Standing

TARGETS: Mobility of the glenohumeral joint to increase external rotation with anterosuperior capsule stretch

INSTRUCTION: Patient stands in a doorway with a staggered stance and trunk straight, scapula retracted and depressed slightly, elbow tucked into the side and flexed to 90 degrees, placing the hand on the door jamb. Patient slowly twists the body away from the affected arm until stretch felt in the anterior glenohumeral joint. Hold and return slowly.

SUBSTITUTIONS: Encourage scapular retraction and depression to minimize subacromial irritation

PARAMETERS: 15 to 30 seconds at end range, 3 to 5 repetitions, 1 set, 1 to 3 times per day

5.05.13 SELF-JOINT MOBILIZATION/STRETCH: ANTEROLATERAL DISTRACTION

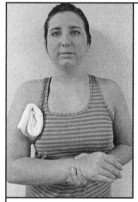

POSITION: Standing

TARGETS: Mobility of the glenohumeral joint to increase internal rotation with anterolateral capsule stretch

INSTRUCTION: Place a towel roll under the axilla to distract glenohumeral joint and have patient place the affected arm across the stomach while the other hand grasps the affected wrist. Patient then pulls the affected arm across the front of the body. The towel serves as a fulcrum to lever the humeral head, distracting it away from the socket. Hold and return slowly.

SUBSTITUTIONS: Encourage scapular retraction and depression to minimize subacromial irritation

PARAMETERS: 15 to 30 seconds at end range, 3 to 5 repetitions, 1 set, 1 to 3 times per day

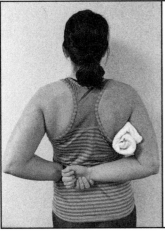

5.05.14 SELF-JOINT MOBILIZATION/STRETCH: POSTEROLATERAL DISTRACTION

POSITION: Standing

TARGETS: Mobility of the glenohumeral joint to increase internal rotation with posterolateral capsule stretch

INSTRUCTION: Place a towel roll under the axilla to distract glenohumeral joint; have patient place the affected arm behind the back and reach behind the back with the other hand to grasp the affected wrist. Patient then pulls the affected arm across the back. The towel serves as a fulcrum to lever the humeral head distracting it way from the socket. Hold and return slowly. If the patient has difficulty reaching the affected arm far enough to grasp, use a stick or a strap to assist.

SUBSTITUTIONS: Encourage scapular retraction and depression to minimize subacromial irritation

PARAMETERS: 15 to 30 seconds at end range, 3 to 5 repetitions, 1 set, 1 to 3 times per day

Where's the Evidence?

Izumi, Aoki, Muraki, Hidaka, and Miyamoto (2008) in cadaver studies found that large strains on the posterior capsule of the shoulder were obtained at a stretching position of 30 degrees of elevation in the scapular plane with internal rotation for the middle and lower capsule, while a stretching position of 30 degrees of extension with internal rotation was effective for the upper and lower capsule.

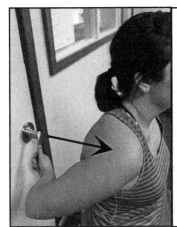

5.05.15 SELF-JOINT MOBILIZATION/STRETCH: ANTEROLATERAL CAPSULE, DOOR KNOB LEAN

POSITION: Standing

TARGETS: Mobility of the glenohumeral joint to increase internal rotation with anterolateral capsule stretch

INSTRUCTION: Patient faces away from the door and grasp the door knob with affected arm behind the back. Patient then leans forward until stretch is felt in shoulder. Hold and return slowly.

SUBSTITUTIONS: Encourage scapular retraction and depression to minimize subacromial irritation

PARAMETERS: 15 to 30 seconds at end range, 3 to 5 repetitions, 1 set, 1 to 3 times per day

---

REFERENCES

Izumi, T., Aoki, M., Muraki, T., Hidaka, E., & Miyamoto, S. (2008). Stretching positions for the posterior capsule of the glenohumeral joint: Strain measurement using cadaver specimens. *American Journal of Sports Medicine, 36*(10), 2014-2022.

Manske, R. C., Meschke, M., Porter, A., Smith, B., & Reiman, M. (2010). A randomized controlled single-blinded comparison of stretching versus stretching and joint mobilization for posterior shoulder tightness measured by internal rotation motion loss. *Sports Health, 2*(2), 94-100.

McClure, P. W., & Flowers, K. R. (1992). Treatment of limited shoulder motion: A case study based on biomechanical considerations. *Physical Therapy, 72*(12), 929-936.

Section 5.06

SHOULDER STRETCHING

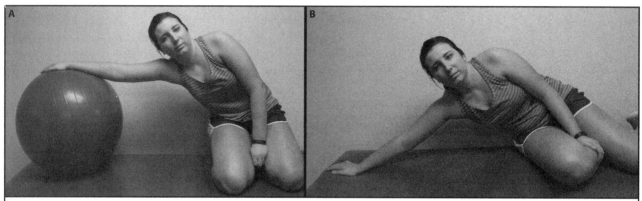

5.06.1 STRETCH: SHOULDER ADDUCTORS, PASSIVE

<u>POSITION</u>: Side-sitting (to affected side with exercise ball on same-side)

<u>TARGETS</u>: Stretch primarily latissimus dorsi with minor stretch also in pectoralis major, subscapularis, teres major, teres minor, coracobrachialis and triceps

<u>INSTRUCTION</u>: Patient places affected arm into abduction with elbow and forearm on exercise ball. Patient leans toward the ball, allowing the ball to roll. Gravity then assists to stretch the shoulder into abduction while stretching adductors (A). This can also be done without the ball by propping up on the affected elbow and leaning into the movement of abduction (B).

<u>SUBSTITUTIONS</u>: Shrugging shoulders

<u>PARAMETERS</u>: Hold for 15 to 30 seconds, 3 to 5 repetitions, 1 to 3 times per day

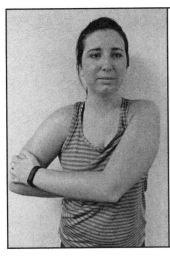

5.06.2 Stretch: Shoulder Internal Rotation, "Chicken Wing", Active Assistive

POSITION: Standing

TARGETS: Mobility of the shoulder into internal rotation; stretching external rotators, infraspinatus, and teres minor.

INSTRUCTION: Patient brings affected arm behind the back. Patient uses the unaffected hand to bring the affected side into more internal rotation by reaching across and pulling the affected elbow closer to the trunk, sliding the affected hand upwards along the torso. Encourage patient to seat the humeral head in the glenoid fossa by retracting and depressing scapula, avoiding excessive anterior head translation.

SUBSTITUTIONS: Encourage scapular retraction to minimize subacromial irritation, avoid jutting chin out, keep slight chin tuck

PARAMETERS: Hold for 15 to 30 seconds, 3 to 5 repetitions, 1 to 3 times per day

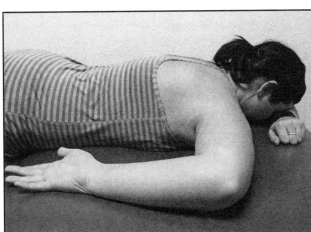

5.06.3 Stretch: Shoulder Internal Rotation, Prone

POSITION: Prone

TARGETS: Mobility of the shoulder into internal rotation; stretching external rotators, infraspinatus, and teres minor.

INSTRUCTION: Patient places involved shoulder at 90 degrees of abduction and elbow at 90 degrees of flexion. With the palm facing up, patient then attempts to bring the elbow toward the supporting surface.

SUBSTITUTIONS: Encourage scapular retraction and depression to minimize subacromial irritation

PARAMETERS: Hold for 15 to 30 seconds, 3 to 5 repetitions, 1 to 3 times per day

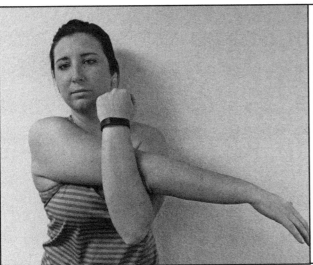

5.06.4 Stretch: Shoulder Horizontal Abductors

POSITION: Seated, standing

TARGETS: Mobility of the scapula into protraction, stretches posterior deltoid and posterior RC, also stretches posterior capsule

INSTRUCTION: With erect posture, patient lifts affected arm to shoulder height, grasps behind the elbow with the unaffected hand and pulls arm across the body. If patient has any pinching or superior shoulder pain, encourage patient to depress the shoulder during the stretch. Stretch should be felt in posterior shoulder only. Chin stays tucked.

SUBSTITUTIONS: Shrugging shoulders, chin juts out

PARAMETERS: Hold for 15 to 30 seconds, 3 to 5 repetitions, 1 to 3 times per day

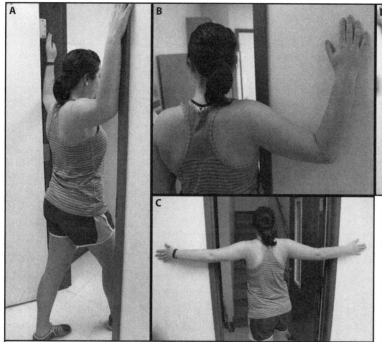

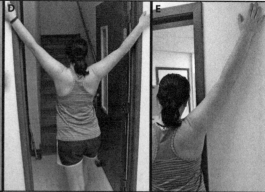

5.06.5 Stretch: Shoulder Horizontal Adductors, Doorway

Position: Standing

Targets: Stretches pectoralis major and minor

Instruction: *Pectoralis major focus*: Patient stands facing doorway with shoulders in 90 degrees of abduction, with elbows flexed 90 degrees or straight, forearms are placed on the door jamb. Patient staggers feet front-to-back and slightly lunges into the doorway until a stretch is felt across the chest. Patient may move feet if needed to avoid leaning forward toward the floor. This can be done bilaterally or unilaterally (A and B). Straightening the elbows adds biceps stretch as well (C). *Pectoralis minor focus*: Patient stands facing doorway and places shoulders in 120 to 150 degrees of abduction with elbows slightly flexed or straight, and forearms placed on the door jamb. Patient staggers feet front-to-back and slightly lunges into the doorway until a stretch is felt anterior to the axilla. Patient may move feet if needed to avoid leaning forward toward the floor. This can be done bilaterally or unilaterally (D and E). Alternatively, both stretches can be done with the elbow extended; therapist should watch for hyperextension of the back.

Substitutions: Shrugging shoulders, jutting chin out, leaning body weight toward floor, trunk should stay upright

Parameters: Hold for 15 to 30 seconds, 3 to 5 repetitions, 1 to 3 times per day

---

Where's the Evidence?

A study by Borstad and Ludewig (2006) compared three different techniques of stretching: the unilateral doorway stretch, a manual stretch in the sitting position, and a supine manual stretch. Electromagnetic motion capture was used to detect changes in muscle length and found that they all produced changes in muscle length, but that the doorway stretch was superior. Lee et al. (2015) studied 15 subjects with tight pectoralis minor and found that stretching the pectoralis minor before scapular posterior tilting exercise (scapular retraction, depression, downward rotation) would be an effective method of modifying scapular alignment and scapular upward rotator activity.

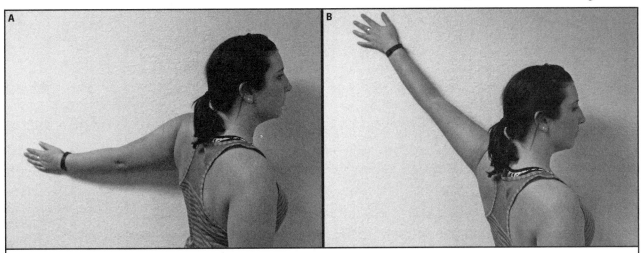

5.06.6 STRETCH: SHOULDER HORIZONTAL ADDUCTORS, WALL

POSITION: Standing

TARGETS: Stretches pectoralis major and minor

INSTRUCTION: *Pectoralis major focus*: Patient stands close to and facing wall and places target shoulder in 90 degrees of abduction with elbow extended and palm against the wall. Patient then rotates the trunk away from the wall toward the opposite side, moving the feet as needed to keep hips neutral (A). *Pectoralis minor focus*: Patient stands close to and facing wall and places target shoulder in 120 to 150 degrees of abduction with elbow extended and palm against the wall. Patient then rotates the trunk away from the wall toward the opposite side, moving the feet as needed to keep hips neutral. Patient slightly lunges into the corner until stretch is felt across anterior to the axilla (B).

SUBSTITUTIONS: Shrugging shoulders, jutting chin out, leaning body weight toward floor, trunk should stay upright

PARAMETERS: Hold for 15 to 30 seconds, 3 to 5 repetitions, 1 to 3 times per day

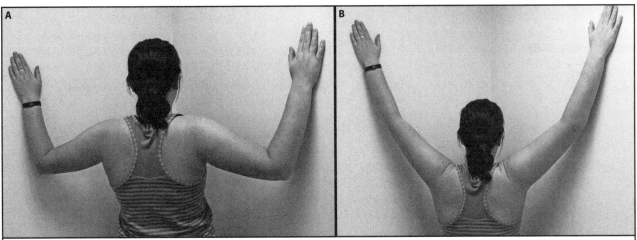

5.06.7 STRETCH: SHOULDER HORIZONTAL ADDUCTORS, CORNER

POSITION: Standing

TARGETS: Stretches pectoralis major and minor

INSTRUCTION: *Pectoralis major focus*: Patient stands facing corner with feet staggered front-to-back and places shoulders in 90 degrees of abduction with elbows flexed 90 degrees. Forearms and palms are placed on the walls. Patient slightly lunges into the corner until stretch is felt across the chest (A). *Pectoralis minor focus*: Patient stands facing corner with feet staggered front-to-back and places shoulders in 120 to 150 degrees of abduction with elbows flexed 30 to 45 degrees. Forearms and palms are placed on the walls. Patient slightly lunges into the corner until stretch is felt across anterior to the axilla (B).

SUBSTITUTIONS: Shrugging shoulders, jutting chin out

PARAMETERS: Hold for 15 to 30 seconds, 3 to 5 repetitions, 1 to 3 times per day

5.06.8 Stretch: Shoulder Horizontal Adductors, Towel Roll and Swiss Ball

Position: Standing

Targets: Stretches pectoralis major and minor

Instruction: *Pectoralis major focus*: Patient lies supine with a long towel roll placed along the spine vertically (A). Patient places shoulders in 90 degrees of abduction with elbows extended and palms up. Patient relaxes and allows gravity to pull into further horizontal abduction until a stretch is felt across the chest (B). For *pectoralis minor focus*: Simply move shoulders to 120 to 150 degrees of abduction and repeat (C). Both of these can also be done reverse table top on exercise ball (D and E).

Substitutions: Shrugging shoulders

Parameters: Hold for up to 5 minutes, 1 repetition, 1 to 3 times per day

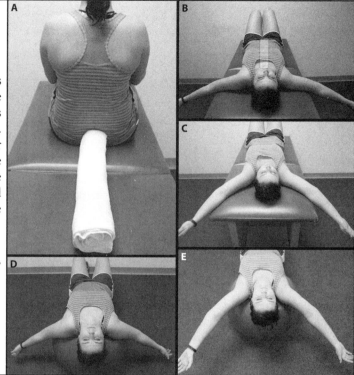

5.06.9 Stretch: Shoulder Horizontal Adductors, Roll-Over

Position: Prone

Targets: Stretches pectoralis major

Instruction: Patient lies face down and places affected shoulder at 90 degrees of abduction then using the unaffected arm to push, slowly rolls the body over bringing unaffected shoulder toward ceiling until a stretch is felt on the affected side across the chest.

Substitutions: Shoulder shrugs

Parameters: 15 to 30 seconds at end range, 3 to 5 repetitions, 1 set, 1 to 3 times per day

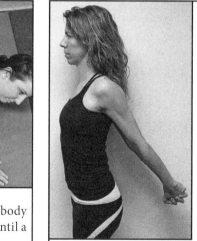

5.06.10 Stretch: Anterior Deltoid and Biceps Hand Clasp

Position: Standing

Targets: Stretch anterior deltoid and biceps brachii

Instruction: Patient clasps hands behind with shoulders and elbows extended. Patient retracts scapula as far as possible, reaching hands out further. Chin stays tucked.

Substitutions: Shrugging shoulders, raising arms too high forcing humeral head into excessive anterior movement, jutting chin out

Parameters: Hold for 15 to 30 seconds, 3 to 5 repetitions, 1 to 3 times per day

References

Borstad, J. D., & Ludewig, P. M. (2006). Comparison of three stretches for the pectoralis minor muscle. *Journal of Shoulder and Elbow Surgery, 15*(3), 324-330.

Lee, J. H., Cynn, H. S., Yoon, T. L., Choi, S. A., Choi, W. J., Choi, B. S., & Ko, C. H. (2015). Comparison of scapular posterior tilting exercise alone and scapular posterior tilting exercise after pectoralis minor stretching on scapular alignment and scapular upward rotators activity in subjects with short pectoralis minor. *Physical Therapy in Sport, 16*(3), 255-261.

Section 5.07

SHOULDER STRENGTHENING

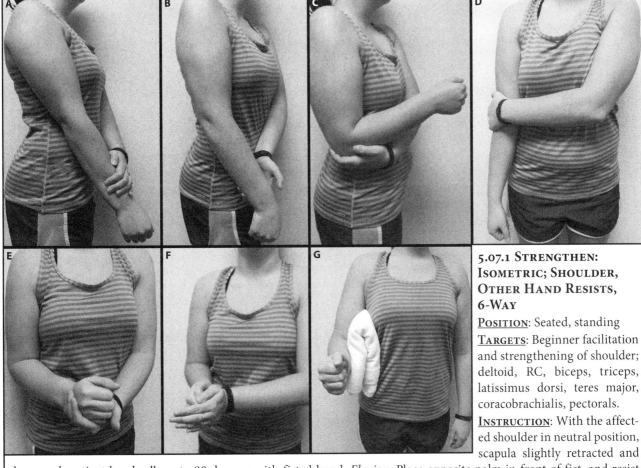

5.07.1 STRENGTHEN: ISOMETRIC; SHOULDER, OTHER HAND RESISTS, 6-WAY

<u>POSITION</u>: Seated, standing

<u>TARGETS</u>: Beginner facilitation and strengthening of shoulder; deltoid, RC, biceps, triceps, latissimus dorsi, teres major, coracobrachialis, pectorals.

<u>INSTRUCTION</u>: With the affected shoulder in neutral position, scapula slightly retracted and depressed, patient bends elbow to 90 degrees with fisted hand. *Flexion*: Place opposite palm in front of fist, and resist flexion of the affected shoulder (A). *Extension*: Place opposite palm behind elbow, and resist extension of the affected shoulder; elbow can be straight or bent (B and C). *Abduction*: Place opposite palm around elbow, and resist abduction of the affected shoulder (D). *Internal rotation*: Place opposite palm medial to fist, and resist internal rotation of the affected shoulder (E). *External rotation*: Place opposite palm lateral to fist, and resist external rotation of the affected shoulder (F). *Adduction*: Place towel or small pillow between elbow and side of body to resist adduction of the affected shoulder (G).

<u>SUBSTITUTIONS</u>: Shrugging shoulder; shoulder not in neutral position.

<u>PARAMETERS</u>: Hold for 6 to 10 seconds with 1 to 2 second ramp up and down, 8 to 12 repetitions, 1 to 3 sets, 1 time per day or every other day

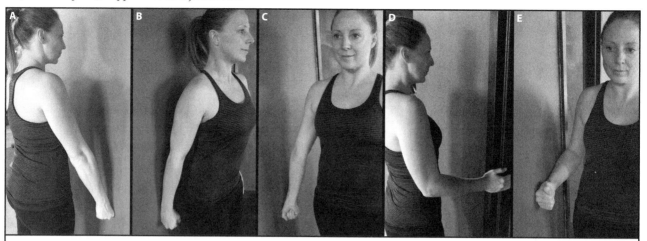

5.07.2 Strengthen: Isometric; Wall Resists, 5-Way

<u>Position</u>: Standing

<u>Targets</u>: Beginner facilitation and strengthening of shoulder; targets deltoid, RC, biceps, triceps, latissimus dorsi, teres major, coracobrachialis, pectorals.

<u>Instruction</u>: With the affected shoulder in neutral position, scapula slightly retracted and depressed, patient bends elbow to 90 degrees with fisted hand. Place a pillow on the wall at elbow height. *Flexion*: Patient faces wall and places fist on pillow. Patient flexes shoulder into the wall, which provides resistance. Watch to make sure patient is not leaning into the wall but attempting to raise arm into the wall (A). *Extension*: Patient faces away from wall and places back of arm and elbow on pillow. Patient extends shoulder into the wall, which provides resistance (B) *Abduction*: Patient stands with affected side toward wall and places lateral elbow on pillow. Patient abducts shoulder into the wall, which provides resistance (C). *Internal rotation*: Standing facing a door jamb, patient places anterior forearm against the wall and internally rotates as wall resists (D). *External rotation*: Standing facing a door jamb, patient places posterior forearm against the wall and externally rotates as wall resists (E).

<u>Substitutions</u>: Shrugging shoulder; shoulder not in neutral position.

<u>Parameters</u>: Hold for 6 to 10 seconds, 1 to 3 sets, 8 to 12 repetitions with 1 to 2 second ramp up and down, 1 time per day or every other day

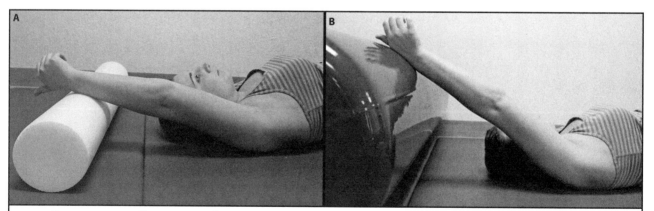

5.07.3 Strengthen: Isometric; Shoulder Flexion Overhead

<u>Position</u>: Supine

<u>Targets</u>: Beginner facilitation and strengthening of shoulder; targets anterior deltoid, coracobrachialis.

<u>Instruction</u>: With the affected shoulder flexed overhead to comfort level, place sturdy bolster or pillows to support the arm. Patient slightly retracts and depresses scapula and flexes shoulder into the bolster, which provides resistance (A and B).

<u>Substitutions</u>: Shrugging shoulder

<u>Parameters</u>: Hold for 6 to 10 seconds, 1 to 3 sets, 8 to 12 repetitions with 1 to 2 second ramp up and down, 1 time per day or every other day

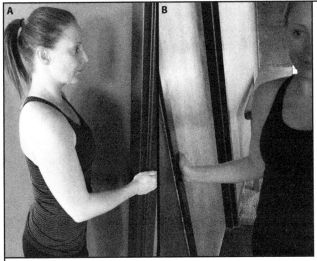

5.07.4 STRENGTHEN: ISOMETRIC; SHOULDER INTERNAL ROTATION MULTI-ANGLE NEUTRAL, DOORWAY

POSITION: Standing

TARGETS: Beginner facilitation and strengthening of shoulder internal rotators; subscapularis, latissimus dorsi, pectoralis major, teres major.

INSTRUCTION: With the affected shoulder in neutral position, scapula slightly retracted and depressed, patient bends elbow to 90 degrees with fisted hand. Place a pillow on the wall at elbow height. Standing facing a door jamb, patient places anterior forearm against the wall. To alter the angle of internal rotation, patient can rotate the trunk toward or away from the door jamb while keeping the elbow tucked into the side. In each position, patient performs a set of isometric internal rotation while the wall resists (A and B).

SUBSTITUTIONS: Shrugging shoulder; elbow should stay tucked into the side (neutral flexion, abduction, extension).

PARAMETERS: Hold for 6 to 10 seconds, 1 to 3 sets, 8 to 12 repetitions with 1 to 2 second ramp up and down, 1 time per day or every other day

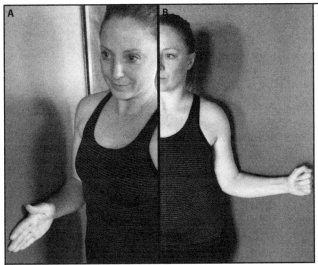

5.07.5 STRENGTHEN: ISOMETRIC; SHOULDER EXTERNAL ROTATION MULTI-ANGLE NEUTRAL, DOORWAY

POSITION: Standing

TARGETS: Beginner facilitation and strengthening of shoulder external rotators; infraspinatus, posterior deltoid, teres minor.

INSTRUCTION: With the affected shoulder in neutral position, scapula slightly retracted and depressed, patient bends elbow to 90 degrees with fisted hand. Place a pillow on the wall at elbow height. Standing facing a door jamb, patient places posterior forearm against the wall. To alter the angle of external rotation, patient can rotate the trunk toward or away from the door jamb while keeping the elbow tucked into the side. In each position, patient performs a set of isometric external rotation while the wall resists (A and B).

SUBSTITUTIONS: Shrugging shoulder; elbow should stay tucked into the side (neutral flexion, abduction, extension).

PARAMETERS: Hold for 6 to 10 seconds, 1 to 3 sets, 8 to 12 repetitions with 1 to 2 second ramp up and down, 1 time per day or every other day

5.07.6 Strengthen: Isometric; Shoulder Internal Rotation Multi-Angle Abduction and Flexion

<u>Position</u>: Standing

<u>Targets</u>: Beginner facilitation and strengthening of shoulder internal rotators; subscapularis, latissimus dorsi, pectoralis major and teres major.

<u>Instruction</u>: With the affected shoulder in neutral position, scapula slightly retracted and depressed, patient bends elbow to 90 degrees with fisted hand. Place a pillow on the wall at elbow height. *In flexion*: Patient faces door jamb so that door jamb is medial to the shoulder, places anterior forearm on pillow and internally rotates as wall resists. This is generally done at 45 degrees, 90 degrees and 120 degrees of flexion (A, B and C). *In abduction*: Patient stands with the side toward,

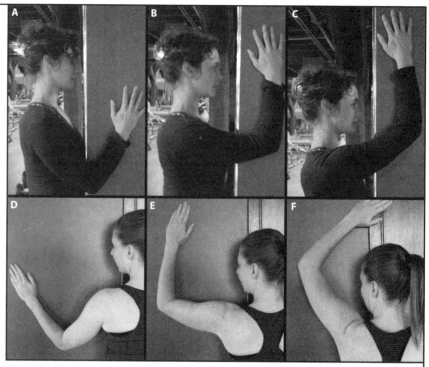

and shoulder slightly behind, door jamb and places forearm on pillow and internally rotates as wall resists. The shoulder begins in a position of external rotation with the abduction multi-angle exercise. This is generally done at 45 degrees, 90 degrees, and 120 degrees of abduction (D, E, and F).

<u>Substitutions</u>: Shrugging shoulder

<u>Parameters</u>: Hold for 6 to 10 seconds, 1 to 3 sets, 8 to 12 repetitions with 1 to 2 second ramp up and down, 1 time per day or every other day

5.07.7 Strengthen: Isometric; Shoulder External Rotation Multi-Angle Abduction and Flexion

<u>Position</u>: Standing

<u>Targets</u>: Beginner facilitation and strengthening of shoulder external rotators; infraspinatus, posterior deltoid, teres minor.

<u>Instruction</u>: With the affected shoulder in neutral position, scapula slightly retracted and depressed, patient bends elbow to 90 degrees with fisted hand. Place a pillow on the wall at elbow height. *In flexion*: Patient faces door jamb so that door jamb is lateral to the shoulder, places posterior forearm on pillow and externally rotates as wall resists. This is generally done at 45 degrees, 90 degrees, and 120 degrees of abduction (A through C). *In abduc-*

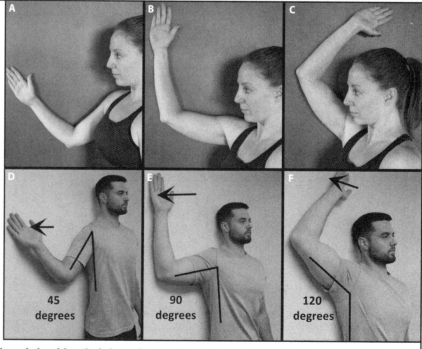

tion: Patient stands with the side toward, and shoulder slightly in front, of door jamb and places forearm on pillow and externally rotates as wall resists. The shoulder begins in a position of external rotation with the abduction multi-angle exercise. This is generally done at 45 degrees, 90 degrees, and 120 degrees of abduction (D through F).

<u>Substitutions</u>: Shrugging shoulder

<u>Parameters</u>: Hold for 6 to 10 seconds, 1 to 3 sets, 8 to 12 repetitions with 1 to 2 second ramp up and down, 1 time per day or every other day

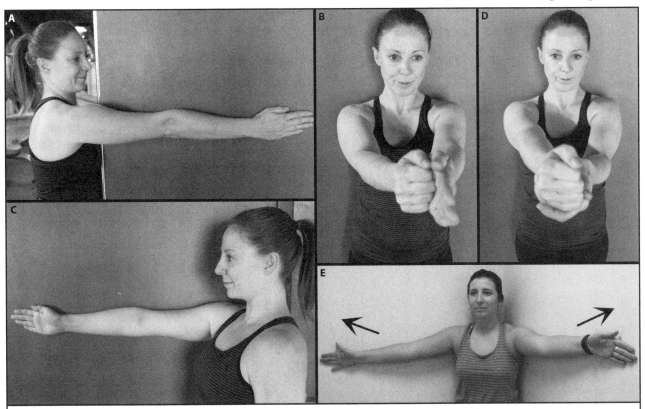

5.07.8 Strengthen: Isometric; Shoulder Horizontal Abduction and Adduction

POSITION: Standing

TARGETS: Beginner facilitation and strengthening of shoulder; horizontal abductors (posterior deltoid, infraspinatus and teres minor), horizontal adductors (anterior deltoid, coracobrachialis, pectoralis major, latissimus dorsi).

INSTRUCTION: With the affected shoulder at 90 degrees of flexion, patient may stand facing a door jamb for wall resistance or resist with the other hand which can be done supine or standing. For *horizontal adduction*, patient presses palm of hand and forearm into the wall (A) or other hand in supine or standing (B). For *horizontal abduction*, patient presses back of hand and forearm into the wall (C) or grasps with opposite hand around the wrist for resistance in supine or standing (D). Patient may also do this in a corner for bilateral horizontal abduction. Both shoulders are raised to 90 degrees scaption and with thumbs up. Dorsum of hand and posterior forearm are in contact with wall as patient pushes outward into horizontal abduction as the wall resists both arms (E).

SUBSTITUTIONS: Shrugging shoulder; shoulders should be in neutral rotation, thumbs up.

PARAMETERS: Hold for 6 to 10 seconds, 1 to 3 sets, 8 to 12 repetitions with 1 to 2 second ramp up and down, 1 time per day or every other day

5.07.9 STRENGTHEN: ISOMETRIC; SHOULDER WALK-OUTS

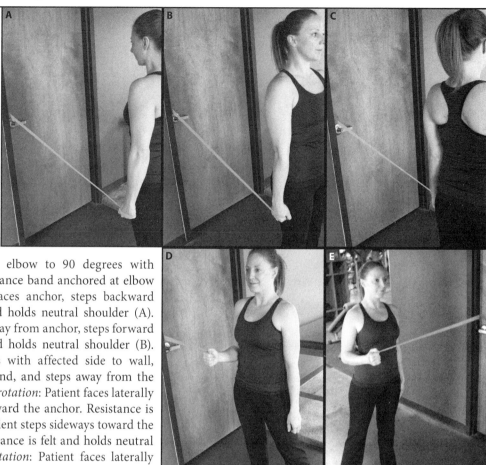

POSITION: Standing

TARGETS: Beginner facilitation and strengthening of shoulder; deltoid, RC, biceps, triceps, latissimus dorsi, teres major, coracobrachialis, pectorals.

INSTRUCTION: With the affected shoulder in neutral position, scapula slightly retracted and depressed, patient bends elbow to 90 degrees with fisted hand, holding resistance band anchored at elbow height. *Flexion*: Patient faces anchor, steps backward until resistance is felt and holds neutral shoulder (A). *Extension*: Patient faces away from anchor, steps forward until resistance is felt and holds neutral shoulder (B). *Adduction*: Patient stands with affected side to wall, holds band in affected hand, and steps away from the wall laterally (C). *Internal rotation*: Patient faces laterally with affected shoulder toward the anchor. Resistance is set at location of hand; patient steps sideways toward the unaffected side until resistance is felt and holds neutral shoulder (D). *External rotation*: Patient faces laterally with unaffected shoulder toward the anchor. Resistance is set at location of hand; patient steps sideways toward the affected shoulder until resistance is felt and holds neutral shoulder (E). To progress, increase resistance by stepping further away from anchor. At the end of the hold, patient steps closer to the anchor in between repetitions.

SUBSTITUTIONS: Shrugging shoulder; shoulder not in neutral position.

PARAMETERS: Hold for 10 seconds, 1 to 3 sets, 8 to 12 repetitions, 1 time per day or every other day

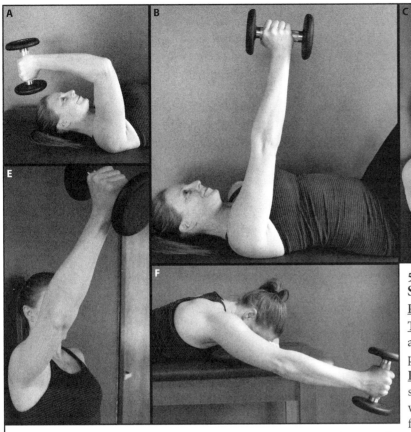

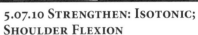

5.07.10 STRENGTHEN: ISOTONIC; SHOULDER FLEXION

POSITION: Supine, progressing to standing

TARGETS: Strengthen anterior deltoid, coracobrachialis, long head biceps brachii, pectoralis major (first 60 degrees)

INSTRUCTION: *Beginner supine*: Patient supine with arm by the sides holding the weight. The patient may start with elbow flexed 90 degrees for a shorter lever arm in the beginning phase, thumb pointing up, and bring the shoulder into flexion (A), progress to elbow extended, thumb leads the way (B). *Beginner standing*: The patient may start with elbow flexed 90 degrees for a shorter lever arm in the beginning phase, thumb pointing up, and bring the shoulder into flexion (C). *Advanced low range*: With the elbow extended for a longer lever arm, thumb pointing up, patient flexes the shoulder to just below 90 degrees. Keeping the range below the impingement range helps strengthen shoulder in the early phases without irritating the subacromial structures. Focus is on form and minimizing upper trapezius compensatory recruitment (D). *Advanced full range*: With the elbow extended for a longer lever arm, thumb pointing up, patient flexes the shoulder as far as possible with proper form. Focus is on form, and minimizing upper trapezius compensatory recruitment, and normal scapulohumeral rhythm (E). Patients also do well with prone flexion, which works the shoulder from 90 to 180 degrees against gravity, but does not work pectoralis major (F).

SUBSTITUTIONS: Shrugging shoulder; arching back, leaning back, forward translation of humeral head, fast movement.

PARAMETERS: 8 to 12 repetitions, 1 to 3 sets, 1 time per day or every other day

5.07.11 STRENGTHEN: ISOTONIC; SCAPTION

<u>POSITION</u>: Seated, standing

<u>TARGETS</u>: Strengthen supraspinatus, anterior deltoid, and middle deltoid

<u>INSTRUCTION</u>: *Full can*: Patient may sit or stand as the arm hangs by the side. With weight in hand and thumb leading the way (shoulder externally rotated), patient brings the arm 30 degrees forward from the coronal plane. The patient may start with elbow flexed 90 degrees for a shorter lever arm in the beginning phase (A). Patient lifts the arm, performing scaption at the shoulder, starting with range less than 90 degrees to avoid subacromial irritation and progressing to full range once strength allows and proper form is main-

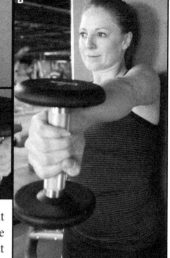

tained. *Emptying can*: Patient may sit or stand as the arm hangs by the side. With weight in hand and thumb leading the way, patient brings the arm 30 degrees forward from the coronal plane. Patient lifts the arm performing scaption at the shoulder to 90 degrees; at this time, the thumb points down with the shoulder internally rotating as if pouring out the can while lowering the arm. This works the supraspinatus eccentrically (B). *Empty can: This particular exercise has been shown to cause subacromial irritation and should be avoided, especially if any underlying shoulder problem exists. It is only mentioned here as it was thought to be a staple exercise for supraspinatus.* With the empty can, the thumb is pointing down and shoulder internally rotated throughout the scaption at the shoulder to 90 degrees. All of these exercises should be focused on minimizing upper trapezius compensatory recruitment and encouraging normal scapulohumeral rhythm.

<u>SUBSTITUTIONS</u>: Shrugging shoulder, arching back, leaning back, forward translation of humeral head, fast movement

<u>PARAMETERS</u>: 8 to 12 repetitions, 1 to 3 sets, 1 time per day or every other day

Where's the Evidence?

Timmons, Ericksen, Yesilyaprak, and Michener (2016) investigated scapular position and scapular muscle activation during the empty can and full can exercises. The empty can exercise has been shown to produce scapular kinematics associated with the mechanism leading to subacromial impingement syndrome. Participants with subacromial impingement syndrome performed 5 consecutive repetitions of full can and empty can exercises. Scapular and clavicular 3-dimensional positions, scapular muscle activity and pain were measured during each exercise. Participants reported greater pain during the empty can exercise vs the full can exercise. During the empty can exercise, participants were in greater scapular upward rotation, internal rotation, and clavicular elevation and less scapular posterior tilt. There was greater activity of upper trapezius, middle trapezius, and serratus anterior during ascent, and during the greater descent of upper trapezius and middle trapezius but less activity of the lower trapezius. They concluded the empty can exercise was associated with more pain and scapular positions that have been reported to decrease the subacromial space. Scapular muscle activity was generally higher with the empty can, which may be an attempt to control the impingement-related scapular motion. The full can exercise of elevation is preferred over the empty can exercise.

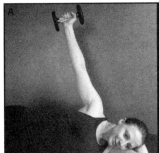
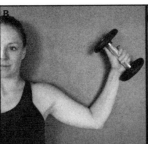
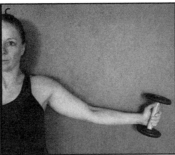
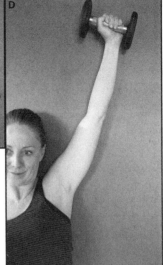

5.07.12 STRENGTHEN: ISOTONIC; SHOULDER ABDUCTION

<u>POSITION</u>: Side-lying (beginner) to standing (progression)

<u>TARGETS</u>: Strengthen middle deltoid, supraspinatus (first 30 degrees)

<u>INSTRUCTION</u>: *Beginner*: Lying on the unaffected side, affected arm by top side holding weight. Patient engages scapular stabilizers by retracting and depressing the scapula while abducting the shoulder with the thumb leading the way (shoulder externally rotated) (A). *Beginner standing*: Patient may start with elbow flexed 90 degrees for a shorter lever arm in the beginning phase, thumb pointing up, and bring the shoulder into abduction (B). *Advanced low range*: With the elbow extended for a longer lever arm, thumb pointing up, patient abducts the shoulder to just below 90 degrees. Keeping the range below the impingement range helps strengthen shoulder in the early phases without irritating the subacromial structures. Focus is on form and minimizing upper trapezius compensatory recruitment (C). *Advanced full range*: With the elbow extended for a longer lever arm, thumb pointing up, patient abducts the shoulder as far as possible with proper form (D). Focus is on form, minimizing upper trapezius compensatory recruitment and normal scapulohumeral rhythm. The standing exercises can be done unilaterally or bilaterally.

<u>SUBSTITUTIONS</u>: Shrugging shoulder; shoulder not in neutral position.

<u>PARAMETERS</u>: 8 to 12 repetitions, 1 to 3 sets, 1 time per day or every other day

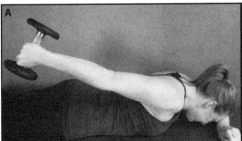
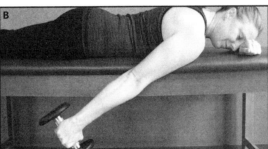

5.07.13 STRENGTHEN: ISOTONIC; SHOULDER EXTENSION

<u>POSITION</u>: Prone, standing

<u>TARGETS</u>: Strengthen posterior deltoid, latissimus dorsi, pectoralis major, teres major and minor, triceps brachii

<u>INSTRUCTION</u>: *Prone*: Patient in prone with small roll under forehead and neck neutral, arms by the sides. With palm facing up, patient raises the arm off the table and extends the shoulder, retracting the scapula. Allowing the palm to face inwards is an alternate position. Both are beneficial (A). Patient may also scoot to the edge of the bed, dropping the arm off the table, and perform the exercise full range (B). *Standing*: Patient starts with arm by the side and, with palm leading, extends the shoulder while retracting the scapula. Focus is on form and minimizing upper trapezius compensatory recruitment and excessive anterior humeral head movement. The standing exercises can be done unilaterally or bilaterally (C).

<u>SUBSTITUTIONS</u>: Shrugging shoulder; shoulder not in neutral position.

<u>PARAMETERS</u>: Hold for 2 to 3 seconds, 1 to 3 sets, 8 to 12 repetitions, 1 time per day or every other day

Where's the Evidence?

De Mey, Cagnie, Danneels, Cools, and Van de Velde (2009) examined the timing of the 3 portions of the trapezius muscle in relation to the posterior deltoidmuscle and in relation to one another during 4 selected shoulder exercises: (1) prone extension, (2) forward flexion in side-lying, (3) external rotation in side-lying, and (4) prone horizontal abduction with external rotation. The timing of muscle activation (based on an activation level of > 10% MVC beyond basic activity of the 3 portions of the trapezius muscle) during 4 exercises were examined by surface EMG in 30 healthy subjects on the dominant side. Differences in timing of the portions of the trapezius muscle were found. The upper trapezius was activated significantly later than the posterior deltoid, and the middle trapezius was activated significantly earlier than the posterior deltoid, during the prone extension exercise. During the horizontal abduction with external rotation exercise, the middle trapezius and the lower trapezius,were activated significantly earlier than the posterior deltoid. During prone extension, side-lying external rotation, and prone horizontal abduction with external rotation, significant differences were found between the upper trapezius and middle trapezius, between the upper trapezius and lower trapezius, but not between the middle trapezius and lower trapezius. In these exercises, the middle trapezius and lower trapezius, were activated significantly earlier than the upper trapezius. During forward flexion in side-lying, no significant timing differences were found between the activation of the portions of the trapezius. They concluded, with the exception of the lower trapezius, during prone extension, the prone extension exercise and the prone horizontal abduction with external rotation exercise promote early activation of the middle trapezius and lower trapezius, in relation to the scapular and glenohumeral prime mover, stating these exercises are potentially promising for the treatment of intermuscular and intramuscular timing disorders of the trapezius muscle.

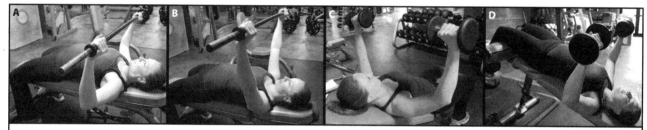

5.07.14 STRENGTHEN: ISOTONIC; SHOULDER, CHEST PRESS, 3 VARIATIONS WITH CANE/BAR OR DUMBBELLS

POSITION: Supine

TARGETS: *Chest press*: Strengthening primarily middle horizontal fibers of pectoralis major. *Incline press*: Strengthening primarily clavicular head pectoralis major. *Decline press*: Strengthening primarily sternal head pectoralis major. All three will also target triceps.

INSTRUCTION: *Chest press*: Patient holds a cane, bar, or dumbbells at chest level. If patient is on a bench, it is important patient does not horizontally abduct past shoulder level. Patient starts with elbow bent 90 degrees and palms facing down toward feet then presses up toward ceiling extending elbows. Patient should not lock elbows (A and B). *Incline press*: Patient is positioned reclining at a 45 degrees angle. Instructions are repeated as for chest press (C). *Decline press*: Patient is positioned with head lower than hips. Instructions are repeated as for chest press (D). Consider precautions and contraindications such as high blood pressure before positioning patient with head below body on decline bench.

SUBSTITUTIONS: Shrugging shoulders, allowing shoulder blades to come off table, patient should keep a natural arch in back and engage the abdominals before doing the exercise; avoid anterior humeral translation by dropping arms below shoulder level.

PARAMETERS: Hold for 1 to 2 seconds, 1 to 3 sets, 8 to 12 repetitions, 1 time per day or every other day

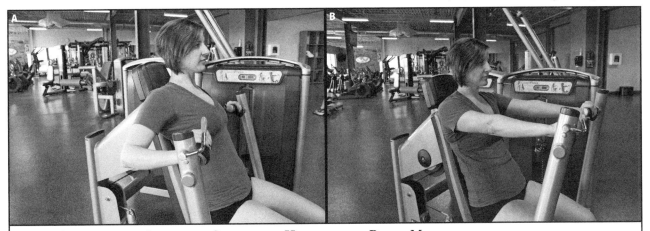

5.07.15 STRENGTHEN: ISOTONIC; SHOULDER, HORIZONTAL PRESS MACHINE

POSITION: Supine

TARGETS: Strengthen primarily middle horizontal fibers of pectoralis major at shoulder and triceps at elbow

INSTRUCTION: Patient sits so that the center of the chest lines up with the center of the horizontal set of handlebars. Patient grips the horizontal handles and pushes forward, straightening the arms without locking the elbows. Patient slowly bends elbows until lined up with shoulders, but no further, and then pushes the handles forward until the arms are straight. Most machines have a foot press that will allow the patient to assist the push during the first repetition so the patient is not pushing from a position of excessive horizontal abduction (A and B).

SUBSTITUTIONS: Shrugging shoulder, patient should keep a natural arch in back and engage the abdominals before doing the exercise, excessive horizontal abduction (elbow are more posterior than shoulder).

PARAMETERS: Hold for 1 to 2 seconds, 1 to 3 sets, 8 to 12 repetitions, 1 time per day or every other day

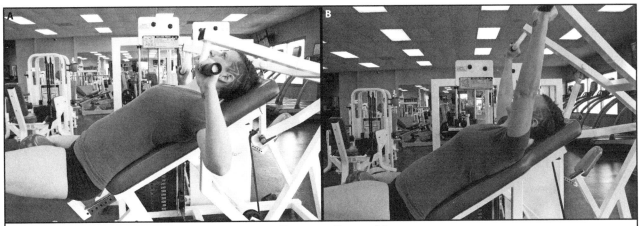

5.07.16 STRENGTHEN: ISOTONIC; SHOULDER, INCLINE PRESS MACHINE

POSITION: Supine

TARGETS: Strengthen primarily clavicular head, pectoralis major at shoulder and triceps at elbow

INSTRUCTION: Patient sits so that the upper portion of the chest lines up with the center of the horizontal set of handlebars. Patient grips the horizontal handles and pushed forward, straightening the arms without locking the elbows. Patient slowly bends elbows until lined up with shoulders, but no further, and then pushes the handles forward until the arms are straight. Most machines have a foot press that will allow the patient to assist the push during the first repetition so the patient is not pushing from a position of excessive horizontal abduction (A and B).

SUBSTITUTIONS: Shrugging shoulder, patient should keep a natural arch in back and engage the abdominals before doing the exercise, excessive horizontal abduction (elbow are more posterior than shoulder).

PARAMETERS: Hold for 1 to 2 seconds, 1 to 3 sets, 8 to 12 repetitions, 1 time per day or every other day

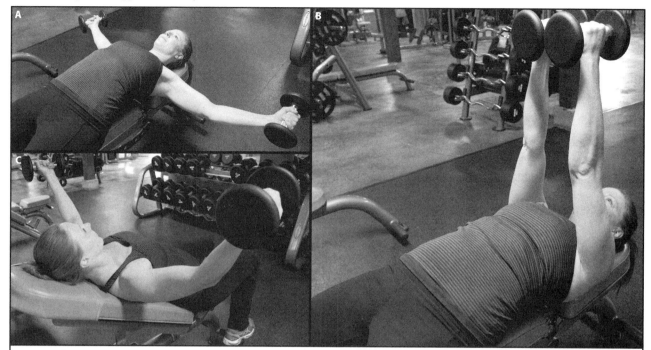

5.07.17 STRENGTHEN: ISOTONIC; SHOULDER, CHEST FLY

POSITION: Supine

TARGETS: Strengthening primarily sternal head, pectoralis major at shoulder (supine), clavicular head, pectoralis major (inclined), triceps at elbow

INSTRUCTION: *Supine*: Patient lies supine or hook-lying and horizontally abducts shoulders, elbows are near fully extended and palms are facing each other. Patient lowers the hands until the elbows are at the same level as the shoulders. Patient then brings the palms into shoulder horizontal adduction while lifting he weights with the hands until the palms/dumbbells touch. Slowly lower and repeat (A and B). *Supine inclined*: Position the bench between 30 to 45 degrees and repeat instructions above. This will target the clavicular portions of the pectoralis major (C).

SUBSTITUTIONS: Shrugging shoulder, patient should keep a natural arch in back and engage the abdominals before doing the exercise, excessive horizontal abduction (elbow are more posterior than shoulder at end range).

PARAMETERS: Hold for 1 to 2 seconds, 1 to 3 sets, 8 to 12 repetitions, 1 time per day or every other day

5.07.18 STRENGTHEN: ISOTONIC; SHOULDER, HORIZONTAL ABDUCTION

POSITION: Prone

TARGETS: Strengthening posterior deltoid, teres major and minor, middle trapezius

INSTRUCTION: Patient places forehead on unaffected forearm or uses towel roll to put neck in neutral. Patient scoots to edge of bed to allow arm to hang off. Holding weight, patient brings arm into horizontal abduction with palm down and elbow slightly flexed to prevent locking. As the arm approaches shoulder height, patient should retract and pinch the scapula to continue to elevate the arm. Do not allow humeral head to excessively translate anteriorly. Slowly lower and repeat (A and B). Patient may also do this with thumb pointed up to promote early activation of the middle and lower trapezius.

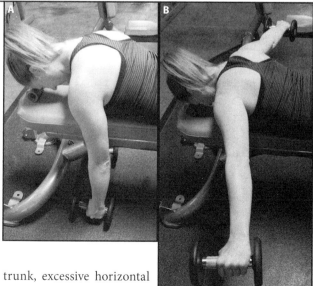

SUBSTITUTIONS: Shrugging shoulder, lifting head, rolling trunk, excessive horizontal abduction pushing humeral head anteriorly

PARAMETERS: Hold for 1 to 2 seconds, 1 to 3 sets, 8 to 12 repetitions, 1 time per day or every other day

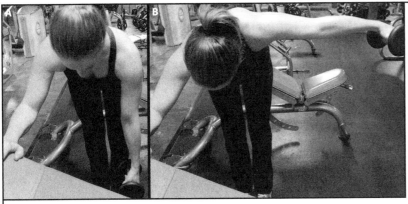

5.07.19 STRENGTHEN: ISOTONIC; SHOULDER, HORIZONTAL ABDUCTION, BENT FORWARD

POSITION: Seated

TARGETS: Strengthen posterior deltoid, teres major and minor, middle trapezius

INSTRUCTION: Patient bends forward at the waist until navel is on the lap. Holding weights, patient lowers arms toward the floor and then brings arm into horizontal abduction with elbow slightly flexed to prevent locking. As the arm approaches shoulder height, patient should retract and pinch the scapula to continue to elevate the arm. Do not allow humeral head to excessively translate anteriorly. Slowly lower and repeat (A and B).

SUBSTITUTIONS: Shrugging shoulder, jutting chin out, rolling trunk, excessive horizontal abduction pushing humeral head anteriorly

PARAMETERS: Hold for 1 to 2 seconds, 1 to 3 sets, 8 to 12 repetitions, 1 time per day or every other day

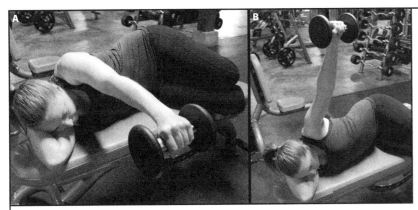

5.07.20 STRENGTHEN: ISOTONIC; SHOULDER, HORIZONTAL ABDUCTION, DECELERATION EMPHASIS

POSITION: Side-lying

TARGETS: Strengthen posterior deltoid, teres major and minor, middle trapezius; focus on eccentric phase.

INSTRUCTION: Patient lies on unaffected side, neck supported, with top shoulder in horizontal adduction, palm down toward table and elbow extended to neutral, but not locked. Patient engages scapula and retracts while lifting arm and horizontally abducting the shoulder. The movement is initiated by the scapula, and it is important to encourage strong scapular retraction throughout the exercise. Once end range is reached, do not allow humeral head to excessively translate anteriorly. The patient continues to keep scapula engaged creating the last few degrees of movement. The patient then slowly lowers the arm back down into horizontal adduction to table (A and B).

SUBSTITUTIONS: Shrugging shoulder, jutting chin out, rolling trunk, excessive horizontal abduction pushing humeral head anteriorly

PARAMETERS: Hold for 1 to 2 seconds, 1 to 3 sets, 8 to 12 repetitions, 1 time per day or every other day

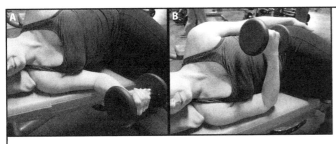

5.07.21 STRENGTHEN: ISOTONIC; SHOULDER INTERNAL ROTATION

POSITION: Side-lying

TARGETS: Strengthen subscapularis, latissimus dorsi, pectoralis major, teres major

INSTRUCTION: Patient lies on affected side, neck supported and trunk slightly rolled toward the back side to take pressure off the glenohumeral joint. With elbow tucked into the side and holding a weight, patient rotates the palm across the stomach. The patient then slowly lowers the arm back down to table. Encourage the patient to engage scapular retractors throughout the movements (A and B).

SUBSTITUTIONS: Shrugging shoulder, rolling trunk

PARAMETERS: Hold for 1 to 2 seconds, 1 to 3 sets, 8 to 12 repetitions, 1 time per day or every other day

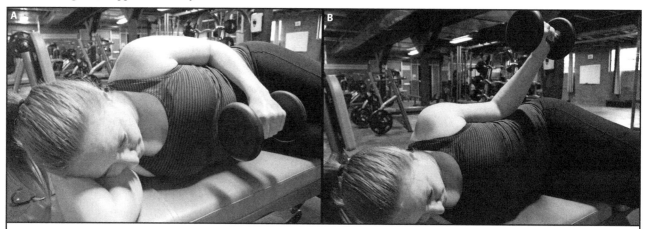

5.07.22 STRENGTHEN: ISOTONIC; SHOULDER EXTERNAL ROTATION

POSITION: Side-lying

TARGETS: Strengthening infraspinatus, posterior deltoid, teres minor

INSTRUCTION: Patient lies on unaffected side, neck supported and affected elbow tucked into the side. Place a towel roll between the elbow and rib cage to squeeze, which helps stay in position. Patient holds a weight and rotates the hand across the body toward the ceiling, squeezing the scapula at end range. Thumb is pointed toward the head throughout the movement. The patient then slowly lowers the arm back down to table. Encourage the patient to engage scapular retractors throughout the movements (A and B).

SUBSTITUTIONS: Shrugging shoulder, rolling trunk

PARAMETERS: Hold for 1 to 2 seconds, 1 to 3 sets, 8 to 12 repetitions, 1 time per day or every other day

---

Where's the Evidence?

De Mey et al. (2013) assessed the effect of conscious correction of scapular orientation on the activation of the 3 sections of the trapezius muscle during shoulder exercises in overhead athletes with scapular dyskinesis. They looked at prone extension, side-lying external rotation, side-lying forward flexion, and prone horizontal abduction with external rotation. Repeated-measures analyses of variance were used to determine if a voluntary scapular orientation correction strategy influenced the activation levels of the different sections of the trapezius during each exercise. With conscious correction of scapular orientation, activation levels of the 3 sections of the trapezius muscle significantly increased during prone extension and side-lying external. There was no difference between conditions for side-lying forward flexion and prone horizontal abduction with external rotation. They concluded conscious correction of scapular orientation during the prone extension and side-lying external rotation exercises can be used to increase the activation level in the three sections of the trapezius in overhead athletes with scapular dyskinesis.

5.07.23 STRENGTHEN: ISOTONIC; SHOULDER EXTERNAL ROTATION 90/90

POSITION: Prone

TARGETS: Strengthen infraspinatus, posterior deltoid, teres minor

INSTRUCTION: Patient places forehead on unaffected forearm or uses towel roll to put neck in neutral. Patient scoots to edge of bed to allow forearm to hang off. Holding weight, patient brings arm into 90 degrees of abduction with elbow flexed 90 degrees. A towel roll

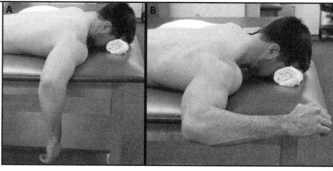

may be placed under the arm to bring the humerus in alignment with the shoulder joint. Patient rotates the top of the hand up toward the ceiling, squeezing the scapula at end range. The patient then slowly lowers the hand back down toward the floor. Encourage the patient to engage scapular retractors throughout the movements (A and B).

SUBSTITUTIONS: Shrugging shoulder, rolling trunk

PARAMETERS: Hold for 1 to 2 seconds, 1 to 3 sets, 8 to 12 repetitions, 1 time per day or every other day

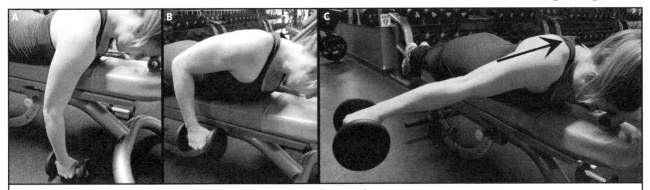

5.07.24 STRENGTHEN: ISOTONIC; SHOULDER, ROW (PRONE)

<u>POSITION</u>: Prone

<u>TARGETS</u>: Strengthen posterior deltoid, rhomboids, and middle trapezius

<u>INSTRUCTION</u>: *Extension (focus to torso only)*: In same position as described above, patient retracts and extends the shoulder while flexing the elbow to align the upper arm with the midline of the torso, then uses scapular retraction only. This prevents forcing humeral head anteriorly. Focus is on strong scapular retraction at the end of the movement (A and B). *Horizontal abduction (focus to shoulder height only)*: Patient places forehead on unaffected forearm or uses towel roll to put neck in neutral. Patient scoots to edge of bed to allow forearm to drop off. Holding weight, patient allows hand to drop toward floor. Patient then pulls up as if pulling a lawn mower cord while retracting scapula, horizontally abducting the shoulder and flexing the elbow. When arm reaches height of shoulder, use only scapular retraction. This prevents forcing humeral head anteriorly. The patient then slowly lowers the hand back down toward the floor. Encourage the patient to engage scapular retractors throughout the movements (C).

<u>SUBSTITUTIONS</u>: Shrugging shoulder, rolling trunk, excessive horizontal abduction, or extension pushing humeral head anteriorly

<u>PARAMETERS</u>: Hold for 1 to 2 seconds, 1 to 3 sets, 8 to 12 repetitions, 1 time per day or every other day

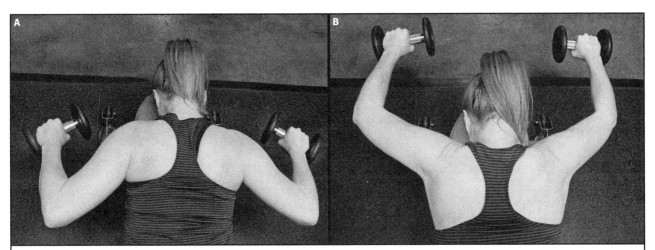

5.07.25 STRENGTHEN: ISOTONIC; SHOULDER, MILITARY PRESS (PRONE)

<u>POSITION</u>: Prone

<u>TARGETS</u>: Strengthening posterior deltoid, rhomboids, upper trapezius, middle and lower trapezius

<u>INSTRUCTION</u>: Patient places forehead on towel roll to put neck in neutral. With arms in the 90/90 position and holding weights palm down, patient retracts the scapula and presses hands directly overhead, keeping elbows in alignment with midline of body and head. The patient then slowly brings elbows back toward the trunk. Encourage the patient to engage scapular retractors throughout the movements (A and B). *Beginner (short arc)* may work the shoulder from 30 to 60 degrees (roughly when hands reach same level as ears) and *progressing (full arc)* to 30 to 160 degrees once patient's strength has improved and normal shoulder mechanics are present.

<u>SUBSTITUTIONS</u>: Shrugging shoulders; elbows should stay at same height as hands at all times.

<u>PARAMETERS</u>: Hold for 1 to 2 seconds, 1 to 3 sets, 8 to 12 repetitions, 1 time per day or every other day

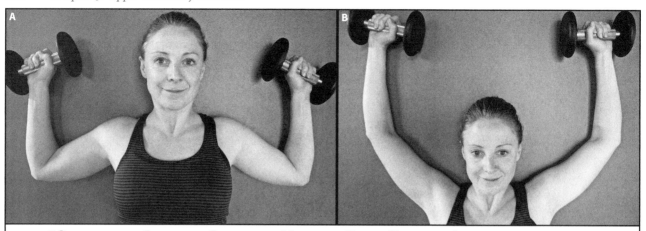

5.07.26 Strengthen: Isotonic; Shoulder, Military Press (Standing)

<u>Position</u>: Standing

<u>Targets</u>: Strengthening middle deltoid, rhomboids, upper trapezius, middle and lower trapezius

<u>Instruction</u>: With arms are in the 90/90 position and holding weights palm forward, patient retracts the scapula and presses hands directly overhead, keeping elbows in alignment with midline of body and head. The patient then slowly brings elbows back toward the trunk. Encourage the patient to engage scapular retractors throughout the movements (A and B). *Beginner (short arc)* may work the shoulder from 30 to 60 degrees (roughly when hands reach height of ears) and *progressing (full arc)* to 30 to 160 degrees once patient's strength has improved and normal shoulder mechanics are present.

<u>Substitutions</u>: Shrugging shoulders; elbows should stay in same coronal plane as hands at all times.

<u>Parameters</u>: Hold for 1 to 2 seconds, 1 to 3 sets, 8 to 12 repetitions, 1 time per day or every other day

---

Where's the Evidence?

A 2013 study compared EMG activity and 1 RM in barbell and dumbbell shoulder presses performed seated and standing. Fifteen healthy men performed 1 RM with a load corresponding to 80% of the 1 RM. EMG activity was measured in the anterior, medial and posterior deotids, and biceps and triceps brachii, and found that presses with dumbbells were significantly higher in muscle recruitment of the deltoid, concluding the exercise with the greatest stability requirement (standing and dumbbells) demonstrated the highest neuromuscular activity of the deltoid muscles (Saeterbakken & Fimland, 2013).

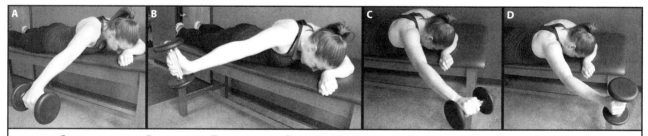

5.07.27 Strengthen: Isotonic; Posterior Cuff, 4-Way

<u>Position</u>: Prone

<u>Targets</u>: Strengthening infraspinatus, supraspinatus, teres minor, posterior deltoid

<u>Instruction</u>: Patient places forehead on unaffected forearm or uses towel roll to put neck in neutral. Patient scoots to edge of bed to allow forearm to drop off. Holding weight, patient completes the following: *90 degrees "T" palm down*: Patient brings arm into horizontal abduction, palm down, to shoulder height level and returns (A). *90 degrees "T" thumb up*: Patient brings arm into horizontal abduction, thumb up, returns (B). *120 degrees "V" palm down*: Patient brings arm into scaption, palm down, returns (C). *120 degrees "V" thumb up*: Patient brings arm into scaption, thumb up, and returns (D). Encourage the patient to engage scapular retractors throughout the movements.

<u>Substitutions</u>: Shrugging shoulder, rolling trunk, lifting trunk

<u>Parameters</u>: Hold for 1 to 2 seconds, 1 to 3 sets, 8 to 12 repetitions, 1 time per day or every other day

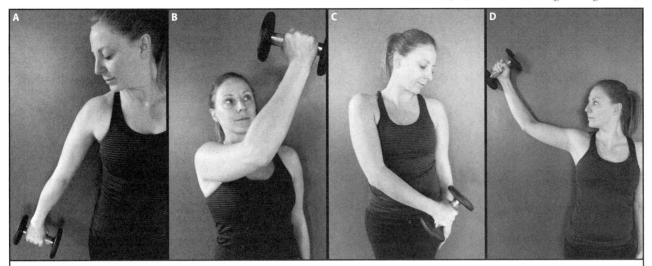

5.07.28 Strengthen: Isotonic; Shoulder, Diagonal Lifts D1 and D2

<u>Position</u>: Standing

<u>Targets</u>: Comprehensive strengthening of shoulder; targets deltoid, RC, biceps, triceps, latissimus dorsi, teres major, coracobrachialis, pectorals.

<u>Instruction</u>: Patient performs movements through combined patterns, strengthening the shoulder in all three movement planes. D1 and D2 patterns may start in the extended position.

Tips:
- Patient should follow the hand movement with the eyes and head.
- Rotational movements should be finished before crossing midline.
- Distal movements at the hand and wrist happen first.

D1: "Throwing salt over opposite shoulder": Starting in a position of arm to the side, palm facing backward (extended D1; scapular retraction, shoulder extension, abduction, internal rotation, forearm pronated, wrist ulnarly deviated, fingers extended) bring so palm is facing back at the end of the motion, as if throwing salt over the opposite shoulder (flexed D1; forearm across the face in shoulder flexion, adduction, external rotation, forearm supinated, wrist radially deviated and fingers flexed). Elbow may remain straight or bent throughout the movement (A and B).

D2: "Unsheath the sword to Tada!": Patient holds the weight with arm across the body, thumb pointing toward hip (extended D2; shoulder extension, abduction, internal rotation across the body, forearm pronated, wrist ulnarly deviated, fingers flexed). Patient lifts weight across the body and up toward the ceiling, turning thumb outwards while crossing trunk midline to end in the "Tada!" position (flexed D2; scapula retracted, shoulder flexed, abducted, externally rotated, forearm pronated, wrist ulnar deviated, fingers extended) (C and D).

<u>Substitutions</u>: Shrugging shoulder; not engaging scapular stabilizers.

<u>Parameters</u>: 8 to 12 repetitions, 1 to 3 sets, 1 time per day or every other day

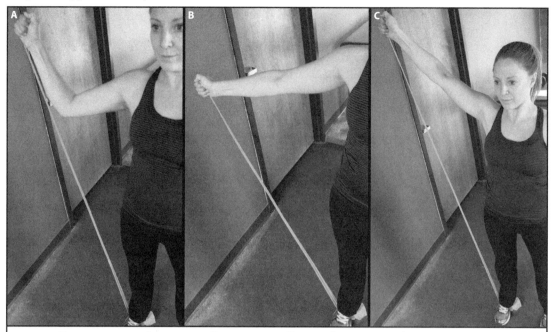

5.07.29 STRENGTHEN: ISOTONIC; RESISTANCE BAND, SHOULDER ABDUCTION

<u>POSITION</u>: Standing

<u>TARGETS</u>: Strengthen middle deltoid, supraspinatus (first 30 degrees)

<u>INSTRUCTION</u>: Resistance band is anchored at the patient's feet. The patient may start with elbow flexed 90 degrees for a shorter lever arm in the beginning phase, thumb pointing up, and brings the shoulder into abduction (A). *Advanced low range*: With the elbow extended for a longer lever arm, thumb pointing up, patient abducts the shoulder to just below 90 degrees. Keeping the range below the impingement range helps strengthening the patient's shoulder in the early phases without irritating the subacromial structures. Focus is on form and minimizing upper trapezius compensatory recruitment (B). *Advanced full range*: With the elbow extended for a longer lever arm, thumb pointing up, patient abducts the shoulder as far as possible with proper form (C). Focus is on form and minimizing upper trapezius compensatory recruitment, and normal scapulohumeral rhythm. The standing exercises can be done unilaterally or bilaterally.

<u>SUBSTITUTIONS</u>: Shrugging or forward shoulder

<u>PARAMETERS</u>: 8 to 12 repetitions, 1 to 3 sets, 1 time per day or every other day

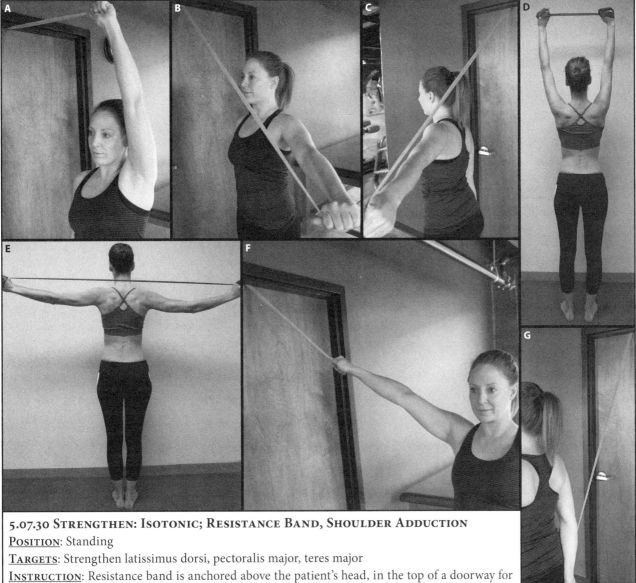

5.07.30 STRENGTHEN: ISOTONIC; RESISTANCE BAND, SHOULDER ADDUCTION

<u>POSITION</u>: Standing

<u>TARGETS</u>: Strengthen latissimus dorsi, pectoralis major, teres major

<u>INSTRUCTION</u>: Resistance band is anchored above the patient's head, in the top of a doorway for example. To achieve resistance for *180 to 90 degrees*, patient stands sideways to wall with unaffected shoulder toward wall. Patient reaches overhead with affected arm and grasps resistance band. Band should have tension on it at start of movement; this can be accomplished by sidestepping away from the wall. Patient pulls band either in front of head or behind to 90 degrees. Pulling behind the head will target the scapular muscles; pulling in front of the head will target the pectoral muscles (A through C). *180 to 90 degrees, no anchor*: This range can also be accomplished by holding a band on each end with both hands overhead; band is not anchored. Patient then pulls ends of band apart while adducting to 90 degrees. This can be done in front of the head for pectoral involvement or behind for scapular and latissimus focus (D and E). To achieve resistance for *90 to 0 degrees,* patient stands sideways to wall with affected shoulder toward wall. Patient reaches with affected arm and grasp resistance band. Band should have tension on it at start of movement with shoulder abducted 90 degrees; this can be accomplished by sidestepping away from the wall. Patient pulls band, bringing palm of hand to thigh (F and G). Focus is on form and minimizing upper trapezius compensatory recruitment, and normal scapulohumeral rhythm. The standing exercises can be done unilaterally or bilaterally.

<u>SUBSTITUTIONS</u>: Shrugging shoulder; shoulder not in neutral position.

<u>PARAMETERS</u>: 8 to 12 repetitions, 1 to 3 sets, 1 time per day or every other day

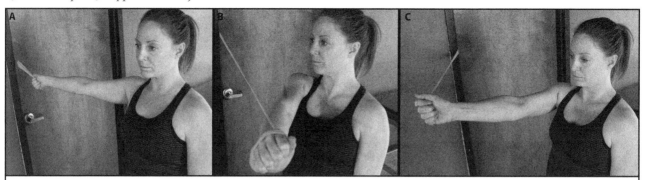

5.07.31 STRENGTHEN: ISOTONIC; RESISTANCE BAND, SHOULDER, HORIZONTAL ADDUCTION, CROSS-OVERS

POSITION: Standing

TARGETS: Strengthen primarily pectoralis major, anterior deltoid, coracobrachialis

INSTRUCTION: Resistance band is anchored at shoulder height. Patient stands sideways to wall with affected shoulder toward wall and lines hand up with anchor, shoulder is abducted to 90 degrees. Band should have tension on it at start of movement; this can be accomplished by sidestepping away from the wall. Patient pulls band across the body into horizontal adduction with the thumb pointed up (A and B). Patient may stop when shoulder is at 90 degrees of flexion, and avoid crossing past this point in the early stages to decrease subacromial irritation and protect healing structures (C).

SUBSTITUTIONS: Shrugging shoulder, twisting body

PARAMETERS: 8 to 12 repetitions, 1 to 3 sets, 1 time per day or every other day

5.07.32 STRENGTHEN: ISOTONIC; RESISTANCE BAND, SHOULDER, HORIZONTAL ABDUCTION

POSITION: Prone

TARGETS: Strengthen posterior deltoid, teres major and minor, middle trapezius

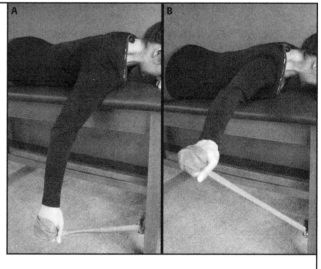

INSTRUCTION: Patient places forehead on unaffected forearm or uses towel roll to put neck in neutral. Patient scoots to edge of bed to allow arm to hang off. Resistance band is anchored to table leg. Grasping band so that resistance starts at beginning of movement, patient brings arm into horizontal abduction with palm down and elbow slightly flexed to prevent locking. As the arm approaches shoulder height, patient should retract and pinch the scapula to continue to elevate the arm. Do not allow humeral head to excessively translate anteriorly. Slowly lower and repeat (A and B).

SUBSTITUTIONS: Shrugging shoulder, lifting head, rolling trunk, excessive horizontal abduction pushing humeral head anteriorly

PARAMETERS: Hold for 1 to 2 seconds, 1 to 3 sets, 8 to 12 repetitions, 1 time per day or every other day

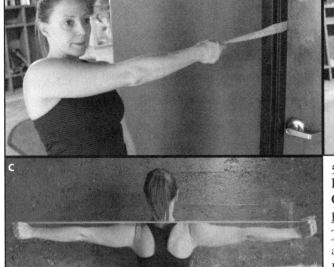

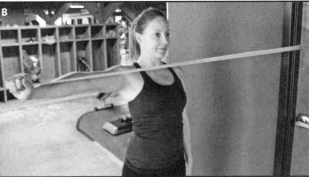

5.07.33 STRENGTHEN: ISOTONIC; RESISTANCE BAND, SHOULDER, HORIZONTAL ABDUCTION, CROSS-OUTS AND PULL-APARTS

POSITION: Standing

TARGETS: Strengthening posterior deltoid, teres major and minor, middle trapezius

INSTRUCTION: *Cross-outs*: Resistance band is anchored at shoulder height. Patient stands sideways to wall with unaffected shoulder toward wall, grasps band and lines hand up with anchor, shoulder flexed to 90 degrees with slight horizontal adduction. Band should have tension on it at start of movement; this can be accomplished by sidestepping away from the wall. Patient pulls band across the body into horizontal abduction, thumb pointed up (A and B) *Pull-aparts*: Patient may also grasp unanchored band with both hands near the middle, thumbs up, patient retracts scapula while horizontally abducting both shoulders, elbow with a slight bend (C).

SUBSTITUTIONS: Shrugging shoulder, twisting body

PARAMETERS: 8 to 12 repetitions, 1 to 3 sets, 1 time per day or every other day

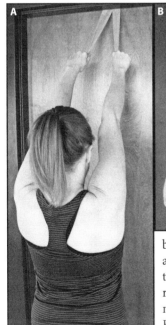

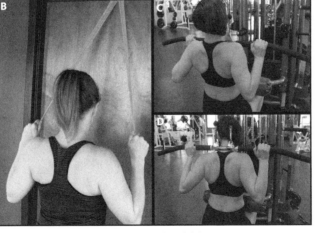

5.07.34 STRENGTHEN: ISOTONIC; RESISTANCE BAND AND MACHINE, SHOULDER, LAT PULL-DOWN

POSITION: Standing, seated

TARGETS: Strengthening latissimus dorsi, rhomboids, lower and middle trapezius, serratus anterior, and biceps brachii

INSTRUCTION: *Resistance band* is anchored overhead with two handles. Patient stands facing wall and grasps bands with both hands overhead. Band should have tension on it at start of movement; this can be accomplished by grasping higher on the band. Patient pulls band down as elbows tuck into the lateral ribs, palms facing forward. Encourage scapular retraction and depression at end range (A and B). This can also be done seated. *Lateral pull-down machine*: Patient sits facing machine. Patient sits tall and reaches for bar with hands spaces wider than shoulder width. Elbows are slightly bent and pointed straight down. Gaze is forward with chin slightly tucked. Patient pulls band down, bar to just below the chin, as elbows tuck in to the lateral ribs, palms facing forward. Encourage scapular retraction and depression at end range. Patient may also pull the bar behind the head to just sitting on top of shoulder but this will require leaning forward slightly. Both in front and behind are beneficial; however, pulling forward to the chest is safest (C and D). It is recommended also to use a pronated grip for increased latissimus dorsi recruitment.

SUBSTITUTIONS: Shrugging shoulder, twisting body, excessive anterior humeral head movement with hyper extension of shoulder, jutting chin out

PARAMETERS: 8 to 12 repetitions, 1 to 3 sets, 1 time per day or every other day

Where's the Evidence?

Sperandei, Barros, Silveira-Júnior, and Oliveira (2009) evaluated the activity of the primary motor muscles during the performance of 3 lateral pull-down techniques through surface EMG. Subjects performed 5 repetitions of behind-the-neck, front-of-the-neck, and V-bar exercises at 80% of 1 RM. EMG signal was registered from the pectoralis major, latissimus dorsi, posterior deltoid, and biceps brachii, then further normalized in respect to that which presented the highest value of all the techniques. During the concentric phase, pectoralis major value showed the front-of-the-neck to be significantly higher than V-bar/behind-the-neck and V-bar higher than behind-the-neck. During the eccentric phase, front-of-the-neck/V-bar was higher than behind-the-neck. For latissimus dorsi, there was no difference between techniques. Posterior deltoid presented behind-the-neck higher than front-of-the-neck/V-bar, with front-of-the-neck higher than V-bar in the concentric phase and behind-the-neck higher than V-bar in the eccentric phase. Biceps brachii exhibited behind-the-neck higher than V-bar/front-of-the-neck and V-bar higher than front-of-the-neck in both concentric and eccentric phases. Considering the main objectives of lateral pull-down, they concluded that front-of-the-neck was the better choice, whereas behind-the-neck is not a good lateral pull-down technique and should be avoided. V-bar was recommended as an alternative.

Lusk, Hale, and Russell (2010) used EMG studies to compare the anterior (to the chest) lateral pull-down with wide-pronated, wide-supinated, narrow-pronated, and narrow-supinated grips. Surface EMG of the latissimus dorsi, middle trapezius, and biceps brachii revealed that a pronated grip elicited greater latissimus dorsi activity than a supinated grip, but had no influence of grip type on the middle trapezius and biceps brachii muscles. Based on these findings, they recommended an anterior lateral pull-down with pronated grip for maximally activating the latissimus dorsi, irrespective of the grip width.

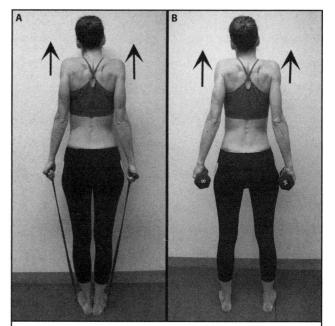

5.07.35 STRENGTHEN: ISOTONIC; RESISTANCE BAND, SHOULDER SHRUGS

POSITION: Standing

TARGETS: Strengthening upper trapezius

INSTRUCTION: Resistance band is anchored under patient's feet so there are two handles. Patient stands with erect posture, scapula retracted slightly and grasps bands with both hands. Band should have tension on it at start of movement. This can be accomplished by grasping lower on the band. Patient shrugs shoulders without involving any elbow flexion (A). This can also be done with weights as resistance (B).

SUBSTITUTIONS: Shrugging shoulder, twisting body, excessive anterior humeral head movement with hyper extension of shoulder, jutting chin out

PARAMETERS: 8 to 12 repetitions, 1 to 3 sets, 1 time per day or every other day

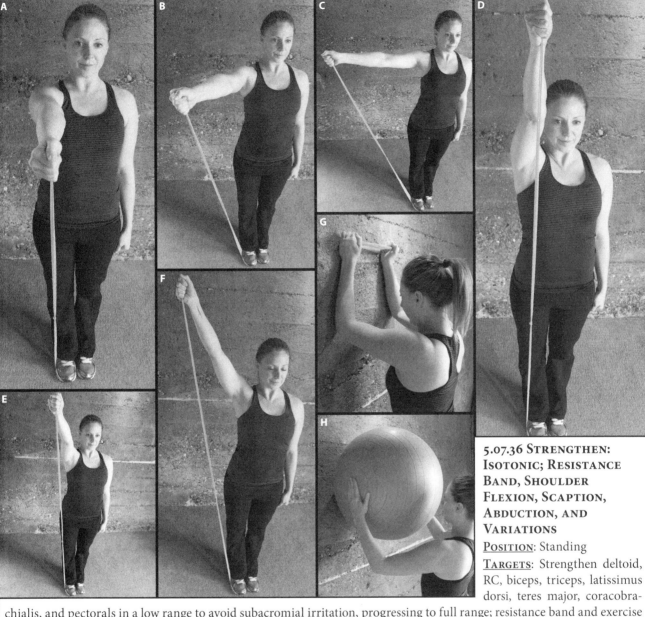

5.07.36 STRENGTHEN: ISOTONIC; RESISTANCE BAND, SHOULDER FLEXION, SCAPTION, ABDUCTION, AND VARIATIONS

POSITION: Standing

TARGETS: Strengthen deltoid, RC, biceps, triceps, latissimus dorsi, teres major, coracobrachialis, and pectorals in a low range to avoid subacromial irritation, progressing to full range; resistance band and exercise ball assist to target upper and lower trapezius and serratus anterior.

INSTRUCTION: *Flexion*: Resistance band is anchored under the feet. The patient grasps band low enough so there is slight tension at the beginning of the movement. With elbow extended, thumb pointing up, patient flexes the shoulder to just below 90 degrees. Keeping the range below the impingement range helps strengthen shoulder in the early phases without irritating the subacromial structures. Focus is on form and minimizing upper trapezius compensatory recruitment. After one set, this is repeated for *scaption and abduction* (A through C). This can also be done bilaterally with two ends free on the resistance band and patient steps on the band in the middle. *Advanced full range*: Patient flexes the shoulder as far as possible with proper form. Repeat for scaption and abduction (D through F). Encourage patient to engage the scapular retractors during the movements. *Flexion with resistance band glenohumeral horizontal abduction load*: Loop band around the wrists so there is resistance to bringing the wrists apart. Patient straightens arms and brings wrists shoulder width apart against the resistance of the band. Patient maintains the tension on the bands and flexes both shoulders as far as possible, then slowly lowers, keeping wrists the same distance apart and repeats (G). *Flexion with exercise ball glenohumeral horizontal abduction load*: Place small exercise ball between wrists so the wrists are shoulder-width apart while patient squeezing pressure to the ball by adducting the shoulders isometrically. Patient maintains the pressure on the ball and flexes both shoulders as far as possible, then slowly lowers, keeping wrists the same distance apart and repeats (H).

SUBSTITUTIONS: Shrugging shoulder, arching back, leaning back, fast movement

PARAMETERS: 8 to 12 repetitions, 1 to 3 sets, 1 time per day or every other day

Where's the Evidence?

Park, Cynn, Yi, and Kwon (2013) studied the effect of isometric horizontal abduction on pectoralis major and serratus anterior EMG activity during three exercises in subjects with scapular winging. The subjects performed the forward flexion, scaption, and wall push-up plus with and without isometric horizontal abduction using resistance band. Surface EMG was used to collect the EMG data of the pectoralis major and serratus anterior during the three exercises. Pectoralis major EMG activity was significantly lower during forward flexion and wall push-up plus with isometric horizontal abduction, and serratus anterior EMG activity was significantly greater with isometric horizontal abduction. Additionally, the pectoralis major/serratus anterior activity ratio was significantly lower during the forward flexion and wall push-up plus with isometric horizontal abduction. The results of this study suggest that isometric horizontal abduction using resistance band can be used as an effective method to facilitate the serratus anterior activity and to reduce excessive pectoralis major activity during exercises for activating the serratus anterior.

Ishigaki et al. (2014) compared the intramuscular balance ratios of the upper trapezius muscle and the lower trapezius muscle, and the intermuscular balance ratios of the upper trapezius muscle and the serratus anterior muscle among prone extension, prone horizontal abduction with external rotation, forward flexion in the side-lying position, side-lying external rotation, shoulder flexion with glenohumeral horizontal abduction load (resistance band), and shoulder flexion with glenohumeral horizontal adduction load (exercise ball) in the standing posture. The EMG activities of the upper trapezius, lower trapezius, and serratus anterior were measured during the tasks. The percentage of maximum voluntary isometric contraction was calculated for each muscle, and the upper trapezius/lower trapezius ratios and the upper trapezius/serratus anterior ratios were compared among the tasks. Their study revealed that the upper trapezius/lower trapezius ratio of the resistance band exercise was not significantly different from those of the 4 exercises performed in the side-lying and prone postures in each phase. Because horizontal abduction load elicits lower trapezius, muscle activity in the resistance band exercise, the resistance band exercise induced balanced intra-scapular muscle activity. The exercise ball exercise elicited a significantly greater upper trapezius/serratus anterior ratio than the other exercises in each phase. Based on these results, they recommend that the resistance band exercise be used to enhance balanced muscle activity between the upper trapezius and lower trapezius, muscles and the exercise ball to enhance balanced upper trapezius/serratus anterior activity in anti-gravity postures.

5.07.37 STRENGTHEN: ISOTONIC; RESISTANCE BAND, SHOULDER FLEXION 90 TO 180 DEGREES

POSITION: Prone

TARGETS: Strengthen anterior deltoid, coracobrachialis, long head biceps brachii

INSTRUCTION: Patient places forehead on unaffected forearm or uses towel roll to put neck in neutral. Patient scoots to edge of bed to allow forearm to hang off. Resistance band is anchored to the table leg under the affected shoulder. The patient grasps band low enough so there is slight tension at the beginning of the movement. With elbow extended ,thumb pointing up, patient flexes the shoulder 90 to 180 degrees against gravity (A and B). Encourage the patient to engage scapular retractors throughout the movements.

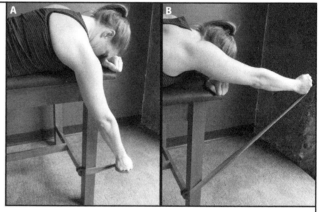

SUBSTITUTIONS: Shrugging shoulder excessively, rolling trunk away, fast movement, moving out of straight flexion

PARAMETERS: 8 to 12 repetitions, 1 to 3 sets, 1 time per day or every other day

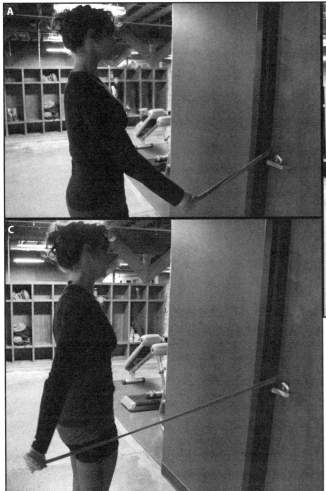

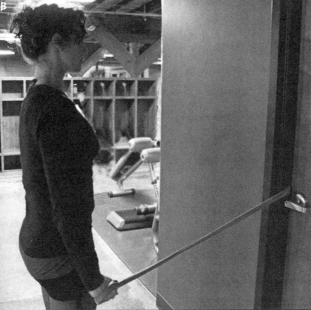

5.07.38 STRENGTHEN: ISOTONIC; RESISTANCE BAND, SHOULDER EXTENSION

<u>POSITION</u>: Standing

<u>TARGETS</u>: Strengthening posterior deltoid, latissimus dorsi, pectoralis major, teres major and minor, triceps brachii

<u>INSTRUCTION</u>: Resistance band is anchored at shoulder height. Patient stands facing wall and grasps band so there is tension at start of movement which is at approximately 90 degrees of flexion; this can be accomplished by grasping closer to wall or stepping backward (A and B). With palm facing inward, patient retracts scapula and extends the shoulder. *Beginner*: Patient stops the movement when the hand reaches the lateral pelvis. This avoids anterior humeral movement and subacromial irritation. *Advanced*: Allow patient to extend beyond the lateral pelvis, as long as patient is retracting scapula along with shoulder extension (C).

<u>SUBSTITUTIONS</u>: Shrugging shoulder, twisting body, excessive anterior humeral head movement with hyperextension of shoulder, jutting chin out

<u>PARAMETERS</u>: 8 to 12 repetitions, 1 to 3 sets, 1 time per day or every other day

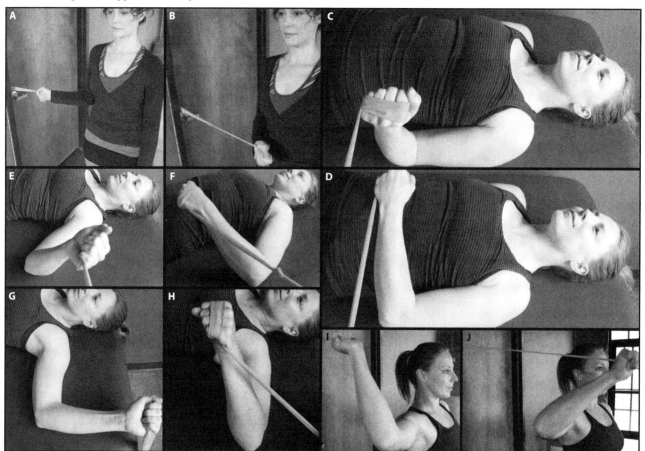

5.07.39 STRENGTHEN: ISOTONIC; RESISTANCE BAND, SHOULDER INTERNAL ROTATION AND VARIATIONS

POSITION: Standing, supine

TARGETS: Strengthening of shoulder internal rotators; subscapularis, latissimus dorsi, pectoralis major, teres major

INSTRUCTION: *0 degrees abduction standing*: Resistance band is anchored at elbow height. Place a small towel between elbow and side, and instruct patient to squeeze throughout exercise. This will help to keep the elbow tucked into the side. Patient stands with affected side toward the anchor and grasps band. Starting position is in external rotation of the shoulder, and patient should sidestep away from the wall so there is tension at start of movement. Patient then internally rotates the shoulder while strongly retracting the scapula to stabilize the base of movement (A and B). *0 degrees abduction supine*: Resistance band is anchored at elbow height or can be held by therapist. Place a small towel between elbow and side, and instruct patient to squeeze throughout exercise. This will help to keep the elbow tucked into the side. Another small towel roll is placed under the humerus shaft to align the shaft with the glenoid fossa and prevent excessive anterior humeral gliding. Starting position is in external rotation of the shoulder. Patient then internally rotates the shoulder while strongly retracting the scapula to stabilize the base of movement (C and D). *45 and 90 degrees abduction supine*: Resistance band is anchored at elbow height and direction to resist internal rotation in abducted position or can be held by therapist. Use a small towel roll under the humerus shaft to align the shaft with the glenoid fossa and prevent excessive anterior humeral gliding. Starting position is in external rotation of the shoulder. Patient then internally rotates the shoulder while strongly retracting the scapula to stabilize the base of movement (45 degrees, E and F; 90 degrees, G and H). For all of the above, consider starting in external rotation and only internally rotating to neutral in the beginner phase. *Pulses*: Pulses are useful for building endurance and can be implemented in any of the positions described above. When performing a pulse, patient moves near the end ranges and returns only 10 to 20 degrees before rotating back again in a pulsing movement. Pulses are performed to fatigue to build endurance. *90 degrees abduction standing*: Resistance band is anchored at height of top of head and direction to resist internal rotation in 90 degrees abducted position. Starting position is in 90 degrees abduction and almost full external rotation of the shoulder. Patient then internally rotates the shoulder while strongly retracting the scapula to stabilize the base of movement (I and J).

SUBSTITUTIONS: Shrugging shoulder, twisting body, excessive anterior humeral head movement with hyperextension of shoulder, jutting chin out

PARAMETERS: 8 to 12 repetitions, 1 to 3 sets, 1 time per day or every other day. *Pulses*: Perform as many as possible to fatigue and repeat 3 to 5 sets, 1 time per day or every other day.

Where's the Evidence?

Hintermeister, Lange, Schultheis, Bey, and Hawkins (1998) looked at muscle activity (measured by EMG) and applied load during 7 shoulder rehabilitation exercises done with an elastic resistance device. Seven exercises were studied: external and internal rotation, forward punch, shoulder shrug, and seated rowing with a narrow, middle, and wide grip. Fine-wire intra-muscular electrodes were inserted into the supraspinatus and subscapularis muscles, and surface electrodes were placed over the anterior deltoid, infraspinatus, pectoralis major, latissimus dorsi, serratus anterior, and trapezius muscles. Ten trials per subject were analyzed for average and peak amplitude. The muscle activity patterns suggest that these shoulder reha-bilitation exercises incorporating elastic resistance, controlled movements, and low initial loading effectively target the RC and supporting musculature and are appropriate for post-injury and postoperative patients.

EMG was recorded in 30 healthy subjects from 16 shoulder girdle muscles/muscles segments during three shoulder inter-nal rotation exercises: standing internal rotation at 0 degrees shoulder abduction, 90 degrees shoulder abduction and 90 degrees abduction in scapular plane. RC, deltoid, middle trapezius and lower trapezius, rhomboid major muscles are highly activated during internal rotation at 90 degrees of abduction. Latissimus dorsi exhibited markedly higher activation during internal rotation in scapular plane abduction, and serratus anterior was most active during internal rotation at 0 degrees abduction (Alizadehkhaiyat, Hawkes, Kemp, & Frostick, 2015).

A 2015 study measured the EMG activity of 16 shoulder girdle muscles/muscle segments during commonly prescribed shoulder internal rotation exercises, looking specifically at activation patterns in order to provide descriptive data regarding their activation. Despite the fact that co-activation of deltoid and RC muscles with standing internal rotation at 90 degrees abduction may provide a functional advantage by mirroring shoulder position and soft tissue mechanics during overhead activities and sports, it can place high levels of stress on shoulder tissues. Hence, internal rotation at 0 degrees abduction, which generates low-to-moderate activation of muscles, may be preferred in the rehabilitation of the individuals at risk for, or affected by, shoulder injuries. Considering the current emphasis on the subscapularis activity during internal rotation exercises, findings revealed markedly higher activation of subscapularis along with low-to-moderate activation of pectora-lis major, latissimus dorsi, and teres major in internal rotation at 90 degrees abduction, supporting the use of this exercise for selective subscapularis activation (Alizadehkhaiyat et al., 2015).

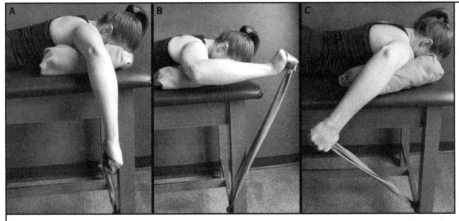

5.07.40 STRENGTHEN: ISOTONIC; RESISTANCE BAND, SHOULDER INTERNAL AND EXTERNAL ROTATION, PRONE

POSITION: Prone

TARGETS: Strengthening infra-spinatus, posterior deltoid, teres minor

INSTRUCTION: Patient lying with shoulder abducted 90 degrees; forearm hangs off table perpen-dicular to the floor. Place a towel under the arm to help align the shoulder joint with a horizontal humerus (A). With resistance band anchored below the hand, patient brings top of hand toward the ceiling into shoulder external rotation (B). This can be repeated, bringing palm up toward ceiling into shoulder internal rotation (C).

SUBSTITUTIONS: Shrugging shoulder, rolling trunk, elbow flexes past 90 degrees

PARAMETERS: Hold for 1 to 2 seconds, 1 to 3 sets, 8 to 12 repetitions, 1 time per day or every other day

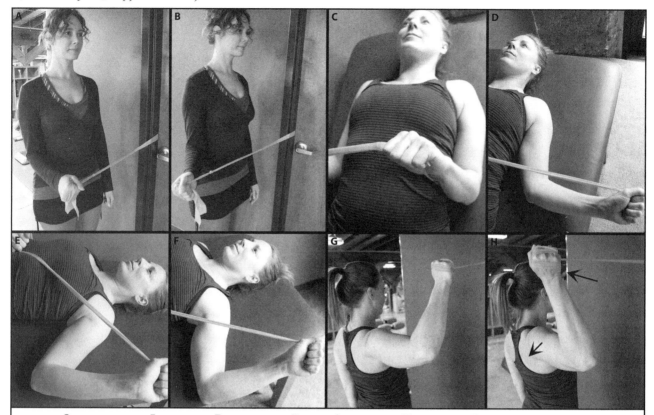

5.07.41 STRENGTHEN: ISOTONIC; RESISTANCE BAND, SHOULDER EXTERNAL ROTATION AND VARIATIONS

POSITION: Standing, supine

TARGETS: Strengthening of shoulder external rotators; infraspinatus, posterior deltoid, teres minor.

INSTRUCTION: *0 degrees abduction standing*: Resistance band is anchored at elbow height. Place a small towel between elbow and side, and instruct patient to squeeze throughout exercise. This will help to keep the elbow tucked into the side. Patient stands with unaffected side toward the anchor and grasps band. Starting position is in internal rotation of the shoulder, and patient should sidestep away from the wall so there is tension at start of movement. Patient then externally rotates the shoulder while strongly retracting the scapula to stabilize the base of movement (A and B). This can also be done bilaterally, holding the band between the hands. *0 degrees abduction supine*: Resistance band is anchored at elbow height or can be held by therapist. Place a small towel between elbow and side, and instruct patient to squeeze throughout exercise. This will help to keep the elbow is tucked into the side. Another small towel roll is placed under the humerus shaft to align the shaft with the glenoid fossa and prevent excessive anterior humeral gliding. Starting position is in internal rotation of the shoulder. Patient then externally rotates the shoulder while strongly retracting the scapula to stabilize the base of movement (C and D). *45 and 90 degrees abduction supine*: Resistance band is anchored at elbow height and direction to resist external rotation in abducted position or can be held by therapist. A small towel roll is placed under the humerus shaft to align the shaft with the glenoid fossa and prevent excessive anterior humeral gliding. Starting position is in internal rotation of the shoulder. Patient then externally rotates the shoulder while strongly retracting the scapula to stabilize the base of movement (E and F). For all of the above, consider starting in internal rotation and only externally rotating to neutral in the beginner phase. *Pulses*: Pulses are useful for building endurance and can be implemented in any of the positions described above. When performing a pulse, patient moves near the end ranges and returns only 10 to 20 degrees before rotating back again in a pulsing movement. Pulses are performed to fatigue to build endurance. *90 degrees abduction standing*: Resistance band is anchored at height of top of head and direction to resist external rotation in 90 degrees abducted position. Starting position is in 90 degrees abduction and almost full internal rotation of the shoulder. Patient then externally rotates the shoulder while strongly retracting the scapula to stabilize the base of movement (G and H).

SUBSTITUTIONS: Shrugging shoulder, twisting body, excessive anterior humeral head movement with hyperextension of shoulder, jutting chin out

PARAMETERS: 8 to 12 repetitions, 1 to 3 sets, 1 time per day or every other day. *Pulses*: Perform as many as possible to fatigue and repeat 3 to 5 sets, 1 time per day or every other day.

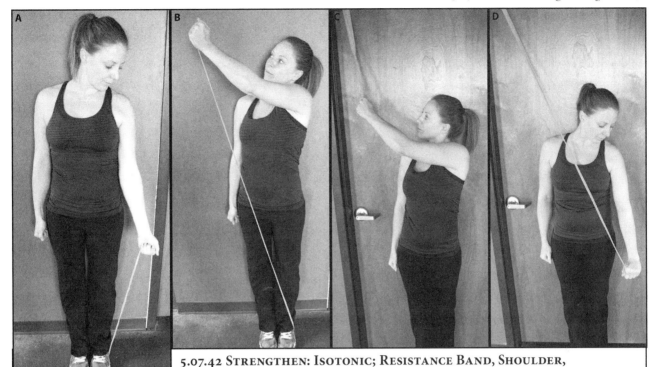

5.07.42 STRENGTHEN: ISOTONIC; RESISTANCE BAND, SHOULDER, COMBINATION MOVEMENTS PNF D1 AND D2

<u>POSITION</u>: Standing

<u>TARGETS</u>: Comprehensive strengthening of the shoulder; targets deltoid, RC, biceps, triceps, latissimus dorsi, teres major, coracobrachialis, pectorals.

Instruction: Patient performs movements through combined patterns, strengthening the shoulder in all three movement planes. D1 and D2 patterns may start in either the flexed or extended position.

Tips:
- Patient should follow the hand movement with the eyes and head.
- Rotational movements should be finished before crossing midline.
- Distal movements at the hand and wrist happen first.

D1 flexion: "Grab the ear to throw the tissue away": Anchor on the affected side knee height or lower; patient holds resistance band, starting in a position of extended D1 (scapular retraction, shoulder extension, abduction, internal rotation, forearm pronated, wrist ulnarly deviated, fingers extended) (A), and brings forearm across the face while moving toward shoulder, ending in flexion, adduction, external rotation, forearm supinated, wrist radially deviated, fingers flexed (B).

D1 extension: "Throw away tissue to grab the ear": Anchor on the unaffected side at head height or higher; patient holds resistance band with arm across the body, starting in a position of flexed D2 (forearm across face in shoulder flexion, adduction, external rotation, forearm supinated, wrist radially deviated, fingers flexed) (C), and pulls down across the body to end in scapular retraction, shoulder extension, abduction, internal rotation, forearm pronates, wrist ulnarly deviates, fingers extend (D). *(continued)*

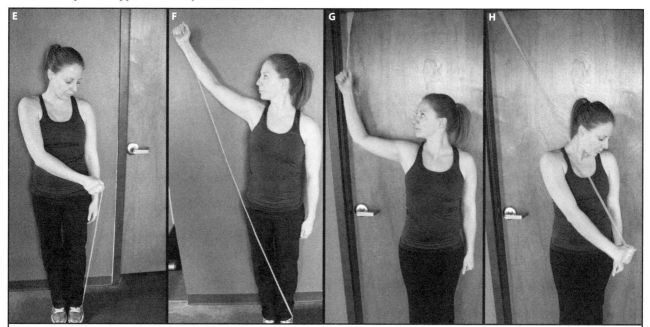

5.07.42 STRENGTHEN: ISOTONIC; RESISTANCE BAND, SHOULDER, COMBINATION MOVEMENTS PNF D1 AND D2 (CONTINUED)

D2 flexion: "Unsheath the sword to Tada!": Anchor on the unaffected side knee height or lower; patient holds the resistance band with arm across the body, thumb pointing toward the hip ending in a position of shoulder extension, abduction and internal rotation across the body, forearm pronated, wrist ulnarly deviated, fingers flexed (E) and then moves across the body and up toward the ceiling, turning thumb outwards while crossing trunk midline, to end in a position of scapula retracted, shoulder flexed, abducted, externally rotated, forearm pronated, wrist ulnarly deviated, fingers extended (F).

D2 extension: "Tada! to sheath the sword": Anchor on the affected side, head height or higher; patient holds the resistance band with arm up toward the ceiling, thumb outwards in a position of scapula retraction, shoulder flexion, abduction, external rotation, forearm pronation, wrist ulnarly deviated and fingers extended (G) then pulls the bands across the body thumb pointing toward the hip, ending in a position of shoulder extension, abduction and internal rotation, forearm pronated, wrist ulnarly deviated, fingers flexed (H).

SUBSTITUTIONS: Encourage scapular stabilization to minimize subacromial irritation, avoid arching back, excessive trunk rotation, chin jutting out, shrugging.

PARAMETERS: 8 to 12 repetitions, 1 to 3 sets, 1 time per day or every other day

5.07.43 STRENGTHEN: ISOTONIC; RESISTANCE BAND, SHOULDER, STANDING MILITARY (OVERHEAD) PRESS

POSITION: Standing

TARGETS: Strengthen primarily middle deltoid and upper trapezius; scapular component strengthens rhomboids, upper, middle and lower trapezius.

INSTRUCTION: Resistance band is anchored under the feet with two ends free (patient steps on the band in the middle). With arms in the "W" or "batwings" position, holding ends of bands and palms forward, patient retracts the scapula and then presses hands directly overhead keeping elbows in alignment with midline of body and head and extends elbows. Then patient slowly brings elbows back down to lateral ribs. Encourage the patient to engage scapular retractors throughout the movements (A and B).

SUBSTITUTIONS: Shrugging shoulders; elbows should stay in same coronal plane as hands at all times.

PARAMETERS: Hold for 1 to 2 seconds, 1 to 3 sets, 8 to 12 repetitions, 1 time per day or every other day

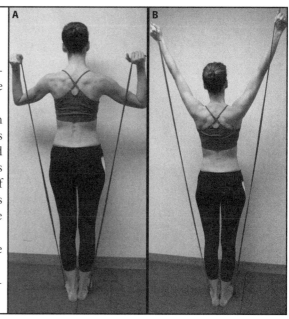

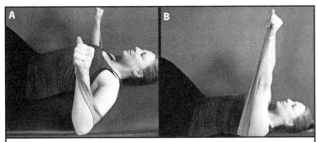

5.07.44 STRENGTHEN: ISOTONIC; RESISTANCE BAND, SHOULDER, CHEST PRESS

POSITION: Supine

TARGETS: Strengthen primarily middle horizontal fibers of pectoralis major

INSTRUCTION: Anchor the middle of the resistance band below the patient at chest level so there are two loose ends. The anchor may attach to base of bench or be situated under the patient's trunk. If patient is on a bench, it is important that patient does not horizontally abduct past shoulder level. Holding both ends of the band, patient starts with elbow bent 90 degrees and palms facing down toward feet, then presses up toward ceiling, extending elbows. Patient should not lock elbows (A and B).

SUBSTITUTIONS: Shrugging shoulder, allowing shoulder blades to come off table, patient should keep a natural arch in back and engage the abdominals before doing the exercise; avoid anterior humeral translation by dropping arms below shoulder level.

PARAMETERS: Hold for 1 to 2 seconds, 1 to 3 sets, 8 to 12 repetitions, 1 time per day or every other day

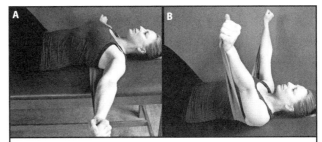

5.07.45 STRENGTHEN: ISOTONIC; RESISTANCE BAND, SHOULDER, CHEST FLY

POSITION: Seated

TARGETS: Strengthen pectoralis major, middle horizontal fibers primarily

INSTRUCTION: Anchor the resistance band at patient's shoulder height, behind patient, leaving two free ends. Patient grasps each end with hands. Patient scoots out until tension is felt when shoulders are abducted 90 degrees. Patient then horizontally adducts shoulders; elbows are near fully extended, and palms are facing each other. Slowly allow arms to come back and repeat (A and B). The anchor may also be lowered to perform an incline fly (targeting upper fibers of pectoralis major) or raise the anchor to perform a decline fly (targeting lower fibers of pectoralis major).

SUBSTITUTIONS: Shrugging shoulder, patient should keep a natural arch in back and engage the abdominals before doing the exercise; excessive horizontal abduction elbow are more posterior than shoulder at end range.

PARAMETERS: Hold for 1 to 2 seconds, 1 to 3 sets, 8 to 12 repetitions, 1 time per day or every other day

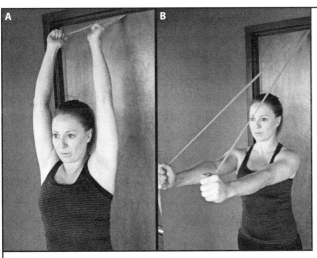

5.07.46 STRENGTHEN: ISOTONIC; RESISTANCE BAND, SHOULDER PULL-OVER

POSITION: Standing or seated

TARGETS: Strengthening latissimus dorsi, teres major, triceps; to a lesser extent pectoralis major and minor.

INSTRUCTION: Anchor the resistance band above patient's head, behind patient, leaving two free ends. Patient stands facing away from the wall with slight bend in hip and knees, feet hip-width apart and grasps each end with hands. Patient walks out (if sitting, scoots chair) until tension is felt when shoulders are flexed fully. Patient then pulls down in front toward extension, hands stopping just above the navel line; elbows are near fully extended and palms are facing each other. Slowly allow arms to come back and repeat (A and B). This can also be unilaterally. Patient may also be seated for entire sequence.

SUBSTITUTIONS: Shrugging shoulder; patient should keep a natural arch in back and engage the abdominals before doing the exercise.

PARAMETERS: Hold for 1 to 2 seconds, 1 to 3 sets, 8 to 12 repetitions, 1 time per day or every other day

5.07.47 STRENGTHEN: ISOTONIC; RESISTANCE BAND, SHOULDER PULL-BACK

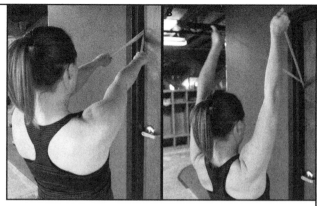

POSITION: Standing, seated

TARGETS: Strengthening latissimus dorsi, teres major, triceps; strong scapular retraction at end range will also strengthen rhomboids, middle and lower trapezius.

INSTRUCTION: Anchor the resistance band at shoulder height with two free ends. Patient grasps both ends with shoulders flexed 90 degrees. Patient then pulls back and overhead into flexion, adding scapular retraction and depression at end range (A and B).

SUBSTITUTIONS: Shrugging shoulder; patient should keep a natural arch in back and engage the abdominals before doing the exercise.

PARAMETERS: Hold for 1 to 2 seconds, 1 to 3 sets, 8 to 12 repetitions, 1 time per day or every other day

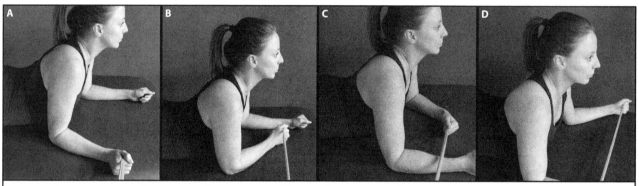

5.07.48 STRENGTHEN: ISOTONIC; RESISTANCE BAND, SHOULDER TRIPOD, INTERNAL ROTATION AND EXTERNAL ROTATION

POSITION: Prone on elbows

TARGETS: Strengthening infraspinatus, posterior deltoid, teres minor (external rotation), subscapularis, latissimus dorsi, teres major (internal rotation); assists to seat the humeral head in the glenoid fossa and promote stability with strengthening movements.

INSTRUCTION: Patient, lying prone props up on elbow, keeping elbow just below the shoulders. Patient holds resistance band in hand, thumb pointed up. *Internal rotation*: Therapist stands on affected side, holding other end of band, and applies tension while patient allows shoulder to externally rotate. Patient then internally rotates across the body bringing hand toward opposite elbow (A and B). *External rotation*: Therapist stands on unaffected side, holding other end of band, and applies tension while patient allows shoulder to internally rotate. Patient then externally rotates across the body, bringing hand toward opposite elbow (C and D). External rotation can also be done bilaterally holding a piece of band between both hands and externally rotating both shoulders simultaneously. Encourage the patient to engage scapular retractors throughout the movements for eccentric control as well. Place a small towel down that will move with the elbow to avoid friction. Eyes should stay focused on mat area between hands.

SUBSTITUTIONS: Shrugging shoulder, sinking into shoulder, lack of active scapular stabilization, hyperextending neck

PARAMETERS: Hold for 1 to 2 seconds, 1 to 3 sets, 8 to 12 repetitions, 1 time per day or every other day

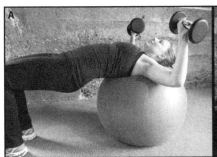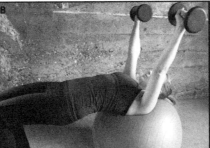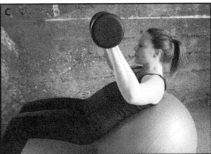

5.07.49 STRENGTHEN: EXERCISE BALL, SHOULDER, CHEST PRESS

POSITION: Table top on ball

TARGETS: Strengthen primarily middle horizontal fibers of pectoralis major while working core (abdominals); lateral epicondylitis (gluteus maximus, hamstring) muscles.

INSTRUCTION: Patient sits and rolls out to table top on an exercise ball while engaging abdominals, gluteals and hamstrings to maintain position. Patient holds dumbbells at chest level in the 90/90 arm position with forearms perpendicular to the floor. It is important that patient does not horizontally abduct past shoulder level. Patient starts with elbows bent 90 degrees and palms facing down toward feet, then presses up toward ceiling, extending elbows. Patient should not lock elbows (A and B). *Incline press*: Patient is positioned reclining at a 45 degrees angle with increased hip and knee flexion, not full table top. Instructions are repeated as for chest press (C).

SUBSTITUTIONS: Shrugging shoulder; allowing shoulder blades to come off ball, patient should keep a natural arch in back and engage the abdominals before doing the exercise, avoid anterior humeral translation by dropping arms below shoulder level, chin should be tucked and head supported by ball.

PARAMETERS: Hold for 1 to 2 seconds, 1 to 3 sets, 8 to 12 repetitions, 1 time per day or every other day

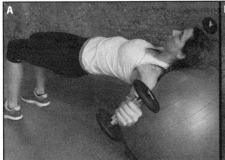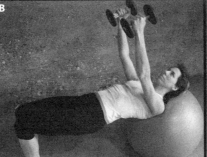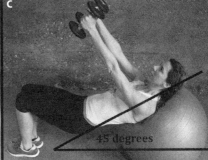

5.07.50 STRENGTHEN: EXERCISE BALL, SHOULDER, CHEST FLY

POSITION: Table top on ball

TARGETS: Strengthen primarily middle horizontal fibers of pectoralis major while working core (abdominals); lateral epicondylitis (gluteus maximus, hamstring) muscles.

INSTRUCTION: *Chest fly*: Patient sits and rolls out to table top on an exercise ball while engaging abdominals, gluteals and hamstrings to maintain position. Patient holds dumbbells and horizontally abducts shoulders; elbows are near fully extended, and palms are facing each other. Lower the hands until the elbows are at the same level as the shoulders. Patient then brings the palms into shoulder horizontal adduction while lifting the weights with the hands until the palms and dumbbells touch. Slowly lower and repeat (A and B). *Incline fly*: Patient is positioned reclining at a 45-degree angle, with increased hip and knee flexion—not full table top. Instructions are repeated as for chest fly (C).

SUBSTITUTIONS: Shrugging shoulder; allowing shoulder blades to come off ball, patient should keep a natural arch in back and engage the abdominals before doing the exercise, avoid anterior humeral translation by dropping arms below shoulder level, chin should be tucked and head supported by ball.

PARAMETERS: Hold for 1 to 2 seconds, 1 to 3 sets 8 to 12 repetitions, 1 time per day or every other day

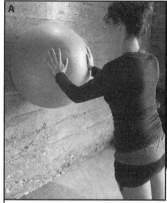
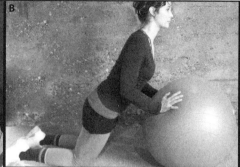
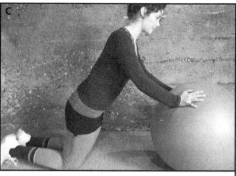

5.07.51 STRENGTHEN: EXERCISE BALL, SHOULDER, PUSH-UP

POSITION: Standing, tall-kneeling

TARGETS: Strengthen pectoralis major, anterior deltoid, triceps, anconeus; protraction at end range will target serratus anterior as well.

INSTRUCTION: *Standing*: Patient stands holding the ball at chest height. Patient places hands at shoulder height and, while holding ball against the wall, steps back, keeping head, spine and pelvis in alignment. Patient lowers chest toward the ball, bending elbows outward followed by pressing away from the ball, straightening elbows but not locking elbows out (A). *Tall-kneeling*: Both of the patient's hands are on the ball while patient leans body weight into the ball. Patient presses up away from ball, extending but not locking elbows and protracts scapula rounding the upper thoracic spine. Keep shoulders depressed (B and C). Gaze is between the hands and chin slightly tucked. Patient may also hold a static plank for isometric training. Triceps focus can be increased by bringing elbows close to the sides (Chaturonga dandasana yoga pose).

SUBSTITUTIONS: Shrugging shoulders; avoid hyperextension at the elbows and jutting chin out or looking up.

PARAMETERS: Hold for 1 to 2 seconds, 1 to 3 sets, 8 to 12 repetitions, 1 time per day or every other day

---

Where's the Evidence?

Tucker, Armstrong, Gribbel, Timmons, and Yeasting (2010) looked at EMG data for muscle activation with standard push-up, push-up on an unstable surface, and shoulder rehabilitation device for overhead athletes with and without shoulder impingement. They found the push-up on an unstable surface had significantly greater activation of serratus anterior, upper trapezius, middle trapezius, and lower trapezius, compared with the standard push-up for the shoulder impingement patients. They also found differences in EMG patterns and recruitment of the 4 muscles with impingement and non-impingement athletes. Their findings suggested that the muscle activation of the middle trapezius differs in overhead athletes with a history of secondary shoulder impingement compared with those who lack this history during closed chain exercise. The levels of muscle activation of the serratus anterior and upper trapezius during these closed chain exercises were similar between the two groups. They supported the use of closed chain exercises in the rehabilitation process of overhead athletes with secondary shoulder impingement.

5.07.52 STRENGTHEN: EXERCISE BALL, SHOULDER, PUSH-UP, HANDS ON BALL

POSITION: Prone, push-up position on ball

Targets: Strengthen pectoralis major, anterior deltoid, triceps, anconeus; protraction at end range will target serratus anterior as well; plank will also strengthen core abdominal muscles and quadriceps.

INSTRUCTION: Patient's hands are on the ball while extending feet out, toes out on the floor in a plank position. Patient should tighten quadriceps to lift knees to straight and engage core abdominal muscles to put lumbar spine in neutral. Patient presses up away from ball, extending but not locking elbows, and protracts scapula, rounding the upper thoracic spine. Keep shoulders depressed (A and B). Gaze is between the hands and chin slightly tucked. Triceps focus can be increased by bringing elbows close to the sides (Chaturonga dandasana yoga pose). Patient may also hold a static plank for isometric training.

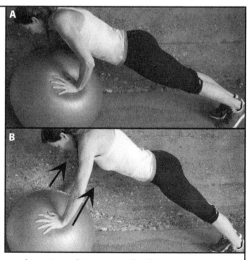

SUBSTITUTIONS: Shrugging shoulders; avoid hyperextension at the elbows and jutting chin out or looking up.

PARAMETERS: Hold for 1 to 2 seconds, 1 to 3 sets, 8 to 12 repetitions, 1 time per day or every other day

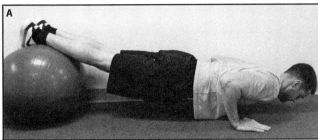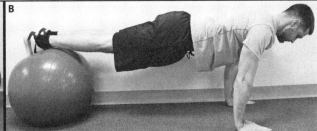

5.07.53 Strengthen: Exercise Ball, Shoulder, Push-Up, Feet on Ball

Position: Prone, plank on ball

Targets: Strengthen pectoralis major, anterior deltoid, triceps, anconeus; protraction at end range will target serratus anterior as well; plank will also strengthen core abdominal muscles and quadriceps.

Instruction: Patient's lower legs are on the ball while extending the legs out into a plank position. Patient should tighten quadriceps to lift knees to straight and engage core abdominal muscles to put lumbar spine in neutral. Patient presses up away from floor, extending but not locking elbows, protracts scapula rounding the upper thoracic spine. Keep shoulders depressed. Gaze is between the hands and chin slightly tucked. Triceps focus can be increased by bringing elbows close to the sides (Chaturonga dandasana yoga pose) (A and B). Patient may also hold a static plank for isometric training.

Substitutions: Shrugging shoulders; avoid hyperextension at the elbows and jutting chin out or looking up.

Parameters: Hold for 1 to 2 seconds, 1 to 3 sets, 8 to 12 repetitions, 1 time per day or every other day

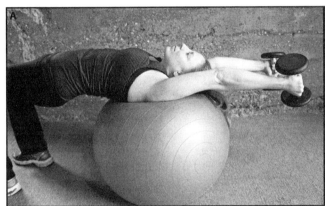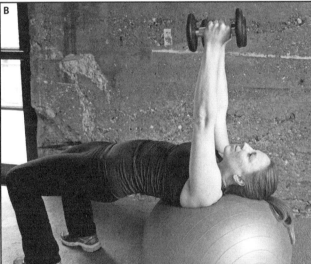

5.07.54 Strengthen: Exercise Ball, Pull-Over (Latissimus Dorsi)

Position: Table top on ball

Targets: Strengthening primarily latissimus dorsi while working core (abdominals); LE (gluteus maximus, hamstring) muscles.

Instruction: Patient sits and rolls out to table top on an exercise ball while engaging abdominals, gluteals and hamstrings to maintain position. Patient holds dumbbells and brings overhead avoiding arching the back, elbows are near fully extended and palms are facing each other. Lower the hands as far as possible without losing form, then lift arms up to perpendicular to floor. Repeat (A and B).

Substitutions: Shrugging shoulder; patient should keep a natural arch in back and engage the abdominals before doing the exercise, chin should be tucked and head supported by ball.

Parameters: Hold for 1 to 2 seconds, 1 to 3 sets, 8 to 12 repetitions, 1 time per day or every other day

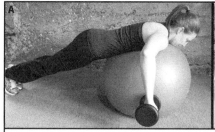
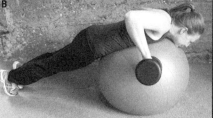
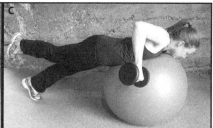

5.07.55 Strengthen: Exercise Ball, Rear Deltoid Rows

POSITION: Quadruped on exercise ball

TARGETS: Strengthen posterior deltoid, rhomboid, middle trapezius

INSTRUCTION: Patient lies face down on the ball with arms stretched forward (just the torso will be on the ball). With feet spaced wide, toes down, knees lifted off the floor, patient tightens abdominal muscles and lifts elbows toward ceiling; elbows are bent to 90 degrees. Patient squeezes scapula while raising arms up and out in a wide arc. This may be done one arm at a time and progressing to both arms (A and B). Adding the exercise ball creates an unstable surface and is more challenging. To further challenge the core, have the patient raise one leg off the floor during the exercise (C).

SUBSTITUTIONS: Shrugging shoulders excessively; thoracic extension rather than retraction, excessive translation of humeral head anteriorly, lifting head.

PARAMETERS: Hold for 1 to 2 seconds, 1 to 3 sets, 8 to 12 repetitions, 1 time per day or every other day

5.07.56 Strengthen: Isotonic; Shoulder, Horizontal Abduction

POSITION: Side-lying over ball

TARGETS: Strengthen posterior deltoid, rhomboid, middle trapezius

INSTRUCTION: Lying on the unaffected side with feet in a wide anterior-to-posterior staggered position, ball just under axilla along lateral trunk, with affected arm holding weight, patient lies in horizontal adduction

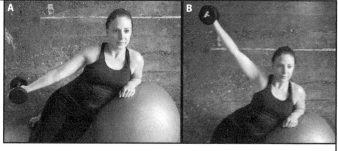

over the ball. Opposite hand supports the head and neck in neutral. Patient engages scapular stabilizers by retracting and depressing the scapula while horizontally abducting the shoulder with the back of the hand leading the way. Focus is on minimizing upper trapezius compensatory recruitment (A and B).

SUBSTITUTIONS: Shrugging shoulder, rolling trunk backward or forward

PARAMETERS: 8 to 12 repetitions, 1 to 3 sets, 1 time per day or every other day

5.07.57 Strengthen: Exercise Ball, Shoulder, Overhead Press

POSITION: Seated on ball

TARGETS: Deltoid, upper trapezius

INSTRUCTION: With arms in the "W" or "batwings" position, holding ends of bands and palm forward, patient retracts the scapula and then presses hands directly overhead, keeping elbows in alignment with midline of body and head, and extending elbows. Then

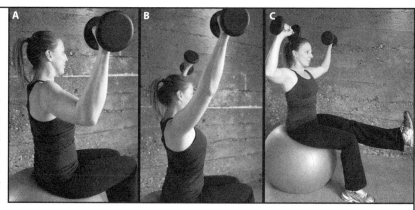

patient slowly brings elbows back down to lateral ribs. Encourage the patient to engage scapular retractors throughout the movements (A and B). Gaze is forward and chin slightly tucked. Additional challenge to core muscles involves lifting one leg for exercise (C).

SUBSTITUTIONS: Shrugging shoulder; elbows should stay in same coronal plane as hands at all times, avoid hyperextension at the elbows and jutting chin out or looking up.

PARAMETERS: 10 times up to 3 sets, 1 time per day or every other day

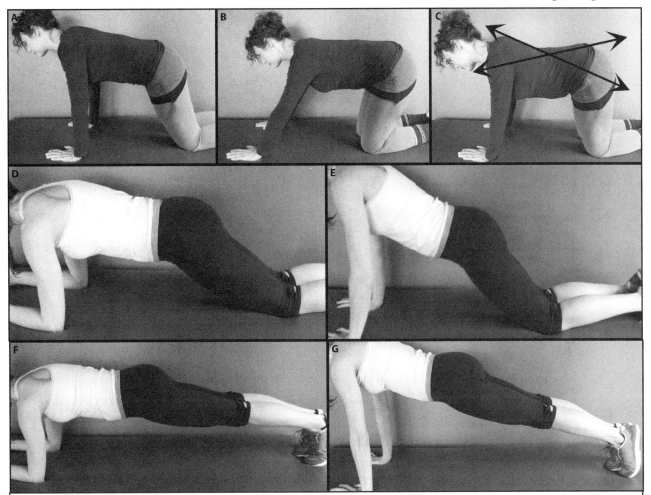

5.07.58 STRENGTHEN: CLOSED KINETIC CHAIN; SHOULDER, WEIGHT SHIFTS

POSITION: Prone on elbows, hands, quadruped

TARGETS: Strengthening global shoulder, particularly latissimus dorsi, deltoid, pectoralis major, teres major, RC, scapular stabilizers, biceps, triceps; assists to seat the humeral head in the glenoid fossa and promote stability with strengthening movements.

INSTRUCTION: Patient in quadruped with hands directly below the shoulders and knees below the hips, patient retracts scapula and slowly rocks forward as far as possible and then backward as far as possible (A and B). This can also be done side-to-side and in diagonal patterns with smaller arcs of movement (C). Progressions include lying prone and propping up on elbows, keeping elbows just below the shoulders. Patient, with knees on table, lifts hips, engaging core muscles and retracts scapula (D). Progression further involves patient moving to plank on hands and knees (E), hands and feet (F), and then hands and feet (G). Gaze is toward floor just in front of hands with chin tucked.

SUBSTITUTIONS: Shrugging shoulder, sinking into shoulder, lack of active scapular stabilization, hyperextending neck

PARAMETERS: Hold each rocking position for 1 to 2 seconds, 1 to 3 sets, 8 to 12 repetitions, 1 time per day or every other day

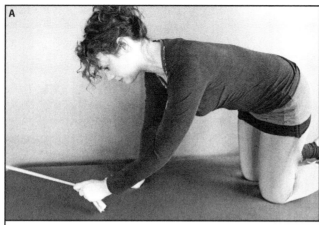

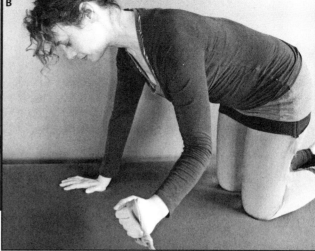

5.07.59 STRENGTHEN: CLOSED KINETIC CHAIN; SHOULDER, RESISTANCE BAND, TRIPOD STABILIZATION

POSITION: Quadruped

TARGETS: Stabilization of shoulder; targets deltoid, RC, biceps, triceps, latissimus dorsi, teres major, coracobrachialis, pectorals; assists to seat the humeral head in the glenoid fossa and promote stability with strengthening movements.

INSTRUCTION: Patient with hands placed just below the shoulders, holds resistance band in the unaffected hand and then shifts weight to the affected UE and both LE with band anchored in front (A) or to the side (B) move the band in short arcs of motion front-to-back or side-to-side. Encourage the patient to engage scapular retractors throughout the movements. Eyes should stay focused on mat area in front of the hands.

SUBSTITUTIONS: Shrugging shoulder, sinking into shoulder, lack of active scapular stabilization, hyperextending neck

PARAMETERS: 10 to 30 short arc movements to fatigue of weightbearing shoulder, 1 to 3 sets, 1 time per day or every other day

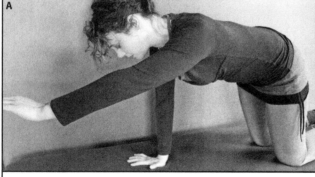

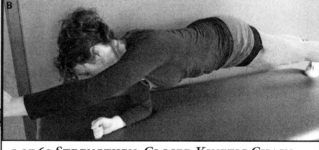

5.07.60 STRENGTHEN: CLOSED KINETIC CHAIN; SHOULDER, ALTERNATING ARM LIFT

POSITION: Quadruped, prone on elbows, prone on elbows and knees, prone on elbows and toes

TARGETS: Strengthening global shoulder, particularly latissimus dorsi, deltoid, pectoralis major, teres major, RC, scapular stabilizers, biceps, triceps; assists to seat the humeral head in the glenoid fossa and promote stability with strengthening movements.

INSTRUCTION: Knees are spaced hip-width apart and hands directly beneath shoulders. Instruct patient to press away from the floor with palms of hands cupping and weight distributed through the fingertips. Shoulders are active and engaged, scapula depressed and retracted slightly. Patient finds neutral spine and holds. Keeping and pelvis level, patient slowly brings one extended arm into shoulder flexion to parallel with to the surface (A). This can also be done prone on elbows (B), prone on elbows and knees (not shown), and prone on elbows and toes (B).

SUBSTITUTIONS: Sagging abdomen, arching lower back, loss of neutral spine, sagging into shoulders or shrugging, hyperextension of the elbows, poor activation of wrist with no cupping, rolling to one side losing pelvis and shoulder level position

PARAMETERS: Hold 3 to 5 seconds, 10 times each up to 3 sets, 1 time per day or every other day

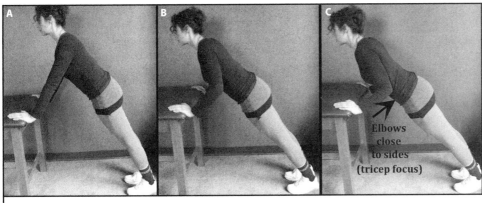

5.07.61 STRENGTHEN: CLOSED KINETIC CHAIN; SHOULDER, BEGINNING WEIGHTBEARING, PROGRESS TO PUSH-UP PARTIAL WEIGHT

POSITION: Standing, modified plantigrade

TARGETS: Strengthen pectoralis major, anterior deltoid, triceps, anconeus; protraction at end range will target serratus anterior. Plank will also strengthen core abdominal muscles and quadriceps; assists to seat the humeral head in the glenoid fossa and promote stability with strengthening movements.

INSTRUCTION: *Beginning weightbearing*: With both hands on table at waist height, patient walks feet away from the table slightly and leans forward so that arms are accepting partial weight. Patient may stay here and work on keeping humeral head seated in the glenoid fossa while weight-shifting side-to-side accepting more weight on each side (A). *Add push-up*: With both hands on table at waist height, patient walks feet away from the table slightly and leans forward so that arms are accepting partial weight. Patient extends feet out, toes on floor, in a plank position. Patient lowers chest toward the table bending elbows outward followed by pressing away from the table straightening but not locking elbows out. Keep shoulders depressed and retracted (B). Gaze is between the hands and chin slightly tucked. Triceps focus can be increased by bringing elbows close to the sides (Chaturonga dandasana yoga pose) (C). Patient may also hold a static modified plantigrade plank for isometric training.

SUBSTITUTIONS: Shrugging shoulders; avoid hyperextension at the elbows and jutting chin out or looking up.

PARAMETERS: Hold for 1 to 2 seconds, 1 to 3 sets, 8 to 12 repetitions, 1 time per day or every other day

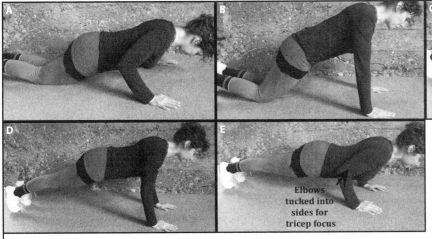

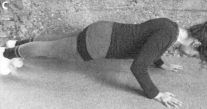

5.07.62 STRENGTHEN: CLOSED KINETIC CHAIN; SHOULDER, PUSH-UP

POSITION: Prone on hands (knees progressing to toes

TARGETS: Strengthen pectoralis major, anterior deltoid, triceps, anconeus; protraction at end range will target serratus anterior as well. Plank will also strengthen core abdominal muscles and quadriceps. Assists to seat the humeral head in the glenoid fossa and promote stability with strengthening movements.

INSTRUCTION: *Modified floor push-up*: Position patient on the hands and knees with head, shoulders, hips and knees in a straight line, elbows slightly bent and scapula in proper position. Patient lowers body toward the floor without letting low back or head sag. Return to the start position. Avoid locking elbows out. Keep shoulders depressed and retracted (A and B). *Floor push-up*: Position patient on hands and toes and follow same instructions as for modified floor push-up (C and D). Gaze is between the hands and chin slightly tucked. Triceps focus can be increased by bringing elbows close to the sides (Chaturonga dandasana yoga pose) (E). Patient may also hold a static plank for isometric training.

SUBSTITUTIONS: Shrugging shoulders; avoid hyperextension at the elbows and jutting chin out or looking up.

PARAMETERS: Hold for 1 to 2 seconds, 1 to 3 sets, 8 to 12 repetitions, 1 time per day or every other day

5.07.63 STRENGTHEN: CLOSED KINETIC CHAIN; SCAPULAR AND SHOULDER DEPRESSION

POSITION: Seated

TARGETS: Strengthen latissimus dorsi, pectoralis major, pectoralis minor, lower trapezius, serratus anterior, and subclavius; assists to seat the humeral head in the glenoid fossa and promote stability with strengthening movements.

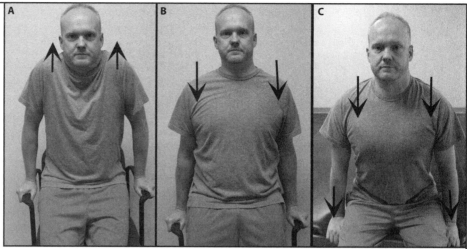

INSTRUCTION: Utilizing a chair with armrests, patient grasps each armrest with hands and maintains the elbows in a straight position, but not locked. Patient raises seat off the chair to start allowing shoulders to be shrugged toward the ears. Patient presses away from armrests, causing scapula to slide down the back, moving the shoulders away from the ears and raising the body up from the chair (A and B). This may also be performed on chair without armrests as shown (C).

SUBSTITUTIONS: Avoid hyperextension at the elbows and jutting chin out or looking up

PARAMETERS: Hold for 1 to 2 seconds, 1 to 3 sets, 8 to 12 repetitions, 1 time per day or every other day

5.07.64 STRENGTHEN: CLOSED KINETIC CHAIN; SHOULDER, TABLE TOP PUSH-PULL

POSITION: Standing, lunge

TARGETS: Strengthen latissimus primarily with assist from posterior deltoid; assists to seat the humeral head in the glenoid fossa and promote stability with strengthening movements.

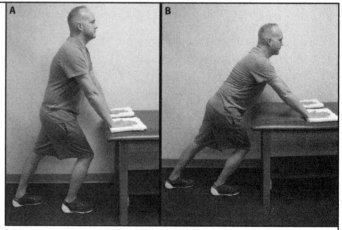

INSTRUCTION: With both hands on a table at waist height, patient staggers feet into a partial forward lunge, positioning feet away from the table slightly, and leans forward so that arms are accepting partial weight. Patient grasps folded-up towel in both hands and pushes down onto the towel with both hands while pushing the towel forward, as if wiping the table, shifting the weight onto the front leg while pushing. Patient then pulls back, returning to the starting position, shifting weight onto the back leg. Keep shoulders depressed and retracted (A and B). Gaze is between the hands and chin slightly tucked.

SUBSTITUTIONS: Shrugging shoulders, jutting chin out or looking up

PARAMETERS: Hold for 1 to 2 seconds, 1 to 3 sets, 8 to 12 repetitions, 1 time per day or every other day

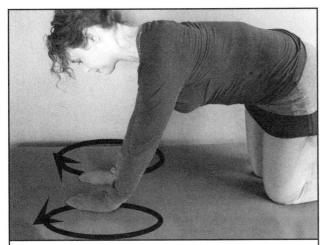

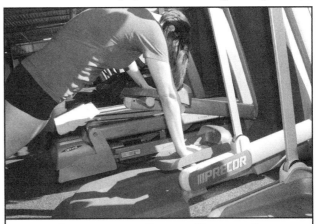

5.07.65 STRENGTHEN: CLOSED KINETIC CHAIN; SHOULDER, FLOOR SCRUBBING

POSITION: Quadruped

TARGETS: Strengthening global shoulder, particularly latissimus dorsi, deltoid, pectoralis major, teres major, RC, scapular stabilizers, biceps, triceps; assists to seat the humeral head in the glenoid fossa and promote stability with strengthening movements.

INSTRUCTION: Place a sock on each of the patient's hands and position so knees are spaced hip-width apart and hands are directly beneath shoulders. Patient slowly moves sternum away from the floor and moves both arms in and out simultaneously, clockwise and then counter-clockwise, initiating the movement with the scapula.

SUBSTITUTIONS: Sagging abdomen, arching lower back, loss of neutral spine, sagging into shoulders or shrugging, rolling to one side losing pelvis, shoulder level position

PARAMETERS: 1 to 3 sets, 8 to 12 repetitions of each movement, 1 time per day or every other day

5.07.66 STRENGTHEN: CLOSED KINETIC CHAIN; STAIRMASTER, SHOULDER

POSITION: Quadruped, prone on hands and knees, prone hands and toes

TARGETS: Strengthening global shoulder particularly latissimus dorsi, deltoid, pectoralis major, teres major, RC, scapular stabilizers, biceps, triceps; assists to seat the humeral head in the glenoid fossa and promote stability with strengthening movements.

INSTRUCTION: Position patient in quadruped for beginner and progress to prone on hands and knees, lifting hips to engage core muscles and retract scapula, then to prone on hands and toes, lifting hips and knees to engage core muscles and retracts scapula. Patient places hands on Stairmaster (Core Health & Fitness) pedals and accepts weight through the UE. At the lower settings, patient climbs using the arms allowing elbows to bend and straighten.

SUBSTITUTIONS: Sagging abdomen, arching lower back, loss of neutral spine, sagging into shoulders or shrugging, rolling to one side losing pelvis and shoulder level position

PARAMETERS: 1 to 5 minutes, 1 time per day or every other day

5.07.67 STRENGTHEN: CLOSED KINETIC CHAIN; BODYBLADE, SHOULDER FLEXION, SCAPTION, AND ABDUCTION

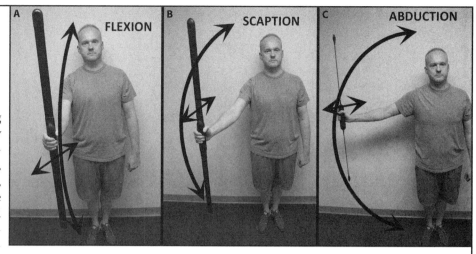

POSITION: Standing

TARGETS: Strengthening global shoulder, particularly latissimus dorsi, deltoid, pectoralis major, teres major, RC, scapular stabilizers, biceps, triceps; assists to seat the humeral head in the glenoid fossa and promote stability with strengthening movements; oscillatory movements provide co-contraction of the muscles surrounding the joint.

INSTRUCTION: Patient stands with feet hip-width apart, slight bend in hip, knees and engaging abdominal core muscles. Hold center of Bodyblade with Bodyblade oriented vertically. Patient makes small movements with the arm to cause the Bodyblade to oscillate front-to-back. Patient then performs flexion **5.07.36** except going full range for each. Focus is on form and minimizing upper trapezius compensatory recruitment. After one set, this is repeated for scaption and abduction. Thumb leads the way for all movements (A through C).

SUBSTITUTIONS: Shrugging shoulder, arching back, leaning back, fast movement, loss of rhythmic oscillation, not engaging scapular stabilizers

PARAMETERS: 8 to 12 repetitions, 1 to 3 sets, 1 time per day or every other day

---

5.07.68 STRENGTHEN: CLOSED KINETIC CHAIN; BODYBLADE, SHOULDER INTERNAL ROTATION AND EXTERNAL ROTATION

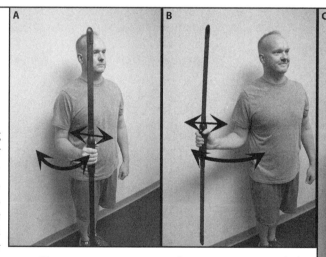

POSITION: Standing

TARGETS: Strengthening global shoulder particularly latissimus dorsi, deltoid, pectoralis major, teres major, RC, scapular stabilizers, biceps, triceps; assists to seat the humeral head in the glenoid fossa and promote stability with strengthening movements; oscillatory movements provide co-contraction of the muscles surrounding the joint.

INSTRUCTION: Patient stands with feet hip-width apart, slight bend in hips knees and engaging abdominal core muscles. Hold center of Bodyblade with Bodyblade oriented vertically. Elbow is tucked into side and flexed 90 degrees. Patient makes small movements with the arm to cause the Bodyblade to oscillate front-to-back. Patient then performs internal rotation bringing the palm and Bodyblade across the stomach, followed by external rotation leading with the back of the hand. The thumb is pointed upward toward the ceiling for the entire sequence (A through C).

SUBSTITUTIONS: Shrugging shoulder, fast movement, loss of rhythmic oscillation, not engaging scapular stabilizers

PARAMETERS: 8 to 12 repetitions, 1 to 3 sets, 1 time per day or every other day

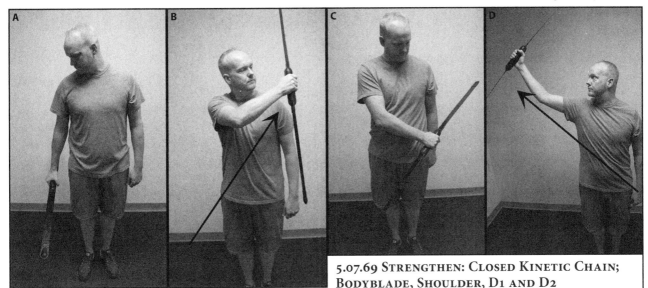

5.07.69 STRENGTHEN: CLOSED KINETIC CHAIN; BODYBLADE, SHOULDER, D1 AND D2

POSITION: Standing

TARGETS: Strengthening global shoulder, particularly latissimus dorsi, deltoid, pectoralis major, teres major, RC, scapular stabilizers, biceps, triceps; assists to seat the humeral head in the glenoid fossa and promote stability with strengthening movements; oscillatory movements provide co-contraction of the muscles surrounding the joint.

INSTRUCTION: Patient stands with feet hip-width apart, slight bend in hips and knees and engaging abdominal core muscles. Hold center of Bodyblade with Bodyblade oriented vertically. Patient performs D1 pattern as described in **5.07.28** for one set (A and B) and follows with D2 pattern as described in **5.07.28** (C and D).

SUBSTITUTIONS: Shrugging shoulder, arching back, leaning back, fast movement, loss of rhythmic oscillation, not engaging scapular stabilizers

PARAMETERS: 8 to 12 repetitions, 1 to 3 sets, 1 time per day or every other day

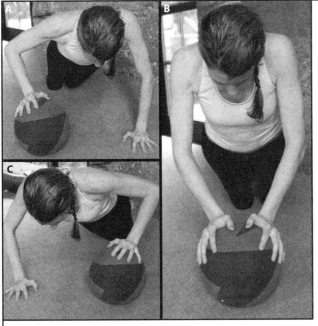

5.07.70 STRENGTHEN: CLOSED KINETIC CHAIN; SHOULDER, PLANK SHUFFLE ON MEDICINE BALL

POSITION: Start in quadruped, move into plank

TARGETS: Strengthen pectoralis major, anterior deltoid, triceps, anconeus; protraction at end range will target serratus anterior; plank will also strengthen core abdominal muscles and quadriceps; assists to seat the humeral head in the glenoid fossa and promote stability with strengthening movements.

INSTRUCTION: Patient takes a medicine ball and kneels on the floor with ball in front. Patient places one hand on top of ball and other hand on floor, slightly wider than shoulder width. Patient then moves into plank with the upper body above hands, floor elbow straight and ball elbow flexed, and feet shoulder-width apart. Keeping body strong and straight, patient picks up floor hand and places on ball as ball hand moves to placement on floor. Repeat, continually swapping hands. Perform at moderate, controlled speed (A through C). Patient may progress to advanced version in full plank.

SUBSTITUTIONS: Shrugging shoulders; avoid hyperextension at the elbows and jutting chin out or looking up, sagging trunk or shoulders.

PARAMETERS: Repeat swapping for 20 to 30 seconds, 1 to 3 sets, 1 time per day or every other day

5.07.71 STRENGTHEN: CLOSED KINETIC CHAIN; SHOULDER, INVERTED ROW

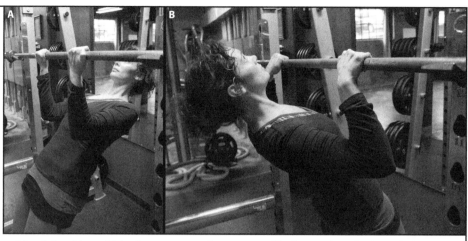

POSITION: Standing

TARGETS: Strengthening biceps brachii, latissimus dorsi, lower trapezius, posterior deltoid, middle trapezius, lumbar multifidus, lumbar thoracic, RA

INSTRUCTION: Patient stands facing a chest-height horizontal bar. Patient grasps bar with wide overhand grip, just outside of shoulder-width elbows outward. Patient walks forward under bar while pulling upper chest close to bar. With heels on floor, patient positions body at angle under bar with legs, hips and spine straight. Patient positions arms perpendicular to body. Patient pulls body toward the bar while trunk stays in straight alignments and upper arms are parallel to the bar (A). This can also be done with an underhand grip (B) and lifting one leg for added challenges (not shown).

SUBSTITUTIONS: Shrugging shoulder, rolling trunk, excessive horizontal abduction or extension pushing humeral head anteriorly

PARAMETERS: Hold for 1 to 2 seconds, 1 to 3 sets 8 to 12 repetitions, 1 time per day or every other day

---

Where's the Evidence?

Youdas, Keith, Noon, Squires, and Hollman (2015) recorded muscle activation, normalized to a MVIC during an inverted row using surface EMG. Analysis conducted on 13 male and 13 female subjects performing 4 inverted row exercises. Four muscles—biceps brachii, latissimus dorsi, lower trapezius, and posterior deltoid—demonstrated very high EMG activation during all four exercise conditions; supinated grip, one and both legs; pronated grip, one and both legs. Three muscles—upper trapezius, middle trapezius, and lumbar multifidus—demonstrated high activation, whereas 2 muscles—lumbar thoracic and RA—demonstrated moderate activation.

5.07.72 FUNCTIONAL: SHOULDER, TIE KNOTS IN TUBING

POSITION: Seated

TARGETS: Functional use of shoulders targeting internal and external rotation

INSTRUCTION: Patient uses resistance band to tie knots and tighten loosely. Patient then unties knots until band is free. The tying of each knot requires internal

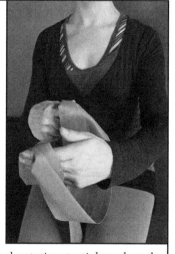

rotation to tie and external rotation to tighten loosely. Untying the knots also demands similar movements. Using strong resistance band makes the exercise more challenging. Encourage good posture and scapular stabilization throughout the activity.

SUBSTITUTIONS: Shrugging shoulders, jutting chin, forward shoulders, slouching

PARAMETERS: 1 to 5 minutes, 1 time per day or every other day

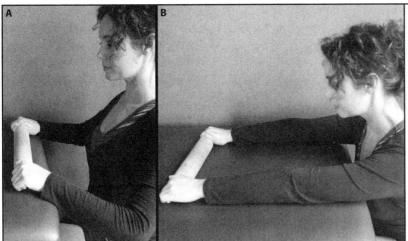

5.07.73 FUNCTIONAL: SHOULDER, ROLLING DOUGH

POSITION: Seated

TARGETS: Functional use of shoulders, elbows

INSTRUCTION: Patient rolls towel or rolling pin out in front to end range reach and back toward chest. Encourage good posture and scapular stabilization throughout the activity (A and B).

SUBSTITUTIONS: Shrugging shoulders, jutting chin, forward shoulders, slouching

PARAMETERS: 1 to 5 minutes, 1 time per day or every other day

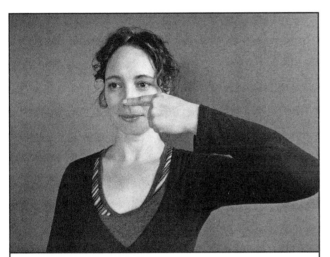

5.07.74 FUNCTIONAL: SHOULDER, RHYTHMIC TOUCH, FINGER TO NOSE/FACE

POSITION: Seated

TARGETS: Functional use of shoulders; elbows focusing on proprioception

INSTRUCTION: Patient starts, the activity with the eyes open and touches the nose several times, with the arm elevated into flexion, scaption or abduction below shoulder level. Then the patient closes the eyes and repeats activity. Therapist can mix it up by having the patient touch the ear, forehead, chin, etc. Work up to changing target and increasing speeds.

SUBSTITUTIONS: Shrugging shoulders, jutting chin, forward shoulders, slouching

PARAMETERS: 1 to 5 minutes, 1 time per day or every other day

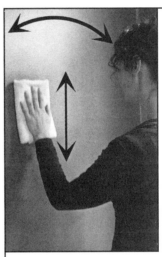

5.07.75 FUNCTIONAL: SHOULDER, WINDOW WASHING

POSITION: Standing

TARGETS: Functional use of shoulders, elbows

INSTRUCTION: Facing close to a wall, patient places palm(s) of hand(s) on wall with a towel under. Patient may "wash the window" up and down (flexion and extension) or in arcs of abduction.

SUBSTITUTIONS: Shrugging shoulders, jutting chin, forward shoulders, slouching

PARAMETERS: 1 to 5 minutes, 1 time per day or every other day

5.07.76 FUNCTIONAL: SHOULDER, PEG BOARD

POSITION: Standing

TARGETS: Functional use of shoulders, elbows

INSTRUCTION: Using a peg board, patient picks peg out of bucket and places in the peg board. Differing heights may be used as well as differing directional movements based on treatment goals. Patient may also move pegs from one location on the board to another to encourage prolonged reach and build endurance above shoulder level.

SUBSTITUTIONS: Shrugging shoulders, jutting chin, forward shoulders, slouching

PARAMETERS: 1 to 5 minutes, 1 time per day or every other day

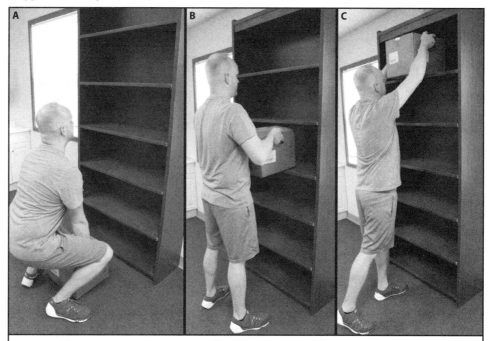

5.07.77 FUNCTIONAL: SHOULDER, LIFTING ITEMS, MULTI-LEVEL SHELF

POSITION: Standing

TARGETS: Functional use of shoulders, elbows

INSTRUCTION: Using a multi-level shelf, patient lifts boxes of differing weights from one shelf to another level above or below. Weight and size of boxes, as well as heights of lifting and setting should be focused on patient's personal demands for daily activities and work (A through C).

SUBSTITUTIONS: Shrugging shoulders, jutting chin, forward shoulders, slouching, using momentum, poor body mechanics, with overhead lifts patient may try to arch upper back

PARAMETERS: 1 to 5 minutes, 1 time per day or every other day

5.07.78 FUNCTIONAL: SHOULDER, FOLDING

POSITION: Standing

TARGETS: Functional use of shoulders, elbows

INSTRUCTION: Using towels to larger items such as a sheet, patient unfolds and folds items. Sheets required larger shoulder movement and should be added as a progression.

SUBSTITUTIONS: Shrugging shoulders, jutting chin, forward shoulders, slouching; using momentum, poor body mechanics, arch upper back when waving larger sheet items.

PARAMETERS: 1 to 5 minutes, 1 time per day or every other day

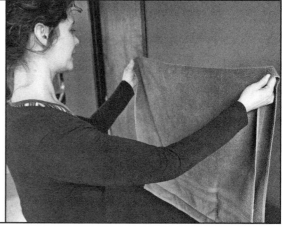

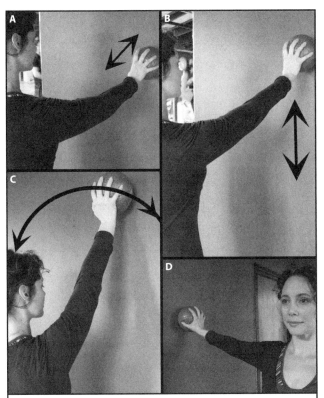

5.07.79 PLYOMETRICS/DYNAMIC: SHOULDER, WALL DRIBBLES

POSITION: Standing

TARGETS: Builds dynamic control, coordination, strength and endurance in the shoulder

INSTRUCTION: Using a small ball, patient holds ball and faces a wall. Patient dribbles the ball on the wall starting at shoulder height to get a feel for it (A). Progress to dribbling overhead in flexion and back down the wall (B). Progress to stationary dribbling overhead (C). To incorporate abduction, patient dribbles the ball outward in a large arc to waist height and back; stationary dribbling can be held at any point in the arc. Patient may also dribble with the shoulder abducted and stand sideways to the wall (D). Speed, rhythm, and hand distance from the wall can all be adjusted based on treatment goals.

SUBSTITUTIONS: Shrugging shoulders, jutting chin, forward shoulders, slouching

PARAMETERS: 1 to 5 minutes, 1 time per day or every other day

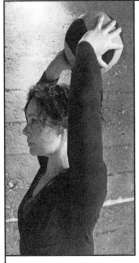

5.07.80 PLYOMETRICS/ DYNAMIC: SHOULDER, BALL TOSS, OVERHEAD

POSITION: Standing, seated

TARGETS: Builds dynamic control, coordination, strength and endurance in the shoulder

INSTRUCTION: Using a small ball to begin, and working up to a weighted medicine ball of small to medium size, patient holds ball and faces therapist or rebounder. Patient brings the ball overhead and throws the ball. Ball then returns to the patient overhead while catching and decelerate the ball with control back overhead. Immediately upon reaching stop, patient contracts quickly to return overhead throw and repeats process to fatigue. Speed, rhythm and force can be adjusted based on treatment goals. This can also be done seated.

SUBSTITUTIONS: Shrugging shoulders, jutting chin, forward shoulders, slouching, poor deceleration

PARAMETERS: 1 to 5 minutes, 1 time per day or every other day

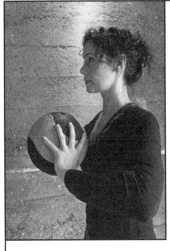

5.07.81 PLYOMETRICS/ DYNAMIC: SHOULDER, CHEST PASS

POSITION: Standing, seated

Targets: Builds dynamic control, coordination, strength and endurance in the shoulder

INSTRUCTION: Using a small ball to begin, and working up to a weighted medicine ball of small to medium size, patient holds ball and faces therapist or rebounder. Patient brings the ball to chest and pushes ball straight in front while throwing the ball. Ball then returns to the patient at chest level reaching out to catch and decelerate the ball back to chest with control. Immediately upon reaching stop, patient contracts quickly to return chest pass and repeats process to fatigue. Speed, rhythm and force can be adjusted based on treatment goals. This can also be done seated.

SUBSTITUTIONS: Shrugging shoulders, jutting chin, forward shoulders, slouching, poor deceleration

PARAMETERS: 1 to 5 minutes, 1 time per day or every other day

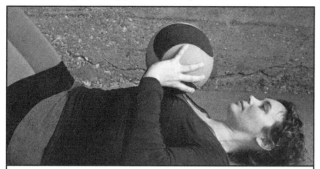

5.07.82 PLYOMETRICS/DYNAMIC: SHOULDER, BENCH PRESS/FLOOR THROWS

POSITION: Standing, seated

TARGETS: Builds dynamic control, coordination, strength and endurance in the shoulder

INSTRUCTION: Using a small ball to begin, and working up to a weighted medicine ball of small to medium size, patient holds ball and lies supine, long ways on a narrow bench. Patient brings the ball to chest and pushes ball straight in front while throwing the ball vertically into the air. Ball then returns to the patient at chest level while reaching out to catch, and patient decelerates the ball back to the chest with control. Immediately upon reaching stop, patient contracts quickly to return the chest pass and repeats process to fatigue. Speed, rhythm, and force can be adjusted based on treatment goals.

SUBSTITUTIONS: Shrugging shoulders, jutting chin, poor deceleration

PARAMETERS: 1 to 5 minutes, 1 time per day or every other day

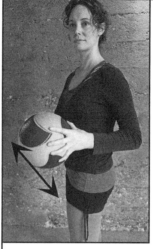

5.07.83 PLYOMETRICS/DYNAMIC: SHOULDER, TWO-HANDED SIDE THROW

POSITION: Standing, seated

TARGETS: Builds dynamic control, coordination, strength and endurance in the shoulder

INSTRUCTION: Using a small ball to begin, and working up to a weighted medicine ball of small to medium size, patient holds ball in front with arms extended. Patient throws the ball sideways. Ball then returns to the patient at chest level while reaching out to catch, and patient decelerates the ball back to the opposite side. Immediately upon reaching stop, patient contracts quickly to return the side throw and repeats process to fatigue. Speed, rhythm, and force can be adjusted based on treatment goals. Repeat to other side. This can also be done seated.

SUBSTITUTIONS: Shrugging shoulders, jutting chin, poor deceleration, twists only through trunk and hips and not using shoulders

PARAMETERS: 1 to 5 minutes, 1 time per day or every other day

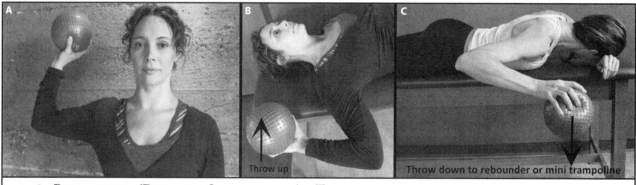

5.07.84 PLYOMETRICS/DYNAMIC: SHOULDER, 90/90 THROW

POSITION: Standing, seated

TARGETS: Builds dynamic control, coordination, strength and endurance in the shoulder; eccentric control of internal rotators.

INSTRUCTION: Using a small ball to begin, and working up to a weighted medicine ball of small size, patient holds ball with the shoulder in the 90/90 position. Patient externally rotates and horizontally abducts to begin and then throws, using internal rotation and slight horizontal adduction of the shoulder. Ball then returns to the patient at the level of the hand while catching, and patient decelerates the ball back by controlling external rotation. Immediately upon reaching stop, patient contracts quickly to return the throw and repeats process to fatigue. Speed, rhythm, and force can be adjusted based on treatment goals (A). This can also be done seated. It is also possible to do this supine by throwing ball into the air and catching (B) or prone with rebounder situated under the hand (C).

SUBSTITUTIONS: Shrugging shoulders, jutting chin, poor deceleration; dropping arm out of 90 degrees abducted shoulder.

PARAMETERS: 1 to 5 minutes, 1 time per day or every other day

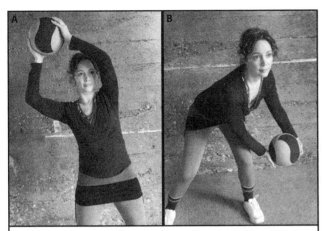

5.07.85 PLYOMETRICS/DYNAMIC: SHOULDER, MULTIDIRECTIONAL CATCH/THROW

POSITION: Standing, seated

TARGETS: Builds dynamic control, coordination, strength, and endurance in the shoulder

INSTRUCTION: Using a small ball to begin, and working up to a weighted medicine ball of small to medium size and even to a larger exercise ball, therapist holds ball and faces patient. Therapist throws the ball to the patient varying location of throw and speed. Patient catches and returns. Speed, rhythm, and force can be adjusted based on treatment goals. Therapist should aim to hit all quadrants (high right, middle right, low right, low, low left, middle left, high left, overhead and chest; A and B). This can also be done seated.

SUBSTITUTIONS: Shrugging shoulders, jutting chin, forward shoulders, slouching, poor deceleration; using trunk only and not shoulders, stepping rather than reaching.

PARAMETERS: 1 to 5 minutes, 1 time per day or every other day

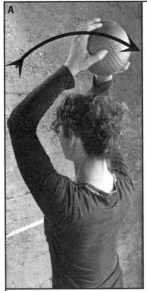

5.07.86 PLYOMETRICS/DYNAMIC: SHOULDER, BALL TOSS, OVERHEAD AND BACKWARDS

POSITION: Standing, seated

TARGETS: Builds dynamic control, coordination, strength, and endurance in the shoulder.

INSTRUCTION: Using a small ball to begin, and working up to a weighted medicine ball of small to medium size, patient holds ball and faces away from therapist or rebounder. Patient brings the ball overhead and throws the ball behind. Ball then returns to the patient from behind and overhead while catching and patient decelerates the ball with control back in front of the face. Immediately upon reaching stop, the patient contracts quickly to return the overhead throw backward and repeats process to fatigue. Speed, rhythm, and force can be adjusted based on treatment goals. This can also be done seated.

SUBSTITUTIONS: Shrugging shoulders, jutting chin, forward shoulders, slouching, poor deceleration

PARAMETERS: 1 to 5 minutes, 1 time per day or every other day

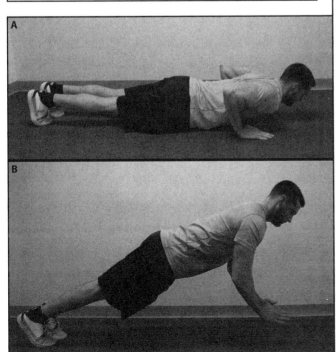

5.07.87 PLYOMETRICS/DYNAMIC: SHOULDER, PUSH-UP

POSITION: Prone on hands and knees, progressing to toes

TARGETS: Strengthen pectoralis major, anterior deltoid, triceps, anconeus; builds dynamic control, coordination, strength and endurance in the shoulder; plank will also strengthen core abdominal muscles and quadriceps.

INSTRUCTION: Position patient on the hands and knees (or advanced hands and toes) with head, shoulders, hips and knees in a straight line, elbows slightly bent and scapula in proper position. Patient lowers body toward the floor without letting low back or head sag, presses up in an explosive movement, hands come slightly off the floor in a hop, and immediately lowers to the floor and repeats. Movement is without any pausing for optimal plyometric benefit and power production. Avoid locking elbows out. Keep shoulders depressed and retracted (A and B). Gaze is between the hands and chin slightly tucked.

SUBSTITUTIONS: Shrugging shoulders, avoid hyperextension at the elbows, jutting chin out or looking up, sagging lower back, pausing before pushing up

PARAMETERS: 1 to 3 sets, 8 to 12 repetitions, 1 time per day or every other day

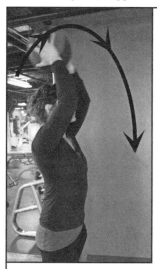

5.07.88 PLYOMETRICS/ DYNAMIC: SHOULDER, SLAMS

POSITION: Standing

TARGETS: Builds dynamic control, coordination, strength and endurance in the shoulder, as well as core trunk muscles

INSTRUCTION: Using a weighted medicine ball of medium to large size, patient holds ball overhead and slams it straight down into the floor in front as hard as possible so that it bounces back up to catch above waist height. Patient brings the ball overhead and repeats. Speed, rhythm, and force can be adjusted based on treatment goals.

SUBSTITUTIONS: Shrugging shoulders, jutting chin, forward shoulders, slouching, poor deceleration

PARAMETERS: 1 to 5 minutes, 1 time per day or every other day

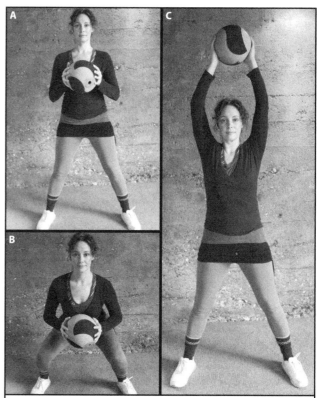

5.07.89 PLYOMETRICS/DYNAMIC: SHOULDER, BALL SQUAT, PUSH-PRESS

POSITION: Standing

TARGETS: Builds dynamic control, coordination, strength and endurance in the shoulder, as well as core trunk and leg muscles

INSTRUCTION: Using a weighted medicine ball of medium to large size, patient holds ball overhead. Patient then begins to squat, bringing ball down toward chest. The back is straight, and the weight is primarily in the heels. Patient then stands back up, pushing ball directly back overhead. Mini-squats will suffice for focusing on shoulder primarily. Speed, rhythm and force can be adjusted based on treatment goals (A through C).

SUBSTITUTIONS: Shrugging shoulders, jutting chin, forward shoulders, slouching; poor deceleration, pausing before pressing back up.

PARAMETERS: 1 to 3 sets 8 to 12 repetitions, 1 time per day or every other day

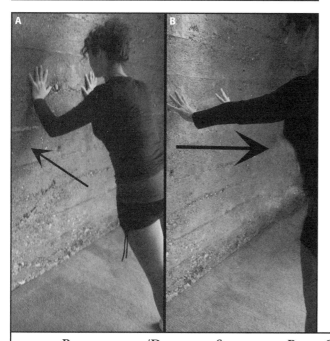

5.07.90 PLYOMETRICS/DYNAMIC: SHOULDER, PUSH-OFFS

POSITION: Standing

TARGETS: Builds dynamic control, coordination, strength, and endurance in the shoulder

INSTRUCTION: Patient stands 6 to 12 inches away from a wall, facing wall. Patient places palms on wall fingers pointed up. Patient then performs a small push-up while pushing off the wall. The trunk is straight with the lower abdominal core engaged. Patient comes off the wall, slowly halts, then returns toward wall. Hands stay in front while landing back on palms, descending into another push-up followed by push off and repeat. Do not allow any pause between push-up to push off (A and B).

SUBSTITUTIONS: Shrugging shoulders, jutting chin, forward shoulders, sagging back; poor deceleration, pausing before pressing back up.

PARAMETERS: 1 to 3 sets, 8 to 12 repetitions, 1 time per day or every other day

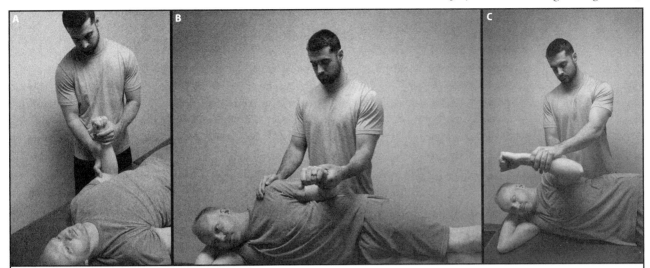

5.07.91 Reactive Neuromuscular Training and Variations, Shoulder

RNT uses outside resistance to neurologically turn on an automatic response. It is often seen as a quick fix to faulty movement patterns and designed to improve functional stability and enhance motor-control skills with an automatic response. As the body reacts to the applied force, instinct to correct the flawed movements is activated. Clinicians can use these techniques to target specific levels of the central nervous system to stimulate appropriate reflex responses promoting functional static and dynamic stability. The RNT program, as part of the functional exercise progression, initially focuses on dynamic stabilization at the spinal level. Rhythmic stabilization exercises in the open chain position encourage co-contraction of the musculature about the shoulder, providing a foundation for dynamic neuromuscular stabilization. Taking advantage of the stretch reflex, rhythmic stabilization activities create a change in the desired length of the muscle, resulting in reflex muscular splinting. Efficient co-activation restores the force couples necessary to balance joint forces and increase joint congruency, thereby reducing the loads imparted onto the static structures. These activities can be performed early in the rehabilitation program, first in protected positions such as 90 degrees of elevation, again at 45 degrees of abduction, and eventually at the ends of the available ROM when the glenohumeral joint is more likely to be unstable (Guido & Stemm, 2007).

Position: Side-lying, supine, standing

Targets: UE neuromuscular control, joint stability, proprioception, and facilitating co-contraction of UE muscles

Instruction: *Rhythmic stabilization internal rotation/external rotation side-lying shoulder neutral*: Patient retracts the scapula with the elbow flexed 90 degrees and by the side. Therapist applies variable resistance to internal and external rotation as well as scapular protraction as patient maintains the position. Resist externally applied forces (A). *Rhythmic stabilization internal rotation/external rotation supine shoulder neutral*: Patient retracts the scapula with the elbow flexed 90 degrees and by the side. Therapist applies variable resistance to internal and external rotation as patient maintains position. Resist externally applied forces (B). *Rhythmic stabilization internal rotation/external rotation side-lying shoulder 30 degrees abducted (scaption plane)*: Patient abducts the shoulder 30 degrees and retracts the scapula with the elbow flexed 90 degrees. Therapist applies variable resistance to internal and external rotation as patient maintains the position. Resist externally applied forces (C). *(continued)*

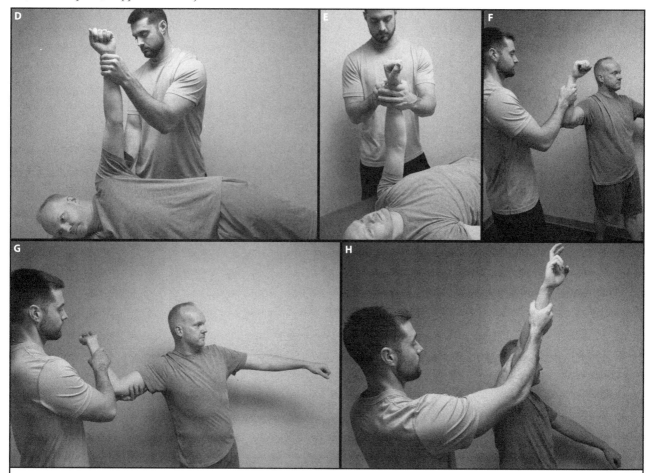

5.07.91 REACTIVE NEUROMUSCULAR TRAINING AND VARIATIONS, SHOULDER (CONTINUED)

Rhythmic stabilization side-lying shoulder abducted: Patient retracts the scapula and abducts the shoulder 90 degrees with the elbow extended. Therapist applies variable resistance to all planes of movement as well as scapular protraction as patient maintains the position. Resist externally applied forces (D). This can be done at differing degrees of flexion depending on treatment goals. *Rhythmic stabilization supine shoulder flexed or in scaption*: Patient retracts the scapula and flexes the shoulder 90 degrees with the elbow extended. Therapist applies variable resistance to all planes of movement as well as scapular protraction as patient maintains the position. Resist externally applied forces (E). This can be done at differing degrees of flexion depending on treatment goals. Alternatively, this can be done in the scapular plane—patient moves 30 degrees forward from full abduction as resistances are applied as described previously. *Rhythmic stabilization standing early cocking position*: Patient retracts the scapula and horizontally abducts the shoulder. Therapist applies variable resistance to all planes of movement as well as scapular protraction as patient maintains the position. Resist externally applied forces (F). *Rhythmic stabilization standing late cocking position*: Patient retracts the scapula, horizontally abducts and fully externally rotates the shoulder. Therapist applies variable resistance to all planes of movement as well as scapular protraction as patient maintains the position. Resist externally applied forces (G). *Rhythmic stabilization standing throwing position*: Patient retracts the scapula, horizontally abducts and fully externally rotates the shoulder, then moves to the "release point" of the throw maneuver at 110 to 120 degrees abduction with external rotation. Therapist applies variable resistance to all planes of movement as well as scapular protraction as patient maintains the position. Resist externally applied forces (H).

SUBSTITUTIONS: Shrugging the shoulders, jutting the chin, forward the shoulders, loss of scapular retraction

PARAMETERS: Clinician must be concerned with the quality of the movement and not necessarily the number of sets and repetitions; however, suggested parameters are 1 to 3 sets, 20 to 30 challenges, 1 time per day or every other day.

5.07.92 SHOULDER, THROWING PROGRESSION
POSITION: Standing
TARGETS: Builds dynamic control, coordination, strength, and endurance in the shoulder
INSTRUCTION: Refer to **8.01.1-A** and **B**

REFERENCES

Alizadehkhaiyat, O., Hawkes, D. H., Kemp, G. J., & Frostick, S. P. (2015). Electromyographic analysis of shoulder girdle muscles during common internal rotation exercises. *International Journal of Sports Physical Therapy, 10*(5), 645-654.

De Mey, K., Cagnie, B., Danneels, L. A., Cools, A. M., & Van de Velde, A. (2009). Trapezius muscle timing during selected shoulder rehabilitation exercises. *Journal of Orthopedic and Sports Physical Therapy, 39*(10), 743-752.

De Mey, K., Danneels, L. A., Cagnie, B., Huyghe, L., Seyns, E., & Cools, A. M. (2013). Conscious correction of scapular orientation in overhead athletes performing selected shoulder rehabilitation exercises: the effect on trapezius muscle activation measured by surface electromyography. *Journal of Orthopedic and Sports Physical Therapy, 43*(1), 3-10.

Guido, J. A., Jr, & Stemm, J. (2007). Reactive neuromuscular training: A multi-level approach to rehabilitation of the unstable shoulder. *North American Journal of Sports Physical Therapy, 2*(2), 97-103.

Hintermeister, R. A., Lange, G. W., Schultheis, J. M., Bey, M. J., & Hawkins, R. J. (1998). Electromyographic activity and applied load during shoulder rehabilitation exercises using elastic resistance. *American Journal of Sports Medicine, 26*(2), 210-220.

Ishigaki, T., Yamanaka, M., Hirokawa, M., Tai, K., Ezawa, Y., Samukawa, M., . . . Sugawara, M. (2014). Rehabilitation exercises to induce balanced scapular muscle activity in an anti-gravity posture. *Journal of Physical Therapy Science, 26*(12), 1871-1874.

Park, K. M., Cynn, H. S., Yi, C. H., & Kwon, O. Y. (2013). Effect of isometric horizontal abduction on pectoralis major and serratus anterior EMG activity during three exercises in subjects with scapular winging. *Journal of Electromyography and Kinesiology, 23*(2), 462-468.

Lusk, S. J., Hale, B. D., & Russell, D. M. (2010). Grip width and forearm orientation effects on muscle activity during the lat pull-down. *Journal of Strength and Conditioning Research, 24*(7), 1895-1900.

Saeterbakken, A. H., & Fimland, M. S. (2013). Effects of body position and loading modality on muscle activity and strength in shoulder presses. *Journal of Strength and Conditioning Research, 27*(7), 1824-1831.

Sperandei, S., Barros, M. A., Silveira-Júnior, P. C., & Oliveira, C. G. (2009). Electromyographic analysis of three different types of lat pull-down. *Journal of Strength and Conditioning Research, 23*(7), 2033-2038.

Timmons, M. K., Ericksen, J. J., Yesilyaprak, S. S., & Michener, L. A. (2016). Empty can exercise provokes more pain and has undesirable biomechanics compared with the full can exercise. *Journal of Shoulder and Elbow Surgery, 25*(4), 548-556.

Tucker, W. S., Armstrong, C. W., Gribble, P. A., Timmons, M. K., & Yeasting, R. A. (2010). Scapular muscle activity in overhead athletes with symptoms of secondary shoulder impingement during closed chain exercises. *Archives of Physical Medicine and Rehabilitation, 91*(4), 550-556.

Youdas, J. W., Keith, J. M., Nonn, D. E., Squires, A. C., & Hollman, J. H. (2015). Activation of spinal stabilizers and shoulder complex muscles during an inverted row using a portable pull-up device and body weight resistance. *Journal of Strength and Conditioning Research, 30*(7), 1933-1941.

Section 5.08

SHOULDER PROTOCOLS AND TREATMENT IDEAS

5.08.1 SUBACROMIAL IMPINGEMENT DISCUSSION

Subacromial impingement is defined as the mechanical compression of subacromial structures between the coracoacromial arch and the humerus during active elevation of the arm above shoulder height (De Strijcker, Drinkard, Van Haver, Lowe, & Brachotte, 2016). Subacromial impingement can be related to structural and/or mechanical impairments. Structural impairments may include bony spurs or compression structural variances in the humeral head or acromion process that decrease the subacromial space. Mechanical factors include decreased control of the humeral head superior translation during humeral elevation. Superior humeral head migration has been observed with RC fatigue, which apparently inhibited the ability of the shoulder musculature to resist upward humeral translation (Chopp, O'Neill, Hurley, & Dickerson, 2010).

> ### Where's the Evidence?
>
> Subacromial impingement symptoms are also associated with altered upper and lower trapezius muscle activity. Symptomatic subjects demonstrate a significantly higher ratio of upper trapezius:lower trapezius activity than the asymptomatic subjects during humeral elevation (Smith, Sparkes, Busse, & Enright, 2009). The lower trapezius has been shown to be delayed in activation during scaption with upper trapezius overfiring in patients with subacromial impingement (Chester, Smith, Hooper, & Dixon, 2010). The serratus anterior muscle activity has also been found to be decreased in this population (Struyf et al., 2014). Scapular kinematics assessments have revealed that subacromial impingement patients present with scapular upward rotation and increased anterior tipping with lower loads elevated in the scapular plane and increased scapular medial rotation under higher load conditions indicating scapular tipping and serratus anterior muscle function are important to consider in the rehabilitation of patients with symptoms of shoulder impingement related to overhead work (Ludewig & Cook, 2000). These alterations in mechanics may lead to decreased space in the subacromial region and lead to inflammation of the structures that therein. A tailored progressive strengthening exercise program for improving shoulder function in subacromial impingement syndrome has been shown to be beneficial (Litchfield, 2013). Additionally, adding manual therapy to an exercise protocol does not necessarily enhance improvements in scapular kinematics, function, and pain in individuals with shoulder impingement syndrome (Camargo et al., 2015). However, altered sagittal mobility in the middle and lower segments of the thoracic spine has been correlated to impingement syndrome of the shoulder implication indicating treatment for the impaired mobility of the thoracic spine should be addressed (Theisen et al., 2010).

Patients that do not respond to conservative management may undergo surgical correction depending on the character and severity of the injury including repair of torn tissues (supraspinatus and long head of the biceps commonly), removal of the subacromial bursa, decompression involving removing bony spurs and/or the coracoacromial ligament and/or part of the acromion (acromioplasty).

Patients with subacromial impingement should be properly assessed and treatment specific to the impairments identified. Clinician's implementing treatment should have a complete understanding of the structures involved and the underlying mechanism causing the impingement presentation. A treatment program should include interventions to address pain, scapular dysfunction and RC weakness. General guidelines are detailed in the protocol that follows.

5.08.2 SUBACROMIAL IMPINGEMENT PROTOCOL

Phase I: Acute

1. Eliminate any activity that causes an increase in symptoms, especially overhead activities
2. Sleeping postures—sleeping on the affected shoulder can aggravate subacromial impingement. Suggested postures include:
   a. 4.04 Bed positioning
      i. Supine
      ii. Side-lying quarter turn supine
      iii. Side-lying both knees flexed (on the unaffected side)
      iv. Side-lying top knee flexed (on the unaffected side)
3. ROM ideas
   a. 5.04.2 ROM: Shoulder, Pendulum, Passive
   b. 5.04.3 ROM: Shoulder, Cradle Rocks, Passive
   c. 5.04.4 ROM: Shoulder, Saws, Active Assistive
   d. 5.04.6 ROM: Pulleys; Shoulder Flexion, Scaption, and Abduction, Passive
   e. 5.04.5 ROM: Shoulder Girdle Circles, Active Assistive
   f. 5.04.9 ROM: Wand/Cane; Shoulder Circles, Active Assistive
   g. 5.04.11 ROM: Wand/Cane; Shoulder Flexion and Scaption, Active Assistive
   h. 5.04.13 ROM: Wand/Cane; Shoulder Internal Rotation, External Rotation, and Combined, Active Assistive (neutral variation only)
   i. 5.04.12 ROM: Wand/Cane; Shoulder Abduction, Active Assistive
   j. 5.04.17 ROM: Wand/Cane; Shoulder Extension, Active Assistive
   k. 5.04.23 ROM: Shoulder Flexion and Abduction, Table Slide, Active Assistive
   l. 5.04.21 ROM: Shoulder Flexion and Abduction, Towel Slide, Active Assistive
   m. 5.04.22 ROM: Shoulder Flexion and Abduction, Wall Walks, Active Assistive
   n. 5.04.20 ROM: Shoulder Flexion, Wall Slide, Active Assistive
   o. 3.01.6 ROM: Thoracic Extension Over Foam Roll, Head Supported
   p. 3.01.8 ROM: Passive—Thoracic Rotation
4. Strengthening ideas (beginner in acute phase)
   a. 5.07.1 Strengthen: Isometric; Shoulder, Other Hand Resists, 6-Way or 5.07.2 Strengthen: Isometric; Shoulder, Wall Resists, 5-Way
   b. 5.03.3 Strengthen: Scapular Retraction and Variations (unilateral side-lying and bilateral seated only)
   c. 5.03.4 Strengthen: Scapular Retraction, Arms by Sides
   d. 2.03.4 Strengthen: Isotonic; Chin Tuck
5. Strengthening ideas (advancing in acute phase)
   a. 5.07.3 Strengthen: Isometric; Shoulder Flexion Overhead
   b. 5.07.4 Strengthen: Isometric; Shoulder Internal Rotation Multi-Angle Neutral, Doorway
   c. 5.07.5 Strengthen: Isometric; Shoulder External Rotation Multi-Angle Neutral, Doorway
   d. 5.07.6 Strengthen: Isometric; Shoulder Internal Rotation Multi-Angle Abduction and Flexion
   e. 5.07.7 Strengthen: Isometric; Shoulder External Rotation Multi-Angle Abduction and Flexion
   f. 5.07.8 Strengthen: Isometric; Shoulder Horizontal Abduction and Adduction
   g. 5.07.9 Strengthen: Isometric—Walk-Outs

Phase II

Begin once pain and symptoms are significantly improved. Watch for normal scapulohumeral mechanics with all activities.

1. Warm-up
   a. 5.04.1 ROM: Shoulder, Warm-Up, Upper Body Ergometer, Active Assistive
2. ROM ideas
   a. 5.04.28 ROM: Shoulder Flexion, Active
   b. 5.04.29 ROM: Shoulder Abduction, Active
   c. 5.04.33 ROM: Shoulder Extension, Active
   d. 5.04.34 ROM: Shoulder Scaption, Active

   e. 5.04.35 ROM: Shoulder Scaption Figure 8s, Active

   f. 5.04.36 ROM: Shoulder Internal Rotation and External Rotation, Active

   g. 5.04.37 ROM: Side-Lying Shoulder Circles, Active

3. Stretching ideas

   a. 2.02.3 Stretch: Self-Assisted Cervical Lateral Flexion

   b. 2.02.7 Stretch: Cervical Flexion and Rotation

   c. 5.06.8 Stretch: Shoulder Horizontal Adductors, Towel Roll and Swiss Ball

4. Self joint mobilization ideas (other mobilizations may be added depending on direction restrictions of the capsule)

   a. 5.05.2 Self-Joint Mobilization/Stretch: Shoulder, Distraction With Weight

   b. 5.05.3 Self-Joint Mobilization/Stretch: Shoulder, Distraction With Chair Pull

5. Strengthening ideas for scapular stabilizers

   a. 5.03.4 Strengthen: Scapular Retraction, Arms by Sides

   b. 5.03.6 Strengthen: Scapular Retraction, Arm Off Table

   c. 5.03.8 Strengthen: Scapular Retraction, "W" or "Batwings"

   d. 5.03.9 Strengthen: Scapular Retraction, Wall Angels

   e. 5.03.11 Strengthen: Resistance Band, Isolated Scapular Retraction

   f. 5.03.12 Strengthen: Resistance Band, Scapular Row and Variations

6. Strengthening ideas for shoulder

   a. 5.07.10 Strengthen: Isotonic; Shoulder Flexion

   b. 5.07.11 Strengthen: Isotonic; Shoulder Scaption

   c. 5.07.12 Strengthen: Isotonic; Shoulder Abduction

   d. 5.07.21 Strengthen: Isotonic; Shoulder Internal Rotation

   e. 5.07.22 Strengthen: Isotonic; Shoulder External Rotation

   f. 5.07.36 Strengthen: Isotonic; Resistance Band, Shoulder Flexion, Scaption, Abduction, and Variations (start by staying below shoulder level/90 degrees)

   g. 5.07.13 Strengthen: Isotonic; Shoulder Extension

   h. 5.07.19 Strengthen: Isotonic; Shoulder, Horizontal Abduction, Bent Forward

   i. 5.07.20 Strengthen: Isotonic; Shoulder, Horizontal Abduction, Deceleration Emphasis

   j. 5.07.24 Strengthen: Isotonic; Shoulder, Row (Prone)

   k. 5.07.27 Strengthen: Isotonic; Posterior Cuff, 4-Way

Phase III

Begin once pain-free. Watch for normal scapulohumeral mechanics with all activities.

1. ROM ideas

   a. 5.04.38 ROM: Shoulder, PNF D1 and D2, Active

2. Stretching ideas

   a. 5.06.5 Stretch: Shoulder Horizontal Adductors, Doorway

3. Joint self-mobilization ideas (other mobilizations may be added depending on direction restrictions of the capsule)

4. Strengthening ideas for scapular stabilizers

   a. 5.03.5 Strengthen: Scapular Retraction, "T", "Y", and "I" and Variations

   b. 5.03.13 Strengthen: Resistance Band, Scapular and Posterior Shoulder, Overhead Pull-down

   c. 5.03.14 Strengthen: Resistance Band, Scapular and Rotator Cuff, Retraction and External Rotation

   d. 5.03.15 Strengthen: Resistance Band, Scapular, Punch

   e. 5.03.16 Strengthen: Resistance Band, Scapular, Dynamic Hug

   f. 5.03.17 Strengthen: Resistance Band, Serratus Wall Slides

   g. 5.03.18 Strengthen: Resistance Band, Scapular Clocks

   h. 5.03.19 Strengthen: Resistance Band, Scapular "Vs"

   i. 5.03.22 Strengthen: Scapular, Arm Lifts

   j. 5.03.21 Strengthen: Scapular, Push-Up Plus (Advanced)

5. Strengthening ideas for shoulder

   a. 5.07.21 Strengthen: Isotonic; Shoulder Internal Rotation

   b. 5.07.22 Strengthen: Isotonic; Shoulder External Rotation

   c. 5.07.23 Strengthen: Isotonic; Shoulder External Rotation 90/90

   d. 5.07.25 Strengthen: Isotonic; Shoulder, Military Press (Prone)

   e. 5.07.28 Strengthen: Isotonic; Shoulder, Diagonal Lifts D1 and D2

   f. 5.07.34 Strengthen: Isotonic; Resistance Band and Machine, Shoulder, Lat Pull-Down

   g. 5.07.38 Strengthen: Isotonic; Resistance Band, Shoulder Extension

   h. 5.07.39 Strengthen: Isotonic; Resistance Band, Shoulder Internal Rotation and Variations

   i. 5.07.41 Strengthen: Isotonic; Resistance Band, Shoulder External Rotation and Variations

   j. 5.07.42 Strengthen: Isotonic; Resistance Band, Shoulder, Combination Movements PNF D1 and D2

k. 5.07.47 Strengthen: Isotonic; Resistance Band, Shoulder Pull-Back

l. 5.07.63 Strengthen: Closed Kinetic Chain; Scapular and Shoulder Depression

m. 5.07.64 Strengthen: Closed Kinetic Chain; Shoulder, Table Top Push-Pull

n. 5.07.62 Strengthen: Closed Kinetic Chain; Shoulder, Push-Up

o. 5.07.61 Strengthen: Closed Kinetic Chain; Shoulder, Beginning Weightbearing, Progress to Push-Up Partial Weight

Phase IV: Dynamic Advanced Strengthening

Begin once pain-free full ROM achieved and strength equal or greater than 75% of unaffected side. Watch for normal scapulohumeral mechanics with all activities.

1. Strengthening ideas

    a. 5.07.66 Strengthen: Closed Kinetic Chain; Stairmaster, Shoulder

    b. 5.07.67 Strengthen: Closed Kinetic Chain; Bodyblade, Shoulder Flexion, Scaption, and Abduction

    c. 5.07.68 Strengthen: Closed Kinetic Chain; Bodyblade, Shoulder Internal Rotation and External Rotation

    d. 5.07.69 Strengthen: Closed Kinetic Chain; Bodyblade, Shoulder, D1 and D2

    e. 5.07.70 Strengthen: Closed Kinetic Chain; Shoulder, Plank Shuffle on Medicine Ball

f. 5.07.71 Strengthen: Closed Kinetic Chain; Shoulder, Inverted Row

g. 5.07.79 Plyometrics/Dynamic: Shoulder, Wall Dribbles

h. 5.07.80 Plyometrics/Dynamic: Shoulder, Ball Toss, Overhead

i. 5.07.81 Plyometrics/Dynamic: Shoulder, Chest Pass

j. 5.07.82 Plyometrics/Dynamic: Shoulder, Bench Press/Floor Throws

k. 5.07.83 Plyometrics/Dynamic: Shoulder, Two-Handed Side Throw

l. 5.07.84 Plyometrics/Dynamic: Shoulder, 90/90 Throw

m. 5.07.85 Plyometrics/Dynamic: Shoulder, Multidirectional Catch/Throw

n. 5.07.86 Plyometrics/Dynamic: Shoulder, Ball Toss, Overhead and Backwards

o. 5.07.87 Plyometrics/Dynamic: Shoulder, Push-Up

p. 5.07.88 Plyometrics/Dynamic: Shoulder, Slams

q. 5.07.89 Plyometrics/Dynamic: Shoulder, Ball Squat, Push-Press

r. 5.07.90 Plyometrics/Dynamic: Shoulder, Push-Offs

s. 5.07.91 Reactive Neuromuscular Training and Variations, Shoulder

t. 5.07.92 Shoulder, Throwing Progression

Phase V

Return to unrestricted, symptom-free activity cleared with physician.

5.08.3 ACROMIOCLAVICULAR RECONSTRUCTION DISCUSSION

Acromioclavicular joint injuries often occur when falling on the shoulder, collision with another player or while being tackled. During the fall, the shoulder will hit the ground and the scapulae will be pushed down. The clavicle can only partially follow this movement and there will be a great deal of strain on the ligaments, causing them to rupture or dislocate (De Dobbeleer, Hennebel, Lowe, Killian, & Pagare, 2016). The acromioclavicular joint injuries are classified as type I: partial injury to the joint capsule; type II: partial tear of the coracoclavicular ligament and rupture of capsule leading to subluxation; type III: complete rupture of the acromioclavicular and coracoclavicular ligaments leading to displacement of the clavicle; type IV: dislocation with posterior dislocation of the clavicle; type V: dislocation with severe upward displacement of the clavicle; and type VI: dislocation of the clavicle inferiorly.

Acromioclavicular joint separations are one of the most common injuries seen in orthopedic and sports medicine practices, accounting for 9% of all injuries to the shoulder girdle. Grade I and II separations seem to respond favorably to conservative management. Conversely, grades IV, V, and VI often require surgical reconstruction. Regardless of the type of injury, rehabilitation as a part of conservative management and postoperative care plays an important role in the management of these injuries (Cote, Wojcik, Gomlinski, & Mazzocca, 2010). An intervention focusing on restoring shoulder strength, ROM, flexibility, and neuromuscular control of the shoulder following a surgical reconstruction of the acromioclavicular joint can lead to a successful functional outcome (Culp & Romani, 2006).

Patients with acromioclavicular separations and postsurgical repairs should be properly assessed and treatment specific to the impairments identified. Clinician's implementing treatment should have a complete understanding of the structures involved and the underlying mechanism causing the impingement presentation. A treatment program should include interventions to address pain, scapular dysfunction, and RC weakness. General guidelines are detailed in the next protocol.

5.08.4 Acromioclavicular Reconstruction Rehabilitation Protocol

General protocol guidelines adapted from Vanderbuilt Sports Medicine Knee and Shoulder Center (n.d.).

During entire course of treatment, watch for any pain that persists for more than 1 hour after exercise or increases in night pain. If this occurs, alter program to avoid aggravating the condition.

Phase I: Immobilization 0 to 6 Weeks

1. The arm must never be unsupported when patient is in the upright position. The weight of the arm and scapula places forces on the ligament reconstruction.
2. Sleeping postures—sleeping on the affected shoulder should avoid for at least 6 weeks. Suggested postures include:
   a. 4.04 Bed Positioning
      i. Semi-reclined with pillow support
      ii. Supine arm supported in sling or immobilizer
      iii. Side-lying quarter turn supine arm supported in sling or immobilizer
3. PROM only restriction in ROM per physician orders. Suggested guideline when orders absent:
   a. 0 to 4 weeks: limit flexion, scaption, and abduction to 70 degrees for the first 4 weeks, then increase as tolerated
   b. No restrictions on glenohumeral internal and external rotation.
   c. No glenohumeral extension; causes the largest amount of stress on the reconstructed ligaments.
4. 4 to 6 weeks: shoulder isometrics in neutral (continue these into Phase II)
   a. 5.07.1 Strengthen: Isometric; Shoulder, Other Hand Resists, 6-Way or 5.07.2 Strengthen: Isometric; Shoulder, Wall Resists, 5-Way

Phase II: Intermediate 7 to 12 Weeks

Aactive assistive motion weeks 7 to 8. Active motion starts week 9. No extension until week 11.

1. ROM ideas weeks 7 to 8
   a. 5.04.2 ROM: Shoulder, Pendulum, Passive
   b. 5.04.3 ROM: Shoulder, Cradle Rocks, Passive
   c. 5.04.6 ROM: Pulleys; Shoulder Flexion, Scaption, and Abduction, Passive
   d. 5.04.5 ROM: Shoulder Girdle Circles, Active Assistive
   e. 5.04.9 ROM: Wand/Cane; Shoulder Circles, Active Assistive
   f. 5.04.11 ROM: Wand/Cane; Shoulder Flexion and Scaption, Active Assistive
   g. 5.04.13 ROM: Wand/Cane; Shoulder Internal Rotation, External Rotation, and Combined, Active Assistive (neutral variation only)

h. 5.04.12 ROM: Wand/Cane; Shoulder Abduction, Active Assistive
i. 5.04.23 ROM: Shoulder Flexion and Abduction, Table Slide, Active Assistive
j. 5.04.21 ROM: Shoulder Flexion and Abduction, Towel Slide, Active Assistive

2. ROM ideas starting week 9
   a. 5.04.28 ROM: Shoulder Flexion, Active
   b. 5.04.29 ROM: Shoulder Abduction, Active
   c. 5.04.34 ROM: Shoulder Scaption, Active
   d. 5.04.35 ROM: Shoulder Scaption Figure 8s, Active
   e. 5.04.36 ROM: Shoulder Internal Rotation and External Rotation, Active
3. ROM ideas starting week 10
   a. 5.04.17 ROM: Wand/Cane; Shoulder Extension, Active Assistive
   b. 5.04.33 ROM: Shoulder Extension, Active
   c. 5.04.38 ROM: Shoulder, PNF D1 and D2, Active

Phase III: Strengthening 12 to 18 Weeks

No pressing activities such as a push-up or pressing up off bed, no lifting from the floor such as a dead lift

1. Warm-up
   a. 5.04.1 ROM: Shoulder, Warm-Up, Upper Body Ergometer, Active Assistive
2. Stretching ideas
   a. 2.02.3 Stretch: Self-Assisted Cervical Lateral Flexion
   b. 2.02.7 Stretch: Cervical Flexion and Rotation
   c. 5.06.8 Stretch: Shoulder Horizontal Adductors, Towel Roll and Swiss Ball
3. Strengthening ideas
   a. 5.03.4 Strengthen: Scapular Retraction, Arms by Sides
   b. 5.07.3 Strengthen: Isometric; Shoulder Flexion Overhead
   c. 5.07.4 Strengthen: Isometric; Shoulder Internal Rotation Multi-Angle Neutral, Doorway
   d. 5.07.5 Strengthen: Isometric; Shoulder External Rotation Multi-Angle Neutral, Doorway
   e. 5.07.6 Strengthen: Isometric; Shoulder Internal Rotation Multi-Angle Abduction and Flexion
   f. 5.07.7 Strengthen: Isometric; Shoulder External Rotation Multi-Angle Abduction and Flexion
   g. 5.07.8 Strengthen: Isometric; Shoulder Horizontal Abduction and Adduction
   h. 5.07.9 Strengthen: Isometric; Shoulder Walk-Outs
   i. 5.07.10 Strengthen: Isotonic; Shoulder Flexion
   j. 5.07.11 Strengthen: Isotonic; Shoulder Scaption

k. 5.07.12 Strengthen: Isotonic; Shoulder Abduction

l. 5.07.36 Strengthen: Isotonic; Resistance Band, Shoulder Flexion, Scaption, Abduction, and Variations (start by staying below shoulder level/90 degrees)

m. 5.07.21 Strengthen: Isotonic; Shoulder Internal Rotation

n. 5.07.22 Strengthen: Isotonic; Shoulder External Rotation

o. 5.07.23 Strengthen: Isotonic; Shoulder External Rotation 90/90

p. 5.07.25 Strengthen: Isotonic; Shoulder, Military Press (Prone)

q. 5.07.28 Strengthen: Isotonic; Shoulder, Diagonal Lifts D1 and D2

r. 5.07.34 Strengthen: Isotonic; Resistance Band and Machine, Shoulder, Lat Pull-Down

s. 5.07.38 Strengthen: Isotonic; Resistance Band, Shoulder Extension

t. 5.07.39 Strengthen: Isotonic; Resistance Band, Shoulder Internal Rotation and Variations

u. 5.07.41 Strengthen: Isotonic; Resistance Band, Shoulder External Rotation and Variations

v. 5.07.42 Strengthen: Isotonic; Resistance Band, Shoulder, Combination Movements PNF D1 and D2

w. 5.07.47 Strengthen: Isotonic; Resistance Band, Shoulder Pull-Back

x. 5.07.13 Strengthen: Isotonic; Shoulder Extension

y. 5.07.19 Strengthen: Isotonic; Shoulder, Horizontal Abduction, Bent Forward

z. 5.07.20 Strengthen: Isotonic; Shoulder, Horizontal Abduction, Deceleration Emphasis

aa. 5.07.24 Strengthen: Isotonic; Shoulder, Row (Prone)

ab. 5.07.27 Strengthen: Isotonic; Posterior Cuff, 4-Way

4. Strengthening ideas for scapular stabilizers

a. 5.03.3 Strengthen: Scapular Retraction and Variations (unilateral side-lying and bilateral seated only)

b. 5.03.4 Strengthen: Scapular Retraction, Arms by Sides

c. 5.03.6 Strengthen: Scapular Retraction, Arm Off Table

d. 5.03.8 Strengthen: Scapular Retraction, "W" or "Batwings"

e. 5.03.9 Strengthen: Scapular Retraction, Wall Angels

f. 5.03.11 Strengthen: Resistance Band, Isolated Scapular Retraction

g. 5.03.12 Strengthen: Resistance Band, Scapular Row and Variations

h. 5.03.5 Strengthen: Scapular Retraction, "T", "Y", and "I" and Variations

i. 5.03.13 Strengthen: Resistance Band, Scapular and Posterior Shoulder, Overhead Pull-down

j. 5.03.14 Strengthen: Resistance Band, Scapular and Rotator Cuff, Retraction and External Rotation

k. 5.03.15 Strengthen: Resistance Band, Scapular, Punch

l. 5.03.16 Strengthen: Resistance Band, Scapular, Dynamic Hug

m. 5.03.17 Strengthen: Resistance Band, Serratus Wall Slides

n. 5.03.18 Strengthen: Resistance Band, Scapular Clocks

o. 5.03.19 Strengthen: Resistance Band, Scapular "Vs"

p. 5.03.22 Strengthen: Scapular, Arm Lifts

Phase IV: 4.5 Months

Return to activity phase: dynamic advanced strengthening phase. Begin once pain-free full ROM achieved and strength equal or >75% of unaffected side. Watch for normal scapulohumeral mechanics with all activities. Power athletes may require 6 to 9 months to return to peak strength.

1. Strengthening ideas

a. 5.07.63 Strengthen: Closed Kinetic Chain; Scapular and Shoulder Depression

b. 5.07.64 Strengthen: Closed Kinetic Chain; Shoulder, Table Top Push-Pull

c. 5.07.62 Strengthen: Closed Kinetic Chain; Shoulder, Push-Up

d. 5.07.61 Strengthen: Closed Kinetic Chain; Shoulder, Beginning Weightbearing, Progress to Push-Up Partial Weight

e. 5.07.66 Strengthen: Closed Kinetic Chain; Stairmaster, Shoulder

f. 5.07.67 Strengthen: Closed Kinetic Chain; Bodyblade, Shoulder Flexion, Scaption, and Abduction

g. 5.07.68 Strengthen: Closed Kinetic Chain; Bodyblade, Shoulder Internal Rotation and External Rotation

h. 5.07.69 Strengthen: Closed Kinetic Chain; Bodyblade, Shoulder, D1 and D2

i. 5.07.70 Strengthen: Closed Kinetic Chain; Shoulder, Plank Shuffle on Medicine Ball

j. 5.07.71 Strengthen: Closed Kinetic Chain; Shoulder, Inverted Row

k. 5.07.79 Plyometrics/Dynamic: Shoulder, Wall Dribbles

l. 5.07.80 Plyometrics/Dynamic: Shoulder, Ball Toss, Overhead

m. 5.07.81 Plyometrics/Dynamic: Shoulder, Chest Pass

n. 5.07.82 Plyometrics/Dynamic: Shoulder, Bench Press/Floor Throws

o. 5.07.83 Plyometrics/Dynamic: Shoulder, Two-Handed Side Throw

p. 5.07.84 Plyometrics/Dynamic: Shoulder, 90/90 Throw

q. 5.07.85 Plyometrics/Dynamic: Shoulder, Multidirectional Catch/Throw

r. 5.07.86 Plyometrics/Dynamic: Shoulder, Ball Toss, Overhead and Backwards

s. 5.07.87 Plyometrics/Dynamic: Shoulder, Push-Up

t. 5.07.88 Plyometrics/Dynamic: Shoulder, Slams

u. 5.07.89 Plyometrics/Dynamic: Shoulder, Ball Squat, Push-Press

v. 5.07.90 Plyometrics/Dynamic: Shoulder, Push-Offs

w. 5.07.91 Reactive Neuromuscular Training and Variations, Shoulder

x. Initiate appropriate interval throwing, pitching, tennis, and golf program as appropriate (**5.07.92** Shoulder, Throwing Progression).

2. Total body conditioning

3. Initiate sport-/work-specific drills or activities

Phase V

Return to unrestricted, symptom-free activity cleared with physician.

5.08.5 SUBACROMIAL DECOMPRESSION REHABILITATION PROTOCOL

General protocol guidelines adapted from South Shore Orthopedics subacromial decompression protocol.

Patients with primary impingements as result of structural deviations who do not respond to conservative treatments may undergo subacromial decompression surgery. This can be done through open or arthroscopic approaches and involve removal of the subacromial bursa, release of the corocoacromial ligaments, removal and resurfacing of the acromion and removal of bony spurs or osteophytes.

Phase I: Acute 0 to 2 Weeks

1. Patient may wear sling for 0 to 2 weeks after surgery; follow physician's specific orders

2. No lifting or active reaching, especially overhead

3. Sleeping postures—sleeping on the affected shoulder should be avoided for 6 weeks. Suggested postures include:
   a. 4.04 Bed Positioning
      i. Semi-reclined with pillow support
      ii. Supine (prop arm on pillows)
      iii. Side-lying quarter turn supine
      iv. Side-lying both knees flexed (on unaffected side)
      v. Side-lying top knee flexed (on unaffected side)

4. ROM ideas 3 to 5 times per day. PROM *only* performed by therapist: flexion, internal rotation, external rotation
   a. 5.04.2 ROM: Shoulder, Pendulum, Passive
   b. 5.04.3 ROM: Shoulder, Cradle Rocks, Passive

5. Strengthening ideas (acute phase) 3 to 5 times per day
   a. 5.03.3 Strengthen: Scapular Retraction and Variations (unilateral side-lying and bilateral seated only)
   b. 5.03.4 Strengthen: Scapular Retraction, Arms by Sides (gentle)
   c. 2.03.4 Strengthen: Isotonic; Chin Tuck

Phase II: 2 to 6 Weeks

Watch for normal scapulohumeral mechanics with all activities.

1. No lifting or carrying, caution with reaching, especially overhead and away from the body

2. Assistive ROM ideas 2 to 3 times per day
   a. 5.04.4 ROM: Shoulder, Saws, Active Assistive
   b. 5.04.6 ROM: Pulleys; Shoulder Flexion, Scaption, and Abduction, Passive
   c. 5.04.5 ROM: Shoulder Girdle Circles, Active Assistive
   d. 5.04.19 ROM: Shoulder Flexion and Saws, Ball Rolls, Active Assistive
   e. 5.04.11 ROM: Wand/Cane; Shoulder Flexion and Scaption, Active Assistive
   f. 5.04.13 ROM: Wand/Cane; Shoulder Internal Rotation, External Rotation, and Combined, Active Assistive (neutral variation only)
   g. 5.04.9 ROM: Wand/Cane; Shoulder Circles, Active Assistive
   h. 5.04.12 ROM: Wand/Cane; Shoulder Abduction, Active Assistive
   i. 5.04.17 ROM: Wand/Cane; Shoulder Extension, Active Assistive
   j. 5.04.20 ROM: Shoulder Flexion, Wall Slide, Active Assistive
   k. 5.04.21 ROM: Shoulder Flexion and Abduction, Towel Slide, Active Assistive
   l. 5.04.22 ROM: Shoulder Flexion and Abduction, Wall Walks, Active Assistive
   m. 5.04.23 ROM: Shoulder Flexion and Abduction, Table Slide, Active Assistive

3. AAROM ideas 2 to 3 times per day
   a. 5.04.33 ROM: Shoulder Extension, Active
   b. 5.07.24 Strengthen: Isotonic; Shoulder, Row (Prone) (no weight)
   c. 5.07.19 Strengthen: Isotonic; Shoulder, Horizontal Abduction, Bent Forward (no weight)
   d. 5.07.22 Strengthen: Isotonic; Shoulder External Rotation (no weight)

4. Strengthening ideas (gentle beginner)
   a. 5.07.1 Strengthen: Isometric; Shoulder, Other Hand Resists, 6-Way or 5.07.2 Strengthen: Isometric; Shoulder, Wall Resists, 5-Way

Phase III: 6 to 12 Weeks

Watch for normal scapulohumeral mechanics with all activities.

1. Warm-up (start with 1 to 2 minutes)
   a. 5.04.1 ROM: Shoulder, Warm-Up, Upper Body Ergometer, Active Assistive
2. AROM ideas 3 to 5 times per week
   a. 5.04.28 ROM: Shoulder Flexion, Active
   b. 5.04.29 ROM: Shoulder Abduction, Active
   c. 5.04.34 ROM: Shoulder Scaption, Active
   d. 5.04.35 ROM: Shoulder Scaption Figure 8s, Active
   e. 5.04.36 ROM: Shoulder Internal Rotation and External Rotation, Active
   f. 5.04.38 ROM: Shoulder, PNF D1 and D2, Active
3. Strengthening ideas (advancing per patient tolerances)
   a. 5.07.3 Strengthen: Isometric; Shoulder Flexion Overhead
   b. 5.07.4 Strengthen: Isometric; Shoulder Internal Rotation Multi-Angle Neutral, Doorway
   c. 5.07.5 Strengthen: Isometric; Shoulder External Rotation Multi-Angle Neutral, Doorway
   d. 5.07.6 Strengthen: Isometric; Shoulder Internal Rotation Multi-Angle Abduction and Flexion
   e. 5.07.7 Strengthen: Isometric; Shoulder External Rotation Multi-Angle Abduction and Flexion
   f. 5.07.8 Strengthen: Isometric; Shoulder Horizontal Abduction and Adduction
   g. 5.07.9 Strengthen: Isometric; Shoulder Walk-Out
   h. 5.07.10 Strengthen: Isotonic; Shoulder Flexion
   i. 5.07.11 Strengthen: Isotonic; Shoulder Scaption
   j. 5.07.12 Strengthen: Isotonic; Shoulder Abduction
   k. 5.07.21 Strengthen: Isotonic; Shoulder Internal Rotation
   l. 5.07.22 Strengthen: Isotonic; Shoulder External Rotation
   m. 5.07.36 Strengthen: Isotonic; Resistance Band, Shoulder Flexion, Scaption, Abduction, and Variations (start by staying below shoulder level/90 degrees)
   n. 5.07.13 Strengthen: Isotonic; Shoulder Extension
   o. 5.07.39 Strengthen: Isotonic; Resistance Band, Shoulder Internal Rotation and Variations (neutral)
   p. 5.07.41 Strengthen: Isotonic; Resistance Band, Shoulder External Rotation and Variations (neutral)
4. Strengthening ideas for scapular stabilizers
   a. 5.03.4 Strengthen: Scapular Retraction, Arms by Sides
   b. 5.03.6 Strengthen: Scapular Retraction, Arm Off Table
   c. 5.03.8 Strengthen: Scapular Retraction, "W" or "Batwings"
   d. 5.03.9 Strengthen: Scapular Retraction, Wall Angels
   e. 5.03.11 Strengthen: Resistance Band, Isolated Scapular Retraction
   f. 5.03.12 Strengthen: Resistance Band, Scapular Row and Variations
   g. 5.07.19 Strengthen: Isotonic; Shoulder, Horizontal Abduction, Bent Forward
   h. 5.07.20 Strengthen: Isotonic; Shoulder, Horizontal Abduction, Deceleration Emphasis
   i. 5.07.24 Strengthen: Isotonic; Shoulder, Row (Prone)
   j. 5.07.27 Strengthen: Isotonic; Posterior Cuff, 4-Way
5. Stretching ideas
   a. 5.06.8 Stretch: Shoulder Horizontal Adductors, Towel Roll and Swiss Ball
   b. 5.06.4 Stretch: Shoulder Horizontal Abductors
   c. 5.06.5 Stretch: Shoulder Horizontal Adductors, Doorway
   d. 2.02.3 Stretch: Self-Assisted Cervical Lateral Flexion
   e. 2.02.7 Stretch: Cervical Flexion and Rotation
6. Joint self-mobilization ideas (other mobilizations may be added depending on direction restrictions of the capsule)
   a. 5.05.2 Self-Joint Mobilization/Stretch: Shoulder, Distraction With Weight
   b. 5.05.3 Self-Joint Mobilization/Stretch: Shoulder, Distraction With Chair Pull

Phase IV: Begin at 12 weeks

Sport-specific and return to activity phase. Watch for normal scapulohumeral mechanics with all activities.

1. Advanced strengthening ideas for shoulder
   a. 5.07.21 Strengthen: Isotonic; Shoulder Internal Rotation
   b. 5.07.22 Strengthen: Isotonic; Shoulder External Rotation
   c. 5.07.23 Strengthen: Isotonic; Shoulder External Rotation 90/90
   d. 5.07.25 Strengthen: Isotonic; Shoulder, Military Press (Prone)
   e. 5.07.28 Strengthen: Isotonic; Shoulder, Diagonal Lifts D1 and D2
   f. 5.07.34 Strengthen: Isotonic; Resistance Band and Machine, Shoulder, Lat Pull-Down
   g. 5.07.38 Strengthen: Isotonic; Resistance Band, Shoulder Extension
   h. 5.07.39 Strengthen: Isotonic; Resistance Band, Shoulder Internal Rotation and Variations
   i. 5.07.41 Strengthen: Isotonic; Resistance Band, Shoulder External Rotation and Variations
   j. 5.07.42 Strengthen: Isotonic; Resistance Band, Shoulder, Combination Movements PNF D1 and D2
   k. 5.07.47 Strengthen: Isotonic; Resistance Band, Shoulder Pull-Back
   l. 5.07.63 Strengthen: Closed Kinetic Chain; Scapular and Shoulder Depression
   m. 5.07.64 Strengthen: Closed Kinetic Chain; Shoulder, Table Top Push-Pull

n. 5.07.61 Strengthen: Closed Kinetic Chain; Shoulder, Beginning Weightbearing, Progress to Push-Up Partial Weight

o. 5.07.62 Strengthen: Closed Kinetic Chain; Shoulder, Push-Up

2. Advanced strengthening ideas for scapular stabilizers

a. 5.03.5 Strengthen: Scapular Retraction, "T", "Y", and "I" and Variations

b. 5.03.13 Strengthen: Resistance Band, Scapular and Posterior Shoulder, Overhead Pull-down

c. 5.03.14 Strengthen: Resistance Band, Scapular and Rotator Cuff, Retraction and External Rotation

d. 5.03.15 Strengthen: Resistance Band, Scapular, Punch

e. 5.03.16 Strengthen: Resistance Band, Scapular, Dynamic Hug

f. 5.03.17 Strengthen: Resistance Band, Serratus Wall Slides

g. 5.03.18 Strengthen: Resistance Band, Scapular Clocks

h. 5.03.19 Strengthen: Resistance Band, Scapular "Vs"

i. 5.03.22 Strengthen: Scapular, Arm Lifts

j. 5.03.21 Strengthen: Scapular, Push-Up Plus (Advanced)

k. 5.07.66 Strengthen: Closed Kinetic Chain; Stairmaster, Shoulder

l. 5.07.67 Strengthen: Closed Kinetic Chain; Bodyblade, Shoulder Flexion, Scaption, and Abduction

m. 5.07.68 Strengthen: Closed Kinetic Chain; Bodyblade, Shoulder Internal Rotation and External Rotation

n. 5.07.69 Strengthen: Closed Kinetic Chain; Bodyblade, Shoulder, D1 and D2

o. 5.07.70 Strengthen: Closed Kinetic Chain; Shoulder, Plank Shuffle on Medicine Ball

p. 5.07.71 Strengthen: Closed Kinetic Chain; Shoulder, Inverted Row

q. 5.07.79 Plyometrics/Dynamic: Shoulder, Wall Dribbles

r. 5.07.80 Plyometrics/Dynamic: Shoulder, Ball Toss, Overhead

s. 5.07.81 Plyometrics/Dynamic: Shoulder, Chest Pass

t. 5.07.82 Plyometrics/Dynamic: Shoulder, Bench Press/Floor Throws

u. 5.07.83 Plyometrics/Dynamic: Shoulder, Two-Handed Side Throw

v. 5.07.84 Plyometrics/Dynamic: Shoulder, 90/90 Throw

w. 5.07.85 Plyometrics/Dynamic: Shoulder, Multidirectional Catch/Throw

x. 5.07.86 Plyometrics/Dynamic: Shoulder, Ball Toss, Overhead and Backwards

y. 5.07.87 Plyometrics/Dynamic: Shoulder, Push-Up

z. 5.07.88 Plyometrics/Dynamic: Shoulder, Slams

aa. 5.07.89 Plyometrics/Dynamic: Shoulder, Ball Squat, Push-Press

ab. 5.07.90 Plyometrics/Dynamic: Shoulder, Push-Offs

ac. 5.07.91 Reactive Neuromuscular Training and Variations, Shoulder

ad. 5.07.92 Shoulder, Throwing Progression

Phase V

Return to unrestricted, symptom-free activity once cleared with physician.

5.08.6 BANKART REPAIR REHABILITATION PROTOCOL

General protocol guidelines adapted from South Shore Orthopedics (2016) Bankart Protocol and The Stone Clinic (2016) Bankart Protocol.

A Bankart lesion is an injury to the anterior-inferior glenoid labrum usually due to glenohumeral dislocation resulting in detachment of the labrum at the anterior glenoid rim. This may result from a traumatic event in which the humeral head is forced into extreme abduction and external rotation or horizontal abduction. Due to the detachment of the labrum anteriorly, patient may also have resultant anterior instability. Surgical correction includes repair of the torn labrum (Bankart repair) and may be in combination with tightening of ligaments that were stretched or torn due to the dislocation (capsular shift). RC tearing may also have occurred during the traumatic dislocation and repair of these may also be performed during surgery. There has been some debate whether patients should be immobilized for several weeks after surgery or begin mobilization post-operative day 1 (considered an accelerated protocol) due to the history of dislocation and possible future instability.

Where's the Evidence?

Early mobilization of the operated shoulder after arthroscopic Bankart repair did not affect recurrence rate in a selected group of patient studies by Kim et al. (2003) as compared to the patients immobilized for 3 weeks after surgery. Kim and colleagues found that final outcomes were approximately the same for both groups whether early mobilization implemented or not; however, patients mobilized early demonstrated less postoperative pain scores.

It is recommended that the clinician understands the specific repairs performed for each patient before implementing a rehabilitation program. The general rehabilitation protocol for a Bankart repair is outlined below. Physician orders regarding patient should supersede this protocol due to the variations in surgical involvement.

Precautions

1. Ensure compliance with sling if prescribed
2. No shoulder extension or external rotation for at least 4 to 6 weeks
3. For posterior repairs: avoid any internal rotation for at least 4 weeks and no forceful internal rotation up to 12 weeks.
4. No passive forceful stretching into external rotation or extension for 12 weeks

Post-Operative Days 1 to 5

1. Eliminate any activity that causes an increase in symptoms
2. Sleeping postures—sleeping on the affected shoulder can aggravate surgery site. Suggested postures include:
   a. 4.04 Bed Positioning
      i. Semi-reclined with pillow support
      ii. Supine (pillow supporting arm as needed)
      iii. Side-lying quarter turn supine
      iv. Side-lying both knees flexed (on unaffected side)
      v. Side-lying top knee flexed (on unaffected side)
3. PROM flexion to 90 degrees by therapist
4. ROM ideas
   a. 5.04.2 ROM: Shoulder, Pendulum, Passive
   b. 5.09.3 ROM: Elbow Flexion and Extension, Active
   c. 5.09.5 ROM: Elbow Pronation and Supination, Passive and Active Assistive
   d. 5.14.1 ROM: Passive and Active Wrist and Finger Movements (active wrist flexion/extension)
5. Stretching ideas
   a. 2.02.3 Stretch: Self-Assisted Cervical Lateral Flexion
   b. 2.02.7 Stretch: Cervical Flexion and Rotation
6. Postural correction
   a. 5.03.4 Strengthen: Scapular Retraction, Arms by Sides
   b. 2.03.4 Strengthen: Isotonic; Chin Tuck
7. Aerobic conditioning throughout the rehabilitation process
   a. Stationary bike
   b. Stairmaster
   c. Elliptical without putting weight on involved arm

Post-Operative Days 6 to 14

1. PROM and AAROM flexion and scaption to 90 degrees
2. Strengthening ideas (beginner in acute phase)
   a. 50% to 60% contraction intensity: 5.07.1 Strengthen: Isometric; Shoulder, Other Hand Resists, 6-Way or 5.07.2 Strengthen: Isometric; Shoulder, Wall Resists, 5-Way

Post-Operative Weeks 2 to 4

1. PROM and AAROM flexion and scaption to 90 degrees

2. Continue isometrics and wrist/forearm exercises
3. Elbow strengthening:
   a. 5.12.10 Strengthen: Isotonic; Elbow Flexion, Curls (high repetitions, low weights)
4. Scapular beginning movement and strengthening
   a. 5.03.3 Strengthen: Scapular Retraction and Variations (unilateral side-lying and bilateral seated only)
   b. 5.01.5 ROM: Scapular Elevation
   c. 5.01.6 ROM: Scapular Depression
5. Early weightbearing
   a. 5.07.61 Strengthen: Closed Kinetic Chain; Shoulder, Beginning Weightbearing, Progress to Push-Up Partial Weight (beginning weightbearing only)

Post-Operative Weeks 4 to 6

1. Warm-up (start with 1 to 2 minutes; watch scapulo-humeral mechanics)
   a. 5.04.1 ROM: Shoulder, Warm-Up, Upper Body Ergometer, Active Assistive (light to no resistance)
2. ROM: PROM and AAROM flexion, scaption, abduction
   a. 5.04.6 ROM: Pulleys; Shoulder Flexion, Scaption, and Abduction, Passive
   b. 5.04.5 ROM: Shoulder Girdle Circles, Active Assistive
   c. 5.04.11 ROM: Wand/Cane; Shoulder Flexion and Scaption, Active Assistive
   d. 5.04.12 ROM: Wand/Cane; Shoulder Abduction, Active Assistive
   e. 5.04.23 ROM: Shoulder Flexion and Abduction, Table Slide, Active Assistive
   f. 5.04.21 ROM: Shoulder Flexion and Abduction, Towel Slide, Active Assistive
   g. 5.04.22 ROM: Shoulder Flexion and Abduction, Wall Walks, Active Assistive
   h. 5.04.20 ROM: Shoulder Flexion, Wall Slide, Active Assistive
3. Continue isometrics at about 75% to 90% contraction intensity and wrist and forearm exercises
4. Start AROM flexion and scaption:
   a. 5.04.28 ROM: Shoulder Flexion, Active
   b. 5.04.34 ROM: Shoulder Scaption, Active
5. Proprioceptive Training:
   a. 5.01.4 ROM: Scapular Circles and Alphabet Ball on Wall

Post-Operative Weeks 6 to 8: Continue With Exercises as Previous Weeks

1. Warm-up
   a. 5.04.1 ROM: Shoulder, Warm-Up, Upper Body Ergometer, Active Assistive (start to add resistance)
2. ROM; may begin light passive and active assistive external and internal rotation and extension.

  a. 5.04.13 ROM: Wand/Cane; Shoulder Internal Rotation, External Rotation, and Combined, Active Assistive (neutral variation only)
  b. 5.04.17 ROM: Wand/Cane; Shoulder Extension, Active Assistive

3. Start AROM abduction and combinations:
  a. 5.04.29 ROM: Shoulder Abduction, Active
  b. 5.04.35 ROM: Shoulder Scaption Figure 8s, Active
  c. 5.04.37 ROM: Side-Lying Shoulder Circles, Active

4. Closed chain for glenohumeral stabilization:
  a. 5.07.67 Strengthen: Closed Kinetic Chain; Bodyblade, Shoulder Flexion, Scaption, and Abduction
  b. 5.07.58 Strengthen: Closed Kinetic Chain; Shoulder, Weight Shifts
  c. 5.07.60 Strengthen: Closed Kinetic Chain; Shoulder, Alternating Arm Lift

5. Shoulder strengthening:
  a. 5.07.10 Strengthen: Isotonic; Shoulder Flexion
  b. 5.07.11 Strengthen: Isotonic; Shoulder Scaption
  c. 5.07.12 Strengthen: Isotonic; Shoulder Abduction
  d. 5.07.36 Strengthen: Isotonic; Resistance Band, Shoulder Flexion, Scaption, Abduction, and Variations (start by staying below shoulder level/90 degrees)
  e. 5.07.19 Strengthen: Isotonic; Shoulder, Horizontal Abduction, Bent Forward
  f. 5.07.20 Strengthen: Isotonic; Shoulder, Horizontal Abduction, Deceleration Emphasis
  g. 5.07.24 Strengthen: Isotonic; Shoulder, Row (Prone)
  h. 5.07.27 Strengthen: Isotonic; Posterior Cuff, 4-Way
  i. 5.03.4 Strengthen: Scapular Retraction, Arms by Sides

6. Aerobic conditioning throughout the rehabilitation process
  a. May start arm resistive exercises in the pool, road cycling, and light jogging

Post-Operative Weeks 8 to 12: Continue With Exercises as Previous Weeks

1. ROM: may begin active external rotation, internal rotation and extension
  a. 5.04.33 ROM: Shoulder Extension, Active
  b. 5.04.36 ROM: Shoulder Internal Rotation and External Rotation, Active

2. Closed chain for glenohumeral stabilization:
  a. 5.07.67 Strengthen: Closed Kinetic Chain; Bodyblade, Shoulder Flexion, Scaption, and Abduction
  b. 5.07.58 Strengthen: Closed Kinetic Chain; Shoulder, Weight Shifts
  c. 5.07.60 Strengthen: Closed Kinetic Chain; Shoulder, Alternating Arm Lift

3. Stretching ideas

  a. 5.06.5 Stretch: Shoulder Horizontal Adductors, Doorway (no anterior movement of the humeral head)

4. Shoulder strengthening:
  a. 5.07.22 Strengthen: Isotonic; Shoulder External Rotation
  b. 5.07.21 Strengthen: Isotonic; Shoulder Internal Rotation
  c. 5.07.13 Strengthen: Isotonic; Shoulder Extension
  d. 5.07.21 Strengthen: Isotonic; Shoulder Internal Rotation
  e. 5.07.22 Strengthen: Isotonic; Shoulder External Rotation
  f. 5.07.91 Reactive Neuromuscular Training and Variations, Shoulder (only variations listed below)
    i. Rhythmic stabilization internal rotation/ external rotation side-lying shoulder neutral
    ii. Rhythmic stabilization internal rotation/ external rotation supine shoulder neutral
    iii. Rhythmic stabilization supine shoulder flexed or in scaption
  g. 5.07.19 Strengthen: Isotonic; Shoulder, Horizontal Abduction, Bent Forward
  h. 5.07.20 Strengthen: Isotonic; Shoulder, Horizontal Abduction, Deceleration Emphasis
  i. 5.07.24 Strengthen: Isotonic; Shoulder, Row (Prone)
  j. 5.07.27 Strengthen: Isotonic; Posterior Cuff, 4-Way
  k. 5.07.25 Strengthen: Isotonic; Shoulder, Military Press (Prone)
  l. 5.07.28 Strengthen: Isotonic; Shoulder, Diagonal Lifts D1 and D2
  m. 5.07.34 Strengthen: Isotonic; Resistance Band and Machine, Shoulder, Lat Pull-Down
  n. 5.07.38 Strengthen: Isotonic; Resistance Band, Shoulder Extension
  o. 5.07.39 Strengthen: Isotonic; Resistance Band, Shoulder Internal Rotation and Variations (neutral)
  p. 5.07.41 Strengthen: Isotonic; Resistance Band, Shoulder External Rotation and Variations (neutral)
  q. 5.07.42 Strengthen: Isotonic; Resistance Band, Shoulder, Combination Movements PNF D1 and D2
  r. 5.07.47 Strengthen: Isotonic; Resistance Band, Shoulder Pull-Back
  s. 5.07.64 Strengthen: Closed Kinetic Chain; Shoulder, Table Top Push-Pull
  t. 5.07.61 Strengthen: Closed Kinetic Chain; Shoulder, Beginning Weightbearing, Progress to Push-Up Partial Weight

5. Scapular strengthening:
  a. 5.03.5 Strengthen: Scapular Retraction, "T", "Y", and "I" and Variations
  b. 5.03.13 Strengthen: Resistance Band, Scapular and Posterior Shoulder, Overhead Pull-down
  c. 5.03.14 Strengthen: Resistance Band, Scapular and Rotator Cuff, Retraction and External Rotation

d. 5.03.15 Strengthen: Resistance Band, Scapular, Punch

e. 5.03.16 Strengthen: Resistance Band, Scapular, Dynamic Hug

f. 5.03.17 Strengthen: Resistance Band, Serratus Wall Slides

g. 5.03.18 Strengthen: Resistance Band, Scapular Clocks

h. 5.03.19 Strengthen: Resistance Band, Scapular "Vs"

i. 5.03.22 Strengthen: Scapular, Arm Lifts

j. 5.03.21 Strengthen: Scapular, Push-Up Plus (Advanced)

6. Aerobic conditioning throughout the rehabilitation process

a. Running may begin, road or mountain biking okay; no ballistic arm movement activities.

Post-Operative Months 3 to 6

1. May begin light throwing and more strenuous exercise; correct faulty mechanics with all activities.

2. Strengthening ideas

a. 5.07.39 Strengthen: Isotonic; Resistance Band, Shoulder Internal Rotation and Variations (move into 45- and 90-degree movements)

b. 5.07.41 Strengthen: Isotonic; Resistance Band, Shoulder External Rotation and Variations (move into 45- and 90-degree movements with caution)

c. 5.07.66 Strengthen: Closed Kinetic Chain; Stairmaster, Shoulder

d. 5.07.67 Strengthen: Closed Kinetic Chain; Bodyblade, Shoulder Flexion, Scaption, and Abduction

e. 5.07.68 Strengthen: Closed Kinetic Chain; Bodyblade, Shoulder Internal Rotation and External Rotation

f. 5.07.69 Strengthen: Closed Kinetic Chain; Bodyblade, Shoulder, D1 and D2

g. 5.07.71 Strengthen: Closed Kinetic Chain; Shoulder, Inverted Row

h. 5.07.79 Plyometrics/Dynamic: Shoulder, Wall Dribbles

i. 5.07.80 Plyometrics/Dynamic: Shoulder, Ball Toss, Overhead

j. 5.07.81 Plyometrics/Dynamic: Shoulder, Chest Pass

k. 5.07.82 Plyometrics/Dynamic: Shoulder, Bench Press/Floor Throws

l. 5.07.83 Plyometrics/Dynamic: Shoulder, Two-Handed Side Throw

m. 5.07.84 Plyometrics/Dynamic: Shoulder, 90/90 Throw (start cautiously!)

n. 5.07.85 Plyometrics/Dynamic: Shoulder, Multidirectional Catch/Throw

o. 5.07.86 Plyometrics/Dynamic: Shoulder, Ball Toss, Overhead and Backwards

p. 5.07.87 Plyometrics/Dynamic: Shoulder, Push-Up

q. 5.07.88 Plyometrics/Dynamic: Shoulder, Slams

r. 5.07.89 Plyometrics/Dynamic: Shoulder, Ball Squat, Push-Press

s. 5.07.90 Plyometrics/Dynamic: Shoulder, Push-Offs

t. 5.07.91 Reactive Neuromuscular Training and Variations, Shoulder

u. 5.07.92 Shoulder, Throwing Progression

Post-Operative Months 6

1. Increase throwing program with focus on return-to-throwing sports as mechanics, conditioning, and strength allow

5.08.7 Superior Labrum (SLAP Lesion) Repair Protocol

General protocol guidelines adapted from Marc Sherry, PT, DPT (2001) and University of Wisconsin Sports Medicine physician group.

Superior labrum extending anterior to posterior tears, or *SLAP lesions*, are associated with a tear at the proximal attachment of the biceps tendon long head. Surgical repair may vary in stabilization and reconstruction procedures due to concomitant uni- or multidirectional instabilities.

Precautions

1. Ensure compliance with immobilization orders—patients may be immobilized in different positions depending on surgical procedure (i.e., additional injuries and issues, anterior or posterior capsule involvement, RC tear)

2. Avoid any positions that places stress on the biceps; elbow extension with shoulder extension for 6 weeks.

3. No active contract of biceps for at least 6 weeks

4. Limit external rotation in neutral abduction to 40 degrees the first 6 weeks.

5. No passive abduction with external rotation combination or extension for 8 to 12 weeks and only then very cautiously

6. No lifting for 8 to 12 weeks

Phase I: 0 to 6 Weeks

1. Sleeping postures—sleeping on the affected shoulder can aggravate surgery site. Suggested postures include:

a. 4.04 Bed Positioning-In immobilizer

i. Semi-reclined with pillow support (**5.08.3**)

ii. Supine (pillow supporting arm as needed)

iii. Side-lying quarter turn supine

2. PROM flexion

a. 0 to 2 weeks to 0 to 60 degrees

b. 2 to 4 weeks 0 to 90 degrees

c. 4 to 6 weeks 0 to 130 degrees

3. ROM ideas
   a. 5.04.2 ROM: Shoulder, Pendulum, Passive
   b. 5.09.3 ROM: Elbow Flexion and Extension, Active
   c. 5.09.5 ROM: Elbow Pronation and Supination, Passive and Active Assistive
   d. 5.14.1 ROM: Passive and Active Assisted Wrist and Finger Movements (active wrist flexion/extension)
4. Stretching ideas
   a. 2.02.3 Stretch: Self-Assisted Cervical Lateral Flexion
   b. 2.02.7 Stretch: Cervical Flexion and Rotation
5. Postural correction
   a. 5.03.3 Strengthen: Scapular Retraction and Variations (unilateral side-lying and bilateral seated only)
   b. 2.03.4 Strengthen: Isotonic; Chin Tuck
6. Aerobic conditioning throughout the rehabilitation process
   a. Stationary bike
   b. Walking (no treadmill)

Phase II: 6 to 12 Weeks

1. ROM ideas
   a. 5.04.6 ROM: Pulleys; Shoulder Flexion, Scaption, and Abduction, Passive
   b. 5.04.19 ROM: Shoulder Flexion and Saws, Ball Rolls, Active Assistive (start in side-lying for flexion ROM as tension lessens on biceps)
   c. 5.04.12 ROM: Wand/Cane; Shoulder Abduction, Active Assistive
   d. 5.04.23 ROM: Shoulder Flexion and Abduction, Table Slide, Active Assistive
   e. 5.01.4 ROM: Scapular Circles and Alphabet Ball on Wall
   f. 5.04.13 ROM: Wand/Cane; Shoulder Internal Rotation, External Rotation, and Combined, Active Assistive (in neutral abduction only; caution with external rotation)
   g. 8 to 10 weeks: 5.04.28 ROM: Shoulder Flexion, Active
   h. 8 to 10 weeks: 5.04.34 ROM: Shoulder Scaption, Active
   i. 8 to 10 weeks: 5.04.29 ROM: Shoulder Abduction, Active
   j. 8 to 10 weeks: 5.04.35 ROM: Shoulder Scaption Figure 8s, Active
   k. 8 to 10 weeks: 5.04.37 ROM: Side-Lying Shoulder Circles, Active
   l. 8 to 10 weeks: 5.01.4 ROM: Scapular Circles and Alphabet Ball on Wall l
2. Strengthening ideas
   a. 5.07.1 Strengthen: Isometric; Shoulder, Other Hand Resists, 6-Way or 5.07.2 Strengthen: Isometric; Shoulder, Wall Resists, 5-Way

b. Progress gradually to 5.07.5 Strengthen: Isometric; Shoulder External Rotation Multi-Angle Neutral, Doorway
c. Progress gradually to 5.07.4 Strengthen: Isometric; Shoulder Internal Rotation Multi-Angle Neutral, Doorway
3. Scapular beginning movement and strengthening ideas
   a. 5.03.4 Strengthen: Scapular Retraction, Arms by Sides
   b. 5.01.5 ROM: Scapular Elevation
   c. 5.01.6 ROM: Scapular Depression
4. Early weightbearing ideas
   a. 5.07.61 Strengthen: Closed Kinetic Chain; Shoulder, Beginning Weightbearing, Progress to Push-Up Partial Weight (beginning weightbearing only)

Post-Operative 12 to 16 Weeks

1. Warm-up (start with 1 to 2 minutes; watch scapulo-humeral mechanics)
   a. 5.04.1 ROM: Shoulder, Warm-Up, Upper Body Ergometer, Active Assistive (light to no resistance)
2. ROM ideas
   a. 5.04.17 ROM: Wand/Cane; Shoulder Extension, Active Assistive
   b. 5.04.33 ROM: Shoulder Extension, Active
   c. 5.04.36 ROM: Shoulder Internal Rotation and External Rotation, Active
3. Closed chain for glenohumeral stabilization ideas
   a. 5.07.67 Strengthen: Closed Kinetic Chain; Bodyblade, Shoulder Flexion, Scaption, and Abduction
   b. 5.07.58 Strengthen: Closed Kinetic Chain; Shoulder, Weight Shifts
   c. 5.07.60 Strengthen: Closed Kinetic Chain; Shoulder, Alternating Arm Lift
4. Shoulder strengthening ideas
   a. 5.07.10 Strengthen: Isotonic; Shoulder Flexion
   b. 5.07.11 Strengthen: Isotonic; Shoulder Scaption
   c. 5.07.12 Strengthen: Isotonic; Shoulder Abduction
   d. 5.07.36 Strengthen: Isotonic; Resistance Band, Shoulder Flexion, Scaption, Abduction, and Variations (start by staying below shoulder level/90 degrees)
   e. 5.07.19 Strengthen: Isotonic; Shoulder, Horizontal Abduction, Bent Forward
   f. 5.07.20 Strengthen: Isotonic; Shoulder, Horizontal Abduction, Deceleration Emphasis
   g. 5.07.24 Strengthen: Isotonic; Shoulder, Row (Prone)
   h. 5.07.27 Strengthen: Isotonic; Posterior Cuff, 4-Way
   i. 5.07.22 Strengthen: Isotonic; Shoulder External Rotation
   j. 5.07.21 Strengthen: Isotonic; Shoulder Internal Rotation
   k. 5.07.13 Strengthen: Isotonic; Shoulder Extension

l. 5.07.91 Reactive Neuromuscular Training and Variations, Shoulder (only variations listed below)

   i. Rhythmic stabilization internal rotation/external rotation side-lying shoulder neutral

   ii. Rhythmic stabilization internal rotation/external rotation supine shoulder neutral

   iii. Rhythmic stabilization internal rotation/external rotation supine shoulder 30 degrees abducted (scaption plan)

   iv. Rhythmic stabilization side-lying shoulder abducted

   v. Rhythmic stabilization supine shoulder flexed or in scaption

m. 5.07.39 Strengthen: Isotonic; Resistance Band, Shoulder Internal Rotation and Variations (neutral)

n. 5.07.38 Strengthen: Isotonic; Resistance Band, Shoulder Extension (keep the humeral head from translating anteriorly)

o. 5.07.41 Strengthen: Isotonic; Resistance Band, Shoulder External Rotation and Variations (neutral)

p. 5.07.79 Plyometrics/Dynamic: Shoulder, Wall Dribbles

5. Scapular strengthening ideas

a. 5.03.4 Strengthen: Scapular Retraction, Arms by Sides

b. 5.03.5 Strengthen: Scapular Retraction, "T", "Y", and "I" and Variations

c. 5.03.13 Strengthen: Resistance Band, Scapular and Posterior Shoulder, Overhead Pull-down

d. 5.03.14 Strengthen: Resistance Band, Scapular and Rotator Cuff, Retraction and External Rotation

e. 5.03.15 Strengthen: Resistance Band, Scapular, Punch

f. 5.03.16 Strengthen: Resistance Band, Scapular, Dynamic Hug

g. 5.03.17 Strengthen: Resistance Band, Serratus Wall Slides

h. 5.03.18 Strengthen: Resistance Band, Scapular Clocks

i. 5.03.19 Strengthen: Resistance Band, Scapular "Vs"

j. 5.03.22 Strengthen: Scapular, Arm Lifts

Postoperative 16 Weeks

1. Stretching ideas

a. 5.06.5 Stretch: Shoulder Horizontal Adductors, Doorway (no anterior movement of the humeral head)

2. Shoulder strengthening ideas

a. 5.07.25 Strengthen: Isotonic; Shoulder, Military Press (Prone)

b. 5.07.28 Strengthen: Isotonic; Shoulder, Diagonal Lifts D1 and D2

c. 5.07.39 Strengthen: Isotonic; Resistance Band, Shoulder Internal Rotation and Variations (move into 45- and 90-degree movements)

d. 5.07.41 Strengthen: Isotonic; Resistance Band, Shoulder External Rotation and Variations (move into 45- and 90-degree movements with caution)

e. 5.07.34 Strengthen: Isotonic; Resistance Band and Machine, Shoulder, Lat Pull-Down

f. 5.07.42 Strengthen: Isotonic; Resistance Band, Shoulder, Combination Movements PNF D1 and D2

g. 5.07.47 Strengthen: Isotonic; Resistance Band, Shoulder Pull-Back

h. 5.07.64 Strengthen: Closed Kinetic Chain; Shoulder, Table Top Push-Pull

i. 5.07.61 Strengthen: Closed Kinetic Chain; Shoulder, Beginning Weightbearing, Progress to Push-Up Partial Weight

j. 5.03.21 Strengthen: Scapular, Push-Up Plus (Advanced)

k. 5.07.66 Strengthen: Closed Kinetic Chain; Stairmaster, Shoulder

l. 5.07.67 Strengthen: Closed Kinetic Chain; Bodyblade, Shoulder Flexion, Scaption, and Abduction

m. 5.07.68 Strengthen: Closed Kinetic Chain; Bodyblade, Shoulder Internal Rotation and External Rotation

n. 5.07.69 Strengthen: Closed Kinetic Chain; Bodyblade, Shoulder, D1 and D2

o. 5.07.71 Strengthen: Closed Kinetic Chain; Shoulder, Inverted Row

p. 5.07.80 Plyometrics/Dynamic: Shoulder, Ball Toss, Overhead

q. 5.07.81 Plyometrics/Dynamic: Shoulder, Chest Pass

r. 5.07.82 Plyometrics/Dynamic: Shoulder, Bench Press/Floor Throws

s. 5.07.83 Plyometrics/Dynamic: Shoulder, Two-Handed Side Throw

t. 5.07.84 Plyometrics/Dynamic: Shoulder, 90/90 Throw (start cautiously!)

u. 5.07.85 Plyometrics/Dynamic: Shoulder, Multidirectional Catch/Throw

v. 5.07.86 Plyometrics/Dynamic: Shoulder, Ball Toss, Overhead and Backwards

w. 5.07.87 Plyometrics/Dynamic: Shoulder, Push-Up

x. 5.07.88 Plyometrics/Dynamic: Shoulder, Slams

y. 5.07.89 Plyometrics/Dynamic: Shoulder, Ball Squat, Push-Press

z. 5.07.90 Plyometrics/Dynamic: Shoulder, Push-Offs

aa. 5.07.91 Reactive Neuromuscular Training and Variations, Shoulder (move into sports positions)

ab. 5.07.92 Shoulder, Throwing Progression

5.08.6 BANKART REPAIR REHABILITATION PROTOCOL

General protocol guidelines adapted from Kevin Wilk, PT, DPT and colleagues (Wilk, Macrina, & Reinold, 2006).

The shoulder is the most frequently dislocated joint in the body. Anterior dislocation accounts for 94% to 98% of shoulder dislocations (Wen, 1999). Anterior shoulder dislocation can be associated with many lesions such as Bankart lesions, RC tears, Hill-Sachs lesions, or greater tuberosity fractures. It has been documented that early management of the associated injury affords better recovery of shoulder function (Atef, El-Tantawy, Gad, & Hefeda, 2016).

Where's the Evidence?

Atef et al. (2016) looked at 240 patients with traumatic anterior glenohumeral dislocations. Associated lesions were reported in 144 of these patients. RC tear was the most common injury (67 cases). It was isolated in 34 patients but combined with other lesions in 33 cases. Axillary nerve injury was encountered in 38 patients: 8 were isolated and 30 were combined. Greater tuberosity fracture was found in 37 patients: 15 were combined with axillary nerve injury and 22 were isolated. All cases with Hill-Sachs and Bankart lesions were combined lesions with no isolated cases. There was a significant relation between the incidence of associated injuries and age, mechanism of injury, and the affected side.

Rehabilitation for patient with a first-time traumatic episode will be progressed based on patient's symptoms with emphasis on early controlled ROM, reduction of muscle spasms and guarding, and relief of pain. A patient presenting with a traumatic instability often presents with a history of repetitive injuries and symptomatic complaints such as a feeling of shoulder laxity or difficulty performing specific tasks. Rehabilitation for this patient should focus on early proprioception training, dynamic stabilization drills, neuromuscular control, scapular muscle exercises, and muscle strengthening exercises to enhance dynamic stability (Wilk, Macrina, & Reinold, 2006). Strength training has demonstrated improvements in joint position sense and better neuromuscular control in the shoulder (Salles et al., 2015). Cools et al.'s (2016) review of scientific evidence stated that depending on the specific characteristics of the instability pattern, the severity, recurrence, and direction, the therapeutic approach may be adapted to the needs and demands of the athlete. In general, attention should go to (1) restoration of RC strength and intermuscular balance, focusing on the eccentric capacity of the external rotators, (2) normalization of rotational ROM with special attention to the internal rotation ROM, (3) optimization of the flexibility and muscle performance of the scapular muscles, and (4) gradually increasing the functional sport-specific load on the shoulder girdle. The functional kinetic chain should be implemented throughout all stages of the rehabilitation

program. Return to play should be based on subjective assessment as well as objective measurements of ROM, strength, and function (Cools et al., 2016).

Strict avoidance of the unstable position of the humeral head for minimum 6 weeks is key to allow structures to tighten and heal without recurrent trauma. Gentle ROM within nonstressful positions and gradual progression of static and dynamic stabilization exercises compose the core of this rehabilitation program. During the early rehabilitation program, caution must be applied in placing the capsule under stress until dynamic joint stability is restored. It is important to refrain from activities in extreme ranges of motion early in the rehabilitation process.

Precautions

1. Ensure compliance with immobilization orders
2. Do *not* stretch injured capsule.
3. Anterior dislocation: Limit external rotation, extension, horizontal abduction
4. Anterior dislocation: Absolutely no combined abduction or external rotation until cleared by physician (8 to 16 weeks)
5. Posterior dislocation: Limit internal rotation and horizontal adduction

Phase I: 0 to 6 Weeks

1. Sleeping postures—no sleeping on the affected shoulder
2. 4.04 Bed Positioning-in immobilizer
   a. Semi-reclined with pillow support (Figure **5.08.3**)
   b. Supine (pillow supporting arm as needed)
   c. Side-lying quarter turn supine
3. Gentle PROM—no stretching
   a. Flexion, scaption, abduction, internal and external rotation in scapular plane (30 degrees abduction)
4. ROM ideas: all movements done in pain-free range
   a. 5.04.2 ROM: Shoulder, Pendulum, Passive
   b. 5.04.6 ROM: Pulleys; Shoulder Flexion, Scaption, and Abduction, Passive (only to tolerance)
   c. 5.09.3 ROM: Elbow Flexion and Extension, Active
   d. 5.09.5 ROM: Elbow Pronation and Supination, Passive and Active Assistive
   e. 5.14.1 ROM: Passive and Active Assisted Wrist and Finger Movements; Active Wrist Flexion/Extension
   f. 5.04.11 ROM: Wand/Cane; Shoulder Flexion and Scaption, Active Assistive
   g. 5.04.12 ROM: Wand/Cane; Shoulder Abduction, Active Assistive

5. Stretching ideas
    a. 2.02.3 Stretch: Self-Assisted Cervical Lateral Flexion (arm neutral)
    b. 2.02.7 Stretch: Cervical Flexion and Rotation (arm neutral)
6. Postural correction
    a. 5.03.3 Strengthen: Scapular Retraction and Variations (unilateral side-lying and bilateral seated only)
    b. 2.03.4 Strengthen: Isotonic; Chin Tuck
7. Strengthening ideas
    a. 5.03.4 Strengthen: Scapular Retraction, Arms by Sides
    b. 5.01.5 ROM: Scapular Elevation
    c. 5.01.6 ROM: Scapular Depression
    d. 5.07.1 Strengthen: Isometric; Shoulder, Other Hand Resists, 6-Way or 5.07.2 Strengthen: Isometric; Shoulder, Wall Resists, 5-Way
    e. Progress gradually to 5.07.5 Strengthen: Isometric; Shoulder External Rotation Multi-Angle Neutral, Doorway (within ROM precautions)
    f. 5.12.2 Strengthen: Isometric; Elbow Flexion
    g. 5.07.91 Reactive Neuromuscular Training and Variations, Shoulder (listed below)
        i. Rhythmic stabilization internal rotation/external rotation supine shoulder 30 degrees abducted (scaption plane) only
        ii. Rhythmic stabilization supine shoulder flexed or in scaption. Do only in scaption and applying only flexion and extension forces
    h. 5.07.61 Strengthen: Closed Kinetic Chain; Shoulder, Beginning Weightbearing, Progress to Push-Up Partial Weight (beginning weightbearing only)

Phase II

Patient may start Phase II when:
- Near full PROM; external rotation may still be limited
- Minimal pain
- Manual muscle tests of shoulder external rotation, internal rotation, flexion, and abduction are 4/5
- Baseline proprioception and dynamic stability

1. Continue gentle PROM—*no* stretching
2. ROM ideas (stay within pain-free range)
    a. 5.04.19 ROM: Shoulder Flexion and Saws, Ball Rolls, Active Assistive
    b. 5.04.23 ROM: Shoulder Flexion and Abduction, Table Slide, Active Assistive
    c. 5.04.13 ROM: Wand/Cane; Shoulder Internal Rotation, External Rotation, and Combined, Active Assistive (neutral variation only)
    d. 5.04.28 ROM: Shoulder Flexion, Active
    e. 5.04.34 ROM: Shoulder Scaption, Active
    f. 5.04.29 ROM: Shoulder Abduction, Active

g. 5.04.33 ROM: Shoulder Extension, Active (prone variation only and to neutral; do not raise arm above midline of torso)
    h. 5.04.36 ROM: Shoulder Internal Rotation and External Rotation, Active
    i. 5.04.35 ROM: Shoulder Scaption Figure 8s, Active
3. Scapular beginning movement and strengthening ideas
    a. 5.04.37 ROM: Side-Lying Shoulder Circles, Active
    b. 5.03.4 Strengthen: Scapular Retraction, Arms by Sides
4. Shoulder strengthening ideas
    a. 5.07.10 Strengthen: Isotonic; Shoulder Flexion
    b. 5.07.11 Strengthen: Isotonic; Shoulder Scaption (full can only)
    c. 5.07.12 Strengthen: Isotonic; Shoulder Abduction (to 90 degrees only)
    d. 5.07.22 Strengthen: Isotonic; Shoulder External Rotation (to 45 degrees only)
    e. 5.07.36 Strengthen: Isotonic; Resistance Band, Shoulder Flexion, Scaption, Abduction, and Variations (start by staying below shoulder level/90 degrees)
    f. 5.07.39 Strengthen: Isotonic; Resistance Band, Shoulder Internal Rotation and Variations (neutral)
    g. 5.07.41 Strengthen: Isotonic; Resistance Band, Shoulder External Rotation and Variations (neutral)
    h. 5.07.19 Strengthen: Isotonic; Shoulder, Horizontal Abduction, Bent Forward
    i. 5.07.61 Strengthen: Closed Kinetic Chain; Shoulder, Beginning Weightbearing, Progress to Push-Up Partial Weight
    j. 5.07.91 Reactive Neuromuscular Training and Variations, Shoulder (listed below)
        i. Rhythmic stabilization side-lying shoulder abducted
        ii. Rhythmic stabilization supine shoulder flexed
5. Elbow strengthening
    a. 5.12.10 Strengthen: Isotonic; Elbow Flexion, Curls
    b. Strengthen: Resistance Band, Tricep Push Down
6. Scapular strengthening ideas
    a. 5.07.24 Strengthen: Isotonic; Shoulder, Row (Prone)
    b. 5.03.6 Strengthen: Scapular Retraction, Arm Off Table
    c. 5.03.12 Strengthen: Resistance Band, Scapular Row and Variations (do not do wide row)
    d. 5.03.17 Strengthen: Resistance Band, Serratus Wall Slides
    e. 5.03.19 Strengthen: Resistance Band, Scapular "Vs"
    f. 5.03.18 Strengthen: Resistance Band, Scapular Clocks
    g. 5.03.5 Strengthen: Scapular Retraction, "T", "Y", and "I" and Variations

7. Advance to these exercises within this phase as patient strength and control improves.
   a. 5.04.1 ROM: Shoulder, Warm-Up, Upper Body Ergometer, Active Assistive
   b. 5.07.27 Strengthen: Isotonic; Posterior Cuff, 4-Way
   c. 5.07.38 Strengthen: Isotonic; Resistance Band, Shoulder Extension (keep humeral head from translating anteriorly; do not pass neutral [mid-line of torso])
   d. 5.03.13 Strengthen: Resistance Band, Scapular and Posterior Shoulder, Overhead Pull-down
   e. 5.03.14 Strengthen: Resistance Band, Scapular and Rotator Cuff, Retraction and External Rotation
   f. 5.03.15 Strengthen: Resistance Band, Scapular, Punch
   g. 5.03.16 Strengthen: Resistance Band, Scapular, Dynamic Hug
   h. 5.03.22 Strengthen: Scapular, Arm Lifts
   i. 5.07.39 Strengthen: Isotonic; Resistance Band, Shoulder Internal Rotation and Variations
   j. 5.07.41 Strengthen: Isotonic; Resistance Band, Shoulder External Rotation and Variations(no external rotation > 90 degrees)
8. Closed chain weightbearing ideas
   a. 5.07.67 Strengthen: Closed Kinetic Chain; Bodyblade, Shoulder Flexion, Scaption, and Abduction
   b. 5.07.58 Strengthen: Closed Kinetic Chain; Shoulder, Weight Shifts
   c. 5.07.60 Strengthen: Closed Kinetic Chain; Shoulder, Alternating Arm Lift
   d. 5.07.52 Strengthen: Exercise Ball, Shoulder, Push-Up, Hands on Ball
9. Core strengthening: abdominals, gluteals, lower back

Phase III

Patient may start Phase III when:
- Full pain-free ROM
- No pain or tenderness
- Good strength, proprioception, and dynamic stability

1. Stretching ideas
   a. 5.06.5 Stretch: Shoulder Horizontal Adductors, Doorway (no anterior movement of humeral head)
2. Shoulder strengthening ideas
   a. 5.07.25 Strengthen: Isotonic; Shoulder, Military Press (Prone)
   b. 5.07.28 Strengthen: Isotonic; Shoulder, Diagonal Lifts D1 and D2
   c. 5.07.39 Strengthen: Isotonic; Resistance Band, Shoulder Internal Rotation and Variations (move into 45- and 90-degree movements)
   d. 5.07.41 Strengthen: Isotonic; Resistance Band, Shoulder External Rotation and Variations (move into 45- and [with caution] 90-degree movements)
   e. 5.07.34 Strengthen: Isotonic; Resistance Band and Machine, Shoulder, Lat Pull-Down
   f. 5.07.42 Strengthen: Isotonic; Resistance Band, Shoulder, Combination Movements PNF D1 and D2
   g. 5.07.47 Strengthen: Isotonic; Resistance Band, Shoulder Pull-Back
   h. 5.07.64 Strengthen: Closed Kinetic Chain; Shoulder, Table Top Push-Pull
   i. 5.03.21 Strengthen: Scapular, Push-Up Plus (Advanced)
   j. 5.07.66 Strengthen: Closed Kinetic Chain; Stairmaster, Shoulder
   k. 5.07.67 Strengthen: Closed Kinetic Chain; Bodyblade, Shoulder Flexion, Scaption, and Abduction
   l. 5.07.68 Strengthen: Closed Kinetic Chain; Bodyblade, Shoulder Internal Rotation and External Rotation
   m. 5.07.69 Strengthen: Closed Kinetic Chain; Bodyblade, Shoulder, D1 and D2
   n. 5.07.71 Strengthen: Closed Kinetic Chain; Shoulder, Inverted Row
   o. 5.07.79 Plyometrics/Dynamic: Shoulder, Wall Dribbles
   p. 5.07.80 Plyometrics/Dynamic: Shoulder, Ball Toss, Overhead
   q. 5.07.81 Plyometrics/Dynamic: Shoulder, Chest Pass
   r. 5.07.82 Plyometrics/Dynamic: Shoulder, Bench Press/Floor Throws
   s. 55.07.83 Plyometrics/Dynamic: Shoulder, Two-Handed Side Throw
   t. 5.07.84 Plyometrics/Dynamic: Shoulder, 90/90 Throw (start cautiously!)
   u. 5.07.85 Plyometrics/Dynamic: Shoulder, Multidirectional Catch/Throw
   v. 5.07.86 Plyometrics/Dynamic: Shoulder, Ball Toss, Overhead and Backwards
   w. 5.07.87 Plyometrics/Dynamic: Shoulder, Push-Up
   x. 5.07.88 Plyometrics/Dynamic: Shoulder, Slams
   y. 5.07.89 Plyometrics/Dynamic: Shoulder, Ball Squat, Push-Press
   z. 5.07.90 Plyometrics/Dynamic: Shoulder, Push-Offs
   aa. 5.07.91 Reactive Neuromuscular Training and Variations, Shoulder (move into sports positions)
   ab. 5.07.92 Shoulder, Throwing Progression

5.08.9 TOTAL SHOULDER ARTHROPLASTY AND REVERSE TOTAL SHOULDER ARTHROPLASTY DISCUSSION

Total shoulder arthroplasty (TSA) is a procedure used to replace the diseased or damaged ball and socket joint of the shoulder with a prosthesis made of polyethylene and metal components. The "ball" is the proximal head of the humerus and the "socket" refers to the concave depression of the scapula referred to as the glenoid. A reverse TSA refers to a similar procedure in which the prosthetic ball and socket that make up the joint are reversed to treat certain complex shoulder problems (Roussel, Kelley, Marek, & Hernandez, n.d.). The reverse TSA offers a salvage-type solution to the problem of failed hemiarthroplasty due to glenoid arthritis and RC deficiency. In cases of severe proximal humeral bone deficiency, reverse TSA with a proximal humeral allograft may improve patient satisfaction (Levy, Frankle, Mighell, & Pupello, 2007). Shoulder replacement surgery is a reliable procedure that provides predictable results in patients with all types of glenohumeral arthritis. When performed by an experienced surgeon for the right indications, and with appropriate physical therapy, dramatic improvements in pain and function are seen in the majority of patients. With the recent availability of the reverse prosthesis, even patients with RC deficiency may have pain relief and restoration of shoulder function after

reverse TSA (Kaback, Green, & Blaine, 2012). Mulieri et al. (2010) found similar outcomes in patients that received a standard physical therapy program as compared to had a home-based, physician-guided physical therapy program after TSA and concluded a home-based, physician-guided therapy program may provide adequate rehabilitation after TSA, allowing for a reduction in cost for the overall procedure (Mulieri et al., 2010). However, the progression of patient through the phases of rehab must be continually modified based on their underlying pathology and clinical presentation. Many protocols will present with time frames between phases which should only be used as a guideline for patient. The physical therapist should continuously work alongside the referring surgeon in developing each patient's specific rehabilitation protocol, with the focus on meeting certain impairment and functional criteria before progressing on to the next stage. Patient education before and after the surgery is vital as patients must know to expect differing levels of postoperative function depending on many factors such as the type of surgical implant, status of the remaining RC, and bone stock of the glenoid and humeral head (Roussel et al., n.d.).

5.08.10 TOTAL SHOULDER ARTHROPLASTY AND REVERSE TOTAL SHOULDER ARTHROPLASTY PROTOCOL

General protocol guidelines adapted from Wilcox et al. (2005).

Precautions: Postoperative

1. Keep incision clean and dry
2. Ensure compliance with sling if prescribed usually 3 to 4 weeks
3. In supine positioning, prop arm with towel roll or pillow to avoid shoulder extension
4. No AROM especially behind the back
5. No lifting
6. No excessive stretching or sudden shoulder movements
7. No supporting weight with the affected shoulder
8. No driving for 3 weeks

Postoperative Day 1

1. Eliminate any activity that causes an increase in symptoms
2. Sleeping postures—sleeping on the affected shoulder can aggravate surgery site. Suggested postures include:
   a. 4.04 Bed Positioning
      i. Semi-reclined with pillow support
      ii. Supine (pillow supporting arm as needed)
      iii. Side-lying quarter turn supine
3. PROM by therapist: flexion to tolerance, external rotation in scapular plane (usually around 30 degrees)—no undue stress on anterior capsule, internal rotation to chest
4. ROM ideas
   a. 5.04.3 ROM: Shoulder, Cradle Rocks, Passive
   b. 5.04.2 ROM: Shoulder, Pendulum, Passive
   c. 5.09.3 ROM: Elbow Flexion and Extension, Active
   d. 5.09.5 ROM: Elbow Pronation and Supination, Passive and Active Assistive
   e. 5.14.1 ROM: Passive and Active Assisted Wrist and Finger Movements (active wrist flexion/extension)
5. Stretching ideas for neck

    a. 2.02.3 Stretch: Self-Assisted Cervical Lateral Flexion (gentle)

    b. 2.02.7 Stretch: Cervical Flexion and Rotation (gentle)

6. Postural correction

    a. 2.03.4 Strengthen: Isotonic; Chin Tuck

Early Phase I (Out of Hospital)

1. Postural correction

    a. 5.03.4 Strengthen: Scapular Retraction, Arms by Sides

2. Continue previous exercises

Late Phase I

1. PROM by therapist goals: flexion and abduction 90 degrees, external rotation in scapular plane (30 degrees abduction) 45 degrees, internal rotation in scapular plane (30 degrees abduction) 70 degrees

Phase II: Early Strengthening—Not to Begin Before 4 to 6 Weeks Postoperative

1. Sling still used for sleeping, removed gradually for short periods throughout the day, eventually weaning off sling over 2 weeks; continue with sleeping position recommendations.

2. Continue no lifting anything heavier than a coffee cup, no supporting body weight with the affected arm and no sudden jerking movements.

3. PROM and AAROM, increasing range as tolerated

4. ROM and AAROM flexion, scaption, abduction

    a. 5.04.6 ROM: Pulleys; Shoulder Flexion, Scaption, and Abduction, Passive

    b. 5.04.5 ROM: Shoulder Girdle Circles, Active Assistive

    c. 5.04.11 ROM: Wand/Cane; Shoulder Flexion and Scaption, Active Assistive

    d. 5.04.12 ROM: Wand/Cane; Shoulder Abduction, Active Assistive

    e. 5.04.13 ROM: Wand/Cane; Shoulder Internal Rotation, External Rotation, and Combined, Active Assistive (neutral variation only)

    f. 5.04.29 ROM: Shoulder Abduction, Active

    g. 5.04.28 ROM: Shoulder Flexion, Active

    h. 5.04.34 ROM: Shoulder Scaption, Active

    i. 5.04.36 ROM: Shoulder Internal Rotation and External Rotation, Active

    j. 5.04.23 ROM: Shoulder Flexion and Abduction, Table Slide, Active Assistive

    k. 5.04.21 ROM: Shoulder Flexion and Abduction, Towel Slide, Active Assistive

    l. 5.04.22 ROM: Shoulder Flexion and Abduction, Wall Walks, Active Assistive

    m. 5.04.20 ROM: Shoulder Flexion, Wall Slide, Active Assistive

    n. 5.04.18 ROM: Wand/Cane; Shoulder, Horizontal Abduction and Adduction, Active Assistive (do not push horizontal abduction)

5. Strengthening ideas (beginner in acute phase)

    a. 5.07.1 Strengthen: Isometric; Shoulder, Other Hand Resists, 6-Way or 5.07.2 Strengthen: Isometric; Shoulder, Wall Resists, 5-Way (sub maximal 50% to 75% contraction intensity)

6. Continue wrist/forearm exercises

7. Elbow strengthening

    a. 5.12.10 Strengthen: Isotonic; Elbow Flexion, Curls (high repetitions, low weights)

8. Scapular beginning movement and strengthening

    a. 5.03.3 Strengthen: Scapular Retraction and Variations (unilateral side-lying and bilateral seated only)

    b. 5.01.5 ROM: Scapular Elevation

    c. 5.01.6 ROM: Scapular Depression

    d. Late Phase II may begin advancing scapular exercises:

        i. 5.03.4 Strengthen: Scapular Retraction, Arms by Sides

        ii. 5.07.24 Strengthen: Isotonic; Shoulder, Row (Prone)

        iii. 5.03.6 Strengthen: Scapular Retraction, Arm Off Table

9. Rhythmic stabilization

    a. Rhythmic stabilization internal rotation/external rotation side-lying shoulder neutral

    b. Rhythmic stabilization internal rotation/external rotation supine shoulder neutral

    c. Rhythmic stabilization supine shoulder flexed or in scaption:

10. Early weightbearing

    a. 5.07.61 Strengthen: Closed Kinetic Chain; Shoulder, Beginning Weightbearing, Progress to Push-Up Partial Weight (beginning weightbearing only)

Phase III: Moderate Strengthening—Not to Begin Before 6 Weeks Postoperative

Patient may start Phase III when:

- Tolerating Phase II program
- PROM flexion 140 degrees
- PROM abduction 120 degrees
- PROM external rotation in scapular plane 60 degrees
- PROM internal rotation in scapular plane 70 degrees
- Active shoulder elevation with good mechanics to 100 degrees

1. Precautions

    a. No lifting more than 3 kg (6 lbs)

    b. No sudden jerking movements

    c. No sudden lifting or pushing movements

2. ROM and AAROM increasing range as tolerated
   a. Early Phase III: initiate gentle
      i. 5.04.14 ROM: Wand/Cane/Strap; Shoulder Internal Rotation Behind Back, Active Assistive
      ii. 5.04.7 ROM: Pulleys; Shoulder Internal Rotation, Passive
   b. Late Phase III: allow patient to actively internal rotate behind the back without assist
      i. 5.04.14 ROM: Wand/Cane/Strap; Shoulder Internal Rotation Behind Back, Active Assistive (modified)
3. Proprioceptive training
   a. 5.01.4 ROM: Scapular Circles and Alphabet Ball on Wall
   b. 5.04.35 ROM: Shoulder Scaption Figure 8s, Active
   c. 5.04.37 ROM: Side-Lying Shoulder Circles, Active
4. Shoulder strengthening
   a. 5.07.10 Strengthen: Isotonic; Shoulder Flexion (beginner supine only 0.5 to 1.5 kg [1 to 3 lbs])
   b. 5.07.39 Strengthen: Isotonic; Resistance Band, Shoulder Internal Rotation and Variations (supine in 30 degrees abduction only)
   c. 5.07.41 Strengthen: Isotonic; Resistance Band, Shoulder External Rotation and Variations (supine in 30 degrees abduction only)
   d. Start in Late Phase III: 5.07.36 Strengthen: Isotonic; Resistance Band, Shoulder Flexion, Scaption, Abduction, and Variations (start by staying below shoulder level/90 degrees)

Phase IV: Advanced Strengthening—Not to Begin Before 6 Weeks Postoperative

Patient may start Phase III when:
- Tolerating Phase III program
- AROM flexion 140 degrees supine
- AROM abduction 120 degrees supine
- AROM external rotation in scapular plane 60 degrees supine
- AROM internal rotation in scapular plane 70 degrees supine
- Active shoulder elevation with good mechanics to 120 degrees

1. Precautions
   a. Avoid exercises and functional activities that place stress on anterior capsule (no combined external rotation with > 80 degrees abduction)
2. Closed chain for glenohumeral stabilization
   a. 5.07.67 Strengthen: Closed Kinetic Chain; Bodyblade, Shoulder Flexion, Scaption, and Abduction
   b. 5.07.58 Strengthen: Closed Kinetic Chain; Shoulder, Weight Shifts
   c. 5.07.60 Strengthen: Closed Kinetic Chain; Shoulder, Alternating Arm Lift

3. Shoulder strengthening ideas
   a. 5.07.10 Strengthen: Isotonic; Shoulder Flexion
   b. 5.07.12 Strengthen: Isotonic; Shoulder Abduction
   c. 5.07.11 Strengthen: Isotonic; Shoulder Scaption
   d. 5.07.22 Strengthen: Isotonic; Shoulder External Rotation
   e. 5.07.21 Strengthen: Isotonic; Shoulder Internal Rotation
   f. 5.07.13 Strengthen: Isotonic; Shoulder Extension
   g. 5.07.19 Strengthen: Isotonic; Shoulder, Horizontal Abduction, Bent Forward
   h. 5.07.20 Strengthen: Isotonic; Shoulder, Horizontal Abduction, Deceleration Emphasis
   i. 5.07.24 Strengthen: Isotonic; Shoulder, Row (Prone)
   j. 5.07.27 Strengthen: Isotonic; Posterior Cuff, 4-Way
   k. 5.07.25 Strengthen: Isotonic; Shoulder, Military Press (Prone) (avoid excessive external rotation)
   l. 5.07.28 Strengthen: Isotonic; Shoulder, Diagonal Lifts D1 and D2
   m. 5.07.36 Strengthen: Isotonic; Resistance Band, Shoulder Flexion, Scaption, Abduction, and Variations (start by staying below shoulder level/90 degrees)
   n. 5.07.39 Strengthen: Isotonic; Resistance Band, Shoulder Internal Rotation and Variations (neutral standing)
   o. 5.07.41 Strengthen: Isotonic; Resistance Band, Shoulder External Rotation and Variations (neutral standing)
   p. 5.07.34 Strengthen: Isotonic; Resistance Band and Machine, Shoulder, Lat Pull-Down
   q. 5.07.38 Strengthen: Isotonic; Resistance Band, Shoulder Extension
   r. 5.07.42 Strengthen: Isotonic; Resistance Band, Shoulder, Combination Movements PNF D1 and D2
   s. 5.07.47 Strengthen: Isotonic; Resistance Band, Shoulder Pull-Back
   t. 5.07.64 Strengthen: Closed Kinetic Chain; Shoulder, Table Top Push-Pull
   u. 5.07.61 Strengthen: Closed Kinetic Chain; Shoulder, Beginning Weightbearing, Progress to Push-Up Partial Weight
4. Scapular strengthening ideas
   a. 5.03.5 Strengthen: Scapular Retraction, "T", "Y", and "I" and Variations
   b. 5.03.13 Strengthen: Resistance Band, Scapular and Posterior Shoulder, Overhead Pull-down
   c. 5.03.14 Strengthen: Resistance Band, Scapular and Rotator Cuff, Retraction and External Rotation
   d. 5.03.15 Strengthen: Resistance Band, Scapular, Punch
   e. 5.03.16 Strengthen: Resistance Band, Scapular, Dynamic Hug

    f. 5.03.17 Strengthen: Resistance Band, Serratus Wall Slides

    g. 5.03.18 Strengthen: Resistance Band, Scapular Clocks

    h. 5.03.19 Strengthen: Resistance Band, Scapular "Vs"

    i. 5.03.22 Strengthen: Arm Lifts

Late Phase IV: Typically 4 to 6 Months Postoperative

- Patient is able to maintain nonpainful AROM
- Maximized functional use of UE
- Maximized muscular strength, power and endurance
- Return to recreational hobbies (i.e., gardening, sports, golf doubles tennis)

5.08.11 ROTATOR CUFF TEARS DISCUSSION

RC tears are a common cause of shoulder pain and disability in adult. Despite varied regional distribution, RC tears have been shown to be prevalent in up to 39% of asymptomatic individuals and 64% of symptomatic individuals. Increasing age, trauma, limb dominance if caused by repetitive use, smoking status, hypercholesterolemia, posture, and occupational demands have all been associated with RC tearing (Sambandam, Khanna, Gul, & Mounasamy, 2015). Additionally, in the older population, RC lesions are a natural correlate and are often present with no clinical symptoms.

Where's the Evidence?

Cadaveric studies of 90 asymptomatic adults aged 30 to 99 years revealed the prevalence of partial- or full-thickness tears increasing markedly after 50 years of age, present in over 50% of dominant shoulders in the seventh decade and in 80% of subjects over 80 years of age (Milgrom, Schaffler, Gilbert, & van Holsbeeck, 1995).

Treatment should be based on clinical findings and not on the results of imaging. Early diagnosis of patients that are asymptomatic and/or have pain and decreasing shoulder strength and function can lead to earlier conservative management. This may prevention early micro tearing and partial tears from progressing to full thickness tearing. Once the tear is full thickness, pathological changes due to muscle retraction, fatty infiltration, and muscle atrophy occur reducing tendon elasticity and viability as well as glenohumeral joint degenerative adaptations. Physical therapy along with activity modifications, anti-inflammatory and analgesic medications form the pillars of nonoperative treatment (Sambandam et al., 2015). While conservative measures are successful in elderly patients with minimal lesions and demands, regular monitoring helps in isolating the surgical candidate. Early surgery should be considered in younger, healthier, active and symptomatic patients. Lower grades of tears do well with debridement alone while more severe lesions warrant a repair. Arthroscopic double-row repairs are superior in patients with massive tears. Satisfactory results are obtained with timely diagnosis and execution of the appropriate treatment modality (Sambandam et al., 2015).

Elderly patients with minimal functional demands may be managed conservatively to avoid unnecessary surgical risks. However, nonoperative treated full-thickness tears tend to increase in size, especially in the older population.

Where's the Evidence?

Maman et al. (2009) assessed 59 shoulders in 54 patients with a mean age of 58.8 years with RC tears on initial MRI who had been managed nonoperatively. All had MRI scans acquired 6 months or more after the initial study. The progression of RC tears was associated with age, anatomical and associated parameters, follow-up time, and structural and other MRI findings. More than one-half of the 33 full-thickness tears increased in size compared with 8% of the 26 partial-thickness tears. Only 17% of the 35 tears in patients who were 60 years old or less deteriorated compared with 54% of the 24 tears in patients who were more than 60 years old (Maman et al., 2009). Safran et al. (2011) evaluated the size change of nonoperatively treated full-thickness RC tears over 2 to 3 years of follow-up for patients 60-years-old or younger who had a full-thickness RC tear equal to or larger than 5 mm. At 2 to 3 years after initial imaging ultrasound examination, a repeat ultrasound examination was performed by the same ultrasonographer looking for change in RC tear size, 43% had not changed and 8% decreased in size. They concluded that full-thickness RC tears tend to increase in size in about half of patients aged 60 years or younger and recommended patients treated nonoperatively should be routinely monitored for tear size increase, especially if they remain symptomatic (Safran et al., 2011).

Regular monitoring helps in isolating patients who require surgical interventions in younger, active and symptomatic, healthy patients.

Arthroscopic repair of small and medium full-thickness RC tears results in reliable improvements in clinical outcomes and a high rate of tendon integrity using a double-row repair technique in patients under the age of 65 years. Surgery is followed by rehabilitation and recommendations for postoperative rehabilitation include; exercise therapy, CPM machines and aquatic therapy. There is no apparent advantage or disadvantage of early PROM compared with immobilization with regard to healing or functional outcome.

Currently, there is uncertainty in the literature as to what constitutes best postsurgical rehabilitation. No one rehabilitation protocol has been found to be superior to another (Thomson, Jukes, & Lewis, 2015; Yi, Villacis, Yalamanchili, & Hatch, 2015). Lee et al.'s (2012) study found that pain, ROM, muscle strength, and function all significantly improved after arthroscopic RC repair, regardless of early postoperative rehabilitation protocols. However, they also found that aggressive early motion may increase the possibility of anatomic failure at the RC. They recommended a gentle rehabilitation protocol with limits in ROM and exercise times after arthroscopic RC repair would be better for tendon healing without taking any substantial risks (Lee et al., 2012).

Numerous rehabilitation protocols for the management of RC disease are based primarily on anecdotal clinical observation. Millett et al. (2006) utilized the available literature on shoulder rehabilitation, in conjunction with clinical observation taking into consideration the underlying tissue quality and structural integrity of the RC, and compiled into a set of rehabilitation guidelines. The four phases of rehabilitation are designed for maintaining and protecting the repair in the immediate postoperative period, followed by progression from early PROM through return to preoperative levels of function. These phases are outlined below (Millett et al., 2006).

5.08.12 ROTATOR CUFF TEARS PROTOCOL

General protocol guidelines adapted from Millet et al. (2006).

Phase I: Immediate Postoperative 0 to 6 Weeks

1. Goals
   a. Maintain and protect integrity of repair
   b. Gradually increase PROM
   c. Diminish pain and inflammation
   d. Prevent muscular inhibition
   e. Become independent with modified ADLs
2. Precautions
   a. Maintain arm in abduction sling or brace; remove only for exercise
   b. No shoulder AROM
   c. No lifting of objects
   d. No shoulder motion behind back (watch donning bra, belt)
   e. No excessive stretching or sudden movements
   f. No supporting of any weight on the affected arm (lifting of body weight by hands)
   g. Keep incision clean and dry

Days 1 to 6

1. Sleeping postures—*no* sleeping on the affected shoulder
   a. 4.04 Bed Positioning-in immobilizer
      i. Semi-reclined with pillow support (**5.08.3**)
      ii. Supine (pillow supporting arm as needed)
      iii. Side-lying quarter turn supine
2. ROM ideas: all movements done in pain-free range
   a. 5.04.2 ROM: Shoulder, Pendulum, Passive
   b. 5.04.3 ROM: Shoulder, Cradle Rocks, Passive
   c. 5.09.3 ROM: Elbow Flexion and Extension, Active
   d. 5.09.5 ROM: Elbow Pronation and Supination, Passive and Active Assistive
   e. 5.14.1 ROM: Passive and Active Assisted Wrist and Finger Movements (active wrist flexion/extension)
3. Postural correction
   a. 5.03.3 Strengthen: Scapular Retraction and Variations (unilateral side-lying and bilateral seated only arm in immobilizer; do not perform for at least 6 weeks if subscapularis tear/repair)
   b. 2.03.4 Strengthen: Isotonic; Chin Tuck

Where's the Evidence?

Based on EMG data in normal volunteers performing scapular clock, elevation, depression, protraction, and retraction exercises, upper subscapularis activity was uniformly high at 40% to 63% MVC. Smith et al. (2006) recommended that all exercises studied should be avoided after subscapularis repair.

---

4. Stretching ideas
   a. 2.02.3 Stretch: Self-Assisted Cervical Lateral Flexion (arm neutral/immobilizer)
   b. 2.02.7 Stretch: Cervical Flexion and Rotation (arm neutral/immobilizer)

Days 7 to 28: Continuing Previous Exercises

1. PROM to tolerance: pain-free performed supine
   a. Flexion to 90 degrees
   b. External rotation in scapular plane < 35 degrees
   c. Internal rotation in scapular plane to chest
2. Overall conditioning
   a. Walking, recumbent bike (no arm use)
   b. Pool therapy (no arm use)

Weeks 5 to 6

1. Discontinue full-time immobilizer between 4 to 6 weeks; slowly wean use for comfort only.
2. PROM to tolerance: pain-free performed supine until near full ROM at week 6 (no aggressive PROM in first 6 weeks); gentle scapular and glenohumeral mobs
3. AAROM
   a. 5.04.6 ROM: Pulleys; Shoulder Flexion, Scaption, and Abduction, Passive
   b. 5.04.11 ROM: Wand/Cane; Shoulder Flexion and Scaption, Active Assistive
   c. 5.04.12 ROM: Wand/Cane; Shoulder Abduction, Active Assistive (supine)
   d. 5.04.13 ROM: Wand/Cane; Shoulder Internal Rotation, External Rotation, and Combined, Active Assistive (supine; neutral variation only)
4. Scapular strengthening
   a. 5.07.24 Strengthen: Isotonic; Shoulder, Row (Prone) (extension focus to torso only)
5. Pool therapy okay for light AROM exercises

Phase II: Protection and Active Motion Postoperative 6 to 12 Weeks

1. Goals
   a. Maintain and protect integrity of repair; allow healing and do not overstress healing tissue
   b. Gradually restore full PROM (weeks 4 to 5)
   c. Diminish pain and inflammation

2. Precautions:
   a. No lifting of objects
   b. No excessive shoulder motion behind back
   c. No sudden jerking movements
   d. No supporting of any weight on the affected arm (lifting of body weight by hands)
   e. No UBE (arm bike)

Weeks 6 to 8

1. PROM
2. AROM ideas (stay within pain-free range)
   a. 5.04.19 ROM: Shoulder Flexion and Saws, Ball Rolls, Active Assistive
   b. 5.04.23 ROM: Shoulder Flexion and Abduction, Table Slide, Active Assistive
   c. 5.04.28 ROM: Shoulder Flexion, Active
   d. 5.04.34 ROM: Shoulder Scaption, Active
   e. 5.04.29 ROM: Shoulder Abduction, Active
   f. 5.04.36 ROM: Shoulder Internal Rotation and External Rotation, Active
   g. 5.04.35 ROM: Shoulder Scaption Figure 8s, Active
3. Strengthening ideas
   a. 5.03.4 Strengthen: Scapular Retraction, Arms by Sides
   b. 5.01.5 ROM: Scapular Elevation
   c. 5.01.6 ROM: Scapular Depression
   d. 5.07.1 Strengthen: Isometric; Shoulder, Other Hand Resists, 6-Way or 5.07.2 Strengthen: Isometric; Shoulder, Wall Resists, 5-Way
   e. 5.12.2 Strengthen: Isometric; Elbow Flexion
   f. 5.07.61 Strengthen: Closed Kinetic Chain; Shoulder, Beginning Weightbearing, Progress to Push-Up Partial Weight (beginning weightbearing only)

Phase III: Early Strengthening

May progress to Phase III once full AROM achieved postoperatively as early as 10 to 16 weeks (overlaps Phase II)

Weeks 10 to 14

1. Goals
   a. Maintain and protect integrity of repair; allow healing and do not overstress healing tissue
   b. Maintain full PROM
   c. Full AROM weeks 10 to 12
   d. Gradually restore strength, power, endurance
   e. Optimize neuromuscular control
   f. Return to functional activities
2. Precautions
   a. No lifting of objects > 2 kg (5 lbs)
   b. No excessive shoulder motion behind back

c. No sudden jerking movements

d. No sudden lifting or pushing movements

e. No overhead lifting

f. No UBE (arm bike)

3. Shoulder strengthening ideas

    a. 5.07.91 Reactive Neuromuscular Training and Variations, Shoulder (listed below)

        i. Rhythmic stabilization internal rotation/external rotation supine shoulder 30 degrees abducted (scaption plane) only

        ii. Rhythmic stabilization supine shoulder flexed or in scaption—do only in scaption and applying only flexion and extension forces

    b. 5.07.10 Strengthen: Isotonic; Shoulder Flexion

    c. 5.07.11 Strengthen: Isotonic; Shoulder Scaption (full can only)

    d. 5.07.12 Strengthen: Isotonic; Shoulder Abduction (to 90 degrees only if able to do without shoulder shrug/hiking)

    e. 5.07.22 Strengthen: Isotonic; Shoulder External Rotation

    f. 5.07.36 Strengthen: Isotonic; Resistance Band, Shoulder Flexion, Scaption, Abduction, and Variations (start by staying below shoulder level/90 degrees)

    g. 5.07.39 Strengthen: Isotonic; Resistance Band, Shoulder Internal Rotation and Variations (neutral)

    h. 5.07.41 Strengthen: Isotonic; Resistance Band, Shoulder External Rotation and Variations (neutral)

4. Elbow strengthening

    a. 5.12.10 Strengthen: Isotonic; Elbow Flexion, Curls

    b. Strengthen: Resistance Band, Tricep Push Down

5. Scapular strengthening ideas

    a. 5.03.6 Strengthen: Scapular Retraction, Arm Off Table

    b. 5.07.24 Strengthen: Isotonic; Shoulder, Row (Prone) (horizontal abduction focus to shoulder height only)

6. Weeks 12 to 14: initiate light functional activities

    a. 5.07.73 Functional: Shoulder, Rolling Dough

    b. 5.07.74 Functional: Shoulder, Rhythmic Touch, Finger to Nose/Face

    c. 5.07.75 Functional: Shoulder, Window Washing

    d. 5.07.76 Functional: Shoulder, Peg Board

    e. 5.07.78 Functional: Shoulder, Folding

7. Week 14 to 16: advance fundamental shoulder exercises

Phase IV: Advanced Strengthening Postoperative Weeks 16 to 22

1. Goals

    a. Maintain full AROM

    b. Improve strength, power, endurance

    c. Advanced conditioning for enhanced functional use

    d. Return to full functional activities

2. Advance to these exercises within this phase as patient strength and control improves

    a. 5.07.24 Strengthen: Isotonic; Shoulder, Row (Prone)

    b. 5.03.12 Strengthen: Resistance Band, Scapular Row and Variations

    c. 5.03.17 Strengthen: Resistance Band, Serratus Wall Slides

    d. 5.03.19 Strengthen: Resistance Band, Scapular "Vs"

    e. 5.03.18 Strengthen: Resistance Band, Scapular Clocks

    f. 5.03.5 Strengthen: Scapular Retraction, "T", "Y", and "I" and Variations

    g. 5.07.27 Strengthen: Isotonic; Posterior Cuff, 4-Way

    h. 5.07.38 Strengthen: Isotonic; Resistance Band, Shoulder Extension (keep humeral head from translating anteriorly; do not pass neutral [midline of torso]).

    i. 5.03.13 Strengthen: Resistance Band, Scapular and Posterior Shoulder, Overhead Pull-down

    j. 5.03.14 Strengthen: Resistance Band, Scapular and Rotator Cuff, Retraction and External Rotation

    k. 5.03.15 Strengthen: Resistance Band, Scapular, Punch

    l. 5.03.16 Strengthen: Resistance Band, Scapular, Dynamic Hug

    m. 5.03.22 Strengthen: Scapular, Arm Lifts

    n. 5.07.39 Strengthen: Isotonic; Resistance Band, Shoulder Internal Rotation and Variations

    o. 5.07.41 Strengthen: Isotonic; Resistance Band, Shoulder External Rotation and Variations

    p. 5.07.91 Reactive Neuromuscular Training and Variations, Shoulder (listed below)

        i. Rhythmic stabilization side-lying shoulder abducted

        ii. Rhythmic stabilization supine shoulder flexed

3. Closed chain weightbearing ideas

    a. 5.07.67 Strengthen: Closed Kinetic Chain; Bodyblade, Shoulder Flexion, Scaption, and Abduction

  b. 5.07.58 Strengthen: Closed Kinetic Chain; Shoulder, Weight Shifts

  c. 5.07.60 Strengthen: Closed Kinetic Chain; Shoulder, Alternating Arm Lift

  d. 5.07.52 Strengthen: Exercise Ball, Shoulder, Push-Up, Hands on Ball

4. Core strengthening: abdominals, gluteals, lower back

  a. 5.06.5 Stretch: Shoulder Horizontal Adductors, Doorway (no anterior movement of humeral head)

  b. 5.05.9 Self-Joint Mobilization/Stretch: Posterior Capsule Stretch, Crossover

5. Shoulder strengthening ideas: advanced dependent on patient age and functional demands.

  a. 5.07.25 Strengthen: Isotonic; Shoulder, Military Press (Prone)

  b. 5.07.28 Strengthen: Isotonic; Shoulder, Diagonal Lifts D1 and D2

  c. 5.07.39 Strengthen: Isotonic; Resistance Band, Shoulder Internal Rotation and Variations (move into 45- and 90-degree movements)

  d. 5.07.41 Strengthen: Isotonic; Resistance Band, Shoulder External Rotation and Variations (move into 45- and [with caution] 90-degree movements)

  e. 5.07.34 Strengthen: Isotonic; Resistance Band and Machine, Shoulder, Lat Pull-Down

  f. 5.07.42 Strengthen: Isotonic; Resistance Band, Shoulder, Combination Movements PNF D1 and D2

  g. 5.07.47 Strengthen: Isotonic; Resistance Band, Shoulder Pull-Back

  h. 5.07.64 Strengthen: Closed Kinetic Chain; Shoulder, Table Top Push-Pull

  i. 5.03.21 Strengthen: Scapular, Push-Up Plus (Advanced)

  j. 5.07.66 Strengthen: Closed Kinetic Chain; Stairmaster, Shoulder

  k. 5.07.67 Strengthen: Closed Kinetic Chain; Bodyblade, Shoulder Flexion, Scaption, and Abduction

  l. 5.07.68 Strengthen: Closed Kinetic Chain; Bodyblade, Shoulder Internal Rotation and External Rotation

  m. 5.07.71 Strengthen: Closed Kinetic Chain; Shoulder, Inverted Row

  n. 5.07.79 Plyometrics/Dynamic: Shoulder, Wall Dribbles

  o. 5.07.80 Plyometrics/Dynamic: Shoulder, Ball Toss, Overhead

  p. 5.07.81 Plyometrics/Dynamic: Shoulder, Chest Pass

  q. 5.07.82 Plyometrics/Dynamic: Shoulder, Bench Press/Floor Throws

  r. 5.07.83 Plyometrics/Dynamic: Shoulder, Two-Handed Side Throw

  s. 5.07.84 Plyometrics/Dynamic: Shoulder, 90/90 Throw (*start cautiously*)

  t. 5.07.85 Plyometrics/Dynamic: Shoulder, Multidirectional Catch/Throw

  u. 5.07.86 Plyometrics/Dynamic: Shoulder, Ball Toss, Overhead and Backwards

  v. 5.07.87 Plyometrics/Dynamic: Shoulder, Push-Up

  w. 5.07.88 Plyometrics/Dynamic: Shoulder, Slams

  x. 5.07.89 Plyometrics/Dynamic: Shoulder, Ball Squat, Push-Press

  y. 5.07.90 Plyometrics/Dynamic: Shoulder, Push-Offs

  z. 5.07.91 Reactive Neuromuscular Training and Variations, Shoulder (move into sports positions)

  aa. 5.07.92 Shoulder, Throwing Progression

REFERENCES

Atef, A., El-Tantawy, A., Gad, H., & Hefeda, M. (2016). Prevalence of associated injuries after anterior shoulder dislocation: A prospective study. *International Orthopedics, 40*(3), 519-524.

Camargo, P. R., Alburquerque-Sendín, F., Avila, M. A., Haik, M. N., Vieira, A., & Salvini, T. F. (2015). Effects of stretching and strengthening exercises, with and without manual therapy, on scapular kinematics, function, and pain in individuals with shoulder impingement: A randomized controlled trial. *Journal of Orthopedic and Sports Physical Therapy, 45*(12), 984-997.

Chester, R., Smith, T. O., Hooper, L., & Dixon, J. (2010). The impact of subacromial impingement syndrome on muscle activity patterns of the shoulder complex: A systematic review of electromyographic studies. *BMC Musculoskeletal Disorders, 11*, 45.

Chopp, J. N., O'Neill, J. M., Hurley, K., & Dickerson, C. R. (2010). Superior humeral head migration occurs after a protocol designed to fatigue the rotator cuff: A radiographic analysis. *Journal of Shoulder and Elbow Surgery, 19*(8), 1137-1144.

Cools, A. M., Borms, D., Castelein, B., Vanderstukken, F., & Johansson, F. R. (2016). Evidence-based rehabilitation of athletes with glenohumeral instability. *Knee Surgery, Sports Traumatology, Arthroscopy, 24*(2), 382-389.

Cote, M. P., Wojcik, K. E., Gomlinski, G., & Mazzocca, A. D. (2010). Rehabilitation of acromioclavicular joint separations: operative and nonoperative considerations. *Clinics in Sports Medicine, 29*(2), 213-228.

Culp, L. B., & Romani, W. A. (2006). Physical therapist examination, evaluation, and intervention following the surgical reconstruction of a grade III acromioclavicular joint separation. *Physical Therapy, 86*(6), 857-869.

De Dobbeleer, M., Hennebel, L., Lowe, R., Killian, B., & Pagare, V. (2016). Acromioclavicular disorders. *Physiopedia.* Retrieved from http://www.physio-pedia.com/Acromioclavicular_Joint_Disorders

De Strijcker, D., Drinkard, D., Van Haver, E., Lowe, R., & Brachotte, F. (2016). Subacromial impingement. *Physiopedia.* Retrieved from http://www.physio-pedia.com/Subacromial_Impingement

Kaback, L. A., Green, A., & Blaine, T. A. (2012). Glenohumeral arthritis and total shoulder replacement. *Medicine and Health, Rhode Island, 95*(4), 120-124.

Keener, J. D., Galatz, L. M., Stobbs-Cucchi, G., Patton, R., & Yamaguchi, K. (2014). Rehabilitation following arthroscopic rotator cuff repair: A prospective randomized trial of immobilization compared with early motion. *Journal of Bone and Joint Surgery, 96*(1), 11-19.

Kim, S. H., Ha, K. I., Jung, M. W., Lim, M. S., Kim, Y. M., & Park, J. H. (2003). Accelerated rehabilitation after arthroscopic Bankart repair for selected cases: A prospective randomized clinical study. *Arthroscopy, 19*(7), 722-731.

Lee, B. G., Cho, N. S., & Rhee, Y. G. (2012). Effect of two rehabilitation protocols on range of motion and healing rates after arthroscopic rotator cuff repair: Aggressive versus limited early passive exercises. *Arthroscopy, 28*(1), 34-42.

Levy, J., Frankle, M., Mighell, M., & Pupello, D. (2007). The use of the reverse shoulder prosthesis for the treatment of failed hemiarthroplasty for proximal humeral fracture. *Journal of Bone and Joint Surgery, 89*(2), 292-300.

Litchfield, R. (2013). Progressive strengthening exercises for subacromial impingement syndrome. *Clinical Journal of Sports Medicine, 23*(1), 86-87.

Ludewig, P. M., & Cook, T. M. (2000). Alterations in shoulder kinematics and associated muscle activity in people with symptoms of shoulder impingement. *Physical Therapy, 80*(3), 276-291.

Maman, E., Harris, C., White, L., Tomlinson, G., Shashank, M., & Boynton, E. (2009). Outcome of nonoperative treatment of symptomatic rotator cuff tears monitored by magnetic resonance imaging. *The Journal of Bone and Joint Surgery, 91*(8), 1898-1906.

Milgrom, C., Schaffler, M., Gilbert, S., & van Holsbeeck, M. (1995). Rotator-cuff changes in asymptomatic adults. The effect of age, hand dominance and gender. *The Journal of Bone and Joint Surgery, 77*(2), 296-298.

Millett, P. J., Wilcox, R. B., 3rd, O'Holleran, J. D., & Warner, J. J. (2006). Rehabilitation of the rotator cuff: An evaluation-based approach. *The Journal of the American Academy of Orthopedic Surgeons, 14*(11), 599-609.

Mulieri, P. J., Holcomb, J. O., Dunning, P., Pliner, M., Bogle, R. K., Pupello, D., & Frankle, M. A. (2010). Is a formal physical therapy program necessary after total shoulder arthroplasty for osteoarthritis? *Journal of Shoulder and Elbow Surgery, 19*(4), 570-579.

Roussel, R., Kelley, D., Marek, A., & Hernandez, J. (n.d.). Total shoulder arthroplasty. *Physiopedia.* Retrieved from http://www.physio-pedia.com/Total_Shoulder_Arthroplasty

Safran, O., Schroeder, J., Bloom, R., Weil, Y., & Milgrom, C. (2011). Natural history of nonoperatively treated symptomatic rotator cuff tears in patients 60 years old or younger. *American Journal of Sports Medicine, 39*(4), 710-714.

Salles, J. I., Velasques, B., Cossich, V., Nicoliche, E., Ribeiro, P., Amaral, M. V., & Motta, G. (2015). Strength training and shoulder proprioception. *Journal of Athletic Training, 50*(3), 277-280.

Sambandam, S., Khanna, V., Gul, A., & Mounasamy, V. (2015). Rotator cuff tears: An evidence based approach. *World Journal of Orthopedics, 6*(11), 902-918.

Sherry, M. (2001). Rehabilitation guidelines for SLAP lesion repair. *University of Wisconsin Sports Medicine.* Retrieved from http://www.uwhealth.org/files/uwhealth/docs/pdf/SM14888_SLAP_Repair6.pdf

Smith, J., Dahm, D. L., Kaufman, K. R., Boon, A. J., Laskowski, E. R., Kotajarvi, B. R., & Jacofsky, D. J. (2006). Electromyographic activity in the immobilized shoulder girdle musculature during scapulothoracic exercises. *Archives of Physical Medicine and Rehabilitation, 87*(7), 923-927.

Smith, M., Sparkes, V., Busse, M., & Enright, S. (2009). Upper and lower trapezius muscle activity in subjects with subacromial impingement symptoms: Is there imbalance and can taping change it? *Physical Therapy in Sport, 10*(2), 45-50.

South Shore Hospital Orthopedic, Spine and Sports Therapy. (n.d.). Subacromial decompression protocol. *South Shore Orthopedics.* Retrieved from https://www.southshorehospital.org/Workfiles/Medical_Services/Orthopedics/Sub-Acromial_Decompression.pdf

South Shore Orthopedic, Spine and Sport Therapy. (2016). Bankart Repair Protocol. *South Shore Orthopedics.* Retrieved from https://www.southshorehospital.org/Workfiles/Medical_Services/Orthopedics/Bankart_Repair.pdf

Struyf, F., Cagnie, B., Cools, A., Baert, I., Brempt, J. V., Struyf, P., & Meeus, M. (2014). Scapulothoracic muscle activity and recruitment timing in patients with shoulder impingement symptoms and glenohumeral instability. *Journal of Electromyography and Kinesiology, 24*(2), 277-284.

The Stone Clinic. (2016). Bankart repair rehabilitation protocol. *The Stone Clinic Orthopedic Surgery and Rehabilitation.* Retrieved from http://www.stoneclinic.com/bankart-Repair-Rehab

Theisen, C., van Wagensveld, A., Timmesfeld, N., Efe, T., Heyse, T. J., Fuchs-Winkelmann, S., & Schofer, M. D. (2010). Co-occurrence of outlet impingement syndrome of the shoulder and restricted range of motion in the thoracic spine--A prospective study with ultrasound-based motion analysis. *BMC Musculoskeletal Disorders, 11*, 135.

Thomson, S., Jukes, C., & Lewis, J. (2015). Rehabilitation following surgical repair of the rotator cuff: A systematic review. *Physiotherapy, 102*(1), 20-28.

Vanderbuilt Sports Medicine Knee Center and Shoulder Center. (n.d.). Post-op guidelines acromioclavicular joint reconstruction. *Vanderbuilt University School of Medicine.* Retrieved from https://www.vumc.org/sports-medicine/files/sports-medicine/public_files/documents/Postoperative%20AC%20Joint%20Reconstruction%20Protocol.pdf

Wen DY. (1999). Current concepts in the treatment of anterior shoulder dislocations. *The American Journal of Emergency Medicine, 17*(4), 401-407.

Wilcox, R. B., Arslanian, L. E., & Millett, P. (2005). Rehabilitation following total shoulder arthroplasty. *Journal of Orthopedic and Sports Physical Therapy, 35*(12), 821-836.

Wilk, K. E., Macrina, L. C., & Reinold, M. M. (2006). Non-operative rehabilitation for traumatic and atraumatic glenohumeral instability. *North American Journal of Sports Physical Therapy, 1*(1), 16-31.

Yi, A., Villacis, D., Yalamanchili, R., & Hatch, G. F., 3rd. (2015). A comparison of rehabilitation methods after arthroscopic rotator cuff repair: A systematic review. *Sports Health, 7*(4), 326-334.

Section 5.09

ELBOW RANGE OF MOTION

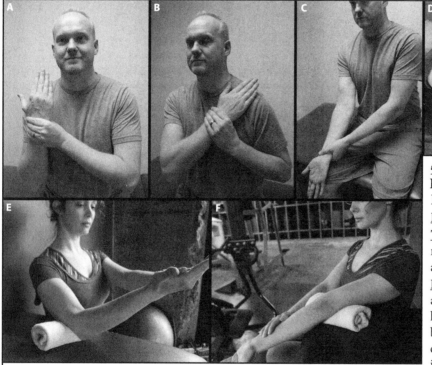

5.09.1 ROM: ELBOW, SELF-FLEXION AND EXTENSION, PASSIVE

POSITION: Seated, supine

TARGETS: Mobility of the humeroulnar joint using unaffected arm to assist in movements

INSTRUCTION: Patient grasps around affected arm's wrist with unaffected hand and assists the affected arm in bringing fingertips toward the shoulder, passively moving elbow into flexion. This can be done toward ipsilateral and contralateral shoulder for variation (A and B). Patient then lets the elbow extend while supporting the forearm, bringing dorsum of hand to top of thigh (C). This can also be done supine, except the hand is lowered to the bed rather than the thigh (D). For more restricted elbows, a table may be used as a surface to prop affected elbow while unaffected hand presses elbow toward extension (E). Aggressive extension involves placing forearm off the edge of a table and pressing forearm into extension with other hand (F).

SUBSTITUTIONS: Active use of target arm; arm remains relaxed while unaffected arm creates the movements, encourage patient to sit up tall with shoulders back.

PARAMETERS: 10 repetitions, holding 3 to 5 seconds at end range, 1 set, 1 to 3 times per day

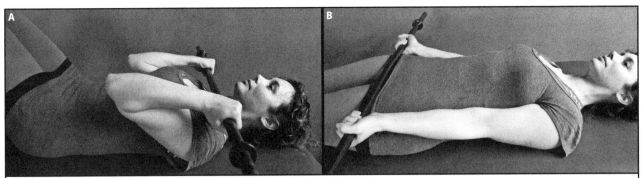

5.09.2 ROM: ELBOW FLEXION AND EXTENSION WITH WAND, ACTIVE ASSISTIVE

<u>POSITION</u>: Supine

<u>TARGETS</u>: Mobility of the humeroulnar joint using unaffected arm to assist in movements

<u>INSTRUCTION</u>: Patient holds the wand with both hands outstretched and palms up. Patient bends the elbows, curling the palms toward the shoulders, and returns to start. At both end range positions, patient uses the unaffected side to assist the affected side (A and B).

<u>SUBSTITUTIONS</u>: Encourage scapular retraction to avoid raising the shoulders.

<u>PARAMETERS</u>: 10 repetitions, holding 3 to 5 seconds at end range, 1 set, 1 to 3 times per day

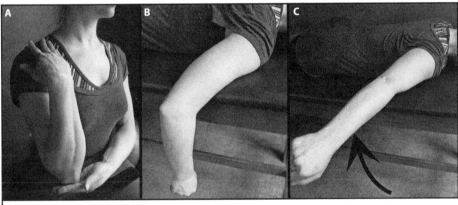

5.09.3 ROM: ELBOW FLEXION AND EXTENSION, ACTIVE

<u>POSITION</u>: Seated, prone

<u>TARGETS</u>: Mobility of the humeroulnar joint

<u>INSTRUCTION</u>: *Flexion seated*: Patient holds hand outstretched, palm up, and bends the elbows, curling the palms toward the shoulder (A). *Extension prone*: Patient drops forearm off table and actively extends the elbow against gravity (B and C).

<u>SUBSTITUTIONS</u>: Encourage scapular retraction to avoid raising the shoulders.

<u>PARAMETERS</u>: 10 repetitions, holding 3 to 5 seconds at end range, 1 set, 1 to 3 times per day

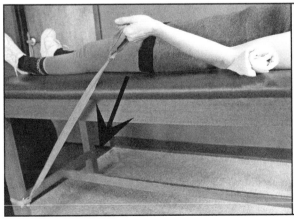

5.09.4 ROM: ELBOW, LOW-LOAD, LONG-DURATION EXTENSION, PASSIVE

<u>POSITION</u>: Supine

<u>TARGETS</u>: Mobility of the humeroulnar joint into extension

<u>INSTRUCTION</u>: Patient lies with forearm off the bed, palm up. Therapist affixes resistance band to a stationary object on the floor; a dumbbell works well for this. The other end is then affixed to the patient's forearm. Move the stationary object to a distance at which a gentle pull is felt in the elbow.

<u>SUBSTITUTIONS</u>: Encourage scapular retraction to avoid raising the shoulders.

<u>PARAMETERS</u>: 5 to 10 minutes, 1 set, 1 to 3 times per day

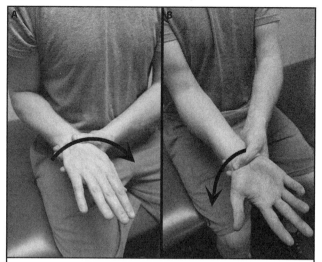

5.09.5 ROM: Elbow Pronation and Supination, Passive and Active Assistive

Position: Seated

Targets: Mobility of the radioulnar joint using unaffected arm to assist in movements

Instruction: Affected shoulder is neutral with elbow flexed 90 degrees. For AAROM, patient turns the palm down (pronation) as far as possible actively and therapist may assist at end range. For self-PROM, patient grasps around affected arm proximal to wrist just with unaffected hand and assists the affected forearm turning the palm down. Repeat for palm up (supination) (A and B).

Substitutions: Encourage patient to sit up tall with shoulders back.

Parameters: 10 repetitions, holding a 3 to 5 seconds at end range, 1 set, 1 to 3 times per day

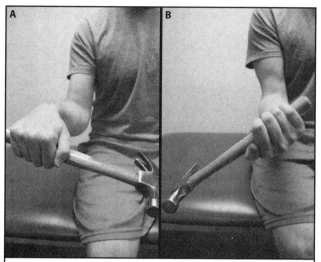

5.09.6 ROM: Elbow Pronation and Supination With Hammer Overload, Active Assistive

Position: Seated

Targets: Mobility of the radioulnar joint using weight of hammer head for assistance

Instruction: Affected shoulder is neutral with elbow flexed 90 degrees. Patient grasps around hammer handle, thumb up, and turns the palm down using the hammer head weight to apply overpressure (pronation). Repeat for palm up (supination) (A and B). The further the hand is down the handle, the more intense the weight assistance. If needed, patient may use other hand to assist in returning to start position.

Substitutions: Encourage patient to sit up tall with shoulders back.

Parameters: 3 to 5 repetitions, holding a 5 to 10 seconds at end range, 1 set, 1 to 3 times per day

5.09.7 ROM: Elbow Pronation and Supination, Active

Position: Seated

Targets: Mobility of the radioulnar joint

Instruction: Affected shoulder is neutral with elbow flexed 90 degrees. Patient turns the palm up, hold 1 to 2 seconds. Repeat for palm down (A and B).

Substitutions: Encourage patient to sit up tall with shoulders back.

Parameters: 1 to 2 repetitions, holding a 5 to 10 seconds at end range, 1 set, 1 to 3 times per day

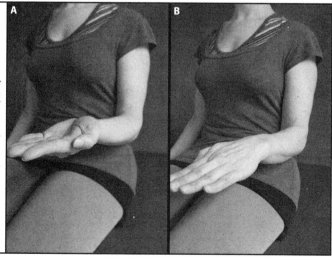

Section 5.10

ELBOW JOINT SELF-MOBILIZATION

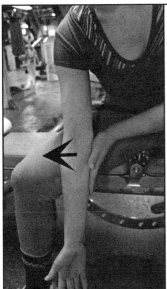

5.10.1 SELF-JOINT MOBILIZATION: ELBOW, LATERAL GAPPING

POSITION: Seated

TARGETS: Mobility of the radioulnar, humeroradial and humeroulnar joints, lateral capsule stretch

INSTRUCTION: Patient starts with affected elbow at the side and braces the anterior surface of the forearm against the inside of ipsilateral knee. With the other hand positioned just below the elbow joint, patient pushes from medical to lateral, feeling joint gapping and stretch along outside of elbow. Hold, release and repeat.

SUBSTITUTIONS: Shrugging shoulder; target arm not relaxed.

PARAMETERS: Hold 3 to 5 seconds, repeat 10 to 20 repetitions, 1 to 3 times per day

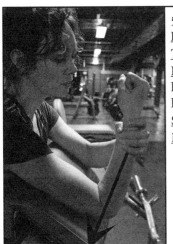

5.10.2 SELF-JOINT MOBILIZATION: ELBOW, POSTERIOR GLIDE

POSITION: Seated

TARGETS: Mobility of the humeroulnar joints, posterior capsule stretch

INSTRUCTION: Place wedge under arm. Patient flexes elbow 90 degrees and uses other hand, grasped firmly around forearm, to drive forearm straight down perpendicular to humerus. Hold, release and repeat.

SUBSTITUTIONS: Shrugging shoulder; target arm not relaxed.

PARAMETERS: Hold 3 to 5 seconds, repeat 10 to 20 repetitions, 1 to 3 times per day

5.10.3 SELF-JOINT MOBILIZATION: ELBOW, DISTRACTION

POSITION: Seated

TARGETS: Mobility of the humeroulnar joints, posterior capsule stretch

INSTRUCTION: Place a towel roll in elbow crease. Patient uses other hand to assist full flexion as towel roll presses outward to distract the elbow joint.

SUBSTITUTIONS: Shrugging shoulder; target arm not relaxed.

PARAMETERS: Hold 3 to 5 seconds, repeat 10 to 20 repetitions, 1 to 3 times per day

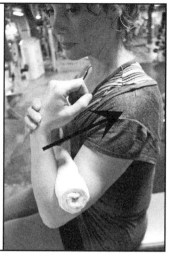

5.10.4 SELF-JOINT MOBILIZATION: ELBOW, RADIAL HEAD

POSITION: Seated

TARGETS: Mobility of the radial head

INSTRUCTION: Place a towel under upper arm and support with opposite hand, shoulder in 90 degrees scaption. Opposite elbow can be supported on table. Patient turns target side palm down and isometrically contracts to extend the elbow. This creates a gapping at the radial head.

SUBSTITUTIONS: Shrugging shoulder; target arm not relaxed.

PARAMETERS: Hold 3 to 5 seconds, repeat 10 to 20 repetitions, 1 to 3 times per day

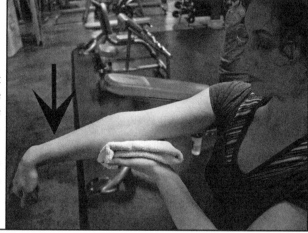

Section 5.11

ELBOW STRETCHING

5.11.1 STRETCH: TRICEPS BEHIND BACK WITH TOWEL

POSITION: Standing

TARGETS: Stretch primarily triceps; beginner stretch.

INSTRUCTION: Patient stands tall with back and neck straight and places towel in hand of affected arm. Patient brings towel over the back of the head, the opposite hand grasps the other end and uses it to pull down. Hand of affected arm slides behind

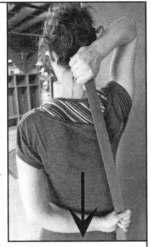

the head and down the back until a stretch is felt in the posterior arm.

SUBSTITUTIONS: Shrugging shoulders, arching back, jutting chin out

PARAMETERS: Hold for 15 to 30 seconds, 3 to 5 repetitions, 1 to 3 times per day

5.11.2 STRETCH: TRICEPS

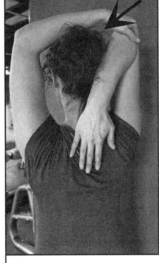

POSITION: Standing

TARGETS: Stretch primarily triceps

INSTRUCTION: Patient stands tall with the back and neck straight and places affected side palm behind the lower neck, other hand on the elbow, while gently pushing elbow backward so hand moves further down spine until a stretch is felt in the posterior arm.

SUBSTITUTIONS: Shrugging shoulders, arching back, jutting chin out

PARAMETERS: Hold for 15 to 30 seconds, 3 to 5 repetitions, 1 to 3 times per day

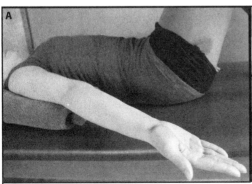
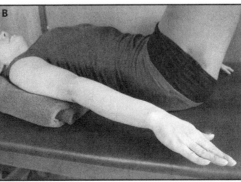

5.11.3 STRETCH: BICEPS USING PILLOW

POSITION: Supine

TARGETS: Stretch primarily biceps

INSTRUCTION: With shoulder propped on pillow, patient reaches away from shoulder to table with arm extended and palm up (A). This can also be done in neutral with thumb up or pronated with palm down (B). Patient should try all positions to find which one gives the best stretch to the anterior arm.

SUBSTITUTIONS: Shoulder rolls forward; active scapular retraction is encouraged.

PARAMETERS: Hold for 15 to 30 seconds, 3 to 5 repetitions, 1 to 3 times per day

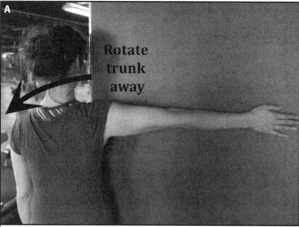
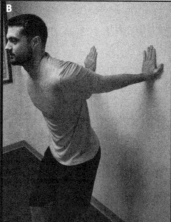
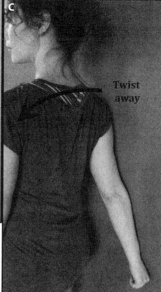

Rotate trunk away

Twist away

5.11.4 STRETCH: BICEPS USING WALL

POSITION: Standing

TARGETS: Stretch pimarily biceps

INSTRUCTION: Patient stands facing wall and raises arm to 90 degrees of abduction, palm on wall then twists the body away from the wall, walking the feet with the trunk, until a stretch is felt in the anterior arm (A). This can be done bilaterally by standing facing away from the wall. Patient bends over and places palms on wall behind with fingers facing up. Patient brings butt toward wall and squats down until a stretch is felt in the anterior arm. This exercise can cause excessive anterior translation of the humerus, thus encouraging scapular retraction is important (B). Keeping the shoulder lowered, patient may also pronate the forearm and place thumb side against the wall at hip height. Patient then twists the body away from the wall, walking the feet with the trunk, until stretch is felt in anterior arm (C).

SUBSTITUTIONS: Shrugging shoulders, slouching, jutting chin out, shoulder rolls forward; active scapular retraction is encouraged.

PARAMETERS: Hold for 15 to 30 seconds, 3 to 5 repetitions, 1 to 3 times per day

5.11.5 STRETCH: BICEPS USING TABLE

POSITION: Standing

TARGETS: Stretch primarily biceps

INSTRUCTION: Patient stands facing away from table that allows arm to be supported behind and above waist height. Palm is facing up. Patient slowly lowers body, allowing arm to move further away from feet, until a stretch is felt in the anterior arm.

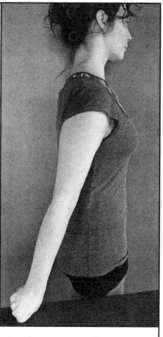

SUBSTITUTIONS: Shrugging shoulders, slouching, jutting chin out, shoulder rolls forward; active scapular retraction is encouraged.

PARAMETERS: Hold for 15 to 30 seconds, 3 to 5 repetitions, 1 to 3 times per day

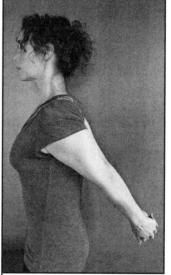

5.11.6 STRETCH: BICEPS, HAND CLASP

POSITION: Standing

TARGETS: Stretch primarily biceps

INSTRUCTION: Patient reaches behind their back and clasps hands together, then straightens arms so palms face each other. Patient then raises arms up until stretch is felt in anterior arm. This exercise can cause excessive anterior translation of the humerus thus encouraging scapular retraction is important.

SUBSTITUTIONS: Shrugging shoulders, slouching, jutting chin out, shoulders rolling forward; active scapular retraction is encouraged.

PARAMETERS: Hold for 15 to 30 seconds, 3 to 5 repetitions, 1 to 3 times per day

5.11.7 STRETCH: BICEPS, OTHER PERSON ASSIST

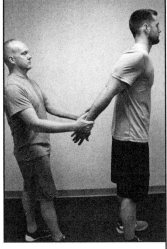

POSITION: Standing

TARGETS: Stretch primarily biceps

INSTRUCTION: Patient reaches behind their back with both arms, then straightens arms so palms face each other. Therapist grasps patient's wrists and gently pulls the arms upwards until stretch is felt in anterior arms. This exercise can cause excessive anterior translation of the humerus, thus encouraging scapular retraction is important.

SUBSTITUTIONS: Shrugging shoulders, slouching, jutting chin out, shoulders rolling forward; active scapular retraction is encouraged.

PARAMETERS: Hold for 15 to 30 seconds, 3 to 5 repetitions, 1 to 3 times per day

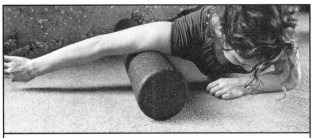

5.11.8 STRETCH: BICEPS, SELF-MASSAGE WITH FOAM ROLLER

POSITION: Side-lying

TARGETS: Deep-tissue release biceps

INSTRUCTION: Patient places the roller under their biceps. Body is supported with the other forearm. Patient uses supporting arm and legs to slowly move body side-to-side allowing the roller to massage biceps muscle. It can be somewhat uncomfortable at the beginning, and therapist should check to ensure patient is not applying excessive pressure.

SUBSTITUTIONS: Shrugging shoulders, slouching, jutting chin out, shoulders rolling forward; active scapular retraction is encouraged.

PARAMETERS: Hold for 15 to 90 seconds, 3 to 5 repetitions, 1 to 3 times per day

Section 5.12

ELBOW STRENGTHENING

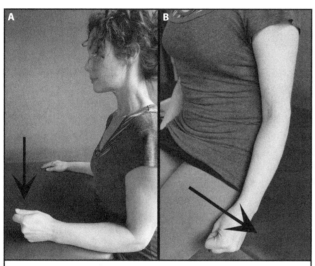

5.12.1 STRENGTHEN: ISOMETRIC; ELBOW EXTENSION

POSITION: Seated

TARGETS: Beginner facilitation and strengthening of elbow; triceps brachii.

INSTRUCTION: *90 degrees table resists*: With the shoulder of affected side in neutral position, scapula slightly retracted and depressed, patient bends elbow to 90 degrees with fisted hand. Patient places pinky side of fist on top of table and pushes down, attempting to extend the elbow (A). *30 degrees seat resists*: With the affected shoulder side in neutral position, scapula slightly retracted and depressed, patient bends elbow roughly 30 to 40 degrees with fisted hand. Patient places pinky side of fist on top of the seat which they are on and pushes down, attempting to extend the elbow (B).

SUBSTITUTIONS: Shrugging shoulder, shoulder not in neutral position; encourage scapular retraction to stabilize origin.

PARAMETERS: Hold for 6 to 10 seconds, 1 to 3 sets, 8 to 12 repetitions with 1 to 2 second ramp up and down, 1 time per day or every other day

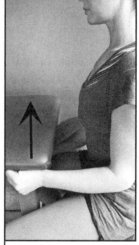

5.12.2 Strengthen: Isometric; Elbow Flexion

POSITION: Seated

TARGETS: Beginner facilitation and strengthening of elbow; biceps brachii.

INSTRUCTION: With the shoulder of affected side in neutral position, scapula slightly retracted and depressed, patient bends elbow to 90 degrees with fisted hand and places just proximal phalanx portion of second digit just under the table in front (this avoids pressure on thumb). Patient attempts to flex elbow with the table providing resistance.

SUBSTITUTIONS: Shrugging shoulder, shoulder not in neutral position; encourage scapular retraction to stabilize origin.

PARAMETERS: Hold for 6 to 10 seconds, 1 to 3 sets, 8 to 12 repetitions with 1 to 2 second ramp up and down, 1 time per day or every other day

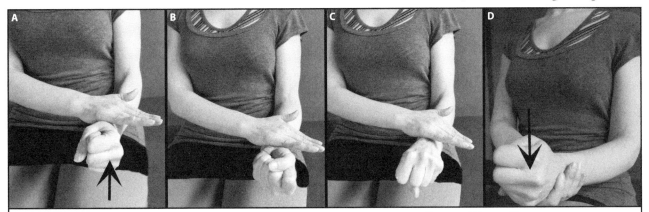

5.12.3 STRENGTHEN: ISOMETRIC; ELBOW FLEXION AND EXTENSION, OTHER HAND RESISTS

<u>POSITION</u>: Seated, standing

<u>TARGETS</u>: Beginner facilitation and strengthening of elbow flexors (biceps brachii, brachialis, brachioradialis) and extensors (triceps brachii)

<u>INSTRUCTION</u>: With shoulder of the affected side in neutral position, scapula slightly retracted and depressed, patient bends elbow to 90 degrees with fisted hand. *For isometric flexion (brachioradialis focus)*: Patient places opposite hand on top of wrist and, as they attempt to flex the elbow, the other hands resists (A). *For isometric flexion (biceps focus)*: Patient places affected hand palm up (B). *For isometric flexion (brachialis focus)*: Patient places affected hand palm down (C). *For isometric extension*: Patient cups opposite hand underneath wrist and, as the patient attempts to extend the elbow, the other hands resist (D). *Multi-angle*: Patient may resist motions at any position of elbow flexion depending on treatment goals (not shown).

<u>SUBSTITUTIONS</u>: Shrugging shoulder, shoulder not in neutral position; encourage scapular retraction to stabilize origin.

<u>PARAMETERS</u>: Hold for 6 to 10 seconds, 1 to 3 sets, 8 to 12 repetitions with 1 to 2 second ramp up and down, 1 time per day or every other day

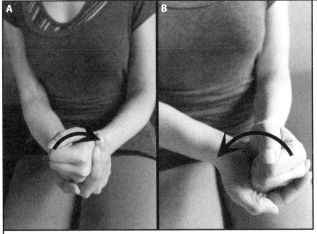

5.12.4 STRENGTHEN: ISOMETRIC; ELBOW PRONATION AND SUPINATION, OTHER HAND RESISTS

<u>POSITION</u>: Seated, standing

<u>TARGETS</u>: Beginner facilitation and strengthening of elbow pronators (pronator teres, pronator quadratus) and supinators (supinator and biceps brachii)

<u>INSTRUCTION</u>: With shoulder of the affected side in neutral position, scapula slightly retracted and depressed, patient bends elbow to 90 degrees with fisted hand. Patient places opposite hand around wrist with thumb resting in the middle of the palm. Patient attempts turn the palm up for supinator strengthening, and then palm down for pronator strengthening, as other hand resists (A and B).

<u>SUBSTITUTIONS</u>: Shrugging shoulder, shoulder not in neutral position; encourage scapular retraction to stabilize origin.

<u>PARAMETERS</u>: Hold for 6 to 10 seconds, 1 to 3 sets, 8 to 12 repetitions with 1 to 2 second ramp up and down, 1 time per day or every other day

5.12.5 Strengthen: Isotonic; Elbow Extension, Overhead With Dumbbell

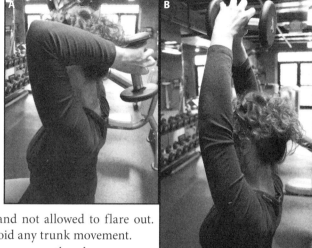

Position: Seated, standing

Targets: Strengthen triceps brachii

Instruction: With the affected shoulder in neutral position, scapula slightly retracted and depressed, patient with dumbbell in hand, instruct patient to keep the back straight and lift arm overhead with thumb down. The opposite arm may rest at the side or may support the extended arm superior to the elbow. Instruct the patient to fully extend the arm, then bend at the elbow joint, bringing the dumbbell to the side of the head in a slow and controlled manner. Return to starting position and repeat (A and B).

Substitutions: Elbow should be kept close to the body and not allowed to flare out. Avoid moving the arm at the shoulder joint. In standing, avoid any trunk movement.

Parameters: 8 to 12 repetitions, 1 to 3 sets, 1 time per day or every other day

5.12.6 Strengthen: Isotonic; Elbow Extension, Bilateral Overhead With Wand/Cane

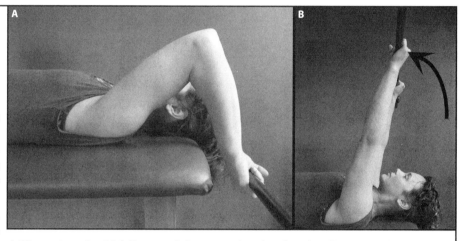

Position: Supine

Targets: Strengthen triceps brachii

Instruction: In sitting or standing with wand/cane in hands and palms of hands facing either away from the body (pronated) or toward the body (supinated), instruct the patient to keep the back straight and lift arms overhead. The patient should fully extend the arms, then bend at the elbow joint, bringing the wand/cane posterior to the head in a slow and controlled manner. Return to starting position and repeat (A and B).

Substitutions: Elbow should be kept close to the body and not allowed to flare out. Avoid moving the arm at the shoulder joint. In standing, avoid any trunk movement.

Parameters: 8 to 12 repetitions, 1 to 3 sets, 1 time per day or every other day

5.12.7 Strengthen: Isotonic; Elbow Extension, Kick-Back

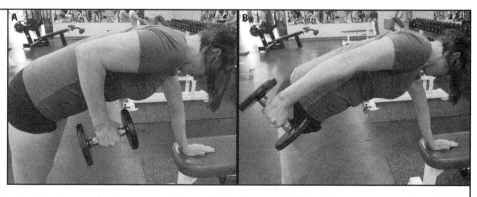

Position: Standing

Targets: Strengthen triceps brachii

Instruction: Patient is bent forward with trunk straight and parallel to the floor, supporting upper body with opposite arm on table or bench. Patient brings shoulder into extension so that upper arm is parallel to floor and elbow hangs to approximately 90 degrees. Place weight in hand and have patient extend the elbow fully. Return to starting position and repeat (A and B).

Substitutions: Elbow should be kept close to the body and not allowed to flare out. Avoid moving the arm at the shoulder joint. Upper arm should stay parallel to floor.

Parameters: 8 to 12 repetitions, 1 to 3 sets, 1 time per day or every other day

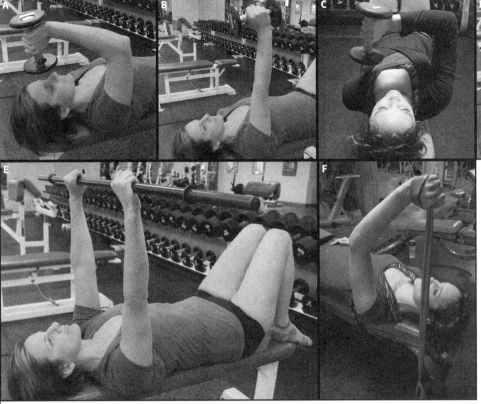

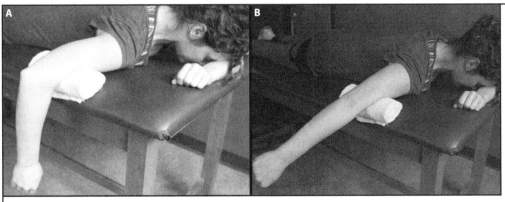

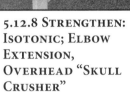

5.12.8 STRENGTHEN: ISOTONIC; ELBOW EXTENSION, OVERHEAD "SKULL CRUSHER"

POSITION: Supine

TARGETS: Strengthen triceps brachii

INSTRUCTION: Patient raises shoulder to 90 degrees of flexion. Place weight in patient's hand and have patient then flex the elbow, bringing the thumb toward the middle of the forehead. Patient then extends the elbow fully. Return to starting position and repeat (A and B). Another option is to orient the forearm to crossing the body at the chest (C). However the internal rotation of the shoulder may cause some aggravation. This can also be done bilaterally with a weighted wand or cane. Patient holds both shoulders to 90 degrees of flexion, palms up, holding the wand. Patient lowers wands directly overhead, bending only at the elbows, followed by pressing up, extending the elbows (D and E). This can also be done with a resistance band (F).

SUBSTITUTIONS: Elbow should be kept directly above the shoulder, upper arm should stay perpendicular to floor.

PARAMETERS: 8 to 12 repetitions, 1 to 3 sets, 1 time per day or every other day

5.12.9 STRENGTHEN: ISOTONIC; ELBOW KICK-OUT

POSITION: Prone

TARGETS: Strengthen triceps brachii

INSTRUCTION: Patient places forehead on unaffected forearm or towel roll to put neck in neutral. Patient scoots to edge of bed to allow forearm to hang off. Holding weight, patient brings arm into 90 degrees of abduction with elbow flexed 90 degrees. A towel roll may be placed under the arm to bring the humerus in alignment with the shoulder joint. Patient extends the elbow, top of hand or pinky side leading the way, then slowly returns to starting position and repeats (A and B).

SUBSTITUTIONS: Lifting shoulder off table, shrugging/tensing shoulder

PARAMETERS: 8 to 12 repetitions, 1 to 3 sets, 1 time per day or every other day

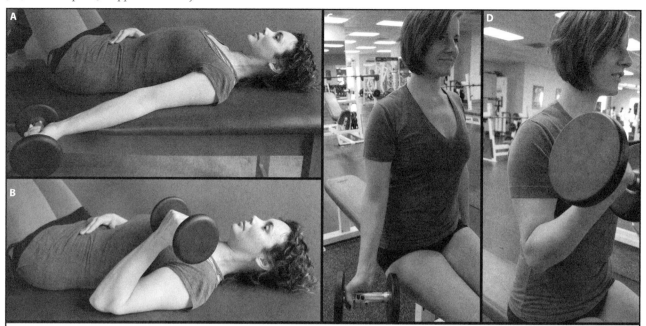

5.12.10 STRENGTHEN: ISOTONIC; ELBOW FLEXION, CURLS

POSITION: Supine, sitting, standing

TARGETS: Strengthen biceps brachii, brachioradialis, brachialis

INSTRUCTION: *In supine*: For beginner phase, with dumbbell in one or both hands, instruct patient to keep back and upper arm(s) flat on surface by retracting scapula while fully extending the arm(s) to the side of the body. The patient flexes elbow(s), bringing the dumbbell(s) toward the shoulder, slowly returning to starting position and repeats (A and B). *Progression to sitting or standing*: With dumbbell in one or both hands, instruct patient to keep back and upper arm(s) straight by retracting scapula and engaging core muscles. Patient fully extends the arm(s) to the side of the body. The patient then flexes elbow(s), bringing the dumbbell(s) toward the shoulder, slowly returns to starting position and repeats (C and D). Alternate curls side-to-side are another option. To target biceps brachii; palms are facing up; brachialis, palms facing down; brachioradialis, palms facing midline.

SUBSTITUTIONS: Elbow should be kept directly aligned with shoulder (horizontally in supine, vertically in seated or standing), shoulder stays in neutral alignment, scapular stabilizers engaged

PARAMETERS: 8 to 12 repetitions, 1 to 3 sets, 1 time per day or every other day

5.12.11 STRENGTHEN: ISOTONIC; ELBOW FLEXION, PREACHER CURLS

POSITION: Sitting

TARGETS: Strengthen biceps brachii primarily, with assist of brachioradialis and brachialis

INSTRUCTION: Patient sits down on the Preacher Curl Machine and selects weight. Patient places the back of the upper arms on the Preacher pad and grabs the handles using an underhand grip. Ensure that when placing arms on pad patient keeps elbows in. Patient lifts

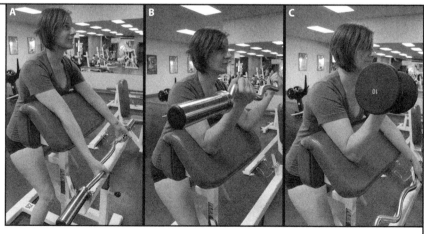

the handles. At the top of the position, ensure patient is holding the contraction for a second. Only the forearms should move; the upper arms should remain stationary and on the pad at all times. Patient lowers the handles slowly back to the starting position and repeat (A and B). *Variations*: Patient can use free weights to perform this exercise on a Preacher bench (C).

SUBSTITUTIONS: Elbow should be kept directly aligned with shoulder, shoulder stays in neutral alignment, scapular stabilizers engaged

PARAMETERS: 8 to 12 repetitions, 1 to 3 sets, 1 time per day or every other day

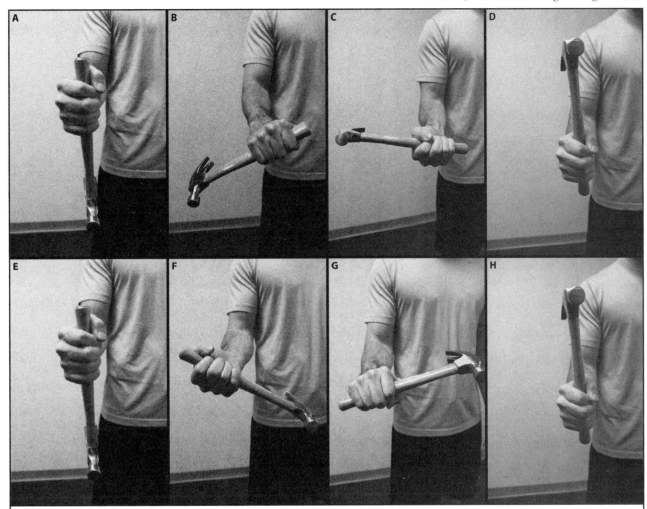

5.12.12 STRENGTHEN: ISOTONIC; ELBOW PRONATION AND SUPINATION WITH HAMMER

<u>POSITION</u>: Seated

<u>TARGETS</u>: Strengthen pronator teres and pronator quadratus using weight of hammer head for resistance

<u>INSTRUCTION</u>: Affected shoulder is neutral, with elbow flexed 90 degrees, thumb up. *Pronation: 0 degrees to full pronation*: Patient grasps around upside-down hammer handle and turns the palm down, using the hammer head weight as resistance (A and B). *Pronation: supinated position to 0 degrees*: With palm up, patient grasps around sideways hammer handle, with hammer head thumb side out, and turns the palm back to neutral, thumb up, using the hammer head weight as resistance (C and D). *Supination: 0 degrees to full supination*: Patient grasps around upside down hammer handle and turns the palm up, using the hammer head weight as resistance (E and F). *Supination: pronated position to 0 degrees*: With palm down, patient grasps around sideways hammer handle, with hammer head thumb side out, and turns the palm back to neutral, thumb up, using the hammer head weight as resistance (G and H). The further the hand is down the handle, the more intense the weight resistance. Adding a cuff weight strapped to end of hammer can also increase resistance.

<u>SUBSTITUTIONS</u>: Encourage patient to sit up tall with shoulders back, elbow stays tucked into side, keep wrist in line with forearm

<u>PARAMETERS</u>: 8 to 12 repetitions, 1 to 3 sets, 1 time per day or every other day

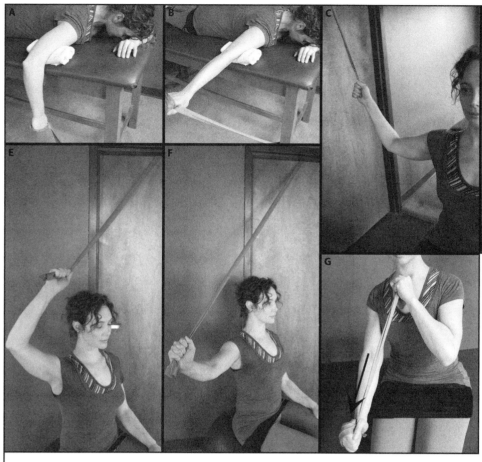

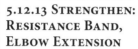

5.12.13 STRENGTHEN: RESISTANCE BAND, ELBOW EXTENSION

POSITION: Prone, seated, standing

TARGETS: Strengthen triceps brachii

INSTRUCTION: *Prone*: Patient places forehead on unaffected forearm or uses towel roll to put neck in neutral. Patient scoots to edge of bed to allow forearm to drop off. Band is anchored to table leg at shoulder level. Patient holds band with shoulder to 90 degrees of abduction and elbow flexed 90 degrees. A towel roll may be placed under the arm to bring the humerus in alignment with the shoulder joint. Patient extends the elbow, top of hand or pinky side leading the way, then slowly returns to starting position and repeats (A and B). *Seated anchored*: With band anchored overhead, patient sits sideways with target arm toward anchor and grasps band high enough so that there is tension at start. Patient extends elbow, bringing palm toward floor (C and D). This can also be done with the affected side away from the anchor reaching overhead to start (E and F). *Seated self-anchor*: With one end of band held at forehead, patient grasps band with target arm high enough so that there is tension at start. Patient extends elbow, bringing palm toward floor (G).

SUBSTITUTIONS: Shrugging or tensing shoulder; encourage tall posture and retracted scapula.

PARAMETERS: 8 to 12 repetitions, 1 to 3 sets, 1 time per day or every other day

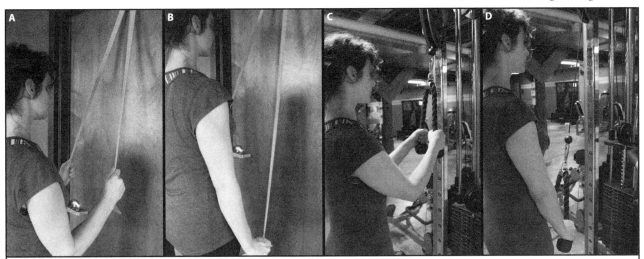

5.12.14 STRENGTHEN: RESISTANCE BAND, TRICEP PUSH DOWN

POSITION: Standing

TARGETS: Strengthen triceps brachii

INSTRUCTION: With band anchored overhead, patient stands close to the wall, facing anchor. With target arm or both arms, patient grasps band high enough so that tension is on band at start and pulls down to align upper arms with trunk. Keeping elbows tucked into sides, patient extends elbow bringing hands toward floor (A and B). Slowly return to starting position by allowing elbow(s) only to flex and repeat. This can be done with both arms. This can also be done with a cable machine (C and D).

SUBSTITUTIONS: Shrugging and tensing shoulder; encourage tall posture and retracted scapula.

PARAMETERS: 8 to 12 repetitions, 1 to 3 sets, 1 time per day or every other day

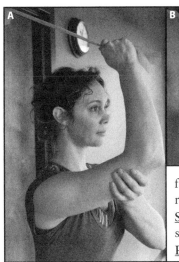

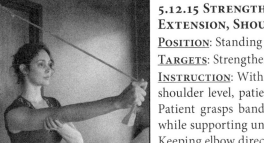

5.12.15 STRENGTHEN: RESISTANCE BAND, ELBOW EXTENSION, SHOULDER FLEXED

POSITION: Standing

TARGETS: Strengthen triceps brachii

INSTRUCTION: With band anchored 6 to 10 inches above shoulder level, patient stands facing away from anchor. Patient grasps band and flexes shoulder to 90 degrees while supporting under the arm with the opposite hand. Keeping elbow directly in front of shoulder, patient steps away from the wall until tension is pulling the elbow into flexion. Patient extends elbow, bringing hands directly out in front (A and B). Slowly return to starting position by allowing elbow only to flex and repeat.

SUBSTITUTIONS: Shrugging or tensing shoulder; encourage tall posture and retracted scapula.

PARAMETERS: 8 to 12 repetitions, 1 to 3 sets, 1 time per day or every other day

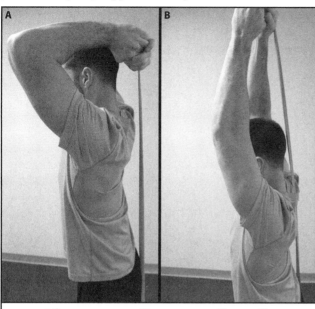

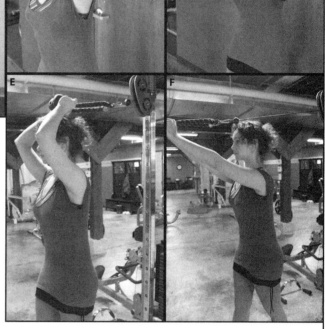

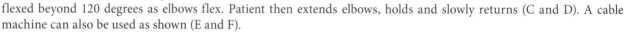

5.12.16 STRENGTHEN: RESISTANCE BAND, ELBOW EXTENSION, OVERHEAD

POSITION: Standing

TARGETS: Strengthen triceps brachii

INSTRUCTION: Anchor one end of band under the patient's foot. With scapula slightly retracted and depressed, patient brings arm overhead into full shoulder flexion with thumb down. Patient grasps other end of band low enough so that tension is on the band at start of movement. Instruct the patient to fully extend the elbow, bringing hand toward ceiling. Return to starting position and repeat (A and B). This can also be done with band anchored behind the patient, overhead. Patient lunges forward, with shoulder flexed beyond 120 degrees as elbows flex. Patient then extends elbows, holds and slowly returns (C and D). A cable machine can also be used as shown (E and F).

SUBSTITUTIONS: Elbow should be directly over the shoulder and not allowed to flare out; avoid shrugging or tensing shoulder, encourage tall posture and retracted scapula, moving the arm at the shoulder joint and any trunk movement.

PARAMETERS: 8 to 12 repetitions, 1 to 3 sets, 1 time per day or every other day

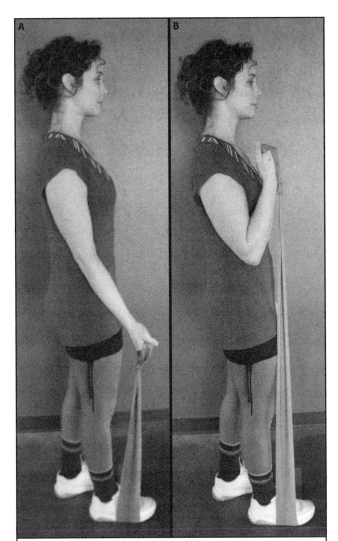

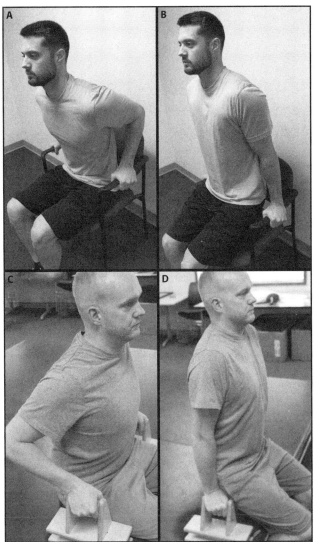

5.12.17 STRENGTHEN: RESISTANCE BAND, ELBOW FLEXION

POSITION: Standing

TARGETS: Strenghten biceps brachii, brachioradialis, brachialis

INSTRUCTION: Anchor one end of band under the patient's foot. With scapula slightly retracted and depressed, patient grasps other end of band low enough so that tension is on the band at start of movement with elbow fully extended. Instruct the patient to fully flex the elbow, bringing palm toward ceiling. Return to starting position and repeat (A and B). To target biceps brachii, palm faces up: brachialis, palm faces down, brachioradialis: palm faces midline.

SUBSTITUTIONS: Shoulder should be directly over the elbow and not allowed to flare out. Avoid shrugging or tensing shoulder, encourage tall posture and retracted scapula, moving the arm at the shoulder joint and any trunk movement.

PARAMETERS: 8 to 12 repetitions, 1 to 3 sets, 1 time per day or every other day

5.12.18 STRENGTHEN: CLOSED KINETIC CHAIN; ELBOW, SEATED DIP/CHAIR PUSH-UPS

POSITION: Seated

TARGETS: Strengthen triceps brachii

INSTRUCTION: Patient places hands beside the hips with fingers facing forward and presses down, lifting buttock off seat of chair, then slowly lowers trunk by bending elbows, keeping elbows aligned with shoulders. Arm rests (A and B) or push-up handles (C and D) can be used for greater range.

SUBSTITUTIONS: Shoulders should be directly over elbows and not allowed to flare out. Avoid shrugging or tensing shoulders, encourage tall posture and retracted scapula. Avoid locking elbows out.

PARAMETERS: 8 to 12 repetitions, 1 to 3 sets, 1 time per day or every other day

5.12.19 STRENGTHEN: CLOSED KINETIC CHAIN; ELBOW, LEAN-BACK DIP

POSITION: Hook-lying

TARGETS: Strengthen triceps brachii

INSTRUCTION: Patient props up on hands, elevating trunk to 45 degrees. Patient's hands are 6 inches behind buttocks and lateral to pelvis on each side, fingertips facing toward feet. Patient slowly lowers trunk by bending elbows to 90 degrees, keeping elbows aligned with shoulders, and then presses up to fully extend the elbows while lifting the trunk.

SUBSTITUTIONS: Shoulders should be directly over elbows and not allowed to flare out. Avoid shrugging or tensing shoulder, encourage tall posture and retracted scapula. Avoid locking elbows out.

PARAMETERS: 8 to 12 repetitions, 1 to 3 sets, 1 time per day or every other day

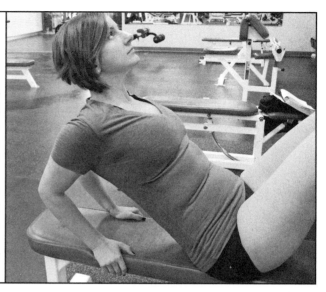

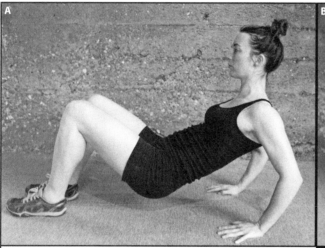
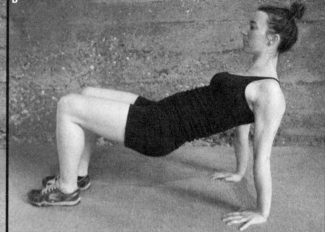

5.12.20 STRENGTHEN: CLOSED KINETIC CHAIN; ELBOW, "CRAB" DIP

POSITION: Hook-lying

TARGETS: Strengthen triceps brachii

INSTRUCTION: Patient props up on hands and lifts buttocks off the surface into a "crab" position; hands are 6 inches behind buttocks and lateral to pelvis on each side, fingertips facing toward feet. Patient slowly lowers trunk by bending elbows to 90 degrees, keeping elbows aligned with shoulders, and then presses up to fully extend the elbows while lifting the trunk. Patient's buttock stays lifted the entire sequence (A and B). To advance, have the patient cross one leg over the other, increasing intensity by increasing the amount of weight arms are accepting (C).

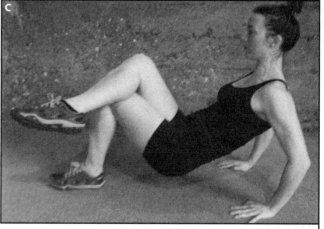

SUBSTITUTIONS: Shoulder should be directly over elbow and not allowed to flare out. Avoid shrugging or tensing shoulder, jutting chin forward, encourage tall posture and retracted scapula. Do not let hips sag. Avoid locking elbow out.

PARAMETERS: 8 to 12 repetitions, 1 to 3 sets, 1 time per day or every other day

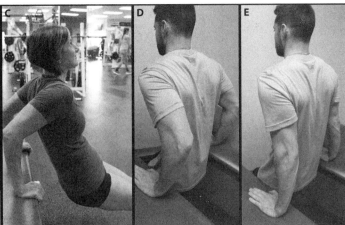

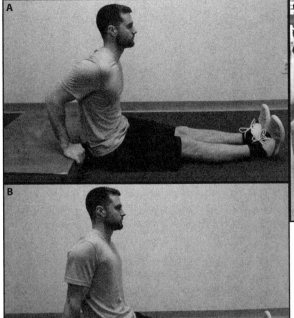

5.12.21 STRENGTHEN: CLOSED KINETIC CHAIN; ELBOW, DIP

POSITION: Long-sitting to standing

TARGETS: Strengthen triceps brachii

INSTRUCTION: *Bench/chair—long-sitting*: Position palms shoulder-width apart with fingers forward on a secured bench or stable chair. Patient slides buttocks off the front of the bench with legs extended out in front, straightens arms, maintaining a slight bend in elbows to keep tension on triceps and off elbow joints. Patient slowly bends elbows to lower body toward floor until elbows are at about a 90 degrees of flexion, keeping back close to the bench. Once patient reaches bottom of the movement, have patient press down into the bench to straighten elbows, returning to the starting position (A and B). Patient may also be allowed to bend knees as needed. *Standing arms behind*: Position with palms on table behind, patient walks feet out while accepting weight into the arms, keeping a slight bend in the elbows. Patient then slowly lowers body, allowing elbows and knees to bend. Once reaching 90 degrees of elbow flexion, patient presses up to straighten elbows (C). *Standing between two tables*: Patient positions palm son either side table and walks feet out while accepting weight into the arms, keeping slight bend in the elbows. Patient then slowly lowers body, allowing elbows and knees to bend. Once reaching 90 degrees of elbow flexion, patient presses up to straighten elbows (D and E).

SUBSTITUTIONS: Elbow should stay aligned in sagittal plane with shoulder and not allowed to flare out. Avoid shrugging or tensing shoulder, jutting chin forward, encourage tall posture and retracted scapula. Avoid locking elbow out.

PARAMETERS: 8 to 12 repetitions, 1 to 3 sets, 1 time per day or every other day

5.12.22 STRENGTHEN: CLOSED KINETIC CHAIN; ELBOW, BODY PRESS

POSITION: Standing

TARGETS: Strengthen triceps brachii

INSTRUCTION: Position bar below chest height. Patient grasps bar with palms down and steps back 3 to 5 feet while leaning on the bar with shoulders at 90 degrees flexion. Trunk is straight in a plank-like position. Patient bends elbows, lowering body toward the floor until elbows flexed 90 degrees. Patient pauses and then reverses, extending elbows to press body away from the floor (not shown).

SUBSTITUTIONS: Elbows should stay aligned in sagittal plane with shoulders and not allowed to flare out. Avoid shrugging or tensing shoulder, jutting chin forward, encourage straight trunk with no sagging hips and retracted scapula. Avoid locking elbow out.

PARAMETERS: 8 to 12 repetitions, 1 to 3 sets, 1 time per day or every other day

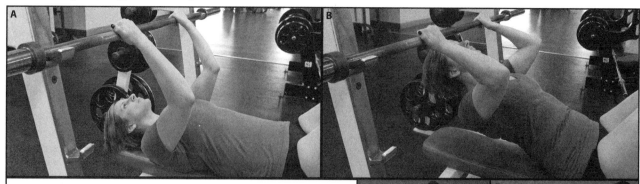

5.12.23 Strengthen: Closed Kinetic Chain; Elbow, Pull-Up

Position: Supine, standing

Targets: Strengthen biceps brachii primarily, with palms up, brachialis with palms down with brachioradialis assist

Instruction: *Beginner/partial weight*: Patient lies supine on a bench with long bar rack at shoulder level. Patient grasps long bar, palms up, hands and elbows aligned in same plane as shoulder. Patient tucks chin and stabilizes trunk while pulling trunk toward the bar, holds and slowly lowers (A and B). This can also be done palms down. *Advanced/full weight*: Patient stands just in front of overhead pull-up bar and grasps bar, palms up or down, hands and elbows aligned in same plane as shoulder. Patient then pulls body weight directly upwards toward the bar, flexing elbows and extending shoulders, holds and slowly lowers (C and D).

Substitutions: Elbow should be directly over the shoulder and not allowed to flare out; avoid shrugging or tensing shoulder, encourage tall posture and retracted scapula.

Parameters: 1 to 12 repetitions, depending on patient fatigue, 1 to 3 sets, 1 time per day or every other day

5.12.24 Functional: Elbow, Velcro Roller for Pronation and Supination Tasks

Position: Seated

Targets: Functional use of forearms and strengthening for turning keys, doorknobs

Instruction: Patient simulates turning key and doorknob while rolling across double Velcro surfaces to provide resistance. Patient should keep elbow at 90 degrees of flexion to isolate pronation and supination movements.

Substitutions: Elbow not allowed to flare out; avoid shrugging or tensing shoulder, encourage tall posture and retracted scapula.

Parameters: To fatigue, 1 to 3 sets, 1 time per day or every other day

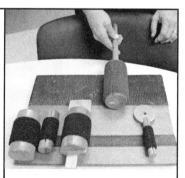

5.12.25 Functional: Elbow, Pouring for Pronation and Supination Tasks

Position: Seated

Targets: Functional use of forearms for pouring movements

Instruction: With two glasses, one full of water, patient sits with elbows bent 90 degrees and pours water from one glass into the other and repeats. A pitcher may also be used.

Substitutions: Elbow not allowed to flare out. Avoid shrugging or tensing shoulder; encourage tall posture and retracted scapula.

Parameters: 10 to 20 pours, 1 to 3 sets, 1 time per day or every other day

5.12.26 Functional: Elbow, Screwdriver

Position: Seated

Targets: Functional use of forearms for turning screwdriver

Instruction: With a bolt and screw box, patient uses screwdriver to put in (supination) and remove screws (pronation).

Substitutions: Avoid shrugging or tensing shoulder; encourage tall posture and retracted scapula.

Parameters: 10 to 20 screws, 1 to 3 sets, 1 time per day or every other day

Section 5.13

ELBOW PROTOCOLS AND TREATMENT IDEAS

5.13.1 LATERAL EPICONDYLITIS/EPICONDALGIA DISCUSSION

Lateral epicondylalgia, epicondylitis, or tennis elbow is a musculoskeletal disorder characterized by pain over the lateral elbow that is typically aggravated by gripping activities. The syndrome is most prevalent in jobs requiring repetitive manual tasks, results in restricted function, and it is one of the most costly of all work-related illnesses. The peak incidence of this condition occurs between the ages of 35 and 50 years and usually affects the dominant arm (Vincenzio, Cleland, & Bisset, 2007). Evidence indicates that the disorder does not involve an inflammatory process, but rather a result from tendinous micro-tearing followed by an incomplete reparative response in the structure of both the extensor carpi radialis brevis muscle and tendon (Rineer & Rush, 2009). Although the most efficient management approach remains controversial, there is a growing body of literature reporting the effects and underlying mechanisms of joint manipulation in the management of lateral epicondylalgia. Evidence exists demonstrating that joint manipulation directed at the elbow and wrist, as well as at the cervical and thoracic spinal regions, results in clinical alterations in pain and the motor system (Vicenzio et al., 2007; Hoogvliet, Randsdrop, Dingemanse, Koes, & Huisstede, 2013).

Where's the Evidence?

Ultrasound therapy and exercise have been shown to be beneficial in the treatment of lateral epicondylitis compared with corticosteroid injection. Murtezani et al. (2015) performed a randomized controlled trial of 12 weeks duration in patients with chronic lateral epicondylitis. They randomly assigned 49 subjects to ultrasound and exercise, *(continued)*

or corticosteroid injection. Outcomes measures used were pain intensity with VAS, functional disability with the patient-rated tennis elbow evaluation questionnaire, and pain-free grip strength. All subjects were evaluated before treatment and at weeks 6 and 12. In the exercise group, significant improvements were demonstrated for VAS, patient-rated tennis elbow evaluation pain and function scores, and pain-free grip strength, compared to the control group. The exercise group reported a significantly greater increase in all variables at 12 weeks than did the control group.

Ultrasound alone has been shown to enhance the recovery of most patients with lateral epicondylitis (Binder, Hodge, Greenwood, Hazelman, & Page Thomas, 1985). However, no strong evidence was presented in any experimental study to suggest that adding a drug to the coupling medium (phonophoresis) produced additional benefits compared with the use of ultrasound alone (Hoppenrath & Ciccone, 2006). Mulligan's mobilization of the elbow with movements can also provide benefits, as well as manipulative therapy to the spine (Herd & Meserve, 2008). Manipulation of the wrist has also been found to offer significant benefit for these patients (Struijs et al., 2003). Kinsiotaping techniques also demonstrate a positive effect on wrist extension force and grip strength of patients with lateral epicondylitis while also reducing pain at the lateral aspect of the elbow in these patients (Shamsoddini & Hollisaz, 2013). (Kouhzad Mohammadi et al., 2014). One study suggests Astym therapy as an effective treatment option for patients with lateral epicondylitis, as an initial treatment, and after an eccentric exercise program has failed. Eccentric exercise is emerging as a first line conservative treatment for lateral epicondylitis and along with Astym therapy is among the few treatment options aiming to improve the degenerative pathophysiology of the tendon (Sevier & Stegnik-Janesen, 2015). Eccentric graded exercise reduces pain and increases muscle strength in chronic tennis elbow more effectively than concentric graded exercise (Peterson, Butler, Ericksson, & Svärdsudd, 2014). Transverse cross friction massage has often been used in conjunction with other treatments, yet reviews of current evidence have not found sufficient evidence to determine the effects of deep transverse friction on pain, improvement in grip strength, or functional status for patients with lateral elbow tendinitis as no evidence of clinically important benefits was found (Loew et al., 2014). Additionally, moderate evidence for the short-term effectiveness was found in favor of stretching plus strengthening exercises vs ultrasound plus friction massage (Hoogvliet, Randsrop, Dingemanse, Koes,

& Huisstede, 2013). Additionally, it has been assessed that physical therapy is needed 3 days per week for 3 weeks in patients with acute lateral epicondylitis. After three weeks, 6 days per week is the most effective treatment frequency (Lee, Ko, & Lee, 2014). Management of lateral epicondylitis also often includes application of a counterforce brace. The most common brace design consists of a single strap wrapped around the proximal forearm. A variation of this brace is the use of an additional strap that wraps above the elbow, which aims to provide further unloading to the injured tissue. Both types of counterforce braces have been reported to have immediate positive effect in participants with lateral epicondylitis, and therefore may be helpful in managing immediate symptoms related to lateral epicondylitis. The choice of which brace to use may be more a function of patient preference, comfort, and cost (Bisset, Collins, & Offord, 2014; Jafarian, Demneh, & Tyson, 2009; Sadeghi-Demneh & Jafarian, 2013).

5.13.2 LATERAL EPICONDYLITIS/EPICONDALGIA PROTOCOL

General protocol guidelines loosely adapted from Virginia Sports Medicine Institute (2001) tennis elbow protocol and current research as outlined in discussion.

Acute Phase 1 to 2 Weeks

1. Pain relief, ice massage, compression, NSAIDs, anti-inflammatory creams, ultrasound, kinesiotaping
2. Avoidance of activities that increase or aggravate pain, modify intensity, duration, and technique of forearm activities "relative rest"
3. Counterforce bracing: place 1 thumb-width distance just below where the pain is (over proximal wrist extensors generally near common extensor tendon over muscle/tendon junction or muscle bellies). Wear snugly, but watch for fingers turning purple or white or numbness tingling presents in forearm/hand. If this happens, loosen the brace immediately.
4. Wrist cock-up splint for more severe cases, remove as needed.
5. Trained therapist may begin cervical, thoracic and wrist mobilization and Mulligan's mobilization of the elbow with movements.
6. AROM
   a. 5.09.3 ROM: Elbow Flexion and Extension, Active
   b. 5.09.7 ROM: Elbow Pronation and Supination, Active
   c. 5.09.1 ROM: Elbow, Self-Flexion and Extension, Passive
      i. Active wrist flexion/extension
      ii. Active wrist radial/ulnar deviation
7. Stretching ideas

   a. 5.15.1 Stretch: Wrist Flexor and Finger Flexor Variation, Self-Assisted
   b. 5.15.2 Stretch: Wrist Flexor Using Wall and Table
   c. 5.15.3 Stretch: Wrist Extensor and Finger Extensor Variation, Self-Assisted
   d. 5.15.4 Stretch: Wrist Extensor Using Wall and Table
   e. 5.15.7 Stretch: Wrist Flexors and Extensors, Self-Massage
   f. 5.06.5 Stretch: Shoulder Horizontal Adductors, Doorway
8. Consider nerve glides
   a. 5.17.1 Nerve Glide: Median Nerve
   b. 5.17.2 Nerve Glide: Radial Nerve
   c. 5.17.3 Nerve Glide: Ulnar Nerve

Strengthening Phase I: 3 to 6 Weeks

   a. 5.16.1 Strengthen: Isometric; Wrist, 4-Way With Variations Using Self, Table, Wall, and Resistance Band
   b. 5.16.2 Strengthen: Isometric and Isotonic; Ball Grip Squeezes
   c. 5.14.6 Strengthen: Wrist Radial/Ulnar Deviation With Dumbbell
      i. Extension elbow flexed
      ii. Eccentric focus extension elbow flexed (heavier weight)

iii. Radial deviation

iv. Ulnar Deviation

d. 5.03.3 Strengthen: Scapular Retraction and Variations

e. 5.01.5 ROM: Scapular Elevation

f. 5.01.6 ROM: Scapular Depression

g. 2.03.4 Strengthen: Isotonic; Chin Tuck

h. 2.02.3 Stretch: Self-Assisted Cervical Lateral Flexion Stretch

i. 2.02.7 Stretch: Cervical Flexion and Rotation

Strengthening Phase II: 7 to 12 Weeks

a. 5.16.6 Strengthen: Isotonic; Wrist, All Planes
   i. Extension elbow extended
   ii. Eccentric focus extension elbow extended

b. 5.16.8 Strengthen: Wrist Roller (focus on extension, palms up)

c. 5.16.10 Strengthen: Resistance Band, Wrist Flexion

d. 5.16.9 Strengthen: Resistance Band, Wrist Extension

e. 5.16.10 Strengthen: Resistance Band, Wrist Flexion

f. 5.16.9 Strengthen: Resistance Band, Wrist Extension

g. 5.16.13 Strengthen: Putty and Gripmaster (Accu Net, LLC) Pro For Hand and Fingers
   i. Double finger grip
   ii. Ball hook grip
   iii. Ball flat grip
   iv. Extension loop
   v. Single extension loop
   vi. Extension spread
   vii. Extension spread variation with rubber band

h. Consider adding additional scapular strengthening and postural correction exercises

i. Consider ideas using web and functional tasks
   i. 5.16.14 Strengthen: Web and Variations For Hand and Fingers
   ii. 5.16.15 Functional, Wrist/Hand and Finger Activities

5.13.3 MEDIAL EPICONDYLITIS/EPICONDALGIA DISCUSSION

Medial epicondylitis, often referred to as golfer's elbow, is another common pathology in the elbow. Flexor-pronator tendon degeneration occurs with repetitive forced wrist extension and forearm supination during activities involving wrist flexion and forearm pronation. A staged process of pathologic change in the tendon can result in structural breakdown and irreparable fibrosis or calcification. Patients typically report persistent medial-side elbow pain that is exacerbated by daily activities. Athletes may be particularly symptomatic during the late cocking or early acceleration phases of the throwing motion. Nonsurgical supportive care includes activity modification, NSAIDs, and corticosteroid injections. Once the acute symptoms are alleviated, focus is turned to flexor-pronator mass rehabilitation and injury prevention. Surgical treatment via open techniques is typically reserved for patients with persistent symptoms (Amin, Kumar, & Schickendantz, 2015). Careful evaluation is important to differentiate medial epicondylitis from other causes of medial elbow pain. A less common cause of medial elbow pain is medial UCL injury. Repetitive valgus stress placed on the joint can lead to micro-traumatic injury and valgus instability (Field & Savoiee, 1988). Nonetheless, medial stress injuries occur in the throwing athlete and can cause inflammation of the adjacent anterior capsule flexor pronator mass, the UCL, and the ulnar nerve (Grana, 2001).

Many of the same treatment principles discussed above under lateral epicondylitis apply to medial epicondylitis with similar treatments focusing on the wrist flexors and common wrist flexor tendon as opposed to the common wrist extensor tendon. The majority of the research focuses on lateral epicondylitis as it is more prevalent. One can infer that graded eccentric exercise, Astym therapy, counterforce bracing, stretching, mobilization of the cervical spine, thoracic spine and wrist, and Mulligan's mobilization of the elbow with movements at the elbow all may potentially assist in rehabilitation of the medial epicondylitis patient.

5.13.4 MEDIAL EPICONDYLITIS/EPICONDALGIA PROTOCOL

General protocol modified from Virginia Sports Medicine Institute (2001) tennis elbow protocol to address the medial epicondylitis/golfer's elbow patient and current research as outlined in discussion.

Acute Phase: 1 to 2 Weeks

1. Pain relief, ice, compression, NSAIDs, anti-inflammatory creams, ultrasound, kinesiotaping
2. Avoidance of activities that increase or aggravate pain, modify intensity, duration, and technique of forearm activities
3. Counterforce bracing: place 1 thumb-width distance just below where the pain is (over proximal wrist flexors generally near common flexor tendon over muscle/tendon junction or muscle bellies). Wear snugly but watch for fingers turning purple or white or numbness or tingling presents in forearm/hand. If this happens, loosen the brace immediately.
4. Trained therapist may begin cervical, thoracic and wrist mobilization and Mulligan's mobilization of the elbow with movements.
5. AROM
    a. 5.09.3 ROM: Elbow Flexion and Extension, Active
    b. 5.09.7 ROM: Elbow Pronation and Supination, Active
    a. 5.14.1 ROM: Wrist and Finger Movements, Passive and Active
        i. Active wrist flexion/extension
        ii. Active wrist radial/ulnar deviation
6. Stretching
    a. 5.15.3 Stretch: Wrist Extensor and Finger Extensor Variation, Self-Assisted
    b. 5.15.4 Stretch: Wrist Extensor Using Wall and Table
    c. 5.15.1 Stretch: Wrist Flexor and Finger Flexor Variation, Self-Assisted
    d. 5.15.2 Stretch: Wrist Flexor Using Wall and Table
    e. 5.13.7 Stretch: Self-Massage Wrist Flexors/Extensors
    f. 5.06.5 Stretch: Shoulder Horizontal Adductors, Doorway
7. Consider nerve glides
    a. 5.17.1 Nerve Glide: Median Nerve
    b. 5.17.2 Nerve Glide: Radial Nerve
    c. 5.17.3 Nerve Glide: Ulnar Nerve

Strengthening Phase I: 3 to 6 Weeks

    a. 5.16.1 Strengthen: Isometric; Wrist, 4-Way With Variations Using Self, Table, Wall, and Resistance Band
    b. 5.16.2 Strengthen: Isometric and Isotonic; Ball Grip Squeezes
    c. 5.16.6 Strengthen: Isotonic; Wrist, All Planes
        i. Flexion elbow flexed
        ii. Eccentric focus flexion elbow flexed (heavier weight)
        iii. Radial deviation
        iv. Ulnar deviation
    d. 5.03.3 Strengthen: Scapular Retraction and Variations
    e. 5.01.5 ROM: Scapular Elevation
    f. 5.01.6 ROM: Scapular Depression
    g. 2.03.4 Strengthen: Isotonic; Chin Tuck
    h. 2.02.3 Stretch: Self-Assisted Cervical Lateral Flexion
    i. 2.02.7 Stretch: Cervical Flexion and Rotation

Strengthening Phase II: 7 to 12 Weeks

    a. 5.16.6 Strengthen: Isotonic; Wrist, All Planes
        i. Flexion Elbow Extended
        ii. Eccentric Focus Flexion Elbow Extended
    b. 5.16.8 Strengthen: Wrist Roller (focus on flexion, palm up)
    c. 5.16.10 Strengthen: Resistance Band, Wrist Flexion
    d. 5.16.9 Strengthen: Resistance Band, Wrist Extension
    e. 5.16.10 Strengthen: Resistance Band, Wrist Flexion
    f. 5.16.9 Strengthen: Resistance Band, Wrist Extension
    g. 5.16.13 Strengthen: Putty and Gripmaster Pro For Hand and Fingers
        i. Double finger grip
        ii. Ball hook grip
        iii. Ball flat grip
        iv. Extension loop
        v. Single extension loop
        vi. Extension spread
        vii. Extension spread variation with rubber band
    h. Consider adding additional scapular strengthening and postural correction exercises
    i. Consider ideas using web and functional tasks
        i. 5.16.14 Strengthen: Web and Variations For Hand and Fingers
        ii. 5.16.15 Functional, Wrist/Hand and Finger Activities

5.13.5 Lateral Epicondylectomy or Medial Epicondylectomy Protocol

General protocol adapted from Methodist Sports Medicine Center Department of Physical Therapy (2004) Lateral or Medial Epicondylectomy Rehabilitation Protocol.

Lateral epicondylectomy consists of a lateral incision made approximately 3 to 4 cm, beginning just proximal to the lateral epicondyle and extending distally at the interval between the extensor carpi radialis longus and brevis tendons. The fascia is incised, and the extensor longus muscle is retracted anteriorly exposing the brevis tendon. Abnormal tendon tissue, which appears grayish and gelatinous, is excised by sharp dissection. The lateral epicondyle is debrided down to subchondral bone. Multiple holes are made in the bone to promote a fibroproliferative healing response, and the fascia is repaired (Methodist Sports Medicine Center Department of Physical Therapy, 2004).

Medial epicondylectomy consists of a longitudinal incision made beginning just proximal to the medial epicondyle and extending distally at the interval between the pronator teres and flexor carpi radialis tendon. Dissection is carried down through the subcutaneous tissues, exposing the flexor pronator mass. Abnormal tissue, which is usually present between the pronator teres and flexor carpi radialis tendon, is excised. The medial epicondyle is debrided down to subchondral bone. Multiple holes are made in the bone to promote a fibroproliferative healing response, and the fascia is repaired (Methodist Sports Medicine Center, 2004).

Acute Phase: 1 to 3 Weeks

1. Pain relief, ice, gentle compression for swelling
2. Patient may be in immobilizer/long arm splint; usually worn between exercises and at night, follow physician guidelines.
3. PROM start at 2 weeks
4. AROM 6 times per day
   a. 5.09.3 ROM: Elbow Flexion and Extension, Active
   b. 5.09.7 ROM: Elbow Pronation and Supination, Active
   c. 5.14.1 ROM: Wrist and Finger Movements, Passive and Active
      i. Active wrist flexion/extension
      ii. Active wrist radial/ulnar deviation
      iii. Active fist to finger spread

Phase II: 3 to 6 Weeks

1. Patient may begin to wean off immobilizer/long arm splint at weeks 4 to 5; follow physician guidelines.
2. Continue PROM and AROM 6 times per day
3. Scar massage
4. Continue AROM
5. Stretching
   a. 5.15.3 Stretch: Wrist Extensor and Finger Extensor Variation, Self-Assisted
   b. 5.15.1 Stretch: Wrist Flexor and Finger Flexor Variation, Self-Assisted
   c. 5.06.5 Stretch: Shoulder Horizontal Adductors, Doorway
6. Consider nerve glides
   a. 5.17.1 Nerve Glide: Median Nerve
   b. 5.17.2 Nerve Glide: Radial Nerve
   c. 5.17.3 Nerve Glide: Ulnar Nerve
7. Light strengthening—starts at 5 to 6 weeks:
   a. 5.16.1 Strengthen: Isometric; Wrist, 4-Way With Variations Using Self, Table, Wall, and Resistance Band
   b. 5.16.13 Strengthen: Putty and Gripmaster Pro For Hand and Fingers
   c. 5.16.2 Strengthen: Isometric and Isotonic; Ball Grip Squeezes
   d. 5.16.6 Strengthen: Isotonic; Wrist, All Planes
      i. Flexion elbow flexed light weight 1 to 2 lbs
      ii. Extension elbow flexed light weight 1 to 2 lbs
      iii. Radial deviation light weight 1 to 2 lbs
      iv. Ulnar deviation
   e. 5.12.10 Strengthen: Isotonic; Elbow Flexion, Curls (light weight 1 to 2 lbs)
   f. 5.03.3 Strengthen: Scapular Retraction and Variations
   g. 5.01.5 ROM: Scapular Elevation
   h. 5.01.6 ROM: Scapular Depression
   i. 2.03.4 Strengthen: Isotonic; Chin Tuck
   j. 2.02.3 Stretch: Self-Assisted Cervical Lateral Flexion Stretch
   k. 2.02.7 Stretch: Cervical Flexion and Rotation

Phase III: Strengthening Phase 6 Weeks to 6 Months

1. Wrist and elbow strengthening
   a. 5.16.6 Strengthen: Isotonic; Wrist, All Planes
      i. Flexion elbow extended
      ii. Extension elbow extended
      iii. Eccentric focus flexion elbow extended
      iv. Eccentric focus extension elbow extended
   b. 5.16.8 Strengthen: Wrist Roller (focus on flexion, palm up)
   c. 5.16.10 Strengthen: Resistance Band, Wrist Flexion
   d. 5.16.9 Strengthen: Resistance Band, Wrist Extension

2. RC strengthening
   a. 5.07.36 Strengthen: Isotonic: Resistance Band: Flexion, Scaption, Abduction, and Variations
   b. 5.07.39 Strengthen: Isotonic: Resistance Band: Internal Rotation (Neutral)
   c. 5.07.41 Strengthen: Isotonic: Resistance Band: External Rotation (Neutral)

d. Consider adding additional scapular strengthening and postural correction exercises
e. Consider ideas using web and functional tasks
   i. 5.16.14 Strengthen: Web and Variations For Hand and Fingers
   ii. 5.16.15 Functional, Wrist/Hand and Finger Activities

5.13.6 ULNAR COLLATERAL LIGAMENT INJURY AND RECONSTRUCTION (TOMMY JOHN SURGERY)

Tommy John was a pitcher for the Los Angeles Dodgers who sustained an injury to the ulnar (medial) collateral ligament of the elbow. Dr. Frank Jobe performed an UCL reconstruction on Tommy using a grafted tendon to replace the ligament in 1974 and subsequently named the procedure after his patient. UCL can be torn or ruptured from repetitive throwing due to the valgus stress at the elbow when the shoulder is in the 90 degrees abduction and full external rotation position. UCL injuries are most commonly reported in baseball players (particularly in pitchers) but have also been observed in other overhead athletes including those involved in javelin, softball, tennis, volleyball, water polo, and gymnastics (Dugas, Chronister, Cain, & Andrews, 2014). Younger athletes can also develop this, termed *little league elbow*; however, due to the epiphyseal plate still being open, the force usually results in bony trauma such as stress fractures, avulsion, and apophysitis more often than UCL tears. UCL reconstruction is performed most commonly in collegiate athletes and more specifically baseball athletes with higher incidence in pitchers. UCL reconstruction has

Where's the Evidence?

One study found that out of 147 major league baseball pitchers who underwent UCL reconstruction, 80% returned to pitch in at least one major league baseball game, but only 67% of established pitchers returned to the same level of competition post-operatively, and 57% of established players returned to the disabled list because of injuries to the throwing arm (Makhni et al., 2014). The most common complications of UCL reconstruction are generally associated with the ulnar nerve; however, transition to the muscle-splitting approach has decreased the occurrence of these complications (Purcell, Matava, & Wright, 2007).

a fairly good success rate allowing high school, collegiate and professional athletes to return to sport at the same or higher level of competition within 1 year post-operation (Osbahr et al., 2014).

5.13.7 ULNAR COLLATERAL LIGAMENT RECONSTRUCTION PROTOCOL USING AUTOGENOUS GRAFT

General protocol guidelines adapted from Ellenbecker, Wilk, Altchek, and Andrews post-operative rehabilitation following chronic UCL reconstruction using autogenous graft published in 2009.

Phase I: Immediate Post-Operative 0 to 3 Weeks

1. Goals
   a. Maintain/protect integrity of repair
   b. Gradually increase PROM as detailed
   c. Diminish pain and inflammation; ice, compression.
   d. Prevent muscular inhibition
   e. Become independent with modified ADLs

Week 1

1. Week 0 to 1: Maintain arm in posterior split at 90 degrees elbow flexion
2. AROM wrist
   a. 5.14.1 ROM: Wrist and Finger Movements, Passive and Active
      i. Active wrist flexion/extension
      ii. Active wrist radial/ulnar deviation
   b. 5.16.2 Strengthen: Isometric and Isotonic; Ball Grip Squeezes

3. Shoulder isometrics: no external rotation
   a. 5.07.1 Strengthen: Isometric: Other Hand Resists, 6-Way (no external rotation)
4. Biceps isometrics
   a. 5.12.2 Strengthen: Isometric; Elbow Flexion

Week 2

1. Week 1 to 2: functional brace 30 degrees to 100 degrees
2. Wrist isometrics
   a. 5.16.1 Strengthen: Isometric; Wrist, 4-Way With Variations Using Self, Table, Wall, and Resistance Band
3. Scapular exercises
   a. 5.03.3 Strengthen: Scapular Retraction; only variations listed below.
      i. A: Unilateral side-lying
      ii. B: Bilateral seated
   b. 5.01.5 ROM: Scapular Elevation
   c. 5.01.6 ROM<: Scapular Depression
4. Triceps isometrics
   a. 5.12.1 Strengthen: Isometric; Elbow Extension

Week 3

1. Week 2 to 3: functional brace 15 degrees to 110 degrees

Phase II: Intermediate 4 to 8 Weeks

1. Goals
   a. Gradually increase ROM as detailed
   b. Promote healing of repaired tissue
   c. Regain and improve muscle strength

Week 4

2. Functional brace set 10 degrees to 120 degrees
3. Wrist strengthening
   a. 5.16.6 Strengthen: Isotonic; Wrist, All Planes (1 lb or .5 Kg)
      i. Flexion elbow flexed
      ii. Extension elbow flexed
      iii. Radial deviation
      iv. Ulnar deviation
4. Elbow strengthening
   a. 5.12.10 Strengthen: Isotonic; Elbow Flexion, Curls (1 lbs or 0.5 Kg)
   b. 5.12.7 Strengthen: Isotonic; Elbow Extension, Kick-Back (1 lbs or 0.5 Kg)
   c. 5.12.12 Strengthen: Isotonic; Elbow Pronation and Supination With Hammer (1 lbs or 0.5 Kg)
5. Shoulder strengthening
   a. 5.07.10 Strengthen: Isotonic: Flexion
   b. 5.07.11 Strengthen: Isotonic: Scaption
   c. 5.07.12 Strengthen: Isotonic: Shoulder Abduction
   d. 5.07.21 Strengthen: Isotonic: Internal Rotation

   e. 5.07.22 Strengthen: Isotonic: External Rotation (limit ROM to 45 degrees until week 6)
   f. 5.07.13 Strengthen: Isotonic: Shoulder Extension
   g. 5.07.19 Strengthen: Isotonic; Shoulder, Horizontal Abduction, Bent Forward
   h. 5.07.20 Strengthen: Isotonic; Shoulder, Horizontal Abduction, Deceleration Emphasis

Week 6

1. Functional brace set 0 degrees to 130 degrees, AROM without brace to 140 degrees
2. Discontinue brace at 6 to 8 weeks per physician clearance
3. Wrist strengthening
   a. 5.16.6 Strengthen: Isotonic; Wrist, All Planes (gradually progress weights).
   b. Flexion elbow flexed
   c. Extension elbow flexed
   d. Radial deviation
   e. Ulnar deviation
4. Elbow strengthening
   a. 5.12.10 Strengthen: Isotonic; Elbow Flexion, Curls (gradually progress weights). 5.12.7 Strengthen: Isotonic; Elbow Extension, Kick-Back (gradually progress weights)
   b. 5.12.12 Strengthen: Isotonic; Elbow Pronation and Supination With Hammer (gradually progress weights).
   c. 5.12.13 Strengthen: Resistance Band, Elbow Extension
   d. 5.12.14 Strengthen: Resistance Band, Tricep Push Down
   e. 5.12.9 Strengthen: Isotonic; Elbow Kick-Out
   f. 5.12.15 Strengthen: Resistance Band, Elbow Extension, Shoulder Flexed
   g. 5.12.17 Strengthen: Resistance Band, Elbow Flexion
   h. 5.12.24 Functional: Elbow, Velcro Roller for Pronation and Supination Tasks
5. Shoulder strengthening
   a. 5.07.36 Strengthen: Isotonic: Resistance Band: Flexion, Scaption, Abduction, and Variations (start by staying below shoulder level/90 degrees)
   b. 5.07.22 Strengthen: Isotonic: External Rotation; Full Range Allowed Now.
   c. 5.07.13 Strengthen: Isotonic: Shoulder Extension
   d. 5.07.19 Strengthen: Isotonic; Shoulder, Horizontal Abduction, Bent Forward
   e. 5.07.20 Strengthen: Isotonic; Shoulder, Horizontal Abduction, Deceleration Emphasis
   f. 5.07.24 Strengthen: Isotonic; Shoulder, Row (Prone)
   g. 5.07.25 Strengthen: Isotonic; Shoulder, Military Press (Prone)

   h. 5.07.29 Strengthen: Isotonic; Resistance Band, Shoulder Abduction

   i. 5.07.30 Strengthen: Isotonic; Resistance Band, Shoulder Adduction

   j. 5.07.32 Strengthen: Isotonic; Resistance Band, Shoulder, Horizontal Abduction

   k. 5.07.34 Strengthen: Isotonic; Resistance Band and Machine, Shoulder, Lat Pull-Down

   l. 5.07.36 Strengthen: Isotonic: Resistance Band: Flexion, Scaption, Abduction, And Variations

   m. 5.07.38 Strengthen: Isotonic: Resistance Band: Extension

6. "Thrower's 10"

   a. 5.16.6 Strengthen: Isotonic; Wrist, All Planes (progress weights).

   b. 5.12.12 Strengthen: Isotonic; Elbow Pronation and Supination With Hammer (progress weights).

   c. 5.07.42 Strengthen: Isotonic; Resistance Band, Shoulder, Combination Movements PNF D1 and D2

     i. D2 Flexion: "UnSheath You Sword to Tada"

     ii. D2 Extension: "Tada! To Sheath the Sword"

   d. 5.07.39 Strengthen: Isotonic: Resistance Band: Internal Rotation and Variations

   e. 5.07.41 Strengthen: Isotonic: Resistance Band: External Rotation and Variations

   f. 5.07.22 Strengthen: Isotonic: External Rotation (Already Doing)

   g. 5.07.10 Strengthen: Isotonic: Flexion (Already Doing)

   h. 5.07.11 Strengthen: Isotonic: Scaption (Already Doing)

   i. 5.07.24 Strengthen: Isotonic; Shoulder, Row (Prone)

   j. 5.07.27 Strengthen: Isotonic: Posterior Cuff, 4-Way

   k. 5.07.23 Strengthen: Isotonic; Shoulder External Rotation 90/90

   l. 5.12.16 Strengthen: Resistance Band, Elbow Extension, Overhead (or use cable machine or dumbbell).

   m. 5.07.61 Strengthen: Closed Kinetic Chain: Beginning Weightbearing, Progress To Push-Up Partial Weight

   n. 5.07.62 Strengthen: Closed Kinetic Chain; Shoulder, Push-Up

   o. 5.07.63 Strengthen: Closed Kinetic Chain: Scapular And Shoulder Depression

Phase III: Advanced Strengthening 9 to 13 Weeks

1. Goals

   a. Increase strength, power, and endurance

   b. Maintain full AROM

   c. Initiate sports activities

Week 9

1. Progress previous exercises shoulder, scapula, elbow and wrist strengthening

2. Initiate eccentric elbow flexion/extension

3. Add manual resistance to diagonal patterns

4. Neuromuscular training

   a. 5.07.91 Reactive Neuromuscular Training and Variations, Shoulder

     i. Rhythmic stabilization internal/external rotation side-lying shoulder neutral

     ii. Rhythmic stabilization internal/external rotation supine shoulder neutral

     iii. Rhythmic stabilization internal/external rotation supine shoulder 30 degrees abducted (scaption plane)

     iv. Rhythmic stabilization side-lying shoulder abducted

     v. Rhythmic stabilization supine shoulder flexed or in scaption

   b. 5.07.79 Plyometrics/Dynamic: Shoulder, Wall Dribbles

   c. 5.07.67 Strengthen: Closed Kinetic Chain: Bodyblade Flexion, Scaption, and Abduction

   d. 5.07.68 Strengthen: Closed Kinetic Chain; Bodyblade, Shoulder Internal Rotation and External Rotation

   e. 5.07.69 Strengthen: Closed Kinetic Chain; Bodyblade, Shoulder, D1 and D2

5. Strengthening ideas

   a. 5.07.60 Strengthen: Closed Kinetic Chain; Shoulder, Alternating Arm Lift

   b. 5.07.59 Strengthen: Closed Kinetic Chain; Shoulder, Resistance Band, Tripod Stabilization

   c. 5.07.71 Strengthen: Closed Kinetic Chain; Shoulder, Inverted Row

   d. 5.07.52 Strengthen: Exercise Ball, Shoulder, Push-Up, Hands on Ball

   e. 5.07.52 Strengthen: Exercise Ball, Shoulder, Push-Up, Hands on Ball

   f. 5.07.46 Strengthen: Isotonic; Resistance Band, Shoulder Pull-Over

   g. 5.07.47 Strengthen: Isotonic: Resistance Band: Pull Back

   h. 5.07.45 Strengthen: Isotonic; Resistance Band, Shoulder, Chest Fly

   i. 5.07.43 Strengthen: Isotonic; Resistance Band, Shoulder, Standing Military (Overhead) Press

Week 11

1. Continue progressing previously listed exercises

2. May begin light sport activities (i.e. golf, swimming)

Week 12

1. Initiate plyometrics; *2 hand drills only.*

2. May initiate interval hitting program for baseball players
3. Two hand plyometric drills
   a. 5.07.80 Plyometrics/Dynamic: Ball Toss, Overhead
   b. 5.07.81 Plyometrics/Dynamic: Chest Pass
   c. 5.07.82 Plyometrics/Dynamic: Shoulder, Bench Press/Floor Throws
   d. 5.07.83 Plyometrics/Dynamic: Shoulder, Two-Handed Side Throw
   e. 5.07.86 Plyometrics/Dynamic: Shoulder, Ball Toss, Overhead and Backwards
   f. 5.07.90 Plyometrics/Dynamic: Shoulder, Push-Offs
   g. 5.07.88 Plyometrics/Dynamic: Shoulder, Slams
   h. 5.07.87 Plyometrics/Dynamic: Shoulder, Push-Up
   i. 5.07.89 Plyometrics/Dynamic: Shoulder, Ball Squat, Push-Press

Phase IV: Return to Activity Phase 12 to 26 Weeks

1. Goals
   a. Increase strength, power, and endurance
   b. Return to sports activities

Week 14

1. Address any flexibility concerns and progress previous strengthening program

2. Progress neuromuscular training
   a. 5.07.91 Reactive Neuromuscular Training and Variations, Shoulder
      i. F. Rhythmic stabilization standing early cocking position
      ii. H. Rhythmic stabilization standing late cocking position
      iii. I. Rhythmic stabilization standing late cocking position
   b. 5.07.70 Strengthen: Closed Kinetic Chain; Shoulder, Plank Shuffle on Medicine Ball
3. Begin one hand plyometric drills
   a. 5.07.85 Plyometrics/Dynamic: Shoulder, Multidirectional Catch/Throw
   b. 5.07.84 Plyometrics/Dynamic: Shoulder, 90/90 Throw

Week 16 to 22

1. Continue progressing all of the above
2. Stretch ROM
   a. Refer to 5.06 for shoulder stretching
   b. Refer to 5.10 for elbow stretching
3. Progress to off-the-mound at 16 weeks

6 to 9 Months

1. Return to competitive throwing

5.13.8 ULNAR COLLATERAL LIGAMENT RECONSTRUCTION PROTOCOL USING DOCKING PROCEDURE

General protocol guidelines adapted from Ellenbecker et al. (2009) post-operative rehabilitation following chronic UCL reconstruction using docking procedure published in 2009.

Phase I: Immediate Post-Operative 0 to 3 Weeks

1. Goals
   a. Maintain and protect integrity of repair
   b. Gradually increase PROM as detailed
   c. Diminish pain and inflammation; ice, compression.
   d. Prevent muscular inhibition
   e. Become independent with modified ADLs

Week 1 to 4

1. Brace set at 30 degrees to 90 degrees worn at all times; elbow AROM in brace encouraged.
2. AROM wrist
   a. 5.14.1 ROM: Wrist and Finger Movements, Passive and Active
      i. Active wrist flexion/extension
      ii. Active wrist radial/ulnar deviation

   b. 5.16.2 Strengthen: Isometric and Isotonic; Ball Grip Squeezes
3. Scapular exercises
   a. 5.03.3 Strengthen: Scapular Retraction; Only Variations Listed Below.
      i. A: Unilateral side-lying
      ii. B: Bilateral seated
   b. 5.01.5 ROM: Scapular Elevation
   c. 5.01.6 ROM: Scapular Depression

Phase II: 4 to 6 Weeks

1. Goals
   a. Gradually increase ROM as detailed
   b. Promote healing of repaired tissue
   c. Regain and improve muscle strength
2. Brace limited to 15 degrees to 115 degrees ROM
3. Brace worn at all times
4. No PROM

5. No valgus stress
6. AROM in brace encourage
7. Wrist isometrics
   a. 5.16.1 Strengthen: Isometric; Wrist, 4-Way With Variations Using Self, Table, Wall, and Resistance Band
8. Biceps isometrics
   a. 5.12.2 Strengthen: Isometric; Elbow Flexion
9. Triceps isometrics
   a. 5.12.1 Strengthen: Isometric; Elbow Extension
10. Shoulder isometrics: flexion, abduction, and extension only; no rotation or adduction.
    a. 5.07.1 Strengthen: Isometric; Shoulder, Other Hand Resists, 6-Way; Flexion, Abduction and Extension Only, No Rotation or Adduction.

Phase III: 6 to 12 Weeks

1. Goals
   a. Restore full ROM
   b. Regain and improve muscle strength to 5/5
   c. Restore endurance of UE
2. Minimize valgus stress
3. No PROM by clinician
4. No pain with exercise
5. ROM
   a. 5.09.3 ROM: Elbow Flexion and Extension, Active
   b. 5.09.4 ROM: Elbow, Low-Load, Long-Duration Extension, Passive
6. Wrist strengthening
   a. 5.16.6 Strengthen: Isotonic; Wrist, All Planes (1lb or .5 Kg)
      i. Flexion elbow flexed
      ii. Extension elbow flexed
      iii. Radial deviation
      iv. Ulnar deviation
7. Elbow strengthening
   a. 5.12.10 Strengthen: Isotonic; Elbow Flexion, Curls
   b. 5.12.7 Strengthen: Isotonic; Elbow Extension, Kick-Back
   c. Start at 8 Weeks: 5.12.12 Strengthen: Isotonic; Elbow Pronation and Supination With Hammer
8. Shoulder strengthening
   a. 5.07.10 Strengthen: Isotonic: Flexion
   b. 5.07.11 Strengthen: Isotonic: Scaption
   c. 5.07.12 Strengthen: Isotonic: Shoulder Abduction
   d. 5.07.13 Strengthen: Isotonic: Shoulder Extension
9. Shoulder strengthening start at 8 weeks
   a. 5.07.21 Strengthen: Isotonic: Internal Rotation
   b. 5.07.22 Strengthen: Isotonic: External Rotation
   c. 5.07.19 Strengthen: Isotonic; Shoulder, Horizontal Abduction, Bent Forward
   d. 5.07.20 Strengthen: Isotonic; Shoulder, Horizontal Abduction, Deceleration Emphasis

10. Conditioning
    a. 5.04.1 ROM: Active Assistive: Warm-Up Upper Body Ergometer
11. Neuromuscular training
    a. 5.07.91 Reactive Neuromuscular Training and Variations, Shoulder
       i. Rhythmic stabilization internal/external rotation side-lying shoulder neutral
       ii. Rhythmic stabilization internal/external rotation supine shoulder neutral
       iii. Rhythmic stabilization internal/external rotation supine shoulder 30 degrees abducted (scaption plane)
       iv. Rhythmic stabilization side-lying shoulder abducted
       v. Rhythmic stabilization supine shoulder flexed or in scaption
    b. 5.07.79 Plyometrics/Dynamic: Shoulder, Wall Dribbles
    c. 5.07.67 Strengthen: Closed Kinetic Chain: Bodyblade Flexion, Scaption, and Abduction
    d. 5.07.68 Strengthen: Closed Kinetic Chain; Bodyblade, Shoulder Internal Rotation and External Rotation
    e. 5.07.69 Strengthen: Closed Kinetic Chain; Bodyblade, Shoulder, D1 and D2

Phase IV: Advanced Strengthening: 12 to 16 Weeks

1. Goals
   a. Full strength and flexibility
   b. Restore neuromuscular function
   c. Prepare for return to activity
2. Stretch ROM
   a. Refer to Section **5.06** for shoulder stretching
   b. Refer to Section **5.10** for elbow stretching
3. Wrist strengthening
      i. 5.14.6 Strengthen: Isotonic Wrist All Planes; gradually progress weights.
      ii. Flexion elbow flexed
      iii. Extension elbow flexed
      iv. Radial deviation
      v. Ulnar deviation
4. Elbow strengthening
   a. 5.12.10 Strengthen: Isotonic; Elbow Flexion, Curls (gradually progress weights). 5.12.7 Strengthen: Isotonic; Elbow Extension, Kick-Back (gradually progress weights).
   b. 5.12.13 Strengthen: Resistance Band, Elbow Extension
   c. Strengthen: Resistance Band, Tricep Push Down
   d. 5.12.9 Strengthen: Isotonic; Elbow Kick-Out
   e. 5.12.15 Strengthen: Resistance Band, Elbow Extension, Shoulder Flexed

    f. 5.12.12 Strengthen: Isotonic; Elbow Pronation and Supination With Hammer (gradually progress weights).

    g. 5.12.17 Strengthen: Resistance Band, Elbow Flexion

    h. 5.12.24 Functional: Elbow, Velcro Roller for Pronation and Supination Tasks

5. Shoulder strengthening

    a. 5.07.36 Strengthen: Isotonic: Resistance Band: Flexion, Scaption, Abduction, and Variations (Start By Staying Below Shoulder Level/90 degrees)

    b. 5.07.22 Strengthen: Isotonic: External Rotation; Full Range Allowed Now.

    c. 5.07.13 Strengthen: Isotonic: Shoulder Extension

    d. 5.07.19 Strengthen: Isotonic; Shoulder, Horizontal Abduction, Bent Forward

    e. 5.07.20 Strengthen: Isotonic: Horizontal Abduction, Deceleration Emphasis

    f. 5.07.24 Strengthen: Isotonic; Shoulder, Row (Prone)

    g. 5.07.25 Strengthen: Isotonic; Shoulder, Military Press (Prone)

    h. 5.07.29 Strengthen: Isotonic; Resistance Band, Shoulder Abduction

    i. 5.07.30 Strengthen: Isotonic; Resistance Band, Shoulder Adduction

    j. 5.07.32 Strengthen: Isotonic; Resistance Band, Shoulder, Horizontal Abduction

    k. 5.07.34 Strengthen: Isotonic; Resistance Band and Machine, Shoulder, Lat Pull-Down

    l. 5.07.36 Strengthen: Isotonic: Resistance Band: Flexion, Scaption, Abduction, and Variations

    m. 5.07.38 Strengthen: Isotonic: Resistance Band: Extension

6. "Thrower's 10"

    a. 5.16.6 Strengthen: Isotonic; Wrist, All Planes (progress weights).

    b. 5.12.12 Strengthen: Isotonic; Elbow Pronation and Supination With Hammer (progress weights).

    c. 5.07.42 Strengthen: Isotonic; Resistance Band, Shoulder, Combination Movements PNF D1 and D2

        i. D2 Flexion: "UnSheath Your Sword To Tada!"

        ii. D2 Extension: "Tada! To Sheath The Sword"

    d. 5.07.39 Strengthen: Isotonic: Resistance Band: Internal Rotation and Variations

    e. 5.07.41 Strengthen: Isotonic: Resistance Band: External Rotation and Variations

    f. 5.07.22 Strengthen: Isotonic: External Rotation (already doing)

    g. 5.07.10 Strengthen: Isotonic: Flexion (already doing)

    h. 5.07.11 Strengthen: Isotonic: Scaption (already doing)

    i. 5.07.24 Strengthen: Isotonic; Shoulder, Row (Prone)

    j. 5.07.27 Strengthen: Isotonic: Posterior Cuff, 4-Way

    k. 5.07.23 Strengthen: Isotonic; Shoulder External Rotation 90/90

    l. 5.12.16 Strengthen: Resistance Band, Elbow Extension, Overhead (or use cable machine or dumbbell)

    m. 5.07.61 Strengthen: Closed Kinetic Chain: Beginning Weightbearing, Progress To Push-Up Partial Weight

    n. 5.07.62 Strengthen: Closed Kinetic Chain; Shoulder, Push-Up

    o. 5.07.63 Strengthen: Closed Kinetic Chain: Scapular And Shoulder Depression

7. Strengthening ideas

    a. 5.07.60 Strengthen: Closed Kinetic Chain; Shoulder, Alternating Arm Lift

    b. 5.07.59 Strengthen: Closed Kinetic Chain; Shoulder, Resistance Band, Tripod Stabilization

    c. 5.07.71 Strengthen: Closed Kinetic Chain; Shoulder, Inverted Row

    d. 5.07.52 Strengthen: Exercise Ball, Shoulder, Push-Up, Hands on Ball

    e. 5.07.52 Strengthen: Exercise Ball, Shoulder, Push-Up, Hands on Ball

    f. 5.07.46 Strengthen: Isotonic; Resistance Band, Shoulder Pull-Over

    g. 5.07.47 Strengthen: Isotonic: Resistance Band: Pull Back

    h. 5.07.45 Strengthen: Isotonic; Resistance Band, Shoulder, Chest Fly

    i. 5.07.43 Strengthen: Isotonic; Resistance Band, Shoulder, Standing Military (Overhead) Press

8. Initiate plyometrics (2-hand drills only, pain-free)

    a. 5.07.80 Plyometrics/Dynamic: Ball Toss, Overhead

    b. 5.07.81 Plyometrics/Dynamic: Chest Pass

    c. 5.5.07.82 Plyometrics/Dynamic: Shoulder, Bench Press/Floor Throws

    d. 5.07.83 Plyometrics/Dynamic: Shoulder, Two-Handed Side Throw

    e. 5.07.86 Plyometrics/Dynamic: Shoulder, Ball Toss, Overhead and Backwards

    f. 5.07.90 Plyometrics/Dynamic: Shoulder, Push-Offs

    g. 5.07.88 Plyometrics/Dynamic: Shoulder, Slams

    h. 5.07.87 Plyometrics/Dynamic: Shoulder, Push-Up

    i. 5.07.89 Plyometrics/Dynamic: Shoulder, Ball Squat, Push-Press

9. Progress neuromuscular training; pain-free, late stage of phase IV.

    a. 5.07.91 Reactive Neuromuscular Training and Variations, Shoulder

        i. F. Rhythmic stabilization standing early cocking position

        ii. H. Rhythmic stabilization standing late cocking position

iii. I. Rhythmic stabilization standing late cocking position

b. 5.07.70 Strengthen: Closed Kinetic Chain; Shoulder, Plank Shuffle on Medicine Ball

10. Begin 1-hand plyometric drills; pain-free, late stage of phase IV.

    a. 5.07.85 Plyometrics/Dynamic: Shoulder, Multidirectional Catch/Throw

    b. 5.07.84 Plyometrics/Dynamic: Shoulder, 90/90 Throw

11. Core strengthening; abdominals, lower back, gluteals, LEs.

Phase V: 4 to 9 Months

1. Goals

    a. Increase strength, power, and endurance

    b. Return to sports activities

2. Address any flexibility concerns and progress previous strengthening program

3. Begin interval throwing program 4 months

4. Begin hitting program 5 months

5. Return to competitive sport once cleared by physician

5.13.9 ULNOHUMERAL DISLOCATION DISCUSSION

Uncomplicated Posterior Elbow Dislocation

In children under 10 years of age, posterior elbow dislocations are the most common type of joint dislocation. In adults, the posterior elbow joint is the second most commonly dislocated joint preceded by shoulder dislocations. Approximately 90% of all elbow dislocations are directionally classified as posterior or posterolateral and are more commonly seen in the non-dominant UE and are typically caused by falling on an outstretch hand (Texas State University, 2016). Posterior elbow dislocation occurs when the radius and ulna are forcefully driven posterior to the humerus. Specifically, the olecranon process of the ulna moves into the olecranon fossa of the humerus and the trochlea of the humerus is displaced over the coronoid process of the ulna. Posterior elbow dislocation is classified as either simple or complex and staged according to severity. Axial compression on the elbow in combination with supination and valgus stress primarily result in the rupture of the lateral UCL, which may cause posterolateral subluxation (Englert, Zellner, Koller, Nerlich, & Lenich, 2013). Early reduction of elbow dislocation, by closed or open means, is of paramount importance if good functional results are to be obtained. Closed reduction of an elbow dislocation is unlikely to be successful if attempted later than 21 days after the injury (Bruce, Laing, Dorgan, Klenerman, & 1993). Immobilization and stress deprivation negatively alters the morphologic, biochemical, and biomechanical characteristics of various components of synovial joints (Akeson, Amiel, Abel, Garfin, & Woo, 1987).

Limited immobilization with a posterior splint is encouraged along with active ROM exercises early in the ROM program to decrease pain at the articulation (Blackard & Sampson, 1997). Schippinger and colleagues found that reducing the elbow for 2 weeks enhances patient comfort and does not adversely affect the eventual outcome,

Where's the Evidence?

Mehlhoff, Noble, Bennett, and Tullos (1988) evaluated the long-term results after treatment of simple dislocation of the elbow in 52 adults, comparing with and without prolonged immobilization after closed reduction. Despite the generally favorable prognosis for this injury, 60% of patients reported some symptoms on follow-up. A flexion contracture of more than 30 degrees was documented in 15% of the patients, residual pain in 45%, and pain on valgus stress in 35 %. Prolonged immobilization after injury was strongly associated with an unsatisfactory result. The longer the immobilization had been, the larger the flexion contracture and the more severe the symptoms of pain. The results indicate that early active motion is the key factor in rehabilitation of the elbow after a dislocation.

however, splintage for over 3 weeks may result in worse function (Schippinger, Seilbert, Steinböck, & Kucharczyk, 1999). Once an elbow is stabile after reduction, a plaster cast may be applied for 3 to 5 days to maintain the forearm in supination and the elbow flexed at 90 degrees. The ROM needs to be adjusted according to the injured ligament. Lateral UCL could be set at 0 to 30 to 110 degrees for extension and flexion in weeks 1 and 2, at 0 to 20 to 120 degrees in weeks 3 and 4, and at 0 to 10 to 130 degrees in weeks 5 and 6. After the week 6, free ROM with light weight should be possible. The ROM is then expanded by 10 degrees per week according to a patient's pain symptoms. Physiotherapists can monitor the healing process with its inflammatory reaction (Englert et al., 2013). For posterolateral instability conservative management, it is recommended to avoid flexion and supination combination movement for 6 weeks and immobilization after reduction in full pronation and 90 to 120 degrees of elbow flexion is encouraged to promote stability (Wolff & Hotchkiss, 2006).

Complicated Posterior Elbow Dislocation

Fracture may occur secondary to dislocation; intra-articular bone fragments and fracture position may dictate treatment, requiring open reduction and surgical fixation. Fractures may include the radial head and/or the coronoid process of the ulna. The terrible triad injury of the elbow is a combination of coronoid and radial head fractures with rupture of the lateral UCL and occasionally the medial UCL (Englert et al., 2013). Effective treatment centers on surgically restoring enough of the bony and ligamentous structures to keep the elbow in joint so that recovery can proceed as for a simple elbow dislocation (Ebrahimzadeh, Amadzadeh-Chabock, & Ring, 2010).

Complicated Anterior Elbow Dislocation

This rare complex injury occurs after a direct high-energy blow to the posterior aspect of the forearm with the elbow in 90 degrees of flexion and always involves fractures of the olecranon (Englert et al., 2013). Caution must be taken the first 6 weeks with elbow flexion.

Complications to Consider

Heterotopic ossification of the elbow is a post-traumatic occurrence resulting in limited ROM. Risk factors for heterotopic ossification are the time elapsed between trauma and surgery, as well as the number of days of immobilization after surgery. Stiffness and heterotopic ossification after elbow dislocation are common occurrences and should be treated by controlled early mobilization in braces with limited ROM and, in severe cases, by oral steroid medication (Englert et al., 2013). Signs and symptoms include warm, tender, or firm swelling in the muscle of forearm and excessive ROM loss in the associated joint(s). Heterotopic ossification can result in a variety of complications, including nerve impingement, joint ankylosis, complex regional pain syndrome, osteoporosis, and soft-tissue infection. Management of heterotopic ossification is aimed at limiting its progression and maximizing function of the affected joint. Nonsurgical treatment is appropriate for early heterotopic ossification; however, surgical excision should be considered in cases of joint ankylosis or significantly decreased ROM before complications arise (Cipriano, Pill, & Keenan, 2009).

5.13.10 ULNOHUMERAL DISLOCATION POST-OPERATIVE PROTOCOL

General protocol guidelines adapted from Pho and Godges (n.d.) ulnohumeral dislocation post-operative rehabilitation protocol.

Any specific physician orders should supersede protocol guidelines here, if differing.

Phase I

1. Weeks 1 to 4 Goals
   a. Control edema and pain; elevation, ice.
   b. Monitor for neurovascular symptoms
   c. Early full ROM
   d. Protect injured tissues
   e. Minimize de-conditioning
2. ROM
   a. Gentle PROM; working to get full extension, passive stretching is generally contraindicated at this point.
      i. Splinting as needed
         1. Week 1: Immobilization period after surgery varies depending on the technique. Most often, the elbow is positioned in 90 degrees of flexion and full pronation and is immobilized in a splint for 7 days to 2 weeks (Texas State University, n.d.)
         2. Week 1 to 2: 30 to 110 degrees
         3. Week 3 to 4: 20 to 120 degrees
         4. Week 5 to 6: 10 to 130 degrees
         5. After week 6 and 8, free ROM (per physician clearance)
         6. If olecranon fracture, may have additional limitation of flexion to 90 degrees maximum for 6 to 8 weeks due to triceps attachment.
         7. Soft tissue mobilization if indicated; brachialis.
      ii. 5.08.1 ROM: Passive: Self-Flexion and Extension Within Restrictions
   b. Gentle AAROM/AROM
      i. 5.09.2 ROM: Elbow Flexion and Extension With Wand, Active Assistive
      ii. 5.09.5 ROM: Elbow Pronation and Supination, Passive and Active Assistive
3. General cardiovascular and muscular conditioning program
   a. Recumbent bike, walking, elliptical (no arms)

Phase II

1. Weeks 5 to 8 goals
   a. Control any residual symptoms of edema and pain

b. Full ROM

c. Minimize de-conditioning

d. Continue to monitor for neurovascular compromise

2. ROM

   a. PROM

      i. Splinting as needed

         1. Week 5 to 6: 10 to 130 degrees

         2. After week 6, free ROM

      ii. Joint mobilization

      iii. Soft tissue mobilization

      iv. Gentle passive stretching if indicated

   b. AROM exercises

      i. 5.09.3 ROM: Elbow Flexion and Extension, Active

      ii. 5.09.7 ROM: Elbow Pronation and Supination, Active

      iii. 5.14.1 ROM: Wrist and Finger Movements, Passive and Active

   c. Strengthening

      i. Isometric exercises

         1. 5.12.2 Strengthen: Isometric; Elbow Flexion

         2. 5.12.1 Strengthen: Isometric; Elbow Extension

         3. 5.12.4 Strengthen: Isometric; Elbow Pronation and Supination, Other Hand Resists

         4. 5.12.3 Strengthen: Isometric; Elbow Flexion and Extension, Other Hand Resists

         5. 5.16.1 Strengthen: Isometric; Wrist, 4-Way With Variations Using Self, Table, Wall, and Resistance Band

         6. 5.16.2 Strengthen: Isometric and Isotonic; Ball Grip Squeezes

      ii. Progressing to resisted exercises using tubing or manual resistance or weights

         1. 5.12.5 Strengthen: Isotonic; Elbow Extension, Overhead With Dumbbell

         2. 5.12.6 Strengthen: Isotonic; Elbow Extension, Bilateral Overhead With Wand/Cane

         3. 5.12.7 Strengthen: Isotonic; Elbow Extension, Kick-Back

         4. 5.12.9 Strengthen: Isotonic; Elbow Kick-Out

         5. 5.12.10 Strengthen: Isotonic; Elbow Flexion, Curls

         6. 5.12.11 Strengthen: Isotonic; Elbow Flexion, Preacher Curls

         7. 5.12.12 Strengthen: Isotonic; Elbow Pronation and Supination With Hammer

         8. 5.12.13 Strengthen: Resistance Band, Elbow Extension

         9. Strengthen: Resistance Band, Tricep Push Down

         10. 5.12.16 Strengthen: Resistance Band, Elbow Extension, Overhead

         11. 5.12.15 Strengthen: Resistance Band, Elbow Extension, Shoulder Flexed

         12. 5.12.17 Strengthen: Resistance Band, Elbow Flexion

         13. 5.16.9 Strengthen: Resistance Band, Wrist Extension

         14. 5.16.10 Strengthen: Resistance Band, Wrist Flexion

         15. 5.16.12 Strengthen: Resistance Band, Ulnar Deviation

         16. 5.16.11 Strengthen: Resistance Band, Radial Deviation

      iii. Incorporate sport specific exercises if indicated; generally when strength is within 15% of unaffected side.

3. Consider nerve glides

   a. 5.17.1 Nerve Glide: Median Nerve

   b. 5.17.2 Nerve Glide: Radial Nerve

   c. 5.17.3 Nerve Glide: Ulnar Nerve

4. Modify/progress cardiovascular and muscular conditioning program

Phase III

Weeks 9 to 16 Goals:

1. Full ROM and normal strength

   a. 5.09.4 ROM: Elbow, Low-Load, Long-Duration Extension, Passive (consider if full extension not achieved)

   b. 5.12.18 Strengthen: Closed Kinetic Chain; Elbow, Seated Dip/Chair Push-Ups

   c. 5.12.19 Strengthen: Closed Kinetic Chain; Elbow, Lean-Back Dip

   d. 5.12.25 Functional: Elbow, Pouring for Pronation and Supination Tasks

   e. 5.12.24 Functional: Elbow, Velcro Roller for Pronation and Supination Tasks

   f. 5.12.22 Strengthen: Closed Kinetic Chain; Elbow, Body Press

      i. Shoulder and upper quarter strengthening

   g. 5.07.28 Strengthen: Isotonic; Shoulder, Diagonal Lifts D1 and D2

   h. 5.07.34 Strengthen: Isotonic; Resistance Band and Machine, Shoulder, Lat Pull-Down

   i. 5.07.38 Strengthen: Isotonic: Resistance Band: Extension

   j. 5.07.39 Strengthen: Isotonic: Resistance Band: Internal Rotation and Variations

   k. 5.07.41 Strengthen: Isotonic: Resistance Band: External Rotation and Variations

   l. 5.07.42 Strengthen: Isotonic; Resistance Band, Shoulder, Combination Movements PNF D1 and D2

   m. 5.07.47 Strengthen: Isotonic: Resistance Band: Pull Back

   n. 5.07.36 Strengthen: Isotonic: Resistance Band: Flexion, Scaption, Abduction And

   o. 5.03.11 Strengthen: Resistance Band: Isolated Scapular Retraction

   p. 5.03.12 Strengthen: Resistance Band: Row And Variations

2. Return to pre-injury functional activities
3. Progress sport-specific or job-specific training
4. Strengthening ideas

   a. 5.07.66 Strengthen: Closed Kinetic Chain; Stairmaster, Shoulder

   b. 5.07.67 Strengthen: Closed Kinetic Chain: Bodyblade Flexion, Scaption, and Abduction

   c. 5.07.68 Strengthen: Closed Kinetic Chain; Bodyblade, Shoulder Internal Rotation and External Rotation

   d. 5.07.69 Strengthen: Closed Kinetic Chain; Bodyblade, Shoulder, D1 and D2

   e. 5.07.70 Strengthen: Closed Kinetic Chain; Shoulder, Plank Shuffle on Medicine Ball

   f. 5.07.71 Strengthen: Closed Kinetic Chain; Shoulder, Inverted Row

   g. 5.07.79 Plyometrics/Dynamic: Shoulder, Wall Dribbles

   h. 5.07.80 Plyometrics/Dynamic: Ball Toss, Overhead

   i. 5.07.81 Plyometrics/Dynamic: Chest Pass

   j. 55.07.82 Plyometrics/Dynamic: Shoulder, Bench Press/Floor Throws

   k. 5.07.83 Plyometrics/Dynamic: Shoulder, Two-Handed Side Throw

   l. 5.07.85 Plyometrics/Dynamic: Shoulder, Multidirectional Catch/Throw

   m. 5.07.86 Plyometrics/Dynamic: Shoulder, Ball Toss, Overhead and Backwards

   n. 5.07.87 Plyometrics/Dynamic: Shoulder, Push-Up

   o. 5.07.88 Plyometrics/Dynamic: Shoulder, Slams

   p. 5.07.89 Plyometrics/Dynamic: Shoulder, Ball Squat, Push-Press

   q. 5.07.90 Plyometrics/Dynamic: Shoulder, Push-Offs

   r. 5.07.84 Plyometrics/Dynamic: Shoulder, 90/90 Throw

   s. 5.07.91 Reactive Neuromuscular Training and Variations, Shoulder

   t. 5.07.92 Shoulder, Throwing Progression

5.13.11 Fractures Discussion and Protocol Modifications

Due to the many different types of fractures that may occur a general chart is provided to help guide the clinician in the modifications of the rehabilitation program. Therapist may utilize **5.13.8** following the additional components detailed below (see **5.13.11**).

TABLE 5.13.11	
DISTAL HUMERUS (INTERCONDYLAR) FRACTURES	Type I • Immobilization up to 3 weeks, followed by gentle ROM and strengthening once healed (bone union) Type II, III, IV • During early rehab after removal of immobilizer (4 to 6 weeks), no passive stretching or manipulation. • May use gentle ROM for flexion/extension and pronation/supination. • Only use joint mobilization techniques when bone union is secure. • It is common to have residual loss of motion; keep in mind patient only needs 30 to 130 degrees extension/flexion and 50 degrees pronation/supination for ADLs.
RADIAL HEAD FRACTURES	Type I • Immobilization 5 to 7 days up to 4 weeks • Early ROM once pain subsides Type II or III • ORIF or excision of radial head • Immobilized in hinged splint • Early ROM begins post-operative Type IV • Immobilization with elbow flexed 90 degrees • No PROM until after 8 to 10 weeks. • It is common to have residual loss of flexion at 2 years after surgery.
OLECRANON FRACTURES (NONDISPLACED)	Immobilization 6 to 8 weeks Nondisplaced may start gentle AROM after 3 weeks of immobilization Displaced may not start until 8 weeks usually but you can work on hand, wrist and shoulder ROM at this time. For both displaced and nondisplaced types do not exceed 90 degrees of flexion for first 6 to 8 weeks due to triceps attachment to olecranon.
Table created from information found in *Therapeutic Exercise for Physical Therapist Assistants* (Bandy & Sanders, 2012).	

5.13.12 Distal Tendon Biceps Repair Discussion

Rupture of the distal biceps tendon accounts for 10% of all biceps brachii ruptures. Injuries typically occur in the dominant elbow of men aged 40 to 49 years during eccentric contraction of the biceps. Degenerative changes, decreased vascularity, and tendon impingement may precede rupture. Nonsurgical management is an option, however, healthy, active persons with distal biceps tendon ruptures benefit from early surgical repair, gaining improved strength in forearm supination and elbow flexion. Surgical complications include sensory and motor neurapraxia, infection, and heterotopic ossification (Sutton, Dodds, Ahmad, & Sethi, 2010). Immediate post-operative ROM after repair of the distal biceps tendon leads to early gain of extension and has no deleterious effect on healing or strength (Cheung,

Lazarus, & Taranta, 2005). Cheung et al. (2005) reported that by increasing ROM through the use of a hinged brace with an extension restriction originally set at 60 degrees of flexion and decreasing 20 degrees every 2 weeks, full extension was achieved by week 6, with strengthening of the biceps starting at week 8. After an average duration of follow-up of 38 weeks, the patients had, on the average, no loss of extension, a 5.8 loss of flexion, a 3.5 loss of supination, and an 8.1 loss of pronation compared with the values on the contralateral side; flexion strength was 91.4% of that on the contralateral side, and supination strength was 89.4% of that on the contralateral side (Cheung et al., 2005). Initial treatment focuses on restoring ROM using PROM, stretching, and grades 3 and 4 joint mobilizations and strengthening scapular stabilizing muscles without placing stress on the biceps brachii. As treatment progresses, strengthening focuses on supporting musculature including scapular stabilizers, shoulder RC, and forearm gradually increasing toward complete recovery. After 8 weeks post operation, therapist may begin gentle strengthening of the biceps brachii (Horschig, Sayers, LaFontaine, & Scheussler, 2012).

5.13.13 Distal Tendon Biceps Repair Protocol

Protocol adapted from Washington University Physicians Rehabilitation Program for Distal Biceps Repair protocol as cited in Horschig et al. (2012) case study of 38-year-old male with a surgically repaired right distal biceps tendon.

Any specific physician orders should supersede protocol guidelines here, if differing.

Phase I: 1 to 2 Weeks

1. Goals
   a. Control edema and pain; elevation, ice.
   b. Monitor for neurovascular symptoms
   c. Early full PROM
   d. Protect injured tissues
   e. Minimize de-conditioning
2. Precautions
   a. No active supination or flexion of the elbow
   b. Posterior splint at 90 degrees flexion for 1 week
3. ROM
   a. Gentle PROM; no passive stretching.
   b. Gentle wrist, hand, grip exercises
      i. 5.12.1 Strengthen: Isometric; Elbow Extension
         1. Active wrist flexion/extension
         2. Active wrist radial/ulnar deviation
      ii. 5.14.2 ROM: Flexion And Extension, Radial and Ulnar Deviation With Wand, Active Assistive
4. Scapular exercises
   a. 5.03.3 Strengthen: Scapular Retraction; only variations listed below.
      i. A: Unilateral side-lying
      ii. B: Bilateral seated
   b. 5.01.5 ROM: Scapular Elevation
   c. 5.01.6 ROM: Scapular Depression
5. General cardiovascular and muscular conditioning program

Phase II: 3 to 6 Weeks

1. Goals
   a. Control any residual symptoms of edema and pain
   b. Full PROM by end of week 6
   c. Minimize de-conditioning

   d. Continue to monitor for neurovascular compromise
2. ROM
   a. Splinting as needed
      i. Splint adjusted to increasing extension slowly (follow specific physician orders)
      ii. Week 8 splint usually at full ROM 0 to 145 degrees
   b. Joint mobilization
   c. Soft tissue mobilization
   d. Gentle PROM elbow flexion/extension
      i. Week 3: limit to 20 degrees extension
      ii. Week 4: limit to 10 degrees extension
      iii. Week 5: to full extension as tolerated
   e. Gentle PROM forearm supination/pronation
      i. Full ROM allowed
   f. AROM exercises
      i. 5.09.7 ROM: Elbow Pronation and Supination, Active
3. Strengthening
   a. Triceps isometrics (start week 5 to 6)
      i. 5.12.1 Strengthen: Isometric; Elbow Extension
   b. Shoulder isometrics
      i. 5.07.1 Strengthen: Isometric; Shoulder, Other Hand Resists, 6-Way; (internal and external rotation, abduction, extension) All neutral, no flexion or adduction.

Phase III: 6 to 10 Weeks

1. ROM
   a. Week 8: splint usually at full ROM 0 to 145 degrees
   b. Joint mobilization
   c. Soft tissue mobilization
   d. Gentle PROM elbow
   e. AROM exercises
      i. 5.09.7 ROM: Elbow Pronation and Supination, Active

2. Strengthening
   a. Wrist PRE's; avoid any biceps contraction.
      i. 5.16.6 Strengthen: Isotonic; Wrist, All Planes
   b. Triceps isotonics (start week 8)
      i. 5.12.5 Strengthen: Isotonic; Elbow Extension, Overhead With Dumbbell
      ii. 5.12.6 Strengthen: Isotonic; Elbow Extension, Bilateral Overhead With Wand/Cane
      iii. 5.12.7 Strengthen: Isotonic; Elbow Extension, Kick-Back
      iv. 5.12.9 Strengthen: Isotonic; Elbow Kick-Out
      v. 5.12.13 Strengthen: Resistance Band, Elbow Extension
   c. Shoulder
      i. 5.03.11 Strengthen: Resistance Band: Isolated Scapular Retraction
      ii. 5.07.38 Strengthen: Isotonic: Resistance Band: Extension
      iii. 5.07.39 Strengthen: Isotonic: Resistance Band: Internal Rotation and Variations; 0 Degrees Abduction Standing or Supine Only
      iv. 5.07.41 Strengthen: Isotonic: Resistance Band: External Rotation and Variations; *0 degrees abduction standing or supine only.*

Phase IV: 10 to 16 Weeks

1. Warm-up and conditioning
   a. 5.04.1 ROM: Active Assistive: Warm-Up Upper Body Ergometer (start week 10 to 12)
2. AROM and flexibility
   a. 5.09.3 ROM: Elbow Flexion and Extension, Active
   b. 5.11.3 Stretch: Biceps Using Pillow
   c. 5.11.5 Stretch: Biceps Using Table (gentle)
   d. 5.11.2 Stretch: Triceps
3. Strengthening
   a. Wrist PRE's (avoid any biceps isotonic contraction)
      i. 5.16.9 Strengthen: Resistance Band, Wrist Extension
      ii. 5.16.10 Strengthen: Resistance Band, Wrist Flexion
      iii. 5.16.12 Strengthen: Resistance Band, Ulnar Deviation
      iv. 5.16.11 Strengthen: Resistance Band, Radial Deviation
   b. Biceps isometrics (start week 8 to 10)
      i. 5.12.2 Strengthen: Isometric; Elbow Flexion
      ii. 5.12.3 Strengthen: Isometric; Elbow Flexion and Extension, Other Hand Resists

iii. 5.12.4 Strengthen: Isometric; Elbow Pronation and Supination, Other Hand Resists
   c. Biceps isotonics (light start week 10 to 12)
      i. 5.12.12 Strengthen: Isotonic; Elbow Pronation and Supination With Hammer
      ii. 5.12.10 Strengthen: Isotonic; Elbow Flexion, Curls

Phase V: 16 to 26 Weeks

1. Flexibility
   a. 5.09.4 ROM: Elbow, Low-Load, Long-Duration Extension, Passive (consider if full extension not achieved)
2. Strengthening
   a. Biceps isotonics (started light week 8 to 10, progress)
      i. 5.12.17 Strengthen: Resistance Band, Elbow Flexion
      ii. 5.12.11 Strengthen: Isotonic; Elbow Flexion, Preacher Curls
      iii. 5.12.25 Functional: Elbow, Pouring for Pronation and Supination Tasks
      iv. 5.12.24 Functional: Elbow, Velcro Roller for Pronation and Supination Tasks
   b. Triceps
      i. 5.12.18 Strengthen: Closed Kinetic Chain; Elbow, Seated Dip/Chair Push-Ups
      ii. 5.12.19 Strengthen: Closed Kinetic Chain; Elbow, Lean-Back Dip
      iii. 5.12.22 Strengthen: Closed Kinetic Chain; Elbow, Body Press
   c. Shoulder and upper quarter strengthening
      i. 5.07.28 Strengthen: Isotonic; Shoulder, Diagonal Lifts D1 and D2
      ii. 5.07.34 Strengthen: Isotonic; Resistance Band and Machine, Shoulder, Lat Pull-Down
      iii. 5.07.42 Strengthen: Isotonic; Resistance Band, Shoulder, Combination Movements PNF D1 and D2
      iv. 5.07.47 Strengthen: Isotonic: Resistance Band: Pull Back
      v. 5.07.36 Strengthen: Isotonic: Resistance Band: Flexion, Scaption and Abduction
      vi. 5.03.12 Strengthen: Resistance Band: Row And Variations
      vii. 5.07.67 Strengthen: Closed Kinetic Chain: Bodyblade Flexion, Scaption, and Abduction
      viii. 5.07.68 Strengthen: Closed Kinetic Chain; Bodyblade, Shoulder Internal Rotation and External Rotation

ix. 5.07.69 Strengthen: Closed Kinetic Chain; Bodyblade, Shoulder, D1 and D2 **5.07.61**

x. 5.07.61 Strengthen: Closed Kinetic Chain: Beginning Weightbearing, Progress To Push-Up Partial Weight

xi. 5.07.62 Strengthen: Closed Kinetic Chain; Shoulder, Push-Up

xii. 5.07.63 Strengthen: Closed Kinetic Chain: Scapular and Shoulder Depression

d. Plyometrics

i. 5.07.79 Plyometrics/Dynamic: Shoulder, Wall Dribbles

ii. 5.07.80 Plyometrics/Dynamic: Ball Toss, Overhead

iii. 5.07.81 Plyometrics/Dynamic: Chest Pass

iv. 5.07.82 Plyometrics/Dynamic: Shoulder, Bench Press/Floor Throws

v. 5.07.83 Plyometrics/Dynamic: Shoulder, Two-Handed Side Throw

vi. 5.07.85 Plyometrics/Dynamic: Shoulder, Multidirectional Catch/Throw

vii. 5.07.86 Plyometrics/Dynamic: Shoulder, Ball Toss, Overhead and Backwards

3. Modify/progress cardiovascular and muscular conditioning program

Phase VI: 26 Weeks and Beyond

1. Return to activities (sport specific)
2. Advanced strengthening ideas

a. 5.07.66 Strengthen: Closed Kinetic Chain; Stairmaster, Shoulder

b. 5.07.70 Strengthen: Closed Kinetic Chain; Shoulder, Plank Shuffle on Medicine Ball

c. 5.07.71 Strengthen: Closed Kinetic Chain; Shoulder, Inverted Row

d. 5.07.87 Plyometrics/Dynamic: Shoulder, Push-Up

e. 5.07.88 Plyometrics/Dynamic: Shoulder, Slams

f. 5.07.89 Plyometrics/Dynamic: Shoulder, Ball Squat, Push-Press

g. 5.07.90 Plyometrics/Dynamic: Shoulder, Push-Offs

h. 5.07.84 Plyometrics/Dynamic: Shoulder, 90/90 Throw

i. 5.07.91 Reactive Neuromuscular Training and Variations, Shoulder

j. 5.07.92 Shoulder, Throwing Progression

REFERENCES

Akeson, W. H., Amiel, D., Abel, M. F., Garfin, S. R., & Woo, S. L. (1987). Effects of immobilization on joints. *Clinical Orthopedics and Related Research*, (219), 28-37.

Amin, N. H., Kumar, N. S., & Schickendantz, M. S. (2015). Medial epicondylitis: Evaluation and management. *The Journal of the American Academy of Orthopedic Surgeons, 23*(6), 348-355.

Bandy, W. D., & Sanders, B. (2012). *Therapeutic exercise for physical therapist assistants* (3rd ed.). Philadelphia, PA: Wolters Kluwer/ Lippincott, Williams and Wilkins.

Binder, A., Hodge, G., Greenwood, A. M., Hazleman, B. L., & Page Thomas, D. P. (1985). Is therapeutic ultrasound effective in treating soft tissue lesions? *British Medical Journal, 290*(6467), 512-514.

Bisset, L. M., Collins, N. J., & Offord, S. S. (2014). Immediate effects of 2 types of braces on pain and grip strength in people with lateral epicondylalgia: A randomized controlled trial. *Journal of Orthopedic and Sports Physical Therapy, 44*(2), 120-128.

Blackard, D., & Sampson, J. (1997). Management of an uncomplicated posterior elbow dislocation. *Journal of Athletic Training, 32*(1), 63-67.

Bruce, C., Laing, P., Dorgan, J., & Klenerman, L. (1993). Unreduced dislocation of the elbow: Case report and review of the literature. *The Journal of Trauma, 35*(6), 962-965.

Cheung, E. V., Lazarus, M., & Taranta, M. (2005). Immediate range of motion after distal biceps tendon repair. *Journal of Shoulder and Elbow Surgery, 14*(5), 516-518.

Cipriano, C. A., Pill, S. G., & Keenan, M. A. (2009). Heterotopic ossification following traumatic brain injury and spinal cord injury. *Journal of the American Academy of Orthopedic Surgeons, 17*(11), 689-697.

Dugas, J., Chronister, J., Cain, E. L., Jr, & Andrews, J. R. (2014). Ulnar collateral ligament in the overhead athlete: A current review. *Sports Medicine and Arthroscopy Review, 22*(3), 169-182.

Ebrahimzadeh, M. H., Amadzadeh-Chabock, H., & Ring, D. (2010). Traumatic elbow instability. *The Journal of Hand Surgery, 35*(7), 1220-1225.

Ellenbecker, T. S., Wilk, K. E., Altchek, D. W., & Andrews, J. R. (2009). Current concepts in rehabilitation following ulnar collateral ligament reconstruction. *Sports Health, 1*(4), 301-313.

Englert, C., Zellner, J., Koller, M., Nerlich, M., & Lenich, A. (2013). Elbow dislocations: A review ranging from soft tissue injuries to complex elbow fracture dislocations. *Advances in Orthopedics, 2013,* 951397.

Field, L. D., & Savoie, F. H. (1998). Common elbow injuries in sport. *Sports Medicine, 26*(3), 193-205.

Grana, W. (2001). Medial epicondylitis and cubital tunnel syndrome in the throwing athlete. *Clinical Sports Medicine, 20*(3), 541-548.

Herd, C. R., & Meserve, B. B. (2008). A systematic review of the effectiveness of manipulative therapy in treating lateral epicondylalgia. *Journal of Manual and Manipulative Therapy, 16*(4), 225-237.

Hoogvliet, P., Randsdorp, M. S., Dingemanse, R., Koes, B. W., & Huisstede, B. M. (2013). Does effectiveness of exercise therapy and mobilisation techniques offer guidance for the treatment of lateral and medial epicondylitis? A systematic review. *British Journal of Sports Medicine, 47*(17), 1112-1119.

Hoppenrath, T., & Ciccone, C. D. (2006). Is there evidence that phonophoresis is more effective than ultrasound in treating pain associated with lateral epicondylitis? *Physical Therapy, 86*(1), 136-140.

Horschig, A., Sayers, S. P., LaFontaine, T., & Scheussler, S. (2012). Rehabilitation of a surgically repaired rupture of the distal biceps tendon in an active middle aged male: A case report. *International Journal of Sports Physical Therapy, 7*(6), 663-671.

Jafarian, F. S., Demneh, E. S., & Tyson, S. F. (2009). The immediate effect of orthotic management on grip strength of patients with lateral epicondylosis. *Journal of Orthopedic and Sports Physical Therapy, 39*(6), 484-489.

Kouhzad Mohammadi, H., Khademi Kalantari, K., Naeimi, S. S., Pouretezad, M., Shokri, E., Tafazoli, M., . . . Kardooni, L. (2014). Immediate and delayed effects of forearm kinesio taping on grip strength. *Iranian Red Crescent Medical Journal, 16*(8), e19797.

Lee, S., Ko, Y., & Lee, W. (2014). Changes in pain, dysfunction, and grip strength of patients with acute lateral epicondylitis caused by frequency of physical therapy: A randomized controlled trial. *Journal of Physical Therapy Science, 26*(7), 1037-1040.

Loew, L. M., Brosseau, L., Tugwell, P., Wells, G. A., Welch, V., Shea, B., . . . Rahman, P. (2014). Deep transverse friction massage for treating lateral elbow or lateral knee tendinitis. *Cochrane Database of Systematic Reviews,* CD003528.

Makhni, E., Lee, R. W., Morrow, Z. S., Gualtieri, A. P., Gorroochurn, P., & Ahmad, C. S. (2014). Performance, return to competition, and reinjury after Tommy John surgery in major league baseball pitchers: A review of 147 cases. *American Journal of Sports Medicine, 42*(6), 1323-1332.

Mehlhoff, T. L., Noble, P. C., Bennett, J. B., & Tullos, H. S. (1988). Simple dislocation of the elbow in the adult. Results after closed treatment. *The Journal of Bone and Joint Surgery, 70*(2), 244-249.

Methodist Sports Medicine Center Department of Physical Therapy. (2004). Guidelines epicondylectomy: Lateral or medial epicondylectomy rehabilitation protocol. *American Society of Shoulder and Elbow Therapists.* Retrieved from http://www.asset-usa.org/Guidelines/Epicondylectomy_%20protocol.pdf

Murtezani, A., Pharm, Z. I., Vllasolli, T. O., Sllamniku, S., Krasniqi, S., & Vokrri, L. (2015). Exercise and therapeutic ultrasound compared with corticosteroid injection for chronic lateral epicondylitis: A randomized controlled trial. *Ortopedia, Traumatologia, Rehabilitacja, 17*(4), 351-357.

Osbahr, D. C., Cain, E. L., Jr, Raines, B. T., Fortenbaugh, D., Dugas, J. R., Andrews, J. R. (2014). Long-term outcomes after ulnar collateral ligament reconstruction in competitive baseball players: Minimum 10-year follow-up. *American Journal of Sports Medicine, 42*(6), 1333-1342.

Peterson, M., Butler, S., Eriksson, M., & Svärdsudd, K. (2014). A randomized controlled trial of eccentric vs. concentric graded exercise in chronic tennis elbow (lateral elbow tendinopathy). *Clinical Rehabilitation, 28*(9), 862-872.

Pho, C., & Godges, J. (n.d.). Elbow—Ulnohumeral dislocation and rehabilitation. Retrieved from https://xnet.kp.org/socal_rehabspecialists/ptr_library/03ElbowRegion/16Elbow-UlnohumeralDislocation.pdf

Purcell, D. B., Matava, M. J., & Wright, R. W. (2007). Ulnar collateral ligament reconstruction: A systematic review. *Clinical Orthopedics and Related Research, 455,* 72-77.

Rineer, C. A., & Ruch, D. S. (2009). Elbow tendinopathy and tendon ruptures: Epicondylitis, biceps and triceps ruptures. *The Journal of Hand Surgery, 34*(3), 566-576.

Sadeghi-Demneh, E., & Jafarian, F. (2013). The immediate effects of orthoses on pain in people with lateral epicondylalgia. *Pain Research and Treatment, 2013,* 353597.

Schippinger, G., Seibert, F. J., Steinböck, J., & Kucharczyk, M. (1999). Management of simple elbow dislocations. Does the period of immobilization affect the eventual results? *Langenbeck's Archive of Surgery, 384*(3), 294-297.

Sevier, T. L., & Stegink-Jansen, C. W. (2015). Astym treatment vs. eccentric exercise for lateral elbow tendinopathy: A randomized controlled clinical trial. *PeerJ, 3,* e967.

Shamsoddini, A., & Hollisaz, M. T. (2013). Effects of taping on pain, grip strength and wrist extension force in patients with tennis elbow. *Trauma Monthly, 18*(2), 71-74.

Struijs, P. A., Damen, P. J., Bakker, E. W., Blankevoort, L., Assendelft, W. J., & van Dijk, C. N. (2003). Manipulation of the wrist for management of lateral epicondylitis: A randomized pilot study. *Physical Therapy, 83*(7), 608-616.

Sutton, K. M., Dodds, S. D., Ahmad, C. S., & Sethi, P. M. (2010). Surgical treatment of distal biceps rupture. *Journal of the American Academy of Orthopedic Surgeons, 18*(3), 139-148.

Texas State University Evidence-Based Practice Project. (n.d.). Posterolateral elbow instability. *Physiopedia.* Retrieved from http://www.physio-pedia.com/index.php?title=Postero-Lateral_Elbow_Instability#cite_ref-O.27Driscoll_1999_9-3

Texas State University Evidence-Based Practice Project. (2016). Posterior elbow dislocation. *Physiopedia.* Retrieved from http://www.physio-pedia.com/Posterior_Elbow_Dislocation

Vicenzino, B., Cleland, J. A., & Leanne Bisset, L. (2007). Joint manipulation in the management of lateral epicondylalgia: A clinical commentary. *The Journal of Manual and Manipulative Therapy, 15*(1), 50-56.

Virginia Sports Medicine Institute. (2001). Elbow pain. Retrieved from http://www.nirschl.com/pdf/tennis-Elbow-Rehab.pdf

Wolff, A. L., & Hotchkiss, R. N. (2006). Lateral elbow instability: Nonoperative, operative, and post-operative management. *Journal of Hand Therapy, 19*(2), 238-243.

Section 5.14

Wrist/Hand/Fingers Range of Motion

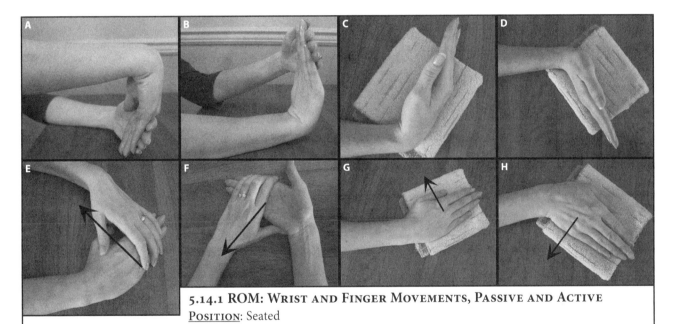

5.14.1 ROM: Wrist and Finger Movements, Passive and Active

Position: Seated

Targets: Mobility of the wrist and finger joints

Instruction: All movements should occur with affect elbow flexed 90 degrees.

Passive wrist flexion/extension: With affected palm up, patient grasps around affected hand as shown to passively move the wrist gently into extension, then flexion (A and B).

Active wrist flexion/extension: With affected thumb up and towel under hypothenar side of hand, patient flexes and extends the wrist as towel slides along table (C and D).

Passive radial/ulnar deviation: With affected palm up, patient grasps around affected hand to passively move the wrist gently into radial and ulnar deviation (E and F).

Active wrist radial/ulnar deviation: With affected palm on towel, patient brings thumb in toward body (radial deviation) and then away from body (ulnar deviation) as towel slides along table (G and H). *(continued)*

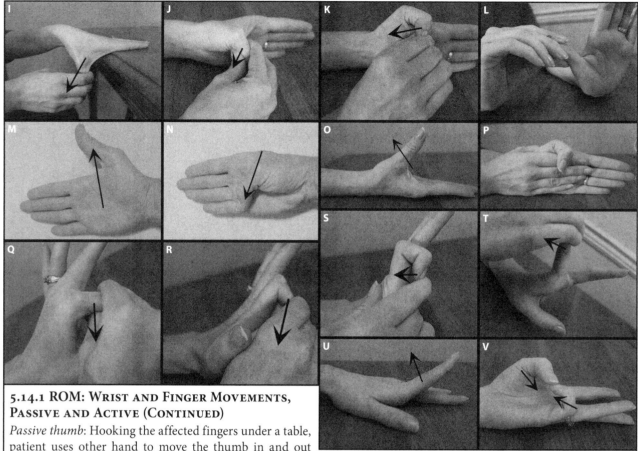

5.14.1 ROM: Wrist and Finger Movements, Passive and Active (Continued)

Passive thumb: Hooking the affected fingers under a table, patient uses other hand to move the thumb in and out (flexion and extension) and up and down (adduction and abduction) (I). Patient then moves to MCP and IP joints, moving into flexion and extension (J through L).

Active thumb: With thumb up, patient lifts thumb toward head (extension) and then down toward table crossing over palm (flexion/opposition) (M and N). With palm up, patient lifts the thumb straight up toward ceiling like a "sock puppet" (abduction) and back down (adduction) (O). For thumb MCP and IP flexion, patient places opposite hand palm to palm and flexes the MCP and IP of the thumb over the second digit of the other hand (P).

Passive Fingers: Patient grasps around each finger, moving MCP, PIP, and DIP joints into flexion and extension. Patient moves each joint separately, then combines flexion and extension of the entire finger (Q through T).

Active fingers: For finger active movements, patient may block proximal joints to isolate each movement and actively flex and extend each MCP, PIP, and DIP separately, and then combines all movements together (not shown).

Active finger lifts: Finger extension can be done with palm down, lifting one finger at a time off the table (U).

Active opposition: Active thumb abduction and finger flexion combination movements are done by having patient touch tip of thumb to tip of each finger. Have patient open hand between each touch for great ROM of thumb (V). *(continued)*

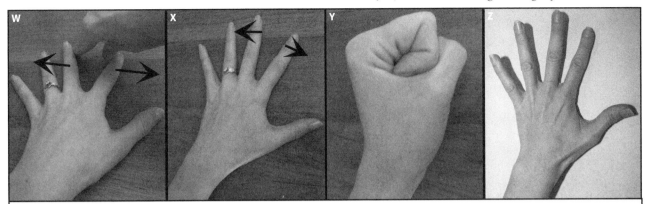

5.14.1 ROM: WRIST AND FINGER MOVEMENTS, PASSIVE AND ACTIVE (CONTINUED)

Passive MCP abduction/adduction: With palm down, use unaffected fingers to spread digits apart one at a time, separating from the digit next to it (W).

Active MCP abduction/adduction: With palm down, open fingers to spread digits apart and back together (X).

Active fist-to-finger spread: Close fingers into palm, making a fist, then open fingers and palm to spread digits apart (Y and Z).

SUBSTITUTIONS: Encourage patient to sit up tall with shoulders back; hand remains relaxed while unaffected hand creates the movements when doing PROM.

PARAMETERS: 10 times holding a 3 to 5 seconds at end range, 1 set, 1 to 3 times per day

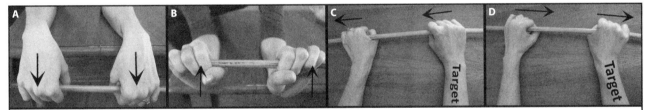

5.14.2 ROM: FLEXION AND EXTENSION, RADIAL AND ULNAR DEVIATION WITH WAND, ACTIVE ASSISTIVE

POSITION: Seated

TARGETS: Mobility of the wrist

INSTRUCTION: *Flexion*: With forearms resting on table, palms down and holding cane, patient moves wrists into flexion, assisting affected hand to go further with the opposite hand (A). *Extension*: With forearms resting on table, palms up and holding cane, patient moves wrists into extension assisting affected hand to go further with the opposite hand (B). *Radial and ulnar deviation*: With forearms resting on table, palms down and holding cane, use unaffected hand to push affected hand into ulnar deviation and then pull toward radial deviation (C and D).

SUBSTITUTIONS: Encourage scapular retraction to avoid raising the shoulders and keel elbows tucked into sides.

PARAMETERS: 10 times holding 3 to 5 seconds at end range, 1 set, 1 to 3 times per day

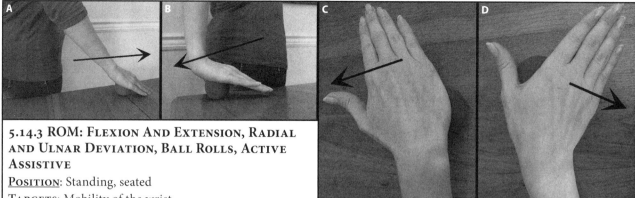

5.14.3 ROM: FLEXION AND EXTENSION, RADIAL AND ULNAR DEVIATION, BALL ROLLS, ACTIVE ASSISTIVE

<u>POSITION</u>: Standing, seated

<u>TARGETS</u>: Mobility of the wrist

<u>INSTRUCTION</u>: *Flexion/extension*: Standing beside a table, waist height or taller, patient rolls ball in front and then alongside and behind (A and B). *Radial/ulnar deviation*: With forearm resting on table, palm down on ball, move hand into radial deviation and then ulnar deviation, rolling the ball side-to-side (C and D).

<u>SUBSTITUTIONS</u>: Encourage scapular retraction to avoid raising the shoulders, and keep elbows tucked into sides.

<u>PARAMETERS</u>: 10 times, holding 3 to 5 seconds at end range, 1 set, 1 to 3 times per day

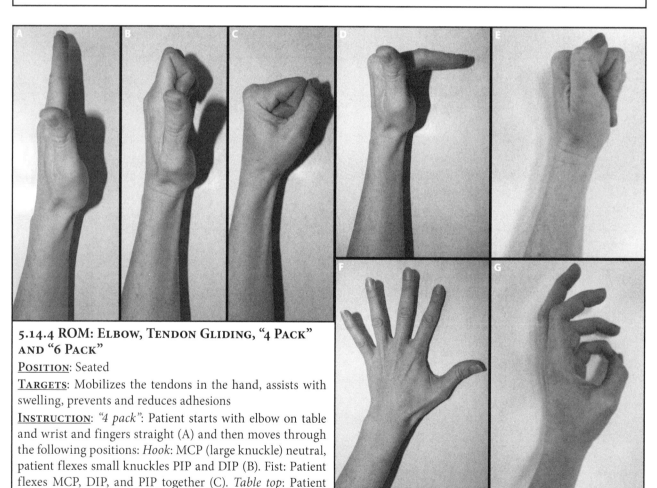

5.14.4 ROM: ELBOW, TENDON GLIDING, "4 PACK" AND "6 PACK"

<u>POSITION</u>: Seated

<u>TARGETS</u>: Mobilizes the tendons in the hand, assists with swelling, prevents and reduces adhesions

<u>INSTRUCTION</u>: *"4 pack"*: Patient starts with elbow on table and wrist and fingers straight (A) and then moves through the following positions: *Hook*: MCP (large knuckle) neutral, patient flexes small knuckles PIP and DIP (B). Fist: Patient flexes MCP, DIP, and PIP together (C). *Table top*: Patient flexes MCP to 90 degrees and keeps DIP and PIP extended (D). *Flat fist*: Patient flexes MCP and PIP 90 degrees, keeping DIP extended (E).

"6 pack": Patient performs "4 pack" with the addition of the following: *Open fingers*: Patient opens hand into full extension of fingers and actively spreads fingers apart (F). *Opposition*: Patient touches the tip of the thumb to the tip of each digit 2 to 5 (G).

<u>SUBSTITUTIONS</u>: Encourage scapular retraction to avoid raising the shoulders, keep elbows tucked into sides.

<u>PARAMETERS</u>: 10 to 30 times, 1 set, 1 to 3 times per day

5.14.5 DESENSITIZATION EXERCISES, UPPER EXTREMITY

<u>POSITION</u>: Seated

<u>TARGETS</u>: After an injury or surgery, it is common for an area to develop increased sensitivity, resulting in discomfort when everyday objects touch the area. Desensitization will assist in decreasing sensitivity by exposing the area to various textures and pressures.

<u>INSTRUCTION</u>: *Rubbing*: Rub the sensitive area with fabrics of various textures. Begin with softer fabrics and progress to rougher fabrics: silk, cotton balls, cotton fabric, flannel, terry cloth, Velcro, hair brush. *Tapping*: Tap along the sensitive area using a fingertips or pencil eraser. Slowly increase the pressure. *Slapping*: Slap lightly around region using anterior surface of fingertips. Slowly increase the pressure. *Rolling*: Roll the area along a foam roll, roll of putty, dough roller or tennis ball. Slowly increase the pressure. *Massager/Vibration*: Using a small massager or electric appliance such as a shaver or toothbrush, massage along the sensitive area. *Hand specific*: If the hand requires desensitization, place patient's hand in a container filled with dry items: rolled oats, rice, sand, and dry beans. Have patient open and close the hand or search for small objects hidden in the substance.

<u>SUBSTITUTIONS</u>: Encourage scapular retraction to avoid raising the shoulders.

<u>PARAMETERS</u>: Each activity can be performed for 1 to 5 minutes as tolerated, 1 to 3 times per day

Section 5.15

WRIST/HAND/FINGERS STRETCHING

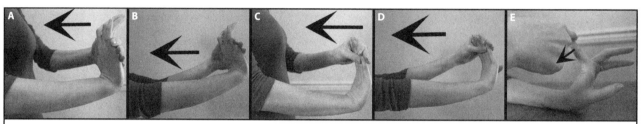

5.15.1 STRETCH: WRIST FLEXOR AND FINGER FLEXOR VARIATION, SELF-ASSISTED

POSITION: Seated

TARGETS: Wrist flexors (flexor digitorum superficialis, flexor digitorum profundus, flexor carpi radialis, flexor carpi ulnaris, palmaris longus, flexor pollicis longus)

INSTRUCTION: *Elbow flexed*: Patient sits tall with back and neck straight, keeping elbow flexed, and uses unaffected palm to spread across affected palm and press the hand into wrist extension until a stretch felt in the anterior forearm (A) This is also done with elbow extended and shoulder flexed to 80 degrees, addressing two joint muscles across wrist and elbow (B). *Adding fingers*: To increase the stretch for the fingers, move opposite hand to across fingers and thumb to add finger and thumb extension to wrist extension (C and D). *Single fingers*: Patient places palms down on table, actively extends the wrist, and pulls one finger into full extension until a stretch is felt. Repeat for all digits including thumb (E).

SUBSTITUTIONS: Shrugging shoulders, hyperextending elbow

PARAMETERS: Hold for 15 to 30 seconds, 3 to 5 repetitions, 1 to 3 times per day

5.15.2 STRETCH: WRIST FLEXOR USING WALL AND TABLE

POSITION: Standing

TARGETS: Wrist flexors (flexor digitorum superficialis, flexor digitorum profundus, flexor carpi radialis, flexor carpi ulnaris, palmaris longus, flexor pollicis longus)

INSTRUCTION: *Wall*: Patient stands facing the wall and flexes shoulder to 80 degrees while placing palm upside down on wall

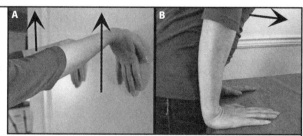

with fingers pointing toward the floor. As patient slides hand up the wall, more extension will occur in the wrist, and patient leans in for overpressure until a stretch is felt in the anterior forearm (A). *Table*: Patient stands in front of a table below waist height and places palms on table fingers facing away. Patient leans over the table, placing slight pressure through wrist, extending wrist until a stretch is felt (B). This can be advanced for increased range by placing the palms facing backward, fingers facing the patient. Patient moves away from the table in a leaning manner as wrist flexes and stretch is felt (not shown).

SUBSTITUTIONS: Shrugging shoulders, hyperextending elbow

PARAMETERS: Hold for 15 to 30 seconds, 3 to 5 repetitions, 1 to 3 times per day

Where's the Evidence?

Yoo (2015) implemented wrist flexor and extensor stretch with the elbow extended and a thenar stretch in a 40-year-old man with pain and progressive tingling in his right hand. His symptoms worsened at night. The numbness increased when he used a computer at work. He had no systemic symptoms and no weakness or muscle-wasting in either hand. There was no evidence of ulnar or radial nerve pathology. On physical examination, he had tingling and numbness over the radial three digits of both hands in the Tinel and Phalen tests. His stretch was held for at least 30 seconds. The subject performed wrist stretches in standing for 30 minutes each, once a day for 2 weeks. In session two, he performed all three exercises in supine for 20 minutes each, once a day for 2 weeks. Before and after each session, the therapist performed the Tinel and Phalen tests 10 times each and measured the pressure pain. Overall, the pressure pain threshold increased progressively and positive Phalen's tests and Tinel signs decreased progressively throughout treatment. Yoo postulated that CTS exercises in the supine position may elevate the wrist more, effectively reducing swelling in the carpal tunnel, thereby enabling the patient to exercise with less pain. Yoo found that these stretching exercises may relieve the symptoms of mild-to-moderate CTS; however, these exercises should be pain-free. If a patient feels pain, numbness, or worse symptoms, it might have a negative effect on the performance of exercises for CTS.

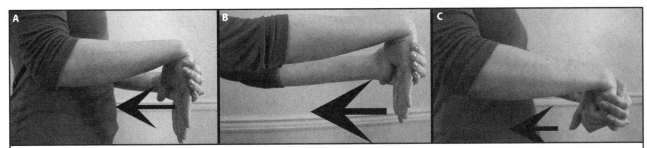

5.15.3 STRETCH: WRIST EXTENSOR AND FINGER EXTENSOR VARIATION, SELF-ASSISTED

POSITION: Seated

TARGETS: Stretch wrist extensors (extensor digitorum, extensor carpi radialis longus and brevis, extensor carpi ulnaris, extensor indicis, extensor digiti minimi, extensor pollicis long and brevis)

INSTRUCTION: *Elbow flexed*: Seated tall with back and neck straight and elbow flexed, patient uses unaffected palm to spread across back of affected hand and press the hand into wrist flexion until a stretch felt in the posterior forearm (A). This is also done with elbow extended and shoulder flexed to 80 degrees, addressing 2 joint muscles across wrist and elbow (B). *Add fingers*: Patient makes a fist during stretch (C).

SUBSTITUTIONS: Shrugging shoulders, hyperextending elbow

PARAMETERS: Hold for 15 to 30 seconds, 3 to 5 repetitions, 1 to 3 times per day

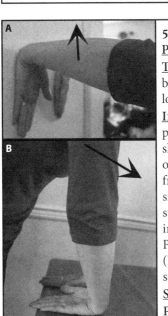

5.15.4 STRETCH: WRIST EXTENSOR USING WALL AND TABLE

POSITION: Standing

TARGETS: Stretch wrist extensors (extensor digitorum, extensor carpi radialis longus and brevis, extensor carpi ulnaris, extensor indicis, extensor digiti minimi, extensor pollicis long and brevis)

INSTRUCTION: *Wall*: Patient stands facing wall and flexes shoulder to 80 degrees while placing back of hand on a wall in front with fingers pointing toward the floor. As patient slides hand up the wall, more flexion will occur in the wrist. Patient gently leans in for overpressure until a stretch is felt in the posterior forearm (A) *Table*: Patient stands in front of a table below waist height and places back of hand on table, fingers facing away, similar to **5.15.2** except palms facing up. Patient leans over the table, placing slight pressure through wrist and wrist is flexed until a stretch is felt. This can be advanced for increased range by placing the back of hands facing backward, fingers facing the patient. Patient moves away from the table in a leaning manner as wrist flexes and stretch is felt (B). Additional stretch can be added making a full fist with the thumb tucked during the stretch.

SUBSTITUTIONS: Shrugging shoulders, hyperextending elbow

PARAMETERS: Hold for 15 to 30 seconds, 3 to 5 repetitions, 1 to 3 times per day

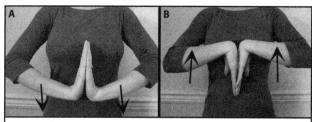

5.15.5 STRETCH: WRIST, PRAYER AND REVERSE PRAYER

<u>POSITION</u>: Seated

<u>TARGETS</u>: *Prayer*: Stretch wrist extensors (extensor digitorum, extensor carpi radialis longus and brevis, extensor carpi ulnaris, extensor indicis, extensor digiti minimi, extensor pollicis long and brevis). *Reverse prayer*: Wrist flexors (flexor digitorum superficialis, flexor digitorum profundus, flexor carpi radialis, flexor carpi ulnaris, palmaris longus, and flexor pollicis longus)

<u>INSTRUCTION</u>: *Prayer*: Patient places palms together in front of the sternum with fingertips pointing up. Patient keeps palms together while lowering hands until stretch felt in anterior forearm and wrist (A). *Reverse prayer*: Patient places dorsum of hand together in front of the sternum with fingertips pointing down. Patient keeps back of hands together while raising hands until stretch felt in posterior forearm and wrist (B).

<u>SUBSTITUTIONS</u>: Shrugging shoulders

<u>PARAMETERS</u>: Hold for 15 to 30 seconds, 3 to 5 repetitions, 1 to 3 times per day

5.15.7 STRETCH: WRIST FLEXORS AND EXTENSORS, SELF-MASSAGE

<u>POSITION</u>: Seated

<u>TARGETS</u>: Soft tissue release wrist extensors and flexors

<u>INSTRUCTION</u>: *Extensors*: Patient sits tall in front of table with elbow flexed and palm down. Patient rolls along small foam rollers forward and back. *Flexors*: Patient sits tall in front of table with elbow flexed and palm down. Patient rolls along small foam rollers forward and back.

<u>SUBSTITUTIONS</u>: Shrugging shoulders; using too much pressure to cause intense pain.

<u>PARAMETERS</u>: Roll each side 1 to 2 minutes, 1 to 3 times per day

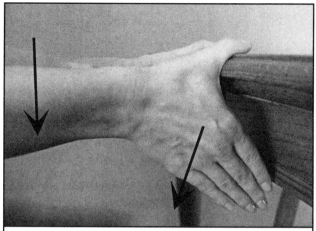

5.15.6 STRETCH: THENAR

<u>POSITION</u>: Seated

<u>TARGETS</u>: Stretch short thumb muscles: flexor pollicis brevis, abductor pollicis brevis, opponens pollicis

<u>INSTRUCTION</u>: Patient sits tall in front of table with elbow flexed and thumbs up. Patient places thumb pads on table edge and presses into the table with body weight for stretch into thumb extension. Patient may also extend wrist and pull thumb toward lateral forearm (not shown).

<u>SUBSTITUTIONS</u>: Shrugging shoulders

<u>PARAMETERS</u>: Hold for 15 to 30 seconds, 3 to 5 repetitions, 1 to 3 times per day

REFERENCE

Yoo, W. G. (2015). Effect of the release exercise and exercise position in a patient with carpal tunnel syndrome. *Journal of Physical Therapy Science, 27*(10), 3345-3346.

Wrist/Hand/Fingers Strengthening

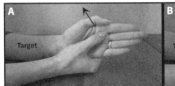
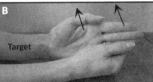
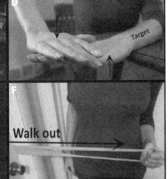

5.16.1 Strengthen: Isometric; Wrist, 4-Way With Variations Using Self, Table, Wall, and Resistance Band

<u>Position</u>: Seated, standing

<u>Targets</u>: Beginner facilitation and strengthening of wrist, all planes. *Extension*: Extensor digitorum, extensor carpi radialis longus and brevis, extensor carpi ulnaris, extensor indicis, extensor digiti minimi, extensor pollicis long and brevis. *Flexion*: Flexor digitorum superficialis, flexor digitorum profundus, flexor carpi radialis, flexor carpi ulnaris, palmaris longus, flexor pollicis longus. *Radial deviation*: extensor carpi radialis longus and brevis, flexor carpi radialis. *Ulnar deviation*: extensor carpi ulnaris, flexor carpi ulnaris

<u>Instruction</u>: Patient sits or stands with shoulder neutral and elbow flexed 90 degrees. Support hand if necessary.

Extension, self-neutral: With affected thumb up, patient places opposite palm under hand, wrapping fingers around dorsum of affected hand. Patient presses dorsum of hand outward, without using shoulder external rotators, as hand resists wrist extension (A). To add finger extensors that cross the wrist, patient to fully extend fingers during exercise (B).

Extension, self-pronated: With palm down, patient places opposite palm over dorsum of hand, wrapping fingers around hypothenar side for support. Patient attempts to extend wrist by trying to lift hand, without using elbow flexion, as other hand resists wrist extension (C). To add wrist finger extensors that cross the wrist; patient to perform with fingers extended (D).

Extension, wall: Standing sideways in a doorway with jamb just lateral to shoulder, patient places dorsum of hand with fingers extended against wall. Patient presses dorsum of hand outward, without using shoulder external rotators, as wall resists wrist extension (E).

Extension resistance band walk-out: Standing with elbow bent 90 degrees and holding resistance band thumb up, unaffected side to anchor and anchor at the level of the hand, patient sidesteps away as band places tension on wrist; band pulls wrist toward flexion as patient resists, holding isometric contraction (F). *(continued)*

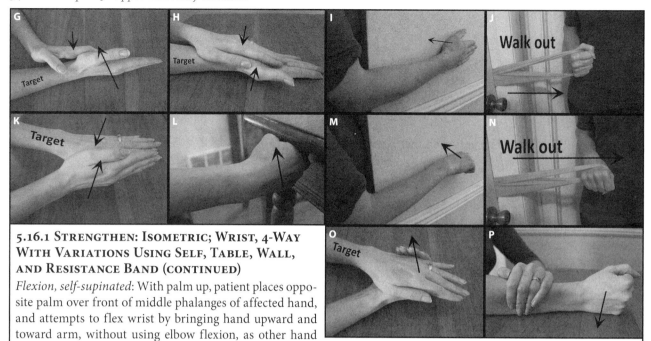

5.16.1 STRENGTHEN: ISOMETRIC; WRIST, 4-WAY WITH VARIATIONS USING SELF, TABLE, WALL, AND RESISTANCE BAND (CONTINUED)

Flexion, self-supinated: With palm up, patient places opposite palm over front of middle phalanges of affected hand, and attempts to flex wrist by bringing hand upward and toward arm, without using elbow flexion, as other hand resists wrist flexion (H).

Flexion, wall: Standing sideways in a doorway with jamb just medial to shoulder, patient places palm of hand with fingers extended against wall. Patient presses palm of hand inward without using shoulder internal rotators, as wall resists wrist flexion (I).

Flexion, resistance band walk-out: Standing with elbow bent 90 degrees and holding resistance band thumb up, affected side to anchor and anchor at the level of the hand, patient sidesteps away as band places tension on wrist; band pulls wrist toward extension as patient resists, holding isometric contraction (J).

Radial deviation, self: Patient places opposite palm over thumb side of hand, wrapping fingers around dorsum and resists wrist radial deviation, attempting to bring thumb side up and toward forearm as hand resists (K).

Radial deviation, table: With thumb inside fist, patient places lateral aspect index finger at proximal phalanx/thumb side under table, resists wrist radial deviation, attempting to bring thumb side up and toward forearm without using elbow flexion as table resists (L).

Radial deviation, wall: With thumb inside fist, patient places thumb side against the wall and resists wrist radial deviation, attempting to bring thumb side up and toward forearm, without using elbow flexion as table resists (M).

Radial deviation, resistance band walk-out: Standing elbow bent 90 degrees and holding resistance band palm down, with affected side to anchor and anchor at the level of the hand, patient sidesteps away as band places tension on wrist. Band pulls wrist toward ulnar deviation as patient resists, holding isometric contraction (N).

Ulnar deviation, self: Patient places opposite palm under hand, wrapping fingers around dorsum of affected hand, and presses pinky side of hand down without using elbow extension, as hand resists ulnar deviation (O).

Ulnar deviation, table: With thumb outside fist, patient places medial aspect pinky finger at proximal phalanx on top of table and attempts to bring pinky side down toward thigh, without using elbow extension, as table resists ulnar deviation (P). *(continued)*

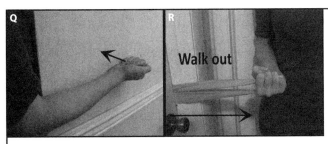

5.16.1 Strengthen: Isometric; Wrist, 4-Way With Variations Using Self, Table, Wall, and Resistance Band (Continued)

Radial deviation, wall: With thumb inside fist, patient places pinky side against the wall. Resist wrist radial deviation (patient attempts to bring thumb side up and toward forearm without using elbow flexion as table resists) (Q).

Ulnar deviation, resistance band: Standing with elbow bent 90 degrees and holding resistance band palm down, unaffected side to anchor and anchor at the level of the hand, patient sidesteps away as band places tension on wrist and pulls toward radial deviation as patient resists, holding isometric contraction (R).

Substitutions: Shrugging shoulder, shoulder should stay in neutral rotation, elbow stays tucked into side, encourage scapular retraction; make sure movement is at the wrist and not shoulder or elbow.

Parameters: Hold for 6 to 10 seconds, with 1 to 2 second ramp up and down, 1 to 3 sets, 8 to 12 repetitions, 1 time per day or every other day

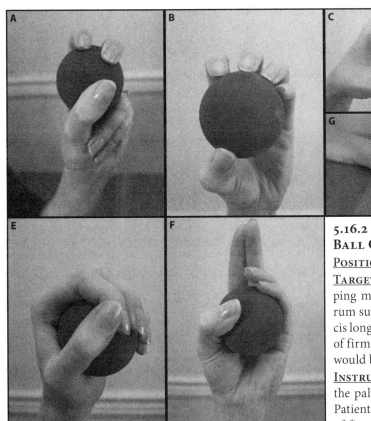

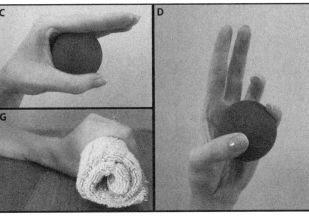

5.16.2 Strengthen: Isometric and Isotonic; Ball Grip Squeezes

Position: Seated

Targets: Beginner facilitation and strengthening of gripping muscles; flexor digitorum profundus, flexor digitorum superficialis, flexor digiti minimi brevis, flexor pollicis longus, lumbricals, interossei and adductor pollicis; use of firm ball makes this more isometric, and an elastic ball would be considered isotonic due to movement allowed.

Instruction: *Double finger grip*: Patient squeezes ball in the palm of the hand with digits 2 and 3 (A). *Hook grip*: Patient squeezes ball in the palm of the hand with tips of fingers hooking into elastic ball (B). *Flat grip*: Patient squeezes ball in the palm of the hand with flat grip, DIPs extended into elastic ball (C). *Ball opposition*: Patient squeezes ball with thumb into palm of the hand with flat grip, DIPs extended into elastic ball (D). *Full grip*: Patient squeezes the ball using a full grip as if trying to make a fist (E). *Lateral grip*: Patient squeezes ball in the palm of the hand with digits 4 and 5 (F). *Towel grip*: A towel can be used for gripping isotonically. Using a small rolled-up towel (size of roll can be adjusted depending on desired grip width) patient squeezes, holds, and releases slowly (G).

Substitutions: Shrugging shoulder; shoulder should stay in neutral rotation and forearm in neutral pronation/supination, elbow stays tucked into side, encourage scapular retraction.

Parameters: *Isometric*: Hold for 6 to 10 seconds with 1 to 2 second ramp up and down; *Isotonic*: Squeeze for 1 to 2 seconds. Both: 1 to 3 sets, 8 to 12 repetitions, 1 time per day or every other day.

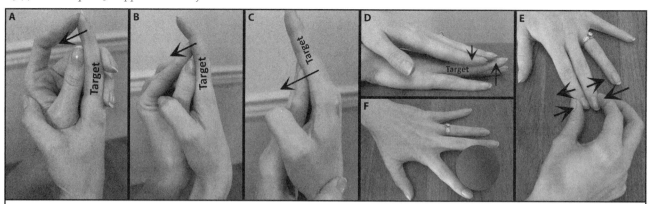

5.16.3 STRENGTHEN: ISOMETRIC; FINGER VARIATIONS

POSITION: Seated

TARGETS: Beginner facilitation and strengthening of finger muscles: *DIP flexion digits 2 to 5,* flexor digitorum profundus; *PIP flexion digits 2 to 5,* flexor digitorum superficialis; *MCP flexion digits 2 to 5 with fingers extended,* lumbricals; *PIP and DIP extension,* extensor digitorum digits 2 to 5, extensor indicis digit 2, extensor digiti minimi digit 5; *Finger adductors,* palmar interossei; *Finger abductors:* dorsal interossei digits 2 to 4 and abductor digiti minimi digit 5.

INSTRUCTION: *DIP flexion digits 2 to 5*: Patient blocks PIP and MCP with opposite hand while using index finger of opposite hand to resist DIP flexion (A). *PIP flexion digits 2 to 5*: Patient blocks MCP with opposite hand while using index finger of opposite hand to resist PIP flexion (B). *MCP flexion digits 2 to 5 with fingers extended*: Keeping affected fingers extended, patient uses opposite index finger to resist MCP flexion (C). *PIP, DIP and MCP extension*: Palm down on table, patient attempts to lift each finger as index finger of opposite hand resists (D). *Finger abductors*: Patient holds two adjacent fingers together with opposite hand as patient attempts to bring them apart (E). *Finger adductors*: Patient opens fingers, places a hard ball between them, and squeeze ball with two fingers (F).

SUBSTITUTIONS: Avoid wrist, elbow and shoulder movements

PARAMETERS: Hold for 6 to 10 seconds, with 1 to 2 second ramp up and down, 1 to 3 sets, 8 to 12 repetitions, 1 time per day or every other day

5.16.4 STRENGTHEN: ISOMETRIC; THUMB VARIATIONS

POSITION: Seated

TARGETS: Beginner facilitation and strengthening of thumb muscles; *thumb flexors* (flexor pollicis longus and brevis; thumb adductors: adductor pollicis) *thumb abductors* (abductor pollicis longus and brevis) thumb extensors (extensor pollicis longus and brevis).

INSTRUCTION: *Thumb flexion CMC*: Patient spreads thumb out from hand, places ball in the web space, and attempts to bring

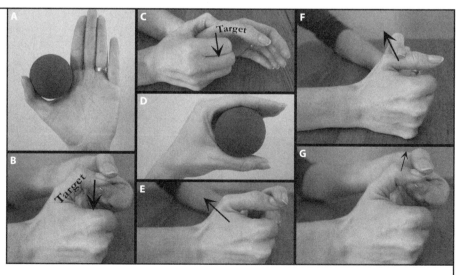

thumb back toward hand as ball resists (A). *Thumb flexion MCP, IP*: Patient curls thumb inward, resisting with fingertips of opposite hand at distal thumb pad (B). *Thumb abduction CMC*: Patient lays hand on table, thumb up, and resists bringing thumb into abduction with the other hand (C). *Thumb adduction CMC*: With thumb abducted and ball in web space, patient resists movement and attempts to adduct the thumb (D). *Thumb extension CMC*: Patient presses thumb outward, resisting with fingertips of opposite hand (E). *Thumb extension MCP*: Patient extends thumb at MCP joint and resists with opposite thumb (F). *Thumb extension IP*: Patient extends thumb at IP joint and resists with opposite thumb (G).

SUBSTITUTIONS: Avoid wrist, elbow and shoulder movements

PARAMETERS: Hold for 6 to 10 seconds, with 1 to 2 second ramp up and down, 1 to 3 sets, 8 to 12 repetitions, 1 time per day or every other day

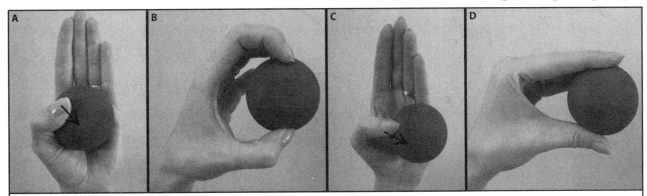

5.16.5 STRENGTHEN: ISOMETRIC AND ISOTONIC; BALL, THUMB VARIATIONS

POSITION: Seated

TARGETS: Beginner facilitation and strengthening of thumb grip and pinching muscles, flexor pollicis longus and brevis, adductor pollicis; use of firm ball makes this more isometric, use elastic ball would be considered isotonic due to movement allowed.

INSTRUCTION: *Thumb opposition*: Patient squeezes ball in the palm of the hand with flat grip, DIPs extended into elastic ball (A). *Thumb MCP and IP flexion*: Patient presses tip of thumb into ball (B). *Thumb claw grip*: Patient squeezes ball between thumb and fingertips (C). *Thumb and finger lumbrical pinch*: Patient squeezes ball between all fingertips and thumb, keeping DIP and PIP of digits 2 and 5 and IP of thumb straight (D).

SUBSTITUTIONS: Shrugging shoulder; shoulder should stay in neutral rotation and forearm in neutral pronation/supination, elbow stays tucked into side, encourage scapular retraction.

PARAMETERS: *Isometric*: Hold for 6 to 10 seconds with 1 to 2 second ramp up and down; *Isotonic*: Squeeze for 1 to 2 seconds; *Both*: 1 to 3 sets, 8 to 12 repetitions, 1 time per day or every other day.

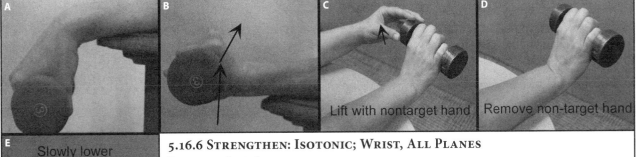

Lift with nontarget hand | Remove non-target hand

Slowly lower

5.16.6 STRENGTHEN: ISOTONIC; WRIST, ALL PLANES

POSITION: Seated

TARGETS: Strengthening of wrist all planes; *Extension*: extensor digitorum, extensor carpi radialis longus and brevis, extensor carpi ulnaris, extensor indicis, extensor digiti minimi, extensor pollicis long and brevis; *Flexion*: flexor digitorum superficialis, flexor digitorum profundus, flexor carpi radialis, flexor carpi ulnaris, palmaris longus, flexor pollicis longus; *Radial deviation*: extensor carpi radialis longus and brevis, flexor carpi radialis; *Ulnar deviation*: extensor carpi ulnaris, flexor carpi ulnaris.

INSTRUCTION: *Extension*: With elbow flexed 90 degrees or straight, anterior forearm resting on table, palm down, and holding a weight, patient allows hand to lower slowly toward floor and then raises weight, bringing back of hand toward them (A and B).

Eccentric focus extension elbow flexed: With forearm resting on table, palm down, and holding a weight, patient uses other hand to raise weight, bringing back of hand toward them. Once at full extension, patient removes the assistance of the other hand and affected hand slowly lowers the weight toward floor (usually in a 10-second count) (C through E).

(continued)

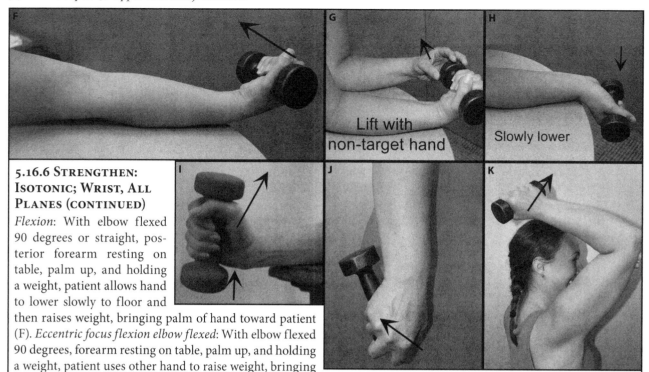

5.16.6 STRENGTHEN: ISOTONIC; WRIST, ALL PLANES (CONTINUED)

Flexion: With elbow flexed 90 degrees or straight, posterior forearm resting on table, palm up, and holding a weight, patient allows hand to lower slowly to floor and then raises weight, bringing palm of hand toward patient (F). *Eccentric focus flexion elbow flexed*: With elbow flexed 90 degrees, forearm resting on table, palm up, and holding a weight, patient uses other hand to raise weight, bringing palm of hand toward them. Once at full flexion, patient removes the assistance of the other hand and affected hand slowly lowers the weight toward floor (usually in a 10-second count) (G and H). *Radial deviation*: With forearm resting on table, thumb up, and holding a weight, patient allows hand to hang off table into ulnar deviation and then radially deviates, lifting the weight up toward the thumb side (I). This can also be done with arm hanging down by side, thumb forward. Patient holds one end of the weight with hand with other end in front and then radially deviates, lifting free end of weight (not shown). This can also be done with hammer (not shown). *Ulnar deviation*: With arm hanging down by side, thumb forward, patient holds one end of the weight with hand, with other end in back and then ulnarly deviates lifting free end of weight up (J). This can also be done with hammer. Another option is to bring the shoulder into 90 degrees of flexion and support the elbow with the other arm. Elbow is bent fully, and weight is in the hand. Patient then ulnarly deviates, bringing pinky side of hand toward the elbow (K).

SUBSTITUTIONS: Shrugging shoulder; shoulder should stay in neutral rotation and forearm in neutral pronation/supination, elbow stays tucked into side, encourage scapular retraction.

PARAMETERS: Squeeze for 1 to 2 seconds, 1 to 3 sets, 8 to 12 repetitions, 1 time per day or every other day

5.16.7 STRENGTHEN: RADIAL AND ULNAR DEVATION, SIDE-LYING

POSITION: Side-lying

TARGETS: Strengthen radial deviation (extensor carpi radialis longus and brevis, flexor carpi radialis); ulnar deviation: (extensor carpi ulnaris, flexor carpi ulnaris).

INSTRUCTION: Patient lies on unaffected side, arm down by side; *Ulnar deviation*: Thumb pointed down, patient holds weight and ulnarly deviates lifting weight up (A). *Radial deviation*: Thumb of affected arm pointed up, patient holds weight and radially deviates, lifting weight up (B).

SUBSTITUTIONS: Rolling arm forward or backward to assist with flexors and extensors.

PARAMETERS: 1 to 3 sets, 8 to 12 repetitions, 1 time per day or every other day

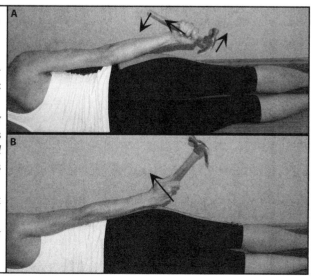

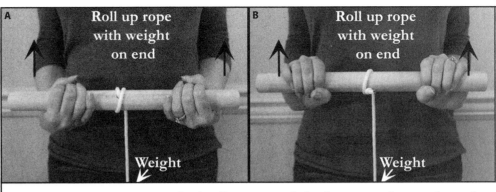

5.16.8 STRENGTHEN: WRIST ROLLER

POSITION: Standing

TARGETS: *Pronated grip*: strengthening extensor carpi radialis longus and brevis, extensor carpi ulnaris, extensor digitorum palm down; *Supinated grip*: strengthening flexor digitorum superficialis, flexor digitorum profundus, flexor carpi radialis, flexor carpi ulnaris, palmaris longus, flexor pollicis longus.

INSTRUCTION: *Pronated grip*: Patient holds wrist roller with palms down, elbows flexed 90 degrees. Starting with weight on the floor, patient rotates one wrist at a time into extension, rolling it up, alternating between sides as they bring the weight up. Once weight reaches roller, patient slowly lowers down by reversing the movements of the wrist in a controlled manner (A). *Supinated grip*: Patient holds wrist roller with palm up, elbows flexed 90 degrees. Repeat instructions for pronated grip (B).

SUBSTITUTIONS: Shrugging shoulders, elbow stays tucked into side, encourage scapular retraction, letting weight pull to unroll; this should be controlled with each movement of the wrist.

PARAMETERS: 1 to 3 sets, 8 to 12 repetitions, 1 time per day or every other day

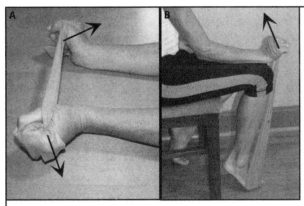

5.16.9 STRENGTHEN: RESISTANCE BAND, WRIST EXTENSION

POSITION: Seated

TARGETS: Strengthen extensor carpi radialis longus and brevis, extensor carpi ulnaris, extensor digitorum

INSTRUCTION: *Bilateral*: With forearms resting to table, thumbs up and band wrapped around dorsum of each hand, patient extends one or both wrists (A). *Stepping on band*: Forearm resting on table, palm down, band wrapped around dorsum of hand and anchored under foot, patient extends wrist. Patient can also do this with hand resting on thigh (B). Patient can also do this with hand holding other end of band underneath affected hand (not shown).

SUBSTITUTIONS: Shrugging shoulder; shoulder should stay in neutral rotation and forearm in neutral pronation/supination, elbow stays tucked into side, encourage scapular retraction.

PARAMETERS: 1 to 3 sets, 8 to 12 repetitions, 1 time per day or every other day

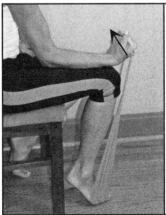

5.16.10 STRENGTHEN: RESISTANCE BAND, WRIST FLEXION

POSITION: Seated

TARGETS: Strengthen flexor digitorum superficialis, flexor digitorum profundus, flexor carpi radialis, flexor carpi ulnaris, palmaris longus, flexor pollicis longus

INSTRUCTION: Forearm resting on table, palm up, band wrapped around palm of hand and anchored under foot, patient flexes wrist (not shown). Patient can also do this with hand resting on thigh. Patient can also do this with hand holding other end of band underneath affected hand (not shown).

SUBSTITUTIONS: Shrugging shoulder; shoulder should stay in neutral rotation and forearm in neutral pronation/supination, elbow stays tucked into side, encourage scapular retraction.

PARAMETERS: 1 to 3 sets, 8 to 12 repetitions, 1 time per day or every other day

5.16.11 STRENGTHEN: RESISTANCE BAND, RADIAL DEVIATION

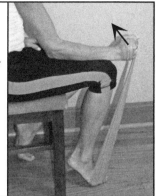

POSITION: Seated

TARGETS: Strengthening extensor carpi radialis longus and brevis, flexor carpi radialis

INSTRUCTION: Forearm resting on table, palm up, band wrapped around thumb side of hand and anchored by holding in other hand, patient radially deviates (not shown). Patient can also do this with hand holding other end of band underneath affected hand; affected hand is thumb up, and patient radially deviates, bringing thumb up (not shown). Patient anchors the band under foot, places medial forearm on thigh, affected hand thumb up in front of the knee. Patient radially deviates bringing thumb up.

SUBSTITUTIONS: Shoulder should stay in neutral rotation.

PARAMETERS: 1 to 3 sets 8 to 12 repetitions, 1 time per day or every other day

5.16.12 STRENGTHEN: RESISTANCE BAND, ULNAR DEVIATION

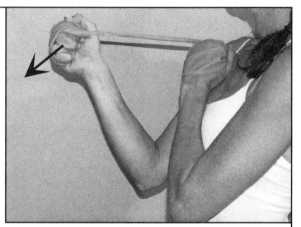

POSITION: Seated

TARGETS: Strengthening extensor carpi ulnaris, flexor carpi ulnaris

INSTRUCTION: Forearm resting on table, palm down, band wrapped around pinky side of hand and anchored by holding in other hand, patient ulnarly deviates (not shown). Patient can also do this with hand holding other end of band. Patient props affected side elbow on table and with band wrapped around hand and anchored by other hand closer to body, patient ulnarly deviates bringing pinky side away from chest (not shown). Patient can also do this with hand holding other end of band above affected hand. Affected hand, is thumb up and patient ulnarly deviates bringing pinky side down.

SUBSTITUTIONS: Shoulder should stay in neutral rotation

PARAMETERS: 1 to 3 sets, 8 to 12 repetitions, 1 time per day or every other day

5.16.13 STRENGTHEN: PUTTY AND GRIPMASTER PRO FOR HAND AND FINGERS

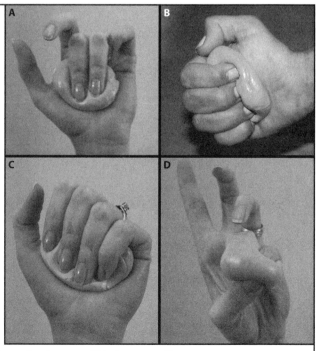

POSITION: Seated

TARGETS: Strengthening hand muscles; *DIP flexion digits 2 to 5*: flexor digitorum profundus; *PIP flexion digits 2 to 5*: flexor digitorum superficialis; *MCP flexion digits 2 to 5 with fingers extended*: lumbricals; *PIP and DIP extension*: extensor digitorum digits 2 to 5, extensor indicis digit 2, extensor digiti minimi digit 5; *finger adductors*: palmar interossei; *finger abductors*: dorsal interossei digits 2 to 4 and abductor digiti minimi digit 5; *thumb flexors*: flexor pollicis longus and brevis; *thumb adductors*: adductor pollicis; *thumb abductors*: abductor pollicis longus and brevis; *thumb extensors*: extensor pollicis longus and brevis.

INSTRUCTION: Forearm resting on table; *Putty double finger grip*: Patient squeezes putty in the palm of the hand with digits 2 and 3 (not shown) or 3 and 4 (A). *Putty hook grip*: Patient squeezes putty in the palm of the hand with tips of fingers hooking into elastic ball (B). *Putty flat grip*: Patient squeezes putty in the palm of the hand with flat grip, DIPs extended into elastic putty (C). *Opposition*: Patient squeezes putty in the palm of the hand with flat grip, DIPs extended into elastic putty (D). *(continued)*

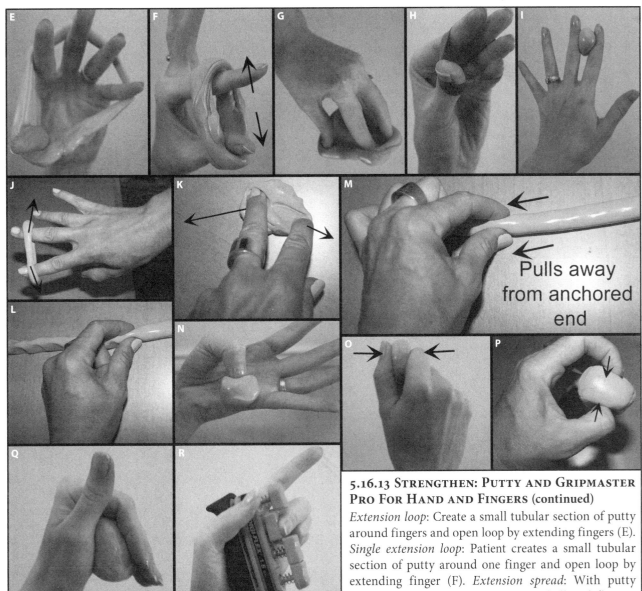

Pulls away from anchored end

5.16.13 STRENGTHEN: PUTTY AND GRIPMASTER PRO FOR HAND AND FINGERS (continued)

Extension loop: Create a small tubular section of putty around fingers and open loop by extending fingers (E). *Single extension loop*: Patient creates a small tubular section of putty around one finger and open loop by extending finger (F). *Extension spread*: With putty rolled in a ball, patient presses into ball and flattens on table, then spreads putty out using finger extension (G). *Extension spread variation with rubber band*: With thumb and fingers in all-finger pinch position, patient places rubber band around fingers and thumb, opens against the resistance of the rubber band using finger extension and thumb abduction (H). *Adduction*: Patient squeezes small rolled up ball of putty between fingers (I). *Abduction loop*: With a small tubular loop around two digits, patient spreads fingers, puling loop apart (J). *Abduction spread*: Patient presses out a small ball of putty then spreads it apart using two fingers (K). *Thumb pinch*: With putty rolled into tubular section, patient pinches putty between thumb and index finger (L). *Thumb pinch pull*: Roll putty into tubular section, patient pinches putty between thumb and index finger and pulls using flexion of IP, PIP, and DIP (M). *Thumb MCP and IP flexion*: Patient presses tip of thumb into putty (N). *Thumb key grip/lateral pinch*: Patient squeezes putty between thumb and lateral aspect of index proximal and middle phalanges (O). *Thumb claw grip*: Patient squeezes putty between thumb and fingertips (P). *Lumbrical grip*: Patient squeezes putty between fingers and palm, keeping DIPs straight (Q). *Grip master Pro: Finger exercise*r: Isolating each finger, use digits 2 to 5 flex to push resistive buttons down, compressing spring as far as it will go. Different colors represent differing levels of resistance (R).

SUBSTITUTIONS: Sitting up straight; active shoulders and scapula but not using shoulder or elbow movements.

PARAMETERS: 1 to 3 sets, 8 to 12 repetitions, 1 time per day or every other day

5.16.14 Strengthen: Web and Variations For Hand and Fingers

Position: Seated

Targets: Strengthening hand muscles; *DIP flexion digits 2 to 5*: flexor digitorum profundus; *PIP flexion digits 2 to 5*: flexor digitorum superficialis; *MCP flexion digits 2 to 5 with fingers extended*: lumbricals; *PIP and DIP extension*: extensor digitorum digits 2 to 5, extensor indicis digit 2, extensor digiti minimi digit 5; *finger adductors*: palmar interossei; *finger abductors*: dorsal interossei digits 2 to 4 and abductor digiti minimi digit 5; *thumb flexors*: flexor pollicis longus and brevis; *thumb adductors*: adductor pollicis; *thumb abductors*: abductor pollicis longus and brevis; *thumb extensors*: extensor pollicis longus and brevis.

Instruction: *4 squares flexing and extending*: With fingers halfway spread and placed in holes, patient brings fingertips together and then opens wide. *Finger weave and wiggle*: Patient weaves finger through and wiggles fingers up and down. *Finger split abduction/adduction*: Patient weaves fingers through and brings index and pinky away from each other, then back together. Patient does this with digits 3 and 4. *Thumbing around*: Patient weaves thumbs through and moves thumbs in and out, up and down and around in circles clockwise and counter-clockwise. *Opposition*: patient places fingers spread apart in web and brings thumb to each digit, 2 to 5, touching tips. *Bend, fold, tap and push*: Patient weaves fingers through, bends all fingers in, folds finger in between each other, pushes each set of fingers each way, taps fingertips and repeats. Good for coordination and endurance. *Single and double finger stepping*: Climbs web with two adjacent fingers for single stepping, or with digits 2 and 5 together followed by 3 and 4 together for double.

Substitutions: Sitting up straight; active shoulders and scapula but not using shoulder or elbow movements.

Parameters: 1 to 3 sets, 8 to 12 repetitions, 1 time per day or every other day

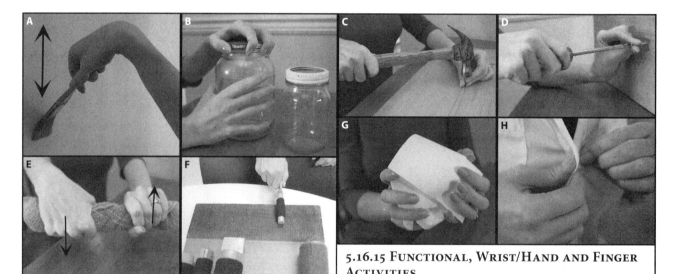

5.16.15 Functional, Wrist/Hand and Finger Activities

Position: Seated, standing

Targets: ROM, coordination, endurance and strengthening of wrist and hand and strengthening wrist.

Instruction:

a: *Painting wrist flexion/extension*: Patient holds painting brush with palm down and "paints" wall, moving wrist into flexion and extension (A).

b: *Screw on/off lids*: Patient uses wrist radial and ulnar deviation to screw on and off lids to jars of multiple sizes (B).

c: *Hammering*: Patient uses wrist radial and ulnar deviation to lightly hammer in nails to a block of wood, then remove nails by prying them out (C).

d: *Screwdriver*: Patient uses screwdriver to put in and remove screws using a block of wood with predrilled holes (D).

e: *Towel/washcloth wrings*: Using washcloth or small towel in soaked water, have patient wring water out (E).

f: *Velcro board*: Patient uses Velcro board to roll objects with differing grips along Velcro strips (F).

g: *Crumpling/uncrumpling pieces of paper*: Patient takes a sheet of paper, crumples into a ball, then opens them back up, smoothing it out (G).

h: *Buttoning/unbuttoning*: Using buttons of different sizes and varied difficulties, have patient button and unbutton (H).

(continued)

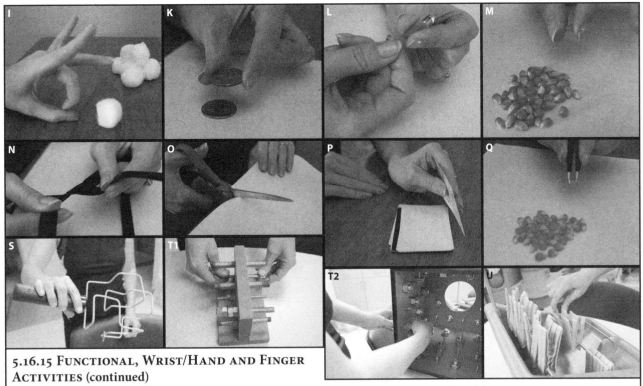

5.16.15 FUNCTIONAL, WRIST/HAND AND FINGER ACTIVITIES (continued)

i: *Flick cotton balls*: Patient picks cotton balls up and flicks across table using each digit (I).

j: *Roll/unroll toilet paper or paper towel*: Have patient unroll toilet paper or paper towel, then re-roll (not shown).

k: *Stacking coins/poker chips*: Patient transfers coins or poker chips from one stack to another, one at a time (K).

l: *Clasp/unclasp safety pins*: Give patient a pile of safety pins and have patient unclasp all, then re-clasp and return to start pile (L).

m: *Picking up small items*: Spread a selection of items—beans, coins, paper clips, marbles, popcorn seeds, dried spaghetti noodles—and have patient pick them up and place in a bucket (M).

n: *Tie knots*: Give patient a shoelace. Using a shoelace or other type of string and have patient tie multiple knots and then untie (N).

o: *Cutting*: Using scissors and multiple items of varying thickness—paper, fabric, cardboard—have patient cut items into tiny pieces (O). Putty can be used if nothing disposable is available.

p: *Card deals*: Patient works through a deck of cards, flipping each card over (P) or sliding cards (not shown).

q: *Tweezers*: Have patient pick up small items such as popcorn kernels or rice and deposit them in a cup (Q).

r: *Finding items in beans or rice*: Bury a variety of items in a large bucket filled with beans or rice and have patient find the items by digging and feeling with hand. Patient may close the eyes to encourage increased use of sensory organs of hand (not shown).

s: *Hand maze*: Using the device shown, patient moves the bead or washer along from start to finish (S).

t: *Bolt box*: Using devices shown, patient tightens and loosens bolts and nuts. This can be used for endurance training and set at multiple levels to work elbows and shoulders as well (T1 and T2).

u: *Clothes pins*: Patient clamps and unclamps clothes pins, using thumb with digits 2 to 3 usually, but can be done with other fingers (U).

<u>SUBSTITUTIONS</u>: Sitting up straight; active shoulders and scapula.

<u>PARAMETERS</u>: Work on each activity for 1 to 5 minutes or until fatigue, 1 time per day or every other day

Section 5.17

UPPER EXTREMITY NERVE GLIDES

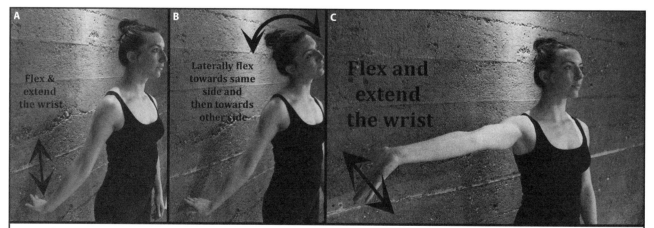

5.17.1 NERVE GLIDE: MEDIAN NERVE

POSITION: Standing

TARGETS: Glides/slides median nerve

INSTRUCTION:

Glide: Patient places affected arm in full elbow extension, shoulder in slight extension and abduction, palm facing forward. Patient extends the wrist until tension is felt anywhere from neck to anterior arm, forearm, wrist, hand. Patient holds 1 to 2 seconds, releases wrist and shoulder, and repeats (A).

Glide: Patient places affected arm in full elbow extension, shoulder in slight extension and abduction, palm facing forward. Patient extends the wrist while side-bending the neck toward ipsilateral side, patient holds 1 to 2 seconds. Patient then flexes the wrist, side-bends the neck toward contralateral side, and repeats (B).

Glide: Patient places affected arm in full elbow extension, shoulder in 90 degrees abduction, palm facing up. Patient extends the wrist, holds 1 to 2 seconds, and repeats (C).

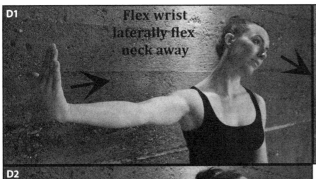

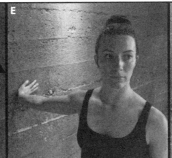

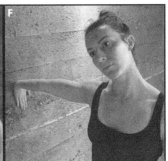

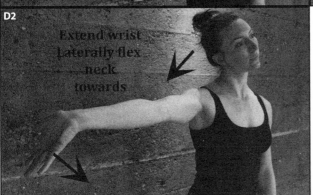

5.17.1 NERVE GLIDE: MEDIAN NERVE (CONTINUED)

Glide: Patient places affected arm in full elbow extension, shoulder in 90 degrees abduction, palm facing up. Patient flexes the wrist and, while side-bending the neck toward contralateral side, holds 1 to 2 seconds. Patient then extends the wrist and side-bends neck to ipsilateral side, holds 1 to 2 seconds, and repeats (D1 and D2).

Tensioning: Patient places affected arm in full elbow extension, shoulder in 90 degrees abduction with palm on wall, fingers facing backward. Patient rotates body away from wall until tension felt, holds 1 to 2 seconds, and repeats (E).

Tensioning: Patient places affected arm in full elbow extension, shoulder in 90 degrees abduction with palm on wall, fingers facing down. Patient side-bends neck toward contralateral side until tension felt, holds 1 to 2 seconds, and repeats (F).

<u>SUBSTITUTIONS</u>: Shrugging shoulder; keep scapula retracted and chin tucked in slightly.

<u>PARAMETERS</u>: 10 to 15 repetitions, repeat 1 to 3 times per day as needed

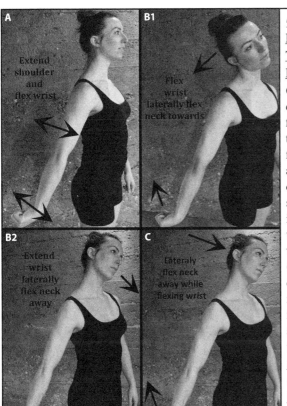

5.17.2 NERVE GLIDE: RADIAL NERVE

<u>POSITION</u>: Standing

<u>TARGETS</u>: Glides/slides radial nerve

<u>INSTRUCTION</u>:

Glide: Patient places affected arm in full elbow extension, shoulder in slight extension and abduction, scapula retracted, palm facing backward, and full fist, thumb inside fist. Patient flexes the wrist until tension felt anywhere from neck to anterior arm, forearm, wrist, hand. Patient holds 1 to 2 seconds, releases wrist and shoulder, and repeats (A). Patient places affected arm in full elbow extension, shoulder in slight extension and abduction, scapula retracted, palm facing backward, with full fist, thumb inside. Patient flexes the wrist and side-bends the neck toward the ipsilateral side. Patient holds 1 to 2 seconds, then extends wrist and side-bends neck toward contralateral side, and repeats (B1 and B2). *Tensioning*: Patient places affected arm in full elbow extension, shoulder in slight extension and abduction, scapula retracted, palm facing backward, full fist thumb inside. Patient flexes the wrist and side-bends the neck toward the contralateral side. Patient holds 1 to 2 seconds, returns wrist and neck to neutral, and repeats (C).

<u>SUBSTITUTIONS</u>: Shrugging shoulder; keep scapula retracted and chin tucked in slightly.

<u>PARAMETERS</u>: 10 to 15 repetitions, repeat 1 to 3 times per day as needed

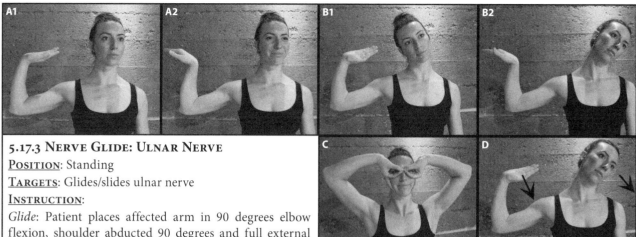

5.17.3 NERVE GLIDE: ULNAR NERVE

<u>POSITION</u>: Standing

<u>TARGETS</u>: Glides/slides ulnar nerve

<u>INSTRUCTION</u>:

Glide: Patient places affected arm in 90 degrees elbow flexion, shoulder abducted 90 degrees and full external rotation, palm facing down and fingers laterally. Patient extends the wrist, bringing fingertips toward ear, holds 1 to 2 seconds, and repeats (A1 and A2).

Glide: Patient places affected arm in 90 degrees elbow flexion, shoulder abducted 90 degrees and full external rotation, palm facing down and fingers laterally. Patient extends the wrist bringing fingertips toward ear while side-bending neck to ipsilateral side. Patient holds 1 to 2 seconds, reverses to flex wrist, and side bend neck toward contralateral side (B1 and B2).

Tensioning: mask: Patient places affected arm in 90 degrees elbow flexion, shoulder abducted 90 degrees and full external rotation, palm facing up. Patient extends wrist with thumb to index fingertips, making a circle that goes around the eye like a mask. Patient extends the wrist bringing fingertips toward ear while side-bending neck to ipsilateral side. Patient holds 1 to 2 seconds and returns to start (C).

Tensioning: waiter/waitress holding tray: Patient places affected arm in 90 degrees elbow flexion, shoulder abducted 90 degrees and full external rotation, palm facing up with fingers toward the head, similar to holding a tray. Patient extends wrist and places palm on ear as they laterally flex the neck toward the contralateral side. Patient holds 1 to 2 seconds and returns to tray-holding position (D).

<u>SUBSTITUTIONS</u>: Shrugging shoulder; keep scapula retracted and chin tucked in slightly.

<u>PARAMETERS</u>: 10 to 15 repetitions, repeat 1 to 3 times per day as needed

REFERENCE

Coppieters, M. W., & Butler, D. S. (2008). Do 'sliders' slide and 'tensioners' tension? An analysis of neurodynamic techniques and considerations regarding their application. *Manual Therapy, 13*(3), 213-221.

Section 5.18

WRIST AND HAND PROTOCOLS AND TREATMENT IDEAS

5.18.1 CARPAL TUNNEL SYNDROME DISCUSSION

CTS is a combination of signs and symptoms due to compression and trapping of the median nerve at the wrist. It is the most commonly reported peripheral nerve entrapment syndrome (Fu et al., 2015). It can lead to pain in the hand, wrist and sometimes arm, and numbness and tingling in the thumb, index, and long finger (Page, Massy-Westropp, O'Connor, & Pitt, 2012). The latest available evidence suggests that CTS should be considered as an occupational disease after certain biomechanical exposures at the workplace results as there is high evidence for an increased risk of CTS in activities requiring a high degree of repetition and forceful exertion (Kozak et al., 2015). Interestingly, computer work was associated with lowered risks of CTS when compared to workers in food processing, manufacturing, service work, construction and other occupations where repeated or sustained exposures to forceful hand exertions pose a strong increased risk. This study does not rule out the possibility that specific biomechanical exposure in some types of computer work may increase the risk for CTS, especially within worker groups without exposure to any other hand-intensive work. It is important to improve any work conditions that place computer workers in sustained awkward postures or lead to other symptoms (Mediouni et al., 2015). Neural and carpal bone mobilizations have often been utilized in the rehabilitation setting. Tendon gliding exercises are also employed; however, the research is somewhat lacking.

Where's the Evidence?

One study by Tal-Akabi and Rushton (2000) investigated the effects of two manual therapy techniques in the treatment of patients experiencing CTS. There were three groups of subjects in three different conditions: two treatment interventions, carpal mobilization and median nerve mobilization, and one control group. Patients in the treatment groups had improved upper limb tension testing with median nerve emphasis, less referral for surgery and decreased pain as compared with the control group; however no difference in outcome was found between the two treatment interventions. Akalin et al. (2002) looked at 36 hands with CTS and randomly assigned them to 2 groups. A custom-made neutral volar wrist splint was given to group one and group two and patients were instructed to wear the splints all night, and during the day as much as possible, for 4 weeks. The patients in group two were instructed to perform a series of nerve and tendon gliding exercises in addition to the splint treatment. At the end of treatment, statistically significant improvement was obtained in all parameters in both groups. The improvement in group two was slightly greater, but the difference between the groups was not significant, except for the lateral pinch strength value. A total of 72% of the patients in group one and 93% of the patients in group two reported good or excellent results (Akalin et al., 2002). A 2012 systematic review of the evidence for exercise and mobilization found limited and very low-quality evidence of benefit for all of a diverse collection of exercise and mobilization interventions for CTS, recommending more high-quality randomized controlled trials to assist the effectiveness and safety of various exercises and mobilization interventions compared to other non-surgical interventions undertaken (Page, O'Connor, Pitt, & Massy-Westropp, 2012). Splinting is usually offered to people with mild to moderate symptoms. Page and colleagues performed a systematic review of the literature in 2012 and found limited evidence that a splint worn at night is more effective than no treatment in the short-term. Ultrasound historically has been used, but current evidence does not support ultrasound as being any better than placebo (Page, O'Connor, Pitt, & Massy-Westropp, 2013). A 2002 systematic review did find evidence to support significant short-term benefit from oral steroids, splinting, ultrasound, yoga and carpal bone mobilization. Other non-surgical treatments did not produce significant benefit (O'Connor, Marshall, & Massy-Westropp, 2003). Another review found local corticosteroid injection for CTS provided greater clinical improvement in symptoms 1 month after injection compared to placebo; however, symptom relief beyond 1 month compared to placebo had not been demonstrated (Marshall, Tardif, & Ashworth, 2002). Alternative delivery systems for corticosteroid may include iontophoresis and phonophoresis. One study in 2013 found phonophoresis of dexamethasone sodium phosphate treatment was more effective than iontophoresis of dexamethasone sodium phosphate for treatment of CTS (Bakhtiary, Fatemi, Emami, & Malek, 2013). Wrist stretching has demonstrated improvement in pain and decreasing positive clinical testing for CTS (Yoo, 2015). Surgical decompression is often implemented. The principle of surgical treatment is to achieve a reduction in intratunnel pressure through increasing the volume of the carpal tunnel, by sectioning the flexor retinaculum. The procedure is done more often unilaterally under local anesthesia, ideally as an outpatient procedure, and frequently using a tourniquet (Chammas, Boretto, Burmann, Ramos, Neto, & Silva, 2014).

5.18.2 CARPAL TUNNEL RELEASE POST-OPERATIVE PROTOCOL

Protocol adapted from University of Virginia School of Medicine Hand Center (n.d.).

First Post-Operative Visit

1. Therapist removes post-operation dressing; wound check.
2. Application of sterile dry dressing (remain over incision at all times until suture removal)
3. Instruct patient on suture site care and edema control
4. Splint: Full time except for exercises (or follow physician orders if different)
5. ROM
   a. 5.09.3 ROM: Elbow Flexion and Extension, Active
   b. 5.09.7 ROM: Elbow Pronation and Supination, Active
   c. 5.14.1 ROM: Wrist and Finger Movements, Passive and Active (no active wrist flexion or extension).
      i. Active wrist radial/ulnar deviation
      ii. Active thumb
      iii. Active fingers
      iv. Active finger lifts
      v. Active opposition
      vi. Active fist to finger spread
6. Tendon glides
   a. 5.14.4 ROM: Elbow, Tendon Gliding, "4 Pack" and "6 Pack"

Second Post-Operative Visit (10 to 14 Days)

1. Surgical follow-up visit with attending surgeon or physician assistant, sutures removed and new dressing applied; keep hand dry up to 14 days post-operation.
2. Splint: Continue to wear splint
3. No heavy lifting

Third Post-Operative Visit (3 Weeks)

1. Ensure proper wound healing, scar mobility, AROM
2. Wean from splint; wear at night for an additional week.
3. Desensitization
   a. 5.14.5 Desensitization Exercises, Upper Extremity
4. ROM
   a. 5.14.1 ROM: Wrist and Finger Movements, Passive and Active (start active wrist extension/flexion).
   b. Active Wrist flexion/extension
   c. Nerve Glides
   d. 5.17.1 Nerve Glide: Median Nerve
5. Grip/pinch strengthening
   a. 5.16.13 Strengthen: Putty and Gripmaster Pro For Hand And Fingers

Home Exercise Program 3 Weeks Post-Operatively

1. Tendon gliding exercises: 5 times per day
2. Scar massage with lotion for 5 minutes, 5 times per day. Use a moderately deep pressure to help flatten the scar and decrease its sensitivity to pressure.

3. Wear the silicone scar pad to soften the scar at night. Patient to make sure skin is clean and dry before applying the scar pad each night followed by washing it each morning with soap and water, and dry it with a cloth towel.
4. Splint: Wear splint at night until 6 weeks post-operation
5. Returning to Activities: Most patients can resume full use of their hand after surgery by about 6 weeks post-operation. Do not repetitively perform activities that cause pain. A gradual return to activities without pain is the goal.
6. If patient feels strength is not returning by week 6 consider adding new exercises to the program.

Week 6: Strengthening if Needed

1. Wrist strengthening ideas
   a. 5.16.5 Strengthen: Isometric and Isotonic; Ball, Thumb Variations
   b. 5.16.6 Strengthen: Isotonic; Wrist, All Planes
   c. 5.16.8 Strengthen: Wrist Roller
   d. 5.16.14 Strengthen: Web and Variations For Hand and Fingers
   e. 5.16.15 Functional, Wrist/Hand and Finger Activities

* Silicone-based products such as sheets and gels are recommended as the gold standard, first-line, noninvasive option for both the prevention and treatment of scars. Other general scar preventative measures include avoiding sun exposure, compression therapy, taping and the use of moisturizers (Meaume, Le Pillouer-Prost, Richert, Roseeuw, & Vadoud, 2014).

REFERENCES

Akalin, E., El, O., Peker, O., Senocak, O., Tamci, S., Gülbahar, S., . . . Oncel, S. (2002). Treatment of carpal tunnel syndrome with nerve and tendon gliding exercises. *American Journal of Physical Medicine and Rehabilitation, 81*(2), 108-113.

Bakhtiary, A. H., Fatemi, E., Emami, M., & Malek, M. (2013). Phonophoresis of dexamethasone sodium phosphate may manage pain and symptoms of patients with carpal tunnel syndrome. *The Clinical Journal of Pain, 29*(4), 348-353.

Chammas, M., Boretto, J., Burmann, L. M., Ramos, R. M., Neto, F. S., & Silva, J. B. (2014). Carpal tunnel syndrome–Part II (treatment). *Revista Brasileira de Ortopedia, 49*(5), 437-445.

Fu, T., Cao, M., Liu, F., Zhu, J., Ye, D., Feng, X., . . . Bai, Y. (2015). Carpal tunnel syndrome assessment with ultrasonography: Value of inlet-to-outlet median nerve area ratio in patients versus healthy volunteers. *PLoS One, 10*(1), e0116777..

Kozak, A., Schedlbauer, G., Wirth, T., Euler, U., Westermann, C., & Nienhaus, A. (2015). Association between work-related biomechanical risk factors and the occurrence of carpal tunnel syndrome: An overview of systematic reviews and a meta-analysis of current research. *BMC Musculoskelet Disorders, 16*, 231.

Marshall, S., Tardif, G., & Ashworth, N. (2002). Local corticosteroid injection for carpal tunnel syndrome. *Cochrane Database of Systematic Reviews,* CD001554.

Meaume, S., Le Pillouer-Prost, A., Richert, B., Roseeuw, D., & Vadoud, J. (2014). Management of scars: Updated practical guidelines and use of silicones. *European Journal of Dermatology, 24*(4), 435-443.

Mediouni, Z., Bodin, J., Dale, A. M., Herquelot, E., Carton, M., Leclerc, A., . . . Descatha, A. (2015). Carpal tunnel syndrome and computer exposure at work in two large complementary cohorts. *BMJ Open,* e008156.

O'Connor, D., Marshall, S., & Massy-Westropp, N. (2003). Non-surgical treatment (other than steroid injection) for carpal tunnel syndrome. *Cochrane Database of Systematic Review,* CD003219.

Page, M. J., Massy-Westropp, N., O'Connor, D., & Pitt, V. (2012). Splinting for carpal tunnel syndrome. *Cochrane Database of Systematic Reviews,* CD010003.

Page, M. J., O'Connor, D., Pitt, V., & Massy-Westropp, N. (2012). Exercise and mobilisation interventions for carpal tunnel syndrome. *Cochrane Database of Systematic Reviews,* CD009899.

Page, M. J., O'Connor, D., Pitt, V., & Massy-Westropp, N. (2013). Therapeutic ultrasound for carpal tunnel syndrome. *Cochrane Database of Systematic Reviews*, CD009601.

Tal-Akabi, A., & Rushton, A. (2000). An investigation to compare the effectiveness of carpal bone mobilisation and neurodynamic mobilisation as methods of treatment for carpal tunnel syndrome. *Manual Therapy, 5*(4), 214-222.

University of Virginia School of Medicine Hand Center. (n.d.). Open carpal tunnel release post-op guidelines. *University of Virginia School of Medicine*. Retrieved from https://med.virginia.edu/orthopaedic-surgery/wp-content/uploads/sites/242/2015/11/copy_of_CTROPENProtocolandHEP.pdf

Yoo, W. G. (2015). Effect of the release exercise and exercise position in a patient with carpal tunnel syndrome. *Journal of Physical Therapy Science, 27*(10), 3345-3346.

Chapter 6

LOWER EXTREMITY EXERCISES

Bryan E. *The Comprehensive Manual of Therapeutic Exercises:*
Orthopedic and General Conditions (pp 359-508).
© 2018 SLACK Incorporated.

Section 6.01

HIP RANGE OF MOTION

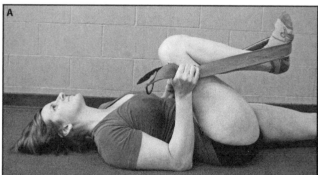

6.01.1 ROM: HIP FLEXION, ACTIVE ASSISTIVE

POSITION: Supine

TARGETS: Mobility of the hip into flexion

INSTRUCTION: Patient places a belt under the arch of the foot and uses belt to pull the hip and knee into flexion (A). Patient may also place a towel behind the knee and use towel to pull the hip into flexion, allowing knee to flex (B). If able, patient may grasp behind the knee and pull the hip into flexion, allowing knee to flex (C).

SUBSTITUTIONS: Lifting pelvis or head off table

PARAMETERS: Hold for 5 seconds, 10 to 15 repetitions, repeat 1 to 3 times per day

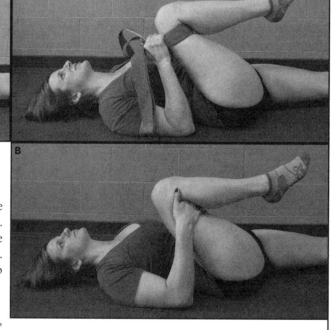

6.01.2 ROM: HIP EXTENSION, LEG DROP, ACTIVE ASSISTIVE

POSITION: Supine

TARGETS: Mobility of the hip into extension using gravity assist

INSTRUCTION: Patient scoots to the side edge of the table and allows leg to drop off, extending the hip. Encourage PPT to protect the lumbar spine.

SUBSTITUTIONS: Anterior tilt of pelvis

PARAMETERS: Allow leg to hang 5 to 15 seconds, 5 repetitions, repeat 1 to 3 times per day

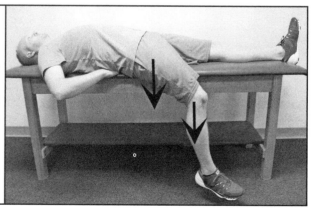

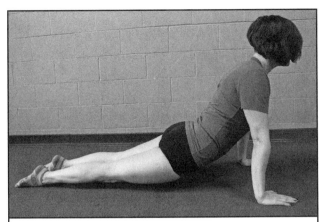

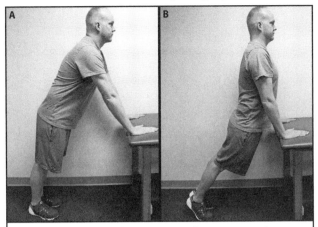

6.01.3 ROM: Hip Extension, Press-Up, Active Assistive

Position: Prone

Targets: Mobility of the hip into extension

Instruction: Patient places hands or elbows under shoulders palms down and presses upper torso upward while maintaining gaze forward. Press far enough so that hip is extending and not just lower back.

Substitutions: Lifting pelvis off table, tensing shoulders, shrugging

Parameters: Hold for 10 seconds, repeat 5 to 15 repetitions, repeat 1 to 3 times per day

6.01.4 ROM: Hip Extension, Standing, Active Assistive

Position: Standing

Targets: Mobility of the hip into extension

Instruction: Patient places hands on table in front and walks feet back. Patient then lets hips drop forward, extending the hips. Look for hip extension not lower back extension; encourage PPT to protect the lumbar spine (A and B).

Substitutions: Lifting pelvis off table, tensing shoulders, shrugging

Parameters: Hold for 5 seconds, 10 to 15 repetitions, repeat 1 to 3 times per day

6.01.5 ROM: Hip Abduction With Belt, Active Assistive

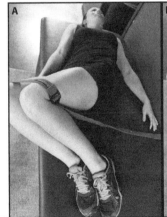

Position: Supine

Targets: Mobility of the hip into abduction

Instruction: Patient hooks belt around ankle or knee and pulls leg outward to abduct the hip.

Substitutions: Anterior tilt of pelvis

Parameters: Allow leg to hang 5 to 15 seconds, 5 repetitions, repeat 1 to 3 times per day

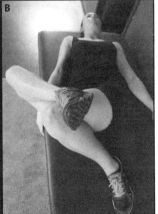

6.01.6 ROM: Hip Rotation, Active Assistive

Position: Hook-lying, 90/90

Targets: Mobility of the hip in the transverse plane (rotation)

Instruction: Start with back flat and feet together flat on mat and belt looped around knees. Patient rotates knees fully to the left and then follows by going to the right. As affected hip externally rotates, top knee can push to gain range. As the hip internally rotates, the opposite knee pulls with belt to assist with internal rotation; movements should be slow. For warm-up only, go part range and the progress to end range rotations. Patient may use hand on ipsilateral side to push hips further as well (A and B). For increasing range, flex hips and knees 90/90. Patient places arms out to the sides and rotates knees fully to the left and then follow by going to the right. Abdominals remain engaged to avoid lumbar extension (C).

Substitutions: Pelvis comes off floor

Parameters: Repeat 10 to 20 times, 1 to 3 times per day

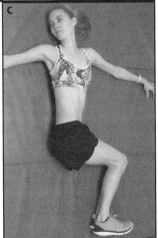

6.01.7 ROM: Hip, Powder Board, Active

<u>Position</u>: Side-lying

<u>Targets</u>: Mobility of the hip in the sagittal plane for patient with difficulty against gravity or friction

<u>Instruction</u>: Start with lying on unaffected side, place stool using sliding board dusted with talcum powder to eliminate friction and optional towel under leg. Patient then flexes hip with knee, bent at first for a shorter lever arm and easier movement. Follow with hip extension. Progress to repeating instructions with knee extended once strength allows. Hold each position 1 to 2 seconds. Repeat (A and B).

<u>Substitutions</u>: Trunk flexion or extension in attempt to use momentum, lumbar flexion/extension; avoid by having patient engage core muscle of trunk to stabilize pelvis.

<u>Parameters</u>: Repeat 10 to 20 times, 1 to 3 times per day

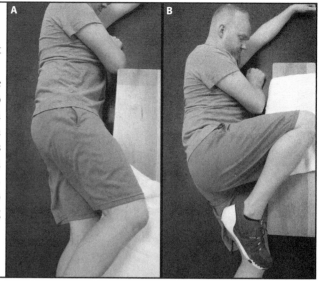

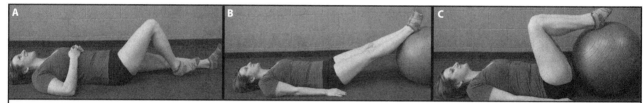

6.01.8 ROM: Hip Flexion and Extension, Heel Slide, Active

<u>Position</u>: Hook-lying

<u>Targets</u>: Mobility of the hip in the sagittal plane

<u>Instruction</u>: Start with back flat and feet together flat on mat. Bring heel toward buttock, bending hip and knee. Hold 1 to 2 seconds and return to full extended. Repeat (A). *Exercise ball:* Use of an exercise ball can assist hip and knee flexion. Patient places calves on ball and rolls ball closer to buttocks so that heels are now on the ball, then returns to start (B and C).

<u>Substitutions</u>: Knee falls in or out

<u>Parameters</u>: Repeat 10 to 20 times, 1 to 3 times per day

6.01.9 ROM: Hip Flexion and Extension, Active

<u>Position</u>: Standing

<u>Targets</u>: Mobility of the hip in the sagittal plane

<u>Instruction</u>: Patient standing with unaffected side near table or wall using hand to balance brings affected hip into extension, followed by flexing hip and knee as if marching in place with only the one leg (A and B).

<u>Substitutions</u>: Knee falls in or out

<u>Parameters</u>: Repeat 10 to 20 times, 1 to 3 times per day

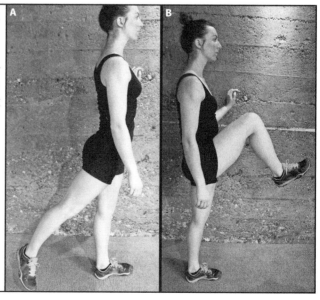

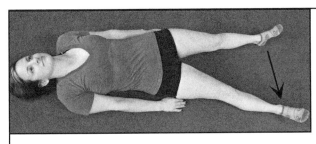

6.01.10 ROM: Hip Abduction and Adduction, Heel Slide, Active

Position: Supine

Targets: Mobility of the hip in coronal plane

Instruction: Patient lies with knees extended to 0 degrees. Patient slides heel out to the side, abducting the hip and then slides back toward the middle, adducting the hip. This can be done bilaterally as well.

Substitutions: Patient flexes or extends hip, rolls trunk forward or backward in side-lying; does not keep toes pointed straight ahead (adding rotation).

Parameters: Repeat 10 to 20 times, 1 to 3 times per day

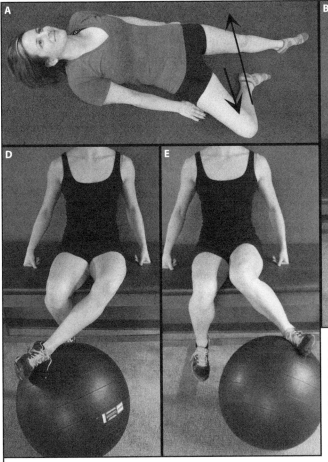

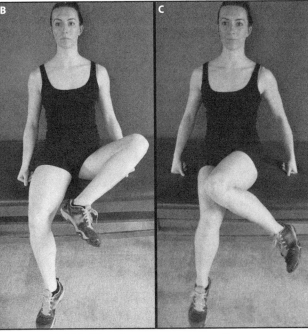

6.01.11 ROM: Hip Abduction and External Rotation, and Adduction and Internal Rotation, Active

Position: Hook-lying, seated

Targets: Mobility of the hip in combined coronal and transverse planes

Instruction: *Hook-lying:* Start with back flat and one hip and knee bent with other leg extended. Patient actively opens bent leg to allow knee to fall out to side (external rotation/abduction). Hold 1 to 2 seconds and return, bringing knee over extended leg (internal rotation/adduction) (A). *Seated:* Patient brings bottom of the foot laterally for internal rotation and then returns to bring the bottom of foot medially for external rotation. For combination movement, allow knee to move inward with internal rotation and outward for external rotation (B and C). *Exercise ball:* Patient places bottom of foot on top of ball and rolls ball to each side as patient rotates the hip (D and E).

Substitutions: Patient lifts hips off table; keep lower abdominals engaged to limit lumbopelvic movements.

Parameters: Repeat 10 to 20 times, 1 to 3 times per day

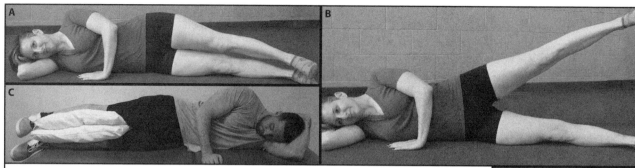

6.01.12 ROM: Hip Abduction, Active

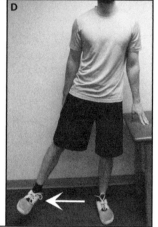

POSITION: Side-lying, standing

TARGETS: Mobility of the hip in coronal plane

INSTRUCTION: Patient lies on unaffected side with hip and knee extended to 0 degrees and lifts leg toward ceiling, keeping toes pointed straight forward. Hold 1 to 2 seconds and return (A and B). If the desire is to avoid crossing midline, place pillows under knee as shown (C). In standing, patient may hold chair or table for balance as patient abducts the hip, keeping hip and knee extended to 0 degrees and toes pointing forward (D).

SUBSTITUTIONS: Patient flexes or extends hip, rolls trunk forward or backward in side-lying; does not keep toes pointed straight ahead (adding rotation). The bottom leg can be bent to help stabilize body.

PARAMETERS: Repeat 10 to 20 times, 1 to 3 times per day

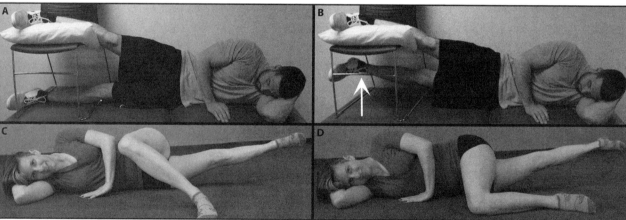

6.01.13 ROM: Hip Adduction, Active

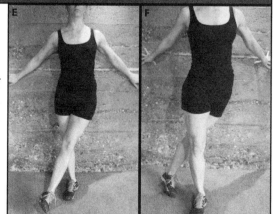

POSITION: Side-lying, standing

TARGETS: Mobility of the hip in coronal plane

INSTRUCTION: Patient lies on affected side with hip and knee extended to 0 degrees. A chair is placed so that top leg can rest on it out of the way. Patient lifts bottom leg toward ceiling, keeping toes pointed straight forward. Hold 1 to 2 seconds and return (A and B). This can also be done without a chair, with top knee and hip flexed 90 degrees and lying in front of bottom leg with knee down or foot down (C and D). In standing, patient may hold chair or table for balance as patient adducts the hip, crossing in front of the other leg or behind and keeping hip and knee extended to 0 degrees and toes pointing forward (E and F).

SUBSTITUTIONS: Patient flexes or extends hip, rolls trunk forward or backward in side-lying; does not keep toes pointed straight ahead (adding rotation).

PARAMETERS: Repeat 10 to 20 times, 1 to 3 times per day

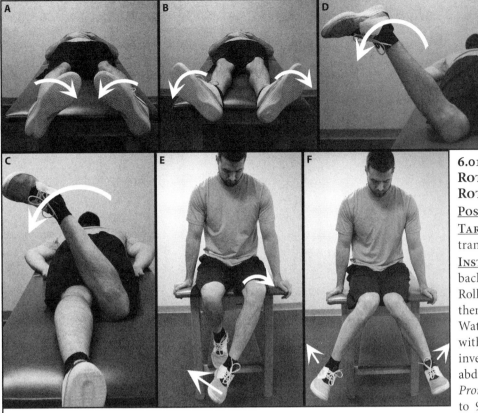

6.01.14 ROM: Hip Internal Rotation and External Rotation, Active

POSITION: Supine, prone, seated

TARGETS: Mobility of the hip in transverse planes

INSTRUCTION: *Supine:* Start with back flat and legs extended. Roll toes toward other foot and then away, causing hip to rotate. Watch that patient is moving with hip and *not* ankle/foot inversion/eversion and forefoot abduction/adduction (A and B). *Prone:* Patient bends one knee to 90 degrees and brings knee together. Patient then bring lower leg across extended leg to externally rotate hip. Hold for 12 seconds and then bring lower leg back across toward outside internally rotating hip (C and D). *Seated:* Keeping knees together, patient brings bottom of foot laterally for internal rotation and then returns to bring bottom of foot medially for external rotation while slightly flexing other knee to clear the path (E and F). This also can be done bilaterally if desired.

SUBSTITUTIONS: Patient lifts hips off table; keep lower abdominals engaged to limit lumbopelvic movements.

PARAMETERS: Repeat 10 to 20 times, 1 to 3 times per day

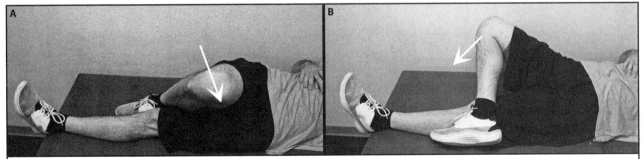

6.01.15 ROM: Hip Internal Rotation and External Rotation Combined With Hip Abduction and Adduction, Active

POSITION: Half hook-lying

TARGETS: Mobility of the hip in transverse planes and coronal planes combined

INSTRUCTION: With unaffected leg extended on mat, place affected foot on mat inside of knee and bring knee across to internally rotate and adduct the hip. Hold 1 to 2 seconds, then lift and bring foot to outside of knee and bring knee outward toward mat to externally rotate and abduct the hip (A and B).

SUBSTITUTIONS: Patient lifts hips off table; keep lower abdominals engaged to limit lumbopelvic movements.

PARAMETERS: Repeat 10 to 20 times, 1 to 3 times per day

6.01.16 ROM: Hip Internal and External Rotation Using Rolling Stool, Active

<u>Position</u>: Half hook-lying

<u>Targets</u>: Mobility of the hip in transverse planes

<u>Instruction</u>: With affected knee on stool, patient keeps knee directly under hip and rotates heel in and out as hip rotates (A and B).

<u>Substitutions</u>: Patient lifts hips off table; keep lower abdominals engaged to limit lumbopelvic movements.

<u>Parameters</u>: Repeat 10 to 20 times, 1 to 3 times per day

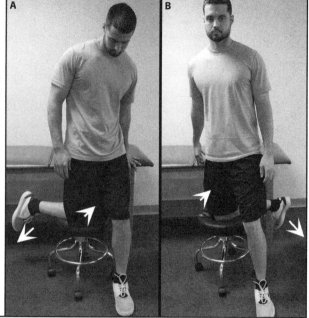

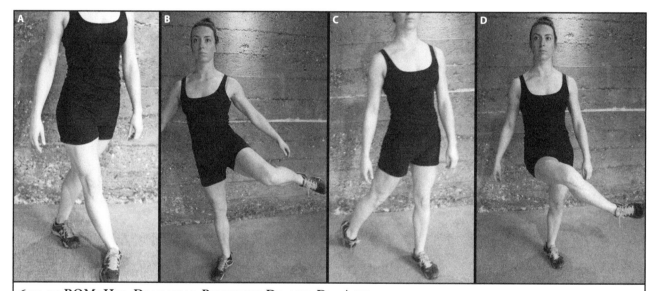

6.01.17 ROM: Hip, Diagonal Patterns D1 and D2, Active

<u>Position</u>: Standing

<u>Targets</u>: Mobility of the hip in combined sagittal, coronal, and transverse planes

<u>Instruction</u>: Patient stands holding onto chair or table for balance, if needed. *D1:* Patient starts with leg behind and hip extended, adducted, and externally rotated. Patient then brings hip into flexion, abduction, and internal rotation, ending with the bottom of the foot facing laterally to affected side. Hold 1 to 2 seconds and return to start. Repeat (A and B). *D2:* Patient starts with leg behind and out to the side and hip extended, abducted, and internally rotated (toes in). Patient then brings hip into flexion, adduction, and internal rotation, ending with the bottom of the foot facing laterally to unaffected side. Hold 1 to 2 seconds and return to start. Repeat (C and D). Patient follows the foot with the eyes.

<u>Substitutions</u>: Keep lower abdominals engaged to limit lumbopelvic movements

<u>Parameters</u>: Repeat 10 to 20 times, 1 to 3 times per day

Section 6.02

HIP JOINT SELF-MOBILIZATION

6.02.1 SELF-JOINT MOBILIZATION: HIP EXTENSION

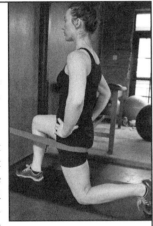

POSITION: Half-kneeling

TARGETS: Mobility of the ischiofemoral joint into extension and anterior capsule stretch

INSTRUCTION: Anchor belt around a stable object. Patient steps into the loop of the band, facing the anchor and slides the loop up into the gluteal fold. Patient moves back to create tension in the belt, pulling the superior femur anteriorly. While keeping the trunk upright, slide knee posteriorly while maintaining a strong PPT. Continue to scoot back so there is a strong pull in the belt.

SUBSTITUTIONS: APT, extending lower back

PARAMETERS: Hold 15 to 30 seconds, 3 to 5 repetitions, 1 to 3 times per day

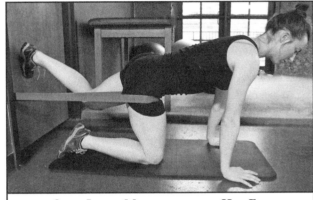

6.02.2 SELF-JOINT MOBILIZATION: HIP FLEXION

POSITION: Seated

TARGETS: Mobility of the ischiofemoral joint into flexion, inferior/posterior capsule stretch

INSTRUCTION: Anchor belt around a stable object. Place one leg into the loop of the band, facing away from anchor in quadruped. Slide loop of the band up to hip crease. Move away from anchor to create tension in the band. Bring the knee forward into further hip flexion on the banded leg. Keep the abdominals activated to keep a neutral spine.

SUBSTITUTIONS: Encourage stabilization of core and gluteal muscles to avoid pelvic tilting posteriorly.

PARAMETERS: Hold 15 to 30 seconds, 3 to 5 repetitions, 1 to 3 times per day

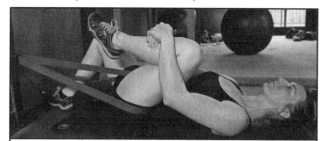

6.02.3 Self-Joint Mobilization: Hip, Knee to Chest

<u>Position</u>: Supine

<u>Targets</u>: Mobility of the ischiofemoral joint into flexion, inferior/posterior capsule stretch

<u>Instruction</u>: Anchor belt around a stable object. Patient slips one leg into loop and places it in the hip crease. Patient scoots back to create tension in the band and pull the knee toward the chest with hands clasped in front of knee. Patient keeps core muscles active during pull to keep pelvis from rotating posteriorly.

<u>Substitutions</u>: Allowing the hip/knee to roll out into external rotation; the hip should move straight into flexion only.

<u>Parameters</u>: Hold 15 to 30 seconds, 3 to 5 repetitions, 1 to 3 times per day

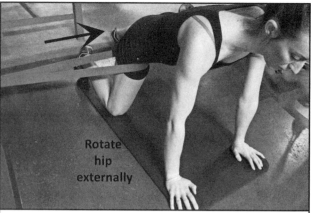

Rotate hip externally

6.02.4 Self-Joint Mobilization: Hip External Rotation

<u>Position</u>: Quadruped

<u>Targets</u>: Mobility of the ischiofemoral joint into external rotation, lateral capsule stretch

<u>Instruction</u>: Anchor belt around a stable object. Patient places one leg in loop and slides band up in the hip crease. Patient moves away from anchor to create tension in the band. Patient externally rotates the leg, keeping tension on the band. Patient keeps core muscles active to ensure a neutral spine throughout the stretch.

<u>Substitutions</u>: Shoulder shrugs; trunk sinks into shoulder or hips.

<u>Parameters</u>: Hold 15 to 30 seconds, 3 to 5 repetitions, 1 to 3 times per day

Section 6.03

HIP STRETCHING

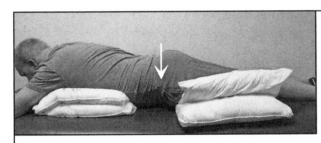

6.03.1 Stretch: Hip Flexor, Gravity and Weight Assist

POSITION: Prone

TARGETS: Stretch iliopsoas

INSTRUCTION: Position patient prone with pillow under stomach and proximal thigh but below the inguinal region. Allow gravity to assist pulling hip into extension. Weight may be added to pelvis to increase passive stretch.

SUBSTITUTIONS: Lateral trunk flexion; pulling bent knee into abduction.

PARAMETERS: Hold for 1 to 5 minutes, 1 repetition, 1 to 3 times per day

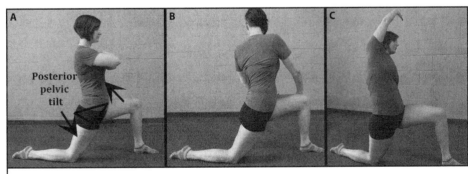

6.03.2 Stretch: Hip Flexor, Kneeling Lunge

POSITION: Half-kneeling

TARGETS: Stretch iliopsoas

INSTRUCTION: Patient places one foot in front into kneeling lunge (keeping knees behind toes) and lets hips melt forward until slight stretch is felt in opposite anterior inguinal region. Patient then performs a PPT to increase the stretch (A). Add trunk twist toward front leg side as forward leg to increase stretch (B). Add trunk lateral flexion arm overhead to front leg side as forward leg to increase stretch (C).

SUBSTITUTIONS: APT, lumbar extension, knees are further forward than toes, knee deviates in or out

PARAMETERS: Hold for 15 to 30 seconds, 3 to 5 repetitions, 1 to 3 times per day

6.03.3 STRETCH: HIP FLEXOR, STANDING LUNGE

POSITION: Standing

TARGETS: Stretch iliopsoas

INSTRUCTION: Patient places one foot in front, lunging forward (keeping knees behind toes), until slight stretch is felt in opposite anterior inguinal region. Patient then performs a PPT to increase the stretch.

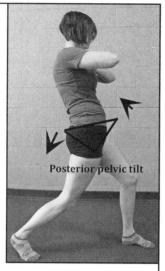

SUBSTITUTIONS: APT, lumbar extension, knees are further forward than toes, knee deviates in or out

PARAMETERS: Hold for 15 to 30 seconds, 3 to 5 repetitions, 1 to 3 times per day

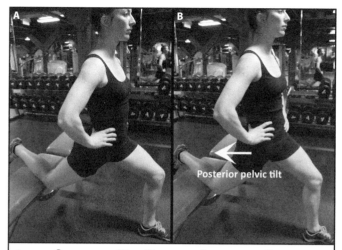

6.03.4 STRETCH: HIP FLEXOR, STANDING LUNGE WITH CHAIR/BENCH

POSITION: Standing

TARGETS: Stretch iliopsoas

INSTRUCTION: Patient places leg behind in a chair or bench with knee on towel for comfort. Patient then places opposite foot in front, lunging forward (keeping knees behind toes) until slight stretch is felt in opposite anterior inguinal region. Patient then performs a PPT to increase the stretch (A and B).

SUBSTITUTIONS: APT, lumbar extension, knees are further forward than toes, knee deviates in or out

PARAMETERS: Hold for 15 to 30 seconds, 3 to 5 repetitions, 1 to 3 times per day

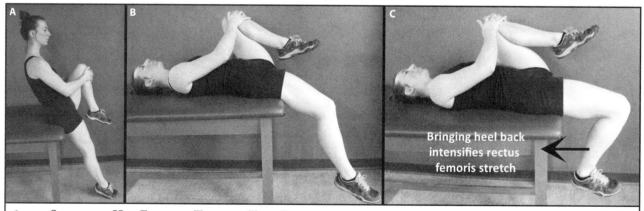

6.03.5 STRETCH: HIP FLEXOR, THOMAS TEST POSITION

POSITION: Seated edge of bed

TARGETS: Stretch iliopsoas

INSTRUCTION: Patient sits on edge of bed so that gluteal crease is just at edge. Patient grasps around unaffected knee with both hands and lies back, allowing affected leg to remain. Patient should perform a PPT to decrease lumbar curve. Hanging leg should feel stretch in inguinal region (A and B). Adding active knee flexion will intensify the rectus femoris stretch (C). This can also be done on a foam roller for patients that cannot tolerate the edge of table. Patient lies supine and bridges to place medium foam roller under pelvis. Patient brings unaffected knee toward chest and then slowly extends target leg. To intensify stretch, patient can actively push extended-side heel into the ground (D).

SUBSTITUTIONS: APT, lumbar extension, deviates in or out

PARAMETERS: Hold for 30 to 60 seconds, 3 to 5 repetitions, 1 to 3 times per day

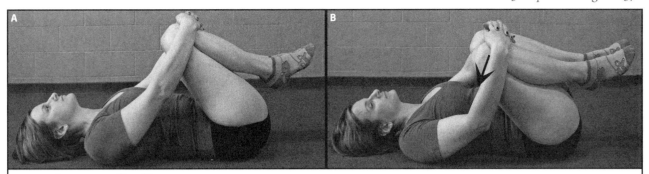

6.03.6 Stretch: Hip Extensor

POSITION: Supine

TARGETS: Stretch gluteus maximus

INSTRUCTION: In supine, patient brings bent knee(s) to chest and holds knee with both hands. Knee should stay aligned in straight sagittal plane toward ipsilateral shoulder (A). To target one side further, patient can pull both knees toward left or right shoulder for increased unilateral stretching (B).

SUBSTITUTIONS: Encourage stabilized pelvis to increase stretch across buttock rather than in lumbar spine.

PARAMETERS: Hold for 15 to 30 seconds, 3 to 5 repetitions, 1 to 3 times per day

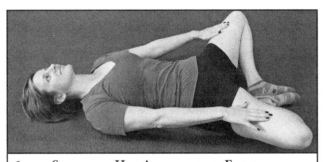

6.03.7 Stretch: Hip Adductors, Frog

POSITION: Hook-lying

TARGETS: Stretch hip adductors: adductor brevis, adductor longus, adductor magnus, adductor minimus, pectineus, and slight obturator externus; this stretch does not affect gracilis, which is also an adductor, but only with knee extended.

INSTRUCTION: Patient allows knees to fall out and actively pulls knees down toward table, adding hands for overpressure until stretch is felt in groin; soles of feet are together.

SUBSTITUTIONS: Excessive pelvic and lumbar movements; keep core engaged to stabilize.

PARAMETERS: Hold for 15 to 30 seconds, 3 to 5 repetitions, 1 to 3 times per day

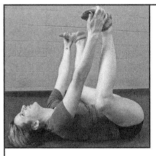

6.03.8 Stretch: Hip Adductors, Happy Baby

POSITION: Hook-lying

TARGETS: Stretch hip adductors: adductor brevis, adductor longus, adductor magnus, adductor minimus, pectineus, slight obturator externus, and gracilis, which is affected with knees extended variation.

INSTRUCTION: Patient flexes hips and knees and grasps around big toes on each foot with thumbs and index and middle fingers. Patient pulls legs into hip abduction, opening hips to bring knees out to sides of body and toward mat. To add gracilis, patient can do this with knees extended, pulling feet out and down toward mat. Grasp can move from toes to medial leg as distal as possible.

SUBSTITUTIONS: Excessive pelvic and lumbar movements; keep core engaged to stabilize.

PARAMETERS: Hold for 15 to 30 seconds, 3 to 5 repetitions, 1 to 3 times per day

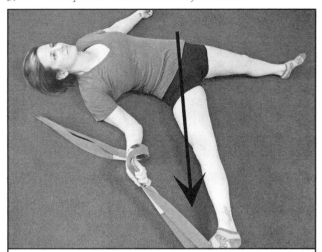

6.03.9 STRETCH: HIP ADDUCTORS WITH BELT

POSITION: Supine

TARGETS: Stretch hip adductors: adductor brevis, adductor longus, adductor magnus, adductor minimus, pectineus, gracilis (with knee extended), slight obturator externus

INSTRUCTION: Patient loops belt around arch of foot and, with knee extended and hip flexed to 90 degrees, pulls leg out to the side into horizontal abduction.

SUBSTITUTIONS: Excessive pelvic and lumbar movements and trunk twisting; keep core engaged to stabilize.

PARAMETERS: Hold for 15 to 30 seconds, 3 to 5 repetitions, 1 to 3 times per day

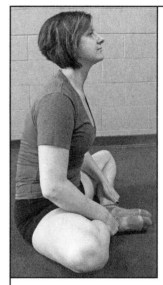

6.03.10 STRETCH: HIP ADDUCTORS, BUTTERFLY

POSITION: Long-sitting

TARGETS: Stretch hip adductors (adductor brevis, adductor longus, adductor magnus, adductor minimus, pectineus, and slight obturator externus); this stretch does not affect gracilis, which is also an adductor, but only with knee extended.

INSTRUCTION: Patient sits tall and allows knees to bend, bringing soles of feet together. Patient grasps around toes and places elbows on inside of distal thigh close to the knee. Patient presses gently into knees to press them down toward the mat. If a stretch is felt in inner thigh, stay there. If not, have patient tighten core and lean forward with chest leading the way. Gaze is toward feet. If patient is having difficulty keeping back straight, try sitting against a wall and pressing knees down.

SUBSTITUTIONS: Excessive pelvic and lumbar movements; keep core engaged to stabilize.

PARAMETERS: Hold for 15 to 30 seconds, 3 to 5 repetitions, 1 to 3 times per day

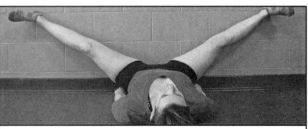

6.03.11 STRETCH: HIP ADDUCTORS ON WALL

POSITION: Supine

TARGETS: Stretch hip adductors: adductor brevis, adductor longus, adductor magnus, adductor minimus, pectineus, gracilis, slight obturator externus

INSTRUCTION: Patient scoots buttocks toward wall until touching and places legs on wall with knees fully extended. Patient slides heels along wall, bringing heels away from each other and down toward the mat. Once patient feels a stretch, hold and return. Patient may assist with hands to return to avoid adductor strain.

SUBSTITUTIONS: Excessive pelvic and lumbar movements and trunk twisting; keep core engaged to stabilize, do not allow toes to turn in or out.

PARAMETERS: Hold for 15 to 30 seconds, 3 to 5 repetitions, 1 to 3 times per day

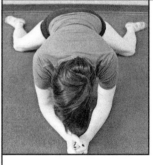

6.03.12 STRETCH: HIP ADDUCTORS, QUAD FROG

POSITION: Quadruped

TARGETS: Stretch hip adductors: adductor brevis, adductor longus, adductor magnus, adductor minimus, pectineus, slight obturator externus

INSTRUCTION: Patient brings knees into as wide a stance as possible and then lowers to placing elbows and forearms on table as patient allows hips to open, feeling stretch at inner thighs.

SUBSTITUTIONS: Excessive pelvic and lumbar movements and trunk twisting; keep core engaged to stabilize.

PARAMETERS: Hold for 15 to 30 seconds, 3 to 5 repetitions, 1 to 3 times per day

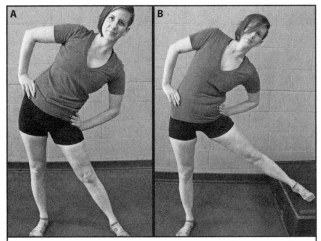

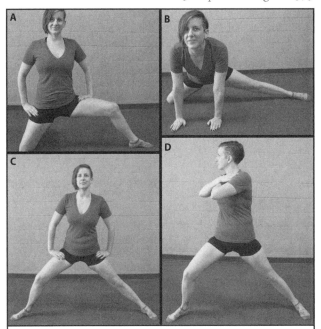

6.03.13 STRETCH: HIP ADDUCTORS, "TEAPOT"

POSITION: Standing

TARGETS: Stretch hip adductors: adductor brevis, adductor longus, adductor magnus, adductor minimus, pectineus, gracilis, slight obturator externus

INSTRUCTION: Patient widens stance and places hands on pelvis with straight spine. Patient lifts pelvis on unaffected side and drop pelvis on affected side as spine stays in alignment with pelvis (moves toward dropped side but staying straight) until stretch is felt on affected inner thigh (A). This can also be done with affected heel propped up on a step (B).

SUBSTITUTIONS: Excessive pelvic and lumbar movements and trunk twisting; keep core engaged to stabilize, do not allow toes to turn in or out.

PARAMETERS: Hold for 15 to 30 seconds, 3 to 5 repetitions, 1 to 3 times per day

6.03.14 STRETCH: HIP ADDUCTORS, SIDE LUNGE

POSITION: Tall-kneeling, quadruped, standing

TARGETS: Stretch hip adductors: adductor brevis, adductor longus, adductor magnus, adductor minimus, pectineus, gracilis (tall-kneeling does not affect gracilis), slight obturator externus

INSTRUCTION: *Tall-kneeling:* Placing target-side knee on foam square or pillow, patient places other foot directly out to the side and sinks into floor with pelvis, and knee bends further until stretch is felt in the inner thigh (A). *Quadruped:* Patient extends target leg out to the side horizontally abducting the hip. Patient sinks hip down with each breath as inner thigh on extended leg is stretched (B). *Standing:* Patient widens stance and places hands on pelvis with straight spine. Patient shifts weight to unaffected side lunging laterally with knee bending, keeping knee behind toes. Patient sinks into stretch of inner thigh on straight leg side (C). *Add twist:* In same position as described above, patient places interlocked fingers on sternum and retracts scapula as patient twists toward the unaffected (bent knee) side, keeping chest up. This increases stretch of inner thigh on straight leg side (D).

SUBSTITUTIONS: Excessive pelvic and lumbar movements; keep core engaged to stabilize, do not allow toes to turn in or out, knee on bent side stays directly aligned with toes and behind toes to avoid knee strain; move foot out further to avoid.

PARAMETERS: Hold for 15 to 30 seconds, 3 to 5 repetitions, 1 to 3 times per day

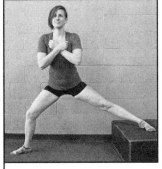

6.03.15 STRETCH: HIP ADDUCTORS, DIP

POSITION: Standing

TARGETS: Advanced stretch hip adductors: adductor brevis, adductor longus, adductor magnus, adductor minimus, pectineus, gracilis, slight obturator externus

INSTRUCTION: Patient places affected leg on chair/table with toes pointed forward. Patient widens stance leg and places hands interlocked in front. Patient bends stance knee and, with straight spine, leans forward at the hips until stretch is felt in the inner thigh of elevated leg.

SUBSTITUTIONS: Excessive pelvic and lumbar movements; keep core engaged to stabilize, do not allow toes to turn up, knee on stance side stays directly aligned with toes and behind toes to avoid knee strain; move foot out further to avoid.

PARAMETERS: Hold for 15 to 30 seconds, 3 to 5 repetitions, 1 to 3 times per day

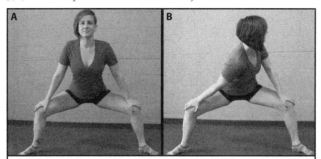

6.03.16 Stretch: Hip Adductors, Horse Stance (Advanced)

Position: Standing

Targets: Advanced stretch hip adductors: adductor brevis, adductor longus, adductor magnus, adductor minimus, pectineus, slight obturator externus

Instruction: Patient widens stance as far as possible with toes pointed out and drops hips down, bringing knees directly over ankles, but not further, so toes are still in front of knees. Patient uses hands to push knees outward, keeping knees over ankles and trunk upright. Patient also focuses on PPT to avoid anterior tilting of pelvis (A). Add trunk twist by bringing one shoulder toward floor as other shoulder rises toward ceiling (B).

Substitutions: Excessive pelvic and lumbar movements; keep core engaged to stabilize, do not allow toes to turn forward, knees stay directly aligned with toes and behind toes to avoid knee strain; move foot out further to avoid.

Parameters: Hold for 15 to 30 seconds, 3 to 5 repetitions, 1 to 3 times per day

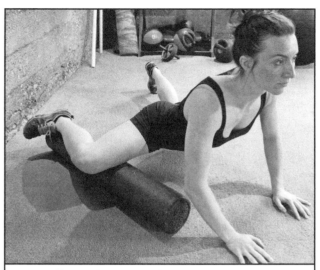

6.03.17 Foam Roller: Hip Adductors

Position: Prone

Targets: Soft tissue release/self-massage hip adductors: adductor brevis, adductor longus, adductor magnus, adductor minimus, pectineus, and gracilis

Instruction: Patient lies with medium-sized foam roller under thigh as shown and uses arms to roll foam roll along the inner thigh down and up as patient massages muscles of inner thigh.

Substitutions: Avoid pressures that are excessively painful; watch that patient is not shrugging shoulders.

Parameters: Massage 2 to 5 minutes, 1 to 3 times per day

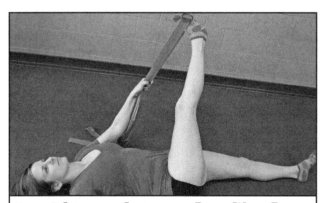

6.03.18 Stretch: Iliotibial Band With Belt

Position: Supine

Targets: Stretch ITB

Instruction: Patient loops belt around arch of foot and, with knee extended and hip flexed to 90 degrees, pulls leg across the body into horizontal adduction until stretch felt on outside of hip or thigh, keeping pelvis on table.

Substitutions: Pelvis rises on affected side, trunk twisting; keep core engaged to stabilize.

Parameters: Hold for 15 to 30 seconds, 3 to 5 repetitions, 1 to 3 times per day

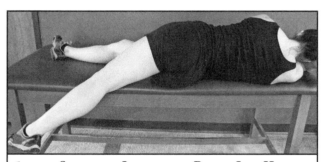

6.03.19 Stretch: Iliotibial Band, Leg Hang

Position: Side-lying

Targets: Stretch ITB

Instruction: Patient lies on unaffected side and brings back of buttock to edge of table while allowing trunk to stay near the middle of table for stability. Patient bends bottom knee and extends top knee as patient brings top leg off table. Patient relaxes and lets gravity pull the leg toward the floor; toes should start facing forward and hip in neutral rotation to best isolate ITB.

Substitutions: Lateral side-bending of trunk; use trunk stabilizers to keep from dropping with leg.

Parameters: Hold for 15 to 30 seconds, 3 to 5 repetitions, 1 to 3 times per day

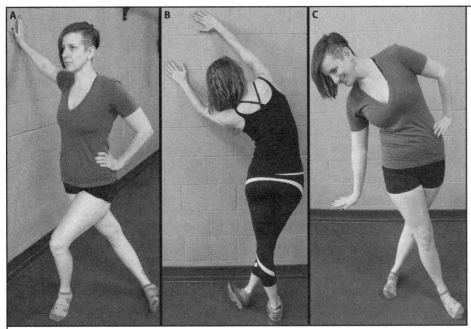

6.03.20 STRETCH: ILIOTIBIAL BAND, STANDING VARIATIONS

POSITION: Standing

TARGETS: Stretch ITB

INSTRUCTION: *Wall sideways:* Patient stands sideways with affected hip toward wall. Patient places hand on wall and brings affected leg behind other leg, adducting the hip and allowing front knee to bend slightly. Patient then pushes pelvis toward wall as patient leans away (A). *Wall in front:* Patient stands facing wall and brings affected leg behind other leg, adducting the hip and allowing front knee to bend slightly. Patient then pushes pelvis toward the affected side as patient uses the wall to pull the body into side-bending as patient leans away from target hip (B). *Free-standing:* Patient brings affected leg behind other leg, adducting the hip and allowing front knee to bend slightly. Patient then pushes pelvis toward the affected side as patient abducts the affected side shoulder overhead and side-bending as patient leans away from target hip (C).

SUBSTITUTIONS: Lateral side-bending of trunk; use trunk stabilizers to keep from dropping with leg.

PARAMETERS: Hold for 15 to 30 seconds, 3 to 5 repetitions, 1 to 3 times per day

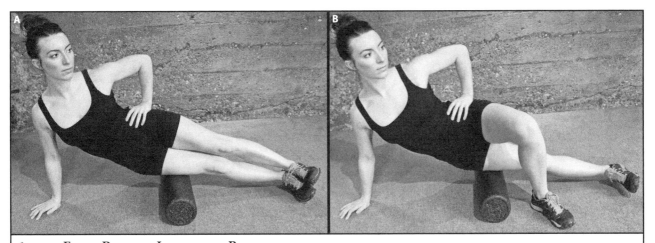

6.03.21 FOAM ROLLER: ILIOTIBIAL BAND

POSITION: Side-lying

TARGETS: Soft tissue release/self-massage ITB

INSTRUCTION: Patient lies with medium-sized foam roller under thigh as shown and uses arms to roll foam roll along the outer thigh up and down as patient massages muscles of outer thigh (A). Patient may put top foot on floor for extra stability (B).

SUBSTITUTIONS: Avoid pressures that are excessively painful; watch that patient is not shrugging shoulders.

PARAMETERS: Massage 2 to 5 minutes, 1 to 3 times per day

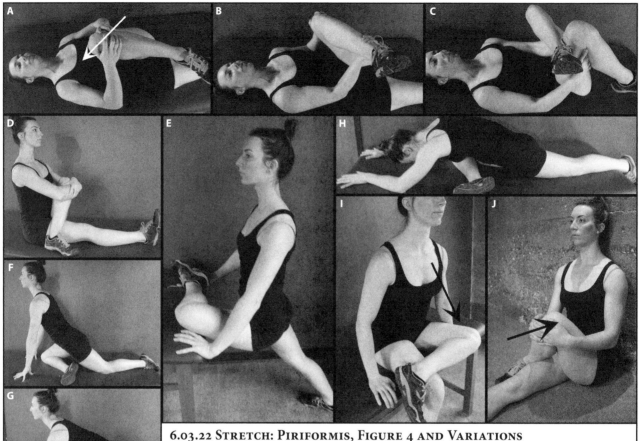

6.03.22 Stretch: Piriformis, Figure 4 and Variations

POSITION: Supine, hook-lying, long-sitting, seated, standing, quadruped

TARGETS: Stretch external rotators (primarily piriformis plus gemelleus superior and inferior, obturator internus and externus, quadratus femoris); some stretch will occur in gluteus medius and minimus as well. Increase hip mobility into external rotation.

INSTRUCTION: *Supine modified:* Patient brings knee to opposite shoulder until stretch is felt across buttock (A). *Hook supine figure 4:* Patient externally rotates the affected hip fully and brings knee toward shoulder while ankle comes toward opposite shoulder. Unaffected leg stays on mat to help stabilize pelvis (B). *Hook-lying figure 4:* Patient externally rotates the affected hip and places lateral ankle on top of unaffected thigh. Patient "threads the needle" by placing hands around unaffected knee and pulls unaffected knee toward ipsilateral shoulder (C). *Long-sitting knee cross:* Patient places target side foot across extended knee of other leg and twists toward affected side while pulling knee further across midline with elbow (D). *Pigeon standing:* Patient places target leg on table with lateral knee and lower leg on edge of table and hip lines up with knee. Patient sinks into stretch across buttock (E). *Pigeon quadruped:* Patient places target leg in front with lateral knee and lower leg on mat table and hip lines up with knee. Encourage knee bend less than 100 degrees. Back leg then slowly extends. To start, patient props on hands, pressing pelvis down toward mat and keeping pelvis level. Also avoid anterior pelvis tilt by engaging lower abdominal core muscles. Patient sinks into stretch across buttock (F). Patient may progress by coming down to elbows (G) and eventually to full pigeon (H) lying over knee. *Seated figure 4:* Patient externally rotates the affected hip, fully crossing target leg over other thigh, laying the lateral mid-lower leg against anterior thigh. Patient straightens back and leans over legs, leading with chest until stretch felt in buttock. Do not allow knee to come up; patient may press down on crossed knee to stabilize in external rotation (I). *Sitting against wall:* Patient scoots buttocks all the way back to the wall and sits upright against the wall. Patient extends unaffected knee and crosses target leg's foot over knee. Patient hugs target knee toward chest as patient slightly rotates the trunk toward the bent leg (J).

SUBSTITUTIONS: Excessive pelvic and lumbar movements; keep core engaged to stabilize.

PARAMETERS: Hold for 15 to 30 seconds, 3 to 5 repetitions, 1 to 3 times per day

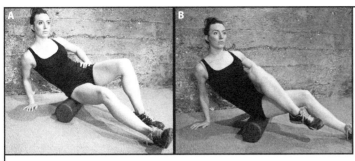

6.03.23 FOAM ROLLER/TENNIS BALL: PIRIFORMIS

POSITION: Standing, side-lying

TARGETS: Soft tissue release/self-massage piriformis

INSTRUCTION: *Tennis ball:* Patient stands sideways alongside a wall with affected side quarter-turned toward wall. Place tennis ball in middle of buttock and have patient push body weight into ball as patient rolls the ball toward sacrum and back toward greater trochanter massaging the piriformis (not shown). *Foam roll:* Patient sits on medium foam roller and leans toward affected side as patient rolls front to back over buttock, massaging the gluteal region (A). Patient can cross target leg over other thigh to assist penetrating to deeper regions (B).

SUBSTITUTIONS: Avoid pressures that are excessively painful; watch that patient is not shrugging shoulders.

PARAMETERS: Massage 2 to 5 minutes, 1 to 3 times per day

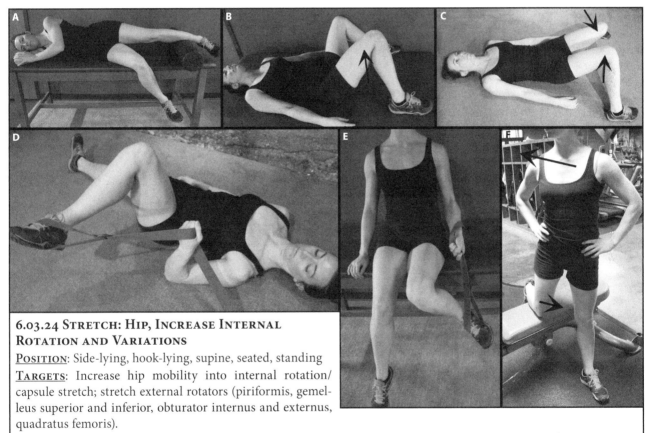

6.03.24 STRETCH: HIP, INCREASE INTERNAL ROTATION AND VARIATIONS

POSITION: Side-lying, hook-lying, supine, seated, standing

TARGETS: Increase hip mobility into internal rotation/capsule stretch; stretch external rotators (piriformis, gemellus superior and inferior, obturator internus and externus, quadratus femoris).

INSTRUCTION: *Side-lying:* Patient lies on affected side, propping top leg with pillows to keep hip in neutral. Patient scoots to edge of mat, allowing bottom lower leg to drop off table until stretch is felt (A). *Hook-lying:* Patient places feet in wide stance and brings affected knee in and down toward mat (B). *Hook-lying bilateral:* Patient places feet in wide stance and brings knees together and down toward mat (C). *Supine with belt:* Patient loops belt around ankle and pulls ankle up and out as hip rotates internally (D). *Seated with belt:* Patient loops belt around ankle and pulls ankle up and out as hip rotates internally (E). *Standing:* Patient stands in front of chair and places affected shin and knee on chair as shown. Place a towel roll under shin for comfort if needed. Patient rotates body toward affected leg (F).

SUBSTITUTIONS: Excessive pelvic and lumbar movements; keep core engaged to stabilize.

PARAMETERS: Hold for 15 to 30 seconds, 3 to 5 repetitions, 1 to 3 times per day

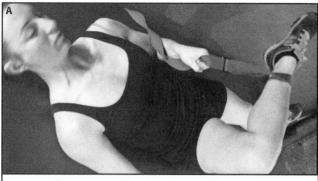

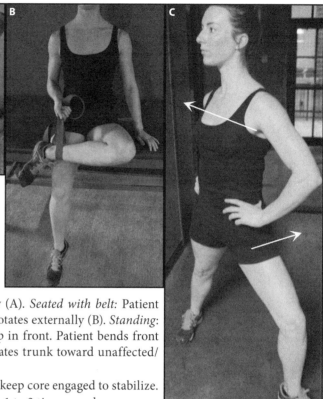

6.03.25 STRETCH: HIP, INCREASE EXTERNAL ROTATION AND VARIATIONS

POSITION: Supine, hook-lying, seated, standing

TARGETS: Increase hip mobility into external rotation/ capsule stretch; stretch internal rotators (TFL, gluteus medius and minimus).

INSTRUCTION: *Supine with belt:* Patient loops belt around ankle and pulls ankle up and in as hip rotates externally (A). *Seated with belt:* Patient loops belt around ankle and pulls ankle up and in as hip rotates externally (B). *Standing:* Patient stands with feet staggered front to back, target hip in front. Patient bends front knee slightly and places hands on pelvis. Patient then rotates trunk toward unaffected/ back leg side while front hip externally rotates (C).

SUBSTITUTIONS: Excessive pelvic and lumbar movements; keep core engaged to stabilize.

PARAMETERS: Hold for 15 to 30 seconds 3 to 5 repetitions, 1 to 3 times per day

6.03.26 STRETCH: SARTORIUS

POSITION: Seated

TARGETS: Stretch sartorius

INSTRUCTION: Patient sits on the side edge of a chair with affected leg hip just slightly overhanging edge of chair. Patient brings target leg behind and, with knee bent, places toes on floor. Patient then turns hip inward, internally rotating and adducting hip. Patient must actively engage core muscles to prevent hip from dropping and tipping anteriorly.

SUBSTITUTIONS: Lateral side-bending of trunk, dropping pelvis on target side, APT; use trunk stabilizers to stabilize pelvis.

PARAMETERS: Hold for 15 to 30 seconds, 3 to 5 repetitions, 1 to 3 times per day

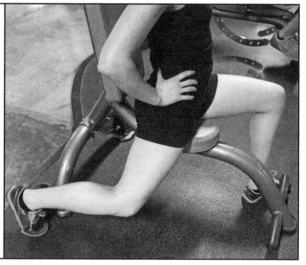

Section 6.04

HIP STRENGTHENING

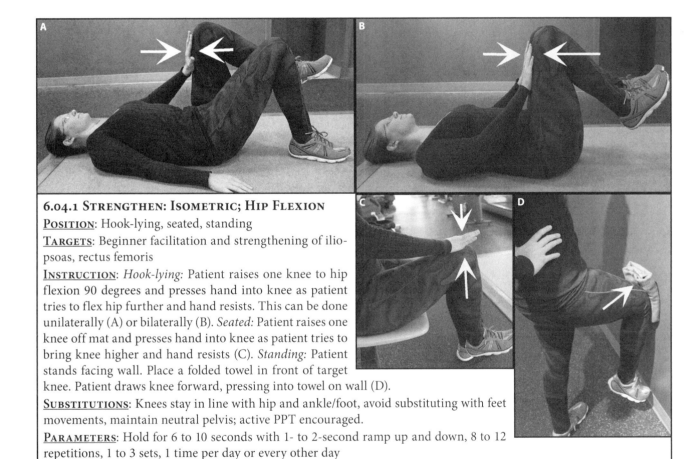

6.04.1 STRENGTHEN: ISOMETRIC; HIP FLEXION

<u>POSITION</u>: Hook-lying, seated, standing

<u>TARGETS</u>: Beginner facilitation and strengthening of iliopsoas, rectus femoris

<u>INSTRUCTION</u>: *Hook-lying:* Patient raises one knee to hip flexion 90 degrees and presses hand into knee as patient tries to flex hip further and hand resists. This can be done unilaterally (A) or bilaterally (B). *Seated:* Patient raises one knee off mat and presses hand into knee as patient tries to bring knee higher and hand resists (C). *Standing:* Patient stands facing wall. Place a folded towel in front of target knee. Patient draws knee forward, pressing into towel on wall (D).

<u>SUBSTITUTIONS</u>: Knees stay in line with hip and ankle/foot, avoid substituting with feet movements, maintain neutral pelvis; active PPT encouraged.

<u>PARAMETERS</u>: Hold for 6 to 10 seconds with 1- to 2-second ramp up and down, 8 to 12 repetitions, 1 to 3 sets, 1 time per day or every other day

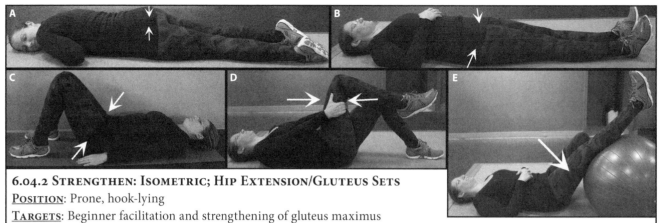

6.04.2 STRENGTHEN: ISOMETRIC; HIP EXTENSION/GLUTEUS SETS

<u>POSITION</u>: Prone, hook-lying

<u>TARGETS</u>: Beginner facilitation and strengthening of gluteus maximus

<u>INSTRUCTION</u>: *Prone*: Patient lies supine or prone and squeezes buttocks by tightening gluteal muscles (A and B). *Hook-lying*: Patient performs gluteal squeeze in hook-lying (C). Patient raises one knee to hip flexion 90 degrees and grasps behind knee. Patient tries to extend hip as hands resist (D). *With ball*: Patient raises target leg onto ball with knee extended. Patient tries to extend hip as ball resists (E).

<u>SUBSTITUTIONS</u>: Knees stay in line with hip and ankle/foot, avoid substituting with feet movements, maintain neutral pelvis; active PPT encouraged.

<u>PARAMETERS</u>: Hold for 6 to 10 seconds with 1- to 2-second ramp up and down, 8 to 12 repetitions, 1 to 3 sets, 1 time per day or every other day

---

Where's the Evidence?

EMG studies comparing exercises for gluteus maximus MVC found gluteus squeezes to be the second best exercise for gluteus maximus recruitment (Boren et al., 2011).

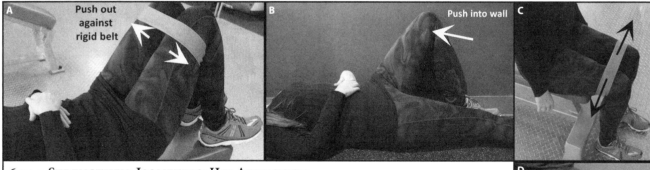

6.04.3 STRENGTHEN: ISOMETRIC; HIP ABDUCTION

<u>POSITION</u>: Supine, hook-lying, seated, standing

<u>TARGETS</u>: Beginner facilitation and strengthening of hip abductors: gluteus medius, gluteus minimus, and TFL

<u>INSTRUCTION</u>: *Hook-lying:* Place rigid belt (not elastic) around thighs with knees and ankles in same sagittal plane as hip. Patient presses outward with one or both hips into belt, trying to separate knees as belt resists (A). *Hook-lying wall press:* Patient lies sideways to wall. Place pillow between knee and wall. Patient pushes knee outward with knee into the wall (B) *Seated:* Place rigid belt (not elastic) around thighs with knees and ankles in same sagittal plane as hip. Patient presses outward with one or both hips into belt trying to separate knees as belt resist. Watch that patient is not using feet (C). *Standing wall press:* Patient stands sideway to wall. Place pillow between knee and wall. Patient flexed hip 45 degrees with knee flexed 90 degrees and pushes knee outward with knee into the wall (D).

<u>SUBSTITUTIONS</u>: Knees stay in line with hip and ankle/foot, avoid substituting with feet movements, maintain neutral pelvis; active PPT encouraged.

<u>PARAMETERS</u>: Hold for 6 to 10 seconds with 1- to 2-second ramp up and down, 8 to 12 repetitions, 1 to 3 sets, 1 time per day or every other day

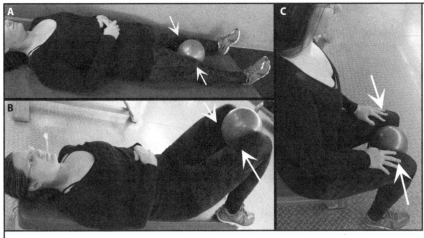

6.04.4 STRENGTHEN: ISOMETRIC; HIP ADDUCTION

POSITION: Supine, hook-lying, seated

TARGETS: Beginner facilitation and strengthening of hip adductors: adductor brevis, adductor longus, adductor magnus, adductor minimus, pectineus, slight obturator externus.

INSTRUCTION: *Supine:* Place pillow or 20- to 25-cm ball between knees and patient squeezes knees together (A). *Hook-lying:* Place pillow between knees and patient squeezes knees together (B). *Seated:* Place pillow or 8- to 10-inch ball between knees and patient squeezes knees together (C).

SUBSTITUTIONS: Knees stay in line with hip and ankle/foot, avoid substituting with feet movements, maintain neutral pelvis; active PPT encouraged.

PARAMETERS: Hold for 6 to 10 seconds with 1- to 2-second ramp up and down, 8 to 12 repetitions, 1 to 3 sets 1 time per day or every other day

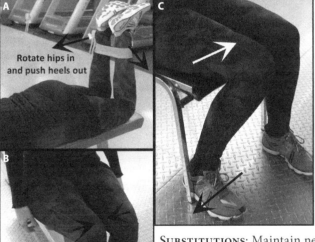

6.04.5 STRENGTHEN: ISOMETRIC; HIP INTERNAL ROTATION

POSITION: Prone, seated

TARGETS: Beginner facilitation and strengthening of hip internal rotators: TFL, gluteus medius, and gluteus minimus

INSTRUCTION: *Prone:* Bend knees to 90 degrees and place rigid belt around ankles. Patient keeps knees together as patient attempts to bring ankles apart (A). *Seated in chair:* Using a rigid belt, place belt around the patient's ankles. Patient then pushes ankles outward into the rigid belt as the knees stay together (B). Patient can also use the chair leg for resistance. Patient keeps knees together as patient attempts to bring lateral foot or feet into legs of chair (C).

SUBSTITUTIONS: Maintain neutral pelvis; active PPT encouraged.

PARAMETERS: Hold for 6 to 10 seconds with 1- to 2-second ramp up and down, 8 to 12 repetitions, 1 to 3 sets 1 time per day or every other day

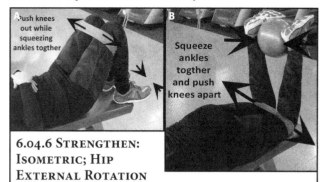

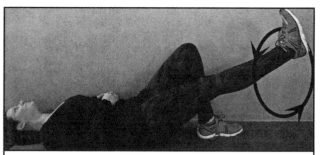

6.04.6 STRENGTHEN: ISOMETRIC; HIP EXTERNAL ROTATION

POSITION: Hook-lying, prone

TARGETS: Beginner facilitation and strengthening of hip external rotators piriformis plus gemelleus superior and inferior, obturator internus and externus, quadratus femoris

INSTRUCTION: *Hook-lying:* Place rigid belt (not elastic) around thighs with feet together and knees further apart. Patient presses outward with both hips into belt trying to separate knees and externally rotating hips as belt resists (A). *Prone:* Bend knees to 90 degrees and place rigid belt around knees. Patient squeezes ball 8- to 10-in ball between ankles (B).

SUBSTITUTIONS: Maintain neutral pelvis; active lower abdominal core encouraged.

PARAMETERS: Hold for 6 to 10 seconds with 1- to 2-second ramp up and down, 8 to 12 repetitions, 1 to 3 sets 1 time per day or every other day

6.04.7 STRENGTHEN: ISOTONIC; HIP, SINGLE-LEG CIRCLES

POSITION: Hook-lying

TARGETS: Beginner facilitation and strengthening of hip flexors (iliopsoas and rectus femoris) with stabilization of hip internal and external rotators to keep toes up. The other quadriceps (VL, vastus medialis, and intermedius) muscles are engaged isometrically to keep knee extended.

INSTRUCTION: With one knee extended, tighten quadriceps and lift leg off mat 6 inches. Patient slowly makes small circles with foot while controlling pelvic movements by holding a PPT. Perform clockwise and counter-clockwise.

SUBSTITUTIONS: Maintain neutral pelvis; active lower abdominal core encouraged, toes stay pointed up, knee fully extended.

PARAMETERS: 8 to 12 repetitions, 1 to 3 sets, 1 time per day or every other day

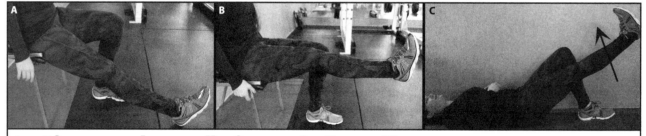

6.04.8 STRENGTHEN: ISOTONIC; HIP, STRAIGHT LEG RAISE, 4-WAY

POSITION: Seated, supine, side-lying, prone

TARGETS: Strengthening of hip flexors (iliopsoas and rectus femoris), extensors (gluteus maximus, hamstrings), abductors (TFL, gluteus medius and minimus), and adductors (adductor brevis, adductor longus, adductor magnus, adductor minimus, pectineus, gracilis, slight obturator externus) with stabilization of hip internal and external rotators to keep leg aligned.

INSTRUCTION: *Flexion (Beginner):* Sitting in edge of chair as shown, patient straightens target knee with dorsiflexion of ankle and tightened quadriceps. Patient raises leg while keeping knee straight to the level of other thigh (A and B). *Supine:* Patient lies supine with unaffected knee bent and foot planted. Patient tightens quadriceps muscle on extended leg and, keeping knee straight, lifts toes straight up toward ceiling until thigh reaches other thigh (C). *(continued)*

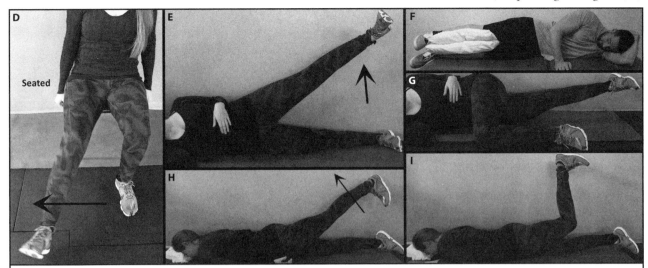

6.04.8 STRENGTHEN: ISOTONIC; HIP, STRAIGHT LEG RAISE, 4-WAY (CONTINUED)

Abduction (Beginner): Sitting on edge of chair as shown, patient straightens target knee with dorsiflexion of ankle and tightened quadriceps. Patient slides heel out, keeping toes up as patient abducts the hip, keeping knee straight (D). *Side-lying:* Patient lies on unaffected side, tightens quadriceps muscle on top leg, and, keeping knee straight, lifts leg up as toes stay pointed forward (E). Pillow can be placed between knees if trying to avoid adduction (F). Bottom leg can be flexed or extended. *Adduction* Patient side-lying on affected side with top leg placed in front allowing bent knee to rest on table or with foot planted, tightens quadriceps muscle on top leg and, keeping knee straight, lifts leg up as toes stay pointed forward (G). *Extension:* Patient lies prone, tightens quadriceps on affected leg, and, keeping knee straight, lifts heel straight up toward ceiling, keeping toes pointed straight down (H). To *isolate gluteus maximus* and remove assist from hamstrings, perform extension with knee flexed 90 degrees, lifting heel toward ceiling and keeping femur in alignment with hip (no rotation) (I).

SUBSTITUTIONS: Maintain neutral pelvis; active lower abdominal core encouraged, knee stays fully extended (except with gluteus maximus knee flexed variation).

PARAMETERS: 8 to 12 repetitions, 1 to 3 sets, 1 time per day or every other day

Where's the Evidence?

In an EMG study to study exercises that targeted gluteus medius activation, straight-leg abduction was found to be optimal for activating the gluteus medius with little activation of the TFL and anterior hip flexors. Additionally, the side plank with dominant leg on bottom (found under lumbar strengthening **4.03.39**) was found to be the most superior exercise at recruiting the gluteus medius, followed by side plank with dominant leg on top while abducting hip top leg (Boren et al., 2011). Distefano, Blackburn, Marshall, and Padua (2009) found similar results in another EMS study, stating the best exercise for the gluteus medius was side-lying hip abduction, while the single-limb squat and single-limb deadlift exercises led to the greatest activation of the gluteus maximus.

6.04.9 STRENGTHEN: ISOTONIC; HIP FLEXION, MARCHING

POSITION: Seated, standing

TARGETS: Strengthening of hip flexor iliopsoas with assist from rectus femoris

INSTRUCTION: These can be done with cuff weights on knee or ankle. *Seated:* Patient lifts knee, bringing thigh off table (A). *Standing:* Patient lifts knee, bringing hip to >90 degrees flexion without allowing pelvis to rotate posteriorly (B).

SUBSTITUTIONS: Maintain neutral pelvis; active core encouraged.

PARAMETERS: Hold 1 to 2 seconds, 8 to 12 repetitions, 1 to 3 sets, 1 time per day or every other day

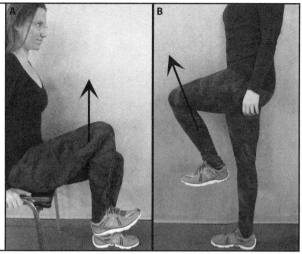

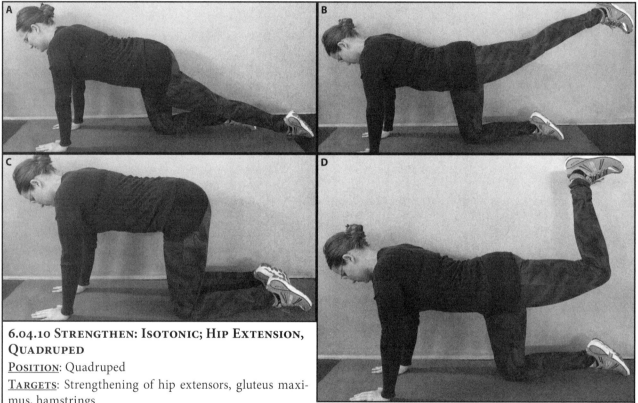

6.04.10 STRENGTHEN: ISOTONIC; HIP EXTENSION, QUADRUPED

POSITION: Quadruped

TARGETS: Strengthening of hip extensors, gluteus maximus, hamstrings

INSTRUCTION: These can be done with cuff weights on knee or ankle. *Knee extended:* Patient places target leg extended with toes on mat. Patient lifts leg toward ceiling to above hip height. Active lower abdominals stabilize pelvis to avoid lumbar extension. Hold and repeat (A and B). *Knee flexed:* Patient keeping knee bent 90 degrees lifts leg toward ceiling to above hip height. Active lower abdominals stabilize pelvis to avoid lumbar extension. Hold and repeat (C and D).

SUBSTITUTIONS: Maintain neutral spine; active core encouraged.

PARAMETERS: Hold 1 to 2 seconds each way, 8 to 12 repetitions, 1 to 3 sets, 1 time per day or every other day

Where's the Evidence?

In an EMG study looking at exercises that targeted gluteus maximus activation, quadruped extension was found to rank 8 out of 22 gluteus maximus-targeted exercises for the hip extending and also 21 out of 22 for the stance side, indicating gluteus maximus is working on both legs regardless of the side lifting, but recruiting significantly more on lifting leg (Boren et al., 2011).

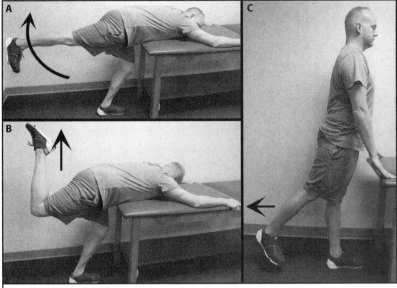

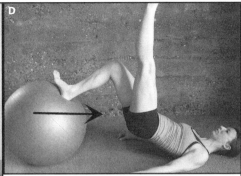

6.04.11 STRENGTHEN: ISOTONIC; HIP EXTENSION, STANDING

POSITION: Standing

TARGETS: Strengthening of hip extensors, gluteus maximus, hamstrings

INSTRUCTION: These can be done with cuff weights on knee or ankle. *Half prone over table, knee extended:* Patient lays trunk over table and lifts extended leg with toes pointing toward the floor. Active lower abdominals stabilize pelvis to avoid lumbar extension. Hold and repeat (A). *Half prone over table, knee flexed:* Repeat instructions for previous exercise with knee bent 90 degrees; this targets gluteus maximus by lessening assist from hamstrings (B). *Standing with hand support:* Patient stands sideways to table on unaffected side. Patient brings extended leg behind, lifting heel toward ceiling, keeping knee straight. Active lower abdominals stabilize pelvis to avoid lumbar extension. Hold and repeat (C). This can be done with knee flexed 90 degrees to target gluteus maximus by lessening assist from hamstrings.

SUBSTITUTIONS: Patient leans forward, hip rotation, maintain neutral spine; active core encouraged.

PARAMETERS: Hold 1 to 2 seconds each way, 8 to 12 repetitions, 1 to 3 sets, 1 time per day or every other day

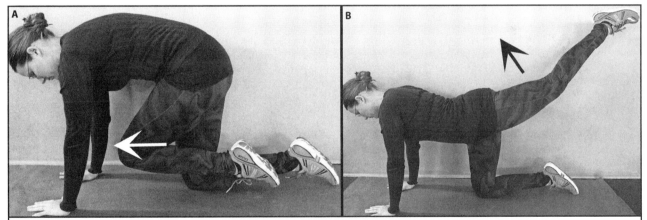

6.04.12 STRENGTHEN: ISOTONIC; HIP FLEXION AND EXTENSION, COMBINATION

POSITION: Quadruped

TARGETS: Strengthening of hip flexors (iliopsoas and rectus femoris) and extensors (gluteus maximus, hamstrings)

INSTRUCTION: These can be done with cuff weights on knee or ankle. Shifting weight to unaffected knee, patient flexes target hip bringing knee to chest, hold, return to pass other leg and extend hip and knee. Hold and repeat (A and B).

SUBSTITUTIONS: Maintain neutral spine; active core encouraged.

PARAMETERS: Hold 1 to 2 seconds each way, 8 to 12 repetitions, 1 to 3 sets, 1 time per day or every other day

6.04.13 STRENGTHEN: ISOTONIC; HIP EXTENSION, MINI-BRIDGE ON TOWEL/BOLSTER

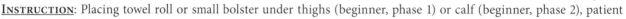

POSITION: Supine

TARGETS: Strengthening of hip extensors; gluteus maximus primarily with assist from hamstrings.

INSTRUCTION: Placing towel roll or small bolster under thighs (beginner, phase 1) or calf (beginner, phase 2), patient lifts buttocks off mat.

SUBSTITUTIONS: Maintain neutral spine; active core encouraged, do not arch back.

PARAMETERS: Hold 1 to 2 seconds, 8 to 12 repetitions, 1 to 3 sets, 1 time per day or every other day

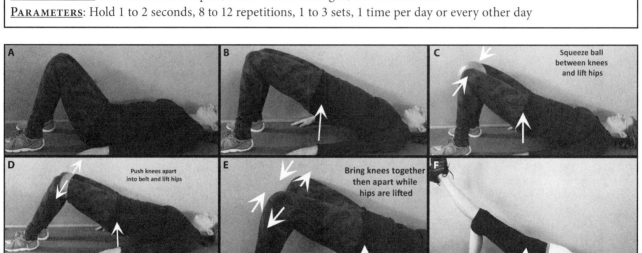

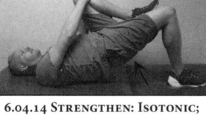

6.04.14 STRENGTHEN: ISOTONIC; HIP EXTENSION, BRIDGE AND VARIATIONS

POSITION: Hook-lying

TARGETS: Strengthening of hip extensors; gluteus maximus primarily with assist from hamstrings.

INSTRUCTION: *Bridge:* Patient with knees and feet hip-width apart tightens lower abdominals and lifts hips up off table until extended to 0 degrees, pelvis should be level (A and B). *Bridge with isometric adduction ball squeeze:* Patient with knees and feet hip-width apart, place 8- to 10-inch ball between knees. Patient squeezes ball, tightens lower abdominals, and lifts hips up off table until extended to 0 degrees, pelvis should be level (C). *Bridge with isometric hip abduction:* Patient with knees and feet hip-width apart, places belt around knees. Patient presses knees outward, tightens lower abdominals, and lifts hips up off table until extended to 0 degrees; pelvis should be level (D). *Bridge in/outs:* Follow instructions for bridge but hold bridge while performing in/out for 8 to 12 repetitions; this involves opening knees out (abduct/externally rotate hip) and bringing back in (adduct/internally rotate) (E). *Single-leg bridge:* Patient extends one leg and raises it off mat so that thighs are aligned. Patient tightens lower abdominals and lifts hips up off table until extended to 0 degrees; pelvis should be level (F). Patient can also do this with knee flexed, bringing one knee to chest and holding with clasped hands around knee, then bridging with opposite hip (G). *Bridge with knee extension:* Patient with knees and feet hip-width apart tightens lower abdominals and lifts hips up off table until extended to 0 degrees, then fully extends one knee, keeping thighs aligned; pelvis should be level (H). For added difficulty, patient places palms together with arms extended in front. Use of a yard stick or wand can help to give feedback to the patient on the pelvic position and cue to correct by raising or lowered pelvis on each side (I).

SUBSTITUTIONS: Maintain neutral spine and pelvis; active core encouraged, do not arch back.

PARAMETERS: Hold 1 to 2 seconds, 8 to 12 repetitions, 1 to 3 sets, 1 time per day or every other day

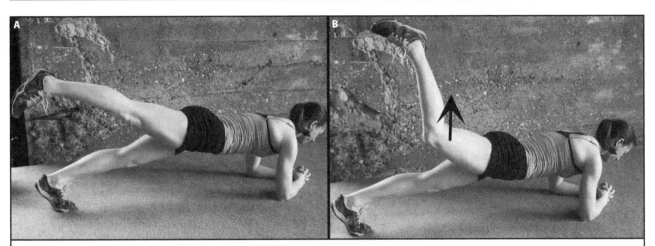

6.04.15 STRENGTHEN: HIP EXTENSION, FOREARM PLANK

POSITION: Prone

TARGETS: Strengthen gluteus maximus and medius

INSTRUCTION: Patient lies facedown with legs extended and elbows bent directly under shoulders and hands clasped or in neutral (thumbs up). Feet should be hip-width apart and elbows should be shoulder-width apart. Patient engages core muscles to maintain a neutral spine while tucking toes and lifting body. Patient should be in a straight line from head to heels. Patient may extend or bend target knee to 90 degrees and lift leg, bringing heel straight toward ceiling (A and B).

SUBSTITUTIONS: Do not allow lower back to extend or body to roll side to side. Neck should remain neutral and tucked slightly, gaze between hands, and chin slightly tucked, breathing normally during entire plank. Shoulders are active and engaged, scapula depressed and retracted slightly.

PARAMETERS: Hold 1 to 2 seconds, 8 to 12 repetitions, 1 to 3 sets, 1 time per day or every other day

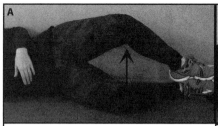

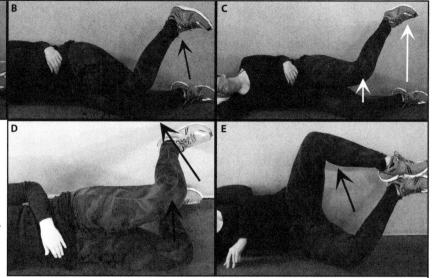

6.04.16 STRENGTHEN: ISOTONIC; HIP ABDUCTION AND EXTERNAL ROTATION, "CLAM" AND VARIATIONS

<u>POSITION</u>: Side-lying

<u>TARGETS</u>: Strengthening of gluteus medius primarily with activation of anterior hip muscles

<u>INSTRUCTION</u>: Patient is lying on unaffected side with hips stacked. *Phase I*: Hips flexed 45 degrees and knees flexed 90 degrees, medial ankles together. Patient lifts top knee, opening hips without rolling trunk (A). *Phase II*: Hips flexed 60 degrees and knees flexed 90 degrees. Patient raises ankle above top hip's height, internally rotating hip followed by opening knees as shown (B). *Phase III*: Hips flexed 60 degrees and knees flexed 90 degrees. Patient raises knee to hip height and then raises ankle above top hip's height, internally rotating hip (C). *Phase IV*: Hips extended to neutral with knees flexed 90 degrees. Patient brings top leg to parallel to mat and lifts ankle, internally rotating hip (D). *Phase V*: Hips flexed 60 degrees and knees flexed 90 degrees medial ankles together. Patient raises ankles off table above top hip's height and lifts top knee, opening hips without rolling trunk (E).

<u>SUBSTITUTIONS</u>: Maintain neutral spine and pelvis; active core encouraged, do not roll trunk back; hip stay stacked.

<u>PARAMETERS</u>: Hold 1 to 2 seconds, 8 to 12 repetitions, 1 to 3 sets, 1 time per day or every other day

Where's the Evidence?

EMG studies comparing clam exercises for gluteus medius activation ranked clams from most activation to least: Phase IV, Phase III, Phase II, Phase I. For gluteus maximus, activation was ranked from most activation to least: Phase I, III, IV, II. Phase V was not studied (Boren et al., 2011). In another EMG study to study exercises that targeted gluteus medius activation, straight leg abduction was found to be optimal for activating the gluteus medius with little activation of the TFL and anterior hip flexors. The clam exercise caused the greatest activation of the anterior hip flexors and very little activation of the gluteus medius. Similarly, the straight leg abduction exercise might induce excess activation and strengthening of the TFL beyond what is desired, depending on the goals of rehabilitation. They concluded straight leg abduction exercise is preferred if targeted activation of the gluteus medius is a goal. Activation of the other muscles in the straight leg abduction with external rotation and clam exercises exceeded that of gluteus medius, which might indicate the exercises are less appropriate when the primary goal is the gluteus medius activation and strengthening (McBeth, Earl-Boehm, Cobb, & Huddleston, 2012).

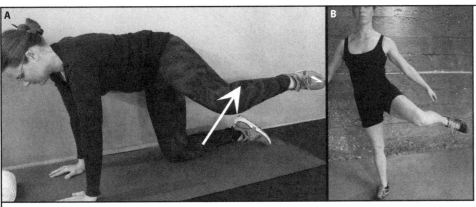

6.04.17 STRENGTHEN: ISOTONIC; HIP ABDUCTION, "FIRE HYDRANTS"

POSITION: Side-lying, quadruped, standing

TARGETS: Strengthening of gluteus medius primarily

INSTRUCTION: *Side-lying:* Lying on unaffected side with hips stacked, hips flexed 60 degrees, and knees flexed 90 degrees. Patient lifts top leg, keeping knee and ankle as one unit (not shown). *Quadruped:* Patient shifts weight to unaffected side and lifts target leg straight into hip horizontal abduction, as dog would lift leg at a fire hydrant (A). *Standing:* Patient stands in front of table or bar to hold for balance. Patient bends slightly forward at the hips, keeping hips level, then bends target knee to 90 degrees and extends hip slightly. Patient then lifts lift leg out to the side and behind (B).

SUBSTITUTIONS: Maintain neutral spine and pelvis; active core encouraged, do not allow trunk to twist or hip hiking.

PARAMETERS: Hold 1 to 2 seconds, 8 to 12 repetitions, 1 to 3 sets, 1 time per day or every other day

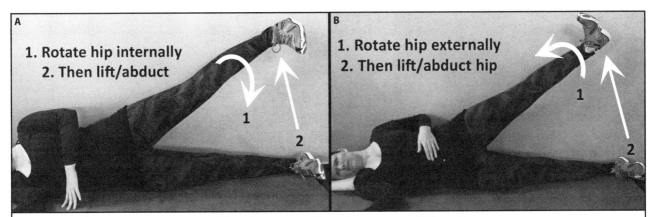

6.04.18 STRENGTHEN: ISOTONIC; HIP, STRAIGHT-LEG ABDUCTION WITH ROTATION

POSITION: Side-lying

TARGETS: *With internal rotation:* Strengthening of gluteus medius. *With external rotation:* Strengthening of TFL.

INSTRUCTION: *Side-lying with internal rotation (gluteus medius):* Lying on unaffected side with hips stacked, knees extended. Patient rolls top hip forward to touch toes to mat in front of other foot then, with tightened quad and straight knee, patient lifts top leg and rolls hip into internal rotation, ending with toes pointed toward bottom foot. Hold return and repeat (A). *Side-lying with external rotation (TFL):* Lying on unaffected side with hips stacked, knees extended. Patient rolls top hip forward to touch toes to mat in front of other foot then, with tightened quad and straight knee, lifts top leg and rolls hip into external rotation, ending with toes pointed toward ceiling. Hold return and repeat (B).

SUBSTITUTIONS: Maintain neutral spine and pelvis; active core encouraged, do not allow trunk to twist.

PARAMETERS: Hold 1 to 2 seconds, 8 to 12 repetitions, 1 to 3 sets, 1 time per day or every other

Where's the Evidence?

Lee and colleagues found gluteus medius EMG activity was significantly greater in side-lying abduction with internal/medial rotation compared with neutral or external rotation. TFL EMG activity was significantly greater in side-lying abduction with external/lateral rotation than in neutral or internal rotation (Lee et al., 2014).

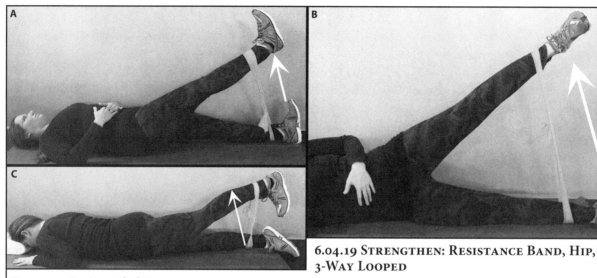

6.04.19 STRENGTHEN: RESISTANCE BAND, HIP, 3-WAY LOOPED

<u>POSITION</u>: Supine, side-lying, prone

<u>TARGETS</u>: Strengthening of hip flexors (iliopsoas and rectus femoris), extensors (gluteus maximus, hamstrings), and abductors (TFL, gluteus medius and minimus) with stabilization of hip internal and external rotators to keep leg aligned

<u>INSTRUCTION</u>: With band looped around both ankles. *Flexion:* Patient tightens quadriceps muscle on extended leg and, keeping knee straight, lifts toes straight up toward ceiling until thigh reaches other thigh against the resistance of the band (A). *Abduction:* Patient lies on unaffected side, tightens quadriceps muscle on top leg, and, keeping knee straight, lifts leg up against the resistance of the band as toes stay pointed forward (B). *Extension:* Patient lies prone, tightens quadriceps on affected leg, and, keeping knee straight, lifts heel straight up toward ceiling against resistance of the band, keeping toes pointed straight down (C).

<u>SUBSTITUTIONS</u>: Maintain neutral pelvis; active lower abdominal core encouraged, knee stays fully extended.

<u>PARAMETERS</u>: 8 to 12 repetitions, 1 to 3 sets, 1 time per day or every other day

---

6.04.20 STRENGTHEN: RESISTANCE BAND, HIP, 4-WAY

<u>POSITION</u>: Standing

<u>TARGETS</u>: Strengthening of hip flexors (iliopsoas and rectus femoris), extensors (gluteus maximus, hamstrings), abductors (TFL, gluteus medius and minimus), and adductors (adductor brevis, adductor longus,

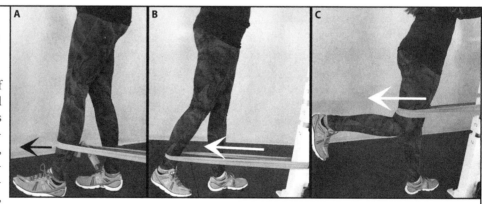

adductor magnus, adductor minimus, pectineus, gracilis, slight obturator externus) with stabilization of hip internal and external rotators to keep leg aligned.

<u>INSTRUCTION</u>: With band anchored at ankle height, loop band around ankle. *Flexion:* Patient faces away from anchor, stands straight up, and tightens quadriceps to keep knee fully extended while bringing leg forward against the resistance of the band (A). *Extension:* Patient faces toward anchor, stands straight up, and tightens quadriceps to keep knee fully extended while bringing leg backward against the resistance of the band (B). *Gluteus maximus isolation:* Patient can slide the band up to distal thigh and flex the knee 90 degrees, then extend hip against resistance band to decrease assist from hamstring and focus target on gluteus maximus (C). *(continued)*

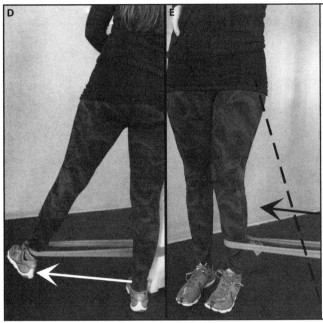

6.04.20 STRENGTHEN: RESISTANCE BAND, HIP, 4-WAY (CONTINUED)

INSTRUCTION: *Abduction:* Patient standing with target side away from anchor steps out so that there is tension on the band. Patient stands straight up and tightens quadriceps to keep knee fully extended while bringing leg away from other leg against the resistance of the band (D). *Adduction:* Patient standing with target side toward anchor steps out so that hip is abducted with tension on the band. Patient stands straight up and tightens quadriceps to keep knee fully extended while bringing leg toward the other leg and crosses in front or behind against the resistance of the band (E). This can also be done with the unaffected leg as the actively moving leg will also challenge the stance leg in all directions.

SUBSTITUTIONS: Maintain neutral pelvis; active lower abdominal core encouraged, knee stays fully extended.

PARAMETERS: 8 to 12 repetitions, 1 to 3 sets, 1 time per day or every other day

Where's the Evidence?

A 2013 study revealed that, although elastic resistance and exercise machine seem equally effective for recruiting muscle activity of the hip adductors, the elastic resistance condition was able to demonstrate greater muscle recruitment than the exercise machine during hip abduction (Brandt, Jakobsen, Thorborg, Sundstrup, Jay, & Andersen, 2013).

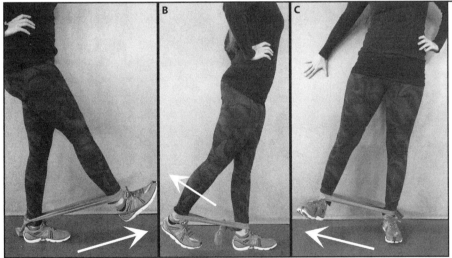

6.04.21 STRENGTHEN: RESISTANCE BAND, HIP, 3-WAY LOOPED, STANDING

POSITION: Standing

TARGETS: Strengthening of hip flexors (iliopsoas and rectus femoris), extensors (gluteus maximus, hamstrings), and abductors (TFL, gluteus medius and minimus) with stabilization of hip internal and external rotators to keep leg aligned

INSTRUCTION: With band looped around both ankles. *Flexion:* Patient stands straight up and tightens quadriceps to keep knee fully extended while bringing leg forward against the resistance of the band (A). *Extension:* Patient stands straight up and tightens quadriceps to keep knee fully extended while bringing leg backward against the resistance of the band (B). *Abduction:* Patient stands straight up and tightens quadriceps to keep knee fully extended while bringing leg away from other leg against the resistance of the band (C).

SUBSTITUTIONS: Maintain neutral pelvis; active lower abdominal core encouraged, knee stays fully extended.

PARAMETERS: 8 to 12 repetitions, 1 to 3 sets, 1 time per day or every other day

6.04.22 STRENGTHEN: RESISTANCE BAND, HIP, SIDESTEPPING

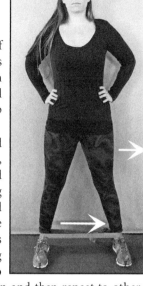

POSITION: Standing

TARGETS: Strengthening of hip abductors (TFL, gluteus medius and minimus) with stabilization of hip internal and external rotators to keep leg aligned

INSTRUCTION: With band looped around both ankles, patient stands straight and steps sideways, abducting the hip with knee extended against the resistance of the band. Patient then brings other leg to meet abducted leg and repeats. Patient can go across the room one direction and then repeat to other side.

SUBSTITUTIONS: Maintain neutral pelvis; active lower abdominal core encouraged, knee stays fully extended.

PARAMETERS: Travel distance to fatigue, 1 to 3 sets, 1 time per day or every other day

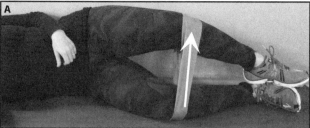

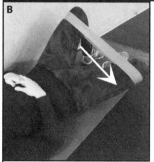

6.04.23 STRENGTHEN: RESISTANCE BAND, HIP, "CLAM"

POSITION: Hook-lying, side-lying

TARGETS: Strengthening of gluteus medius primarily

INSTRUCTION: *Unilateral side-lying*: Patient is lying on unaffected side with hips stacked, hips flexed 45 degrees, and knees flexed 90 degrees medial ankles together. Loop band around knees. Patient lifts top knee, opening hips without rolling trunk against the resistance of the band (A). *Unilateral hook-lying*: Loop band around knees. Patient engages lower abdominals and pelvis tilts posteriorly. Patient brings knees apart, opening hips and keeping feet touching (B).

SUBSTITUTIONS: Maintain neutral spine and pelvis; active core encouraged.

PARAMETERS: Hold 1 to 2 seconds, 8 to 12 repetitions, 1 to 3 sets, 1 time per day or every other day

6.04.24 STRENGTHEN: RESISTANCE BAND, HIP INTERNAL ROTATION AND VARIATIONS

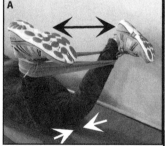
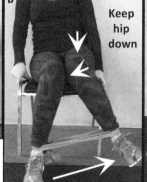
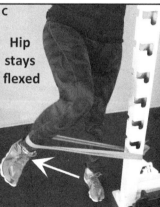

POSITION: Prone, seated, standing

TARGETS: Strengthening of hip internal rotators: TFL, gluteus medius, gluteus minimus

INSTRUCTION: *Prone*: With knees bent to 90 degrees and band looped around ankles. Patient engages core to stabilize pelvis and spine, then slowly pulls the feet apart, keeping knees together (A). *Seated*: Loop band around ankles. Patient engages lower abdominals and gluteus to stabilize pelvis. Patient brings ankles out while keeping knee together (B). For greater ROM, band can be anchored so that tension starts with the hip externally rotated. *Standing*: Anchor band to opposite side of target leg at knee height. Patient brings target hip and knee into 90 degrees flexion. Loop band around ankle. Patient internally rotates hip, bringing ankle out to the side without dropping thigh or moving out of sagittal plane flexion (C).

SUBSTITUTIONS: Maintain neutral spine and pelvis; active core encouraged, avoid hip hiking.

PARAMETERS: Hold 1 to 2 seconds, 8 to 12 repetitions, 1 to 3 sets, 1 time per day or every other day

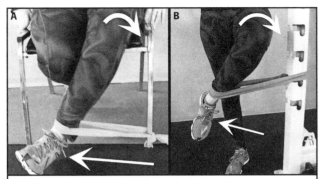

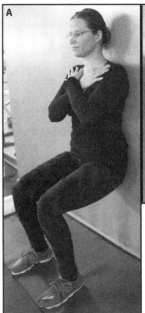

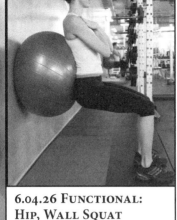

6.04.25 STRENGTHEN: RESISTANCE BAND, HIP EXTERNAL ROTATION AND VARIATIONS

<u>POSITION</u>: Prone, seated, standing

<u>TARGETS</u>: Strengthening of hip external rotators piriformis plus gemelleus superior and inferior, obturator internus and externus, quadratus femoris

<u>INSTRUCTION</u>: *Seated:* Anchor band on target side at ankle height with tension on ankle with hip internally rotated. Patient engages lower abdominals and gluteus to stabilize pelvis. Patient brings ankle toward the other ankle and crosses over the top. Patient pulls unaffected foot back to clear path for target leg. Knee stays in same sagittal plane as hip (A). *Standing:* Anchor band to same side as target leg at knee height. Patient brings target hip and knee into 90 degrees flexion. Loop band around ankle. Patient externally rotates hip, bringing ankle across midline and medial aspect of foot up toward ceiling. Patient should not allow thigh to drop or move out of sagittal plane flexion (B).

<u>SUBSTITUTIONS</u>: Maintain neutral spine and pelvis; active core encouraged.

<u>PARAMETERS</u>: Hold 1 to 2 seconds, 8 to 12 repetitions, 1 to 3 sets, 1 time per day or every other day

6.04.26 FUNCTIONAL: HIP, WALL SQUAT

<u>POSITION</u>: Standing

<u>TARGETS</u>: Strengthening of hip extensors gluteus maximus, hamstrings, and quadriceps, extending the knee

<u>INSTRUCTION</u>: *Wall squat:* Patient crosses arms and leans back against wall with feet hip-width apart and patellas lined up with second toes of feet, which are pointed forward. Patient performs PPT and slides down wall to 90-degree bend at hips and knee. Patient should still be able to see toes in front of knees. Patient then rises back up and repeats (A). *Exercise ball squat:* This can also be done with an exercise ball for added support and decreased friction (B).

<u>SUBSTITUTIONS</u>: Maintain neutral pelvis; active lower abdominal core encouraged, knee stays directly aligned with hip and behind toes.

<u>PARAMETERS</u>: 8 to 12 repetitions, 1 to 3 sets, 1 time per day or every other day

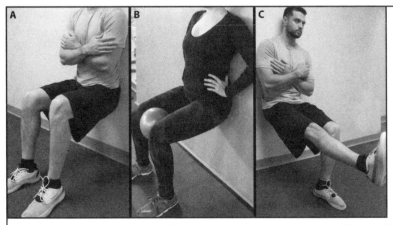

6.04.27 FUNCTIONAL: HIP, WALL SIT

<u>POSITION</u>: Standing

<u>TARGETS</u>: Strengthening of hip extensors (gluteus maximus, hamstrings and quadriceps) extending the knee, ball squeeze brings in isometric contraction of hip adductors. Due to prolonged sitting time, this will build endurance in above muscles.

<u>INSTRUCTION</u>: Patient crosses arms and leans back against a wall with feet hip-width apart and patellas lined up with second toes of feet, which are pointed forward. Patient performs PPT and slides down the wall to 90-degree bend at hips and knee. Patient should still be able to see toes in front of knees. Patient holds position to fatigue (A). This can also be done with a 20- to 25-cm ball between knees; encourage patient to squeeze ball between knees during entire exercise (B). To advance, you may add lifting one foot off floor in a marching movement or extending one knee and then the other (C).

<u>SUBSTITUTIONS</u>: Maintain neutral pelvis; active lower abdominal core encouraged, knee stays directly aligned with hip and behind toes.

<u>PARAMETERS</u>: *Static sit:* Start with 10 seconds and work up to 60 seconds (longer if athlete); *Marching and knee extension variation:* 8 to 12 repetitions, 1 to 3 sets, 1 time per day or every other day

6.04.28 FUNCTIONAL: HIP, FREE-STANDING SQUAT

<u>POSITION</u>: Standing

<u>TARGETS</u>: Strengthening of hip extensors (gluteus maximus, hamstrings) and abductors (TFL, gluteus medius and minimus), stabilization of hip internal and external rotators to keep leg aligned and quadriceps extending the knee.

<u>INSTRUCTION</u>: Patient stands with arms extended out in front at shoulder height. Feet are hip-width apart. Patient engages core and squats down, maintaining neutral spine and pelvis, knee and foot pointed straight forward. Patient keeps knee behind toes and squats as if sitting in a chair. Patient extends hip and knee slowly to return to start and repeats.

<u>SUBSTITUTIONS</u>: Maintain neutral pelvis; active lower abdominal core encouraged, knees stay directly aligned with hip and behind toes.

<u>PARAMETERS</u>: 8 to 12 repetitions, 1 to 3 sets, 1 time per day or every other day

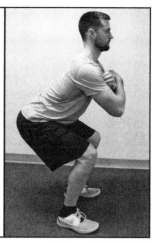

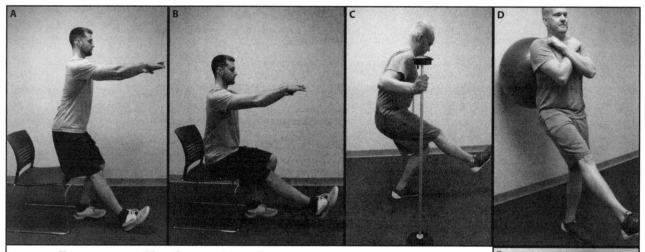

6.04.29 FUNCTIONAL: HIP, SINGLE-LIMB SQUAT

<u>POSITION</u>: Standing

<u>TARGETS</u>: Strengthening of hip extensors (gluteus maximus, hamstrings) and abductors (TFL, gluteus medius and minimus), stabilization of hip internal and external rotators to keep leg aligned, quadriceps extending the knee; this activity should only be initiated after strengthening in side-lying. Patients struggle to maintain balance on one leg, and the deeper the hip and knee position, the more chance of aggravating ITB and patellofemoral joint; excellent control is key.

<u>INSTRUCTION</u>: *Chair:* Patient stands with arms extended out in front at shoulder height. Patient shifts weight to target side and balances on leg with opposite leg extended straight forward as high as possible. Patient squats down, keeping other leg elevated off of floor, back straight, and stance knee and foot pointed straight forward. Patient keeps knee behind toes as patient sits in a chair. Patient reverses to return to standing (A and B). *Poles (beginner):* Poles are placed behind the patient with the ends of the poles at the base of a wall.

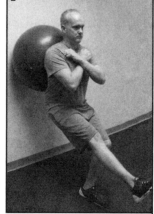

Patient holds poles at the sides and balances on one leg with opposite leg extended straight forward as high as possible. Patient squats down, up to 90 degrees at the knee, while keeping other leg elevated off of floor, no more than 90 degrees flexion at the knee, and using poles for support. Keep back straight and supporting knee pointed same direction as toes. Patient raises body back up to original position until stance hip and knee are extended. Repeat (C). *Exercise ball:* This can also be done with an exercise ball for added support. Make sure patient's feet are forward enough that, as patient squats, the knee will not go in front of the toes (D and E). *(continued)*

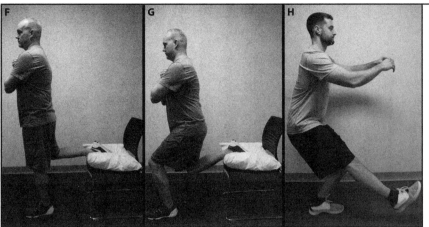

6.04.29 FUNCTIONAL: HIP, SINGLE-LIMB SQUAT (CONTINUED)

INSTRUCTION: *Bench/chair:* Patient stands 3 feet (1 meter) facing away from a bench or chair and places the top of the non-target foot on the bench/chair seat as shown. Patient posteriorly tilts the pelvis by engaging the lower abdominals to prevent anterior tilt of pelvis during squat. Stance leg should be under the patient's torso aligned with hip, toes forward. Patient squats down, up to 90 degrees at the knee, while keeping other leg elevated off of floor. Patient then extends hip and knee to return to start and repeats (F and G). *Free-standing (advanced):* Patient places arms in front with extended elbow and shoulders flexed 90 degrees. Patient balances on one leg with opposite leg extended straight forward as high as possible. Patient squats down up to 90 degrees at the knee while keeping other leg elevated off of floor. Keep back straight and supporting knee pointed the same direction as toes. Patient raises body back up to original position until stance hip and knee are extended. Repeat (H).

SUBSTITUTIONS: Maintain neutral pelvis; active lower abdominal core encouraged, knees stay directly behind toes, focus on keeping hips and knee as controlled as possible and knee over second toe, keep trunk upright.

PARAMETERS: 8 to 12 repetitions, 1 to 3 sets, 1 time per day or every other day

---

Where's the Evidence?

EMG studies comparing exercises for gluteus maximus and medius MVC found 82% MVC for gluteus medius and 70% for gluteus maximus with chair sitting variation (Boren et al., 2011).

Where's the Evidence?

EMG studies comparing exercises for gluteus maximus and medius MVC found 57% MVC for gluteus medius and 37% for gluteus maximus with hip circumduction on a stable surface. Performance on an unstable surface had lower results but still was effective at recruiting both gluteal muscles (Boren et al., 2011).

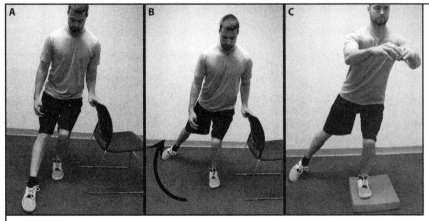

6.04.30 FUNCTIONAL: HIP, SINGLE-LIMB SQUAT, CIRCUMDUCTION

POSITION: Standing

TARGETS: Strengthening of hip extensors (gluteus maximus, hamstrings) and abductors (TFL, gluteus medius and minimus), stabilization of hip internal and external rotators to keep leg aligned and quadriceps extending the knee

INSTRUCTION: Patient performs a single-limb squat on the target leg while drawing an arc with the non-target foot, extending the arc away from the subject for three counts. Patient then returns the foot to the starting position by drawing the foot in, while returning to a standing position for 3 counts. Patient may use hand for balance on table or wall (A and B). This can also be done on an unstable surface such as foam square (C).

SUBSTITUTIONS: Maintain neutral pelvis; active lower abdominal core encouraged, knee on target side stays directly aligned with hip and behind toes.

PARAMETERS: 8 to 12 repetitions, 1 to 3 sets, 1 time per day or every other day

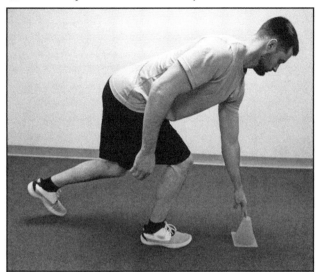

6.04.31 FUNCTIONAL: HIP, SINGLE-LIMB SQUAT, CONE TAPS

<u>POSITION</u>: Standing

<u>TARGETS</u>: Strengthening of hip extensors (gluteus maximus, hamstrings) and abductors (TFL, gluteus medius and minimus), stabilization of hip internal and external rotators to keep leg aligned, and quadriceps extending the knee.

<u>INSTRUCTION</u>: Patient begins in single-leg squat on target side (**6.04.29**), weight through the heel and knee behind toes. Cone is placed 6 inches in front of target-side toes. Arms are abducted 90 degrees at shoulder with elbows extended. Patient focuses gaze on cone while rotating trunk to bring one hand to tap cone.

<u>SUBSTITUTIONS</u>: Maintain neutral pelvis; active lower abdominal core encouraged, knee on target side stays directly aligned with hip and behind toes, focus on keeping hips and knee still and as controlled as possible.

<u>PARAMETERS</u>: 8 to 12 repetitions, 1 to 3 sets, 1 time per day or every other day

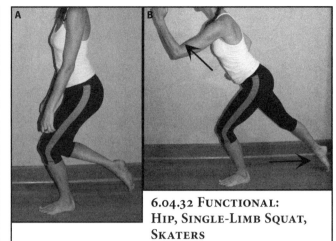

6.04.32 FUNCTIONAL: HIP, SINGLE-LIMB SQUAT, SKATERS

<u>POSITION</u>: Standing

<u>TARGETS</u>: Strengthening of hip extensors (gluteus maximus, hamstrings) and abductors (TFL, gluteus medius and minimus), stabilization of hip internal and external rotators to keep leg aligned, and quadriceps extending the knee.

<u>INSTRUCTION</u>: Patient begins in stance and performs single leg squat on target side for two counts (**6.04.29**). Once single leg squatted down, patient leans forward with the trunk, bringing opposite arm forward as opposite hip extends behind to tap toe behind as far as possible. Patient then returns to standing straight up, extends knee and hip for another two counts, and repeats (A and B).

<u>SUBSTITUTIONS</u>: Maintain neutral pelvis; active lower abdominal core encouraged, knee on target side stays directly aligned with hip and behind toes, focus on keeping hips and knee still and as controlled as possible.

<u>PARAMETERS</u>: 8 to 12 repetitions, 1 to 3 sets, 1 time per day or every other day

Where's the Evidence?

EMG studies comparing exercises for gluteus maximus and medius MVC found 59% MVC for gluteus medius and 66% for gluteus maximus with skater squat (Boren et al., 2011).

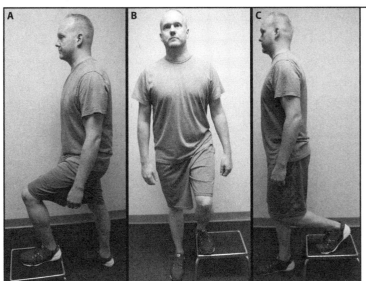

6.04.33 FUNCTIONAL: HIP, STEP-UPS

POSITION: Standing

TARGETS: Strengthening of hip extensors (gluteus maximus, hamstrings) and abductors (TFL, gluteus medius and minimus), stabilization of hip internal and external rotators to keep leg aligned, and quadriceps extending the knee.

INSTRUCTION: *Forward:* Beginning with both feet on the ground, patient steps forward onto a 20-cm step with the target leg for one count. Patient then steps up with the non-target leg during the next count. Patient then lowers the target leg back to the ground for one count followed by the non-target leg during the next count (A). *Lateral:* Patient stands on the edge of a 15-cm step on the target leg and squats slowly to lower the heel of the non-target leg toward floor for one count and then returns to start position during the next count (B). *Retro:* Patient stands in front of a 20-cm step and steps backward onto step with the target leg for one count. Patient then steps up with the non-target leg during the next count. Patient then lowers the target leg back to the ground for one count followed by the non-target leg during the next count (C).

SUBSTITUTIONS: Maintain neutral pelvis; active lower abdominal core encouraged, knee on target side stays directly aligned with hip and behind toes, focus on keeping hips and knee still and as controlled as possible.

PARAMETERS: 8 to 12 repetitions, 1 to 3 sets, 1 time per day or every other day

Where's the Evidence?

EMG studies comparing exercises for gluteus maximus and medius MVC found lateral steps to be superior to forward step-up. The study found 59% MVC for gluteus medius and 63% for gluteus maximus with lateral step-up and 54% MVC for gluteus medius and gluteus maximus with lateral step up (Boren et al., 2011).

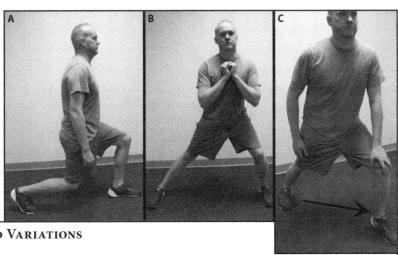

6.04.34 FUNCTIONAL: HIP, LUNGE AND VARIATIONS

POSITION: Standing

TARGETS: Strengthening of hip extensors (gluteus maximus, hamstrings) and abductors (TFL, gluteus medius and minimus), stabilization of hip internal and external rotators to keep leg aligned, and quadriceps extending the knee.

INSTRUCTION: *Beginner:* For forward and lateral lunges, patient may start with large steps and only mini-lunging. Follow instructions for each, but decrease knee flexion to <90 degrees based on patient tolerances and form. *Forward:* Patient takes a large step leg forward and bends both knees to 90 degrees. Keep front knee straight forward alignment with hip and toes pointed forward. Most of body weight is transferred to front leg. Push off of front leg to return to standing (A). *Lateral:* Patient takes a large step laterally and slightly forward. Lunging knee bends to 90 degrees and stance leg stays extended. Keep bent knee in straight forward alignment with toes pointed forward. Most of body weight is transferred to laterally placed leg. Push off of front leg to return to standing (B). *Diagonal:* Patient takes a large step laterally and forward at a 45-degree angle. Lunging knee bends to 90 degrees and stance leg stays extended. Keep bent knee in straight forward alignment with toes pointed forward. Most of body weight is transferred to laterally placed leg. Push off of front leg to return to standing (C).

SUBSTITUTIONS: Maintain neutral pelvis; active lower abdominal core encouraged, knee on target side stays directly behind toes, focus on keeping hips and knee as controlled as possible.

PARAMETERS: 8 to 12 repetitions, 1 to 3 sets, 1 time per day or every other day

6.04.35 Functional: Hip, Dynamic Leg Swing, "Running Man"

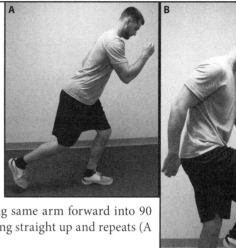

Position: Standing

Targets: Strengthening of hip extensors (gluteus maximus, hamstrings) and abductors (TFL, gluteus medius and minimus), stabilization of hip internal and external rotators to keep leg aligned, and quadriceps extending the knee. Hip flexors are also engaged in hip flexion component; iliopsoas and rectus femoris.

Instruction: Patient begins in stance and brings hip and knee to 90 degrees flexion while opposite arm comes into 90 degrees shoulder and elbow flexion. While simultaneously performing a single-leg squat on the other side, patient then brings leg back to extends behind to tap toe behind as far as possible while bringing same arm forward into 90 degrees shoulder and elbow flexion. Patient then returns to standing straight up and repeats (A and B).

Substitutions: Maintain neutral pelvis; active lower abdominal core encouraged, knees stay directly aligned with hip and on single squat-side behind toes, focus on keeping hips and knee still and as controlled as possible.

Parameters: 8 to 12 repetitions, 1 to 3 sets, 1 time per day or every other day

---

Where's the Evidence?

EMG studies comparing exercises for gluteus maximus and medius MVC found 57% MVC for gluteus medius and 33% for gluteus maximus with dynamic leg swing single-leg squat (Boren et al., 2011).

6.04.36 Functional: Hip, Deadlift and Variations

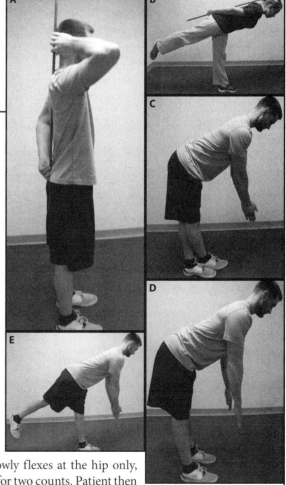

Position: Standing

Targets: Strengthening of hip extensors (gluteus maximus, hamstrings) and abductors (TFL, gluteus medius and minimus), stabilization of hip internal and external rotators to keep leg aligned.

Instruction: *Dowel training:* Patient may struggle with keeping straight spine, and use of a dowel along the spine is a good place to start before beginning other variations of the dead lift. Patient places dowel along the spine so that head, middle and lower back, and sacrum are all touching and works on bending forward only, hinging at the hips. Patient is to keep dowel in contact with all areas entire sequence (A and B). *Cross-legged:* Patient stands heel to toe and slowly flexes at the hip only, keeping the back straight, to touch a step (beginner), the floor (advanced phase I), or beyond feet with patient standing on stool (advanced phase II) with the opposite hand for two counts. Patient then extends at the hip to standing for two counts. Knees may be slightly bent if hamstrings are restricted (C). *Double limb "Romanian dead lift":* Patient slowly flexes at the hips only, keeping the back straight, to touch the floor with the fingertips for two counts. Patient then extends at the hips to standing for two counts. Knees may be slightly bent if hamstrings are restricted (D). *Single limb:* Patient stands on the target leg and slowly flexes at the hip only, keeping the back straight, to touch the floor with the opposite hand for two counts. Patient then extends at the hip to standing for two counts. Knee may be slightly bent if hamstrings are restricted (E).

Substitutions: Maintain neutral pelvis; active lower abdominal core encouraged, knees stay directly aligned with hip and on single squat side behind toes, focus on keeping hips and knee still and as controlled as possible.

Parameters: 8 to 12 repetitions, 1 to 3 sets, 1 time per day or every other day

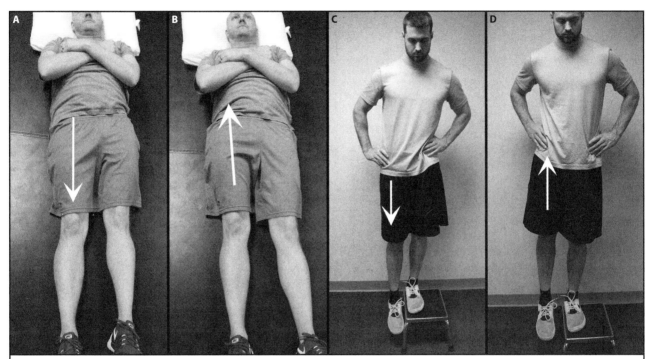

6.04.37 FUNCTIONAL: PELVIC DROP/HIP HIKE

POSITION: Beginner supine, advanced standing

TARGETS: Strengthening of gluteus medius

INSTRUCTION: *Supine (beginner):* Patient slides pelvis down on non-target side, pushing heel away and then hikes the pelvis back toward the shoulder, pulling heel upward along the mat. Avoid lateral bending of the trunk (A and B). *Standing (advanced):* Patient stands on a step stool, straightens spine, and lowers one heel toward floor by dropping pelvis on non-target side. Patient actively engages gluteal muscles on stance side to hike the hip up, bringing foot away from the floor (C and D).

SUBSTITUTIONS: Maintain neutral pelvis; active lower abdominal core encouraged, knees stay directly aligned with hip and on single squat-side behind toes, focus on keeping hips and knee still and as controlled as possible.

PARAMETERS: 8 to 12 repetitions, 1 to 3 sets, 1 time per day or every other day

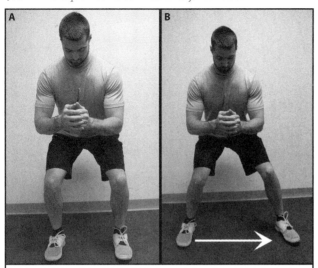

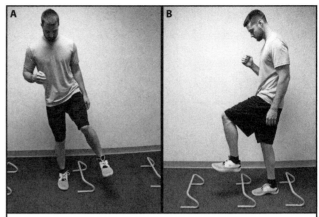

6.04.38 FUNCTIONAL: HIP, SIDESTEPPING WITH MINI-SQUAT

POSITION: Standing

TARGETS: Strengthening of hip abductors (TFL, gluteus medius and minimus) with stabilization of hip internal and external rotators to keep leg aligned; quadriceps are engaged with limiting knee flexion.

INSTRUCTION: Patient with feet hip-width apart performs a mini-squat with hips and knees flexed 30 to 45 degrees and trunk upright. Patient maintains hip and knee flexion and side steps, abducting the hip. Patient follows by adducting the trailing hip and continues over a distance, repeating steps. Patient can go across the room one direction and then repeat to other side (A and B).

SUBSTITUTIONS: Maintain neutral pelvis; active lower abdominal core encouraged, knees stay behind toes and trunk upright.

PARAMETERS: Travel distance to fatigue, 1 to 3 sets, 1 time per day or every other day

6.04.39 FUNCTIONAL: HIP, STEP-OVERS

POSITION: Standing

TARGETS: Strengthening of hip abductors (TFL, gluteus medius and minimus) with stabilization of hip internal and external rotators to keep leg aligned; hip flexors assist with flexing hip to clear hurdle in both forward and sidestepping; quadriceps are engaged on stance legs.

INSTRUCTION: Therapist may set up cones or mini hurdles for this activity. Space hurdles far enough apart to allow moderate-size step and room for both feet to be planted between. *Lateral:* Patient with trunk upright lifts leading leg into hip and knee flexion and abducts to clear hurdle far enough to allow room for the following leg to then adduct at the hip and clear hurdle to plant foot next to leading leg and repeat. Repeat to other side A). *Forward:* This can also be done to increase hip and knee flexion with gait by walking forward and stepping over hurdles or cones. Watch that patient does not use compensatory circumduction to clear objects (B).

SUBSTITUTIONS: Maintain neutral pelvis; active lower abdominal core encouraged, knees stay behind toes and trunk upright.

PARAMETERS: May use multiple hurdles in a row or just one going back and forth; repeat 10 to 12 hurdles each way, 1 to 3 sets, 1 time per day or every other day.

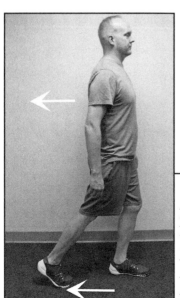

6.04.40 FUNCTIONAL: HIP, BACKWARD WALKING

POSITION: Standing

TARGETS: Strengthening of hip extensors (gluteus maximus, hamstrings) also assists with ROM into hip extension; quadriceps are engaged on stance legs.

INSTRUCTION: Patient takes large steps backward, keeping toes pointed forward.

SUBSTITUTIONS: Leaning forward with trunk, keep trunk upright

PARAMETERS: Travel distance to fatigue, 1 to 3 sets, 1 time per day or every other day

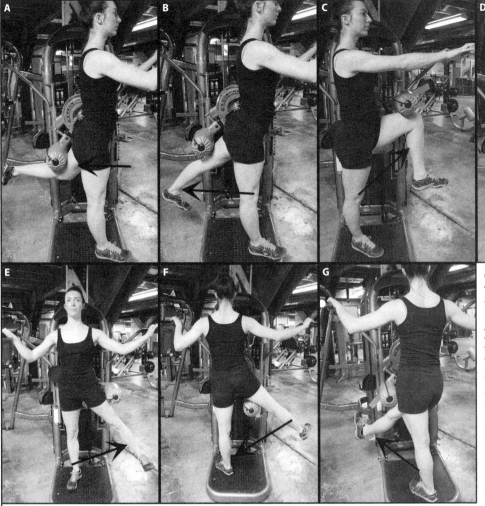

6.04.41 Strengthen: "Multi-Hip" 4-Way on Weight Machines

Position: Standing

Targets: Strengthening of hip flexors (iliopsoas and rectus femoris), extensors (gluteus maximus, hamstrings), abductors (TFL, gluteus medius and minimus), and adductors (adductor brevis, adductor longus, adductor magnus, adductor minimus, pectineus, gracilis, slight obturator externus) with stabilization of hip internal and external rotators to keep leg aligned.

Instruction: Adjust height of the platform so that the hip joint aligns with the axis of the rotation. Adjust height of thigh pad to just above the knee. Using range selector, set up thigh bar to the starting position. Depending on range in which you want the patient to work, this can be neutral hip or further opposite to the desired motion. Patient holds handrails for stability and performs desired movement. Patient should engage core to keep spine and pelvis neutral throughout the movement. Flexion, extension, abduction, and adduction can all be done on this machine (A through G).

Substitutions: Maintain neutral pelvis; active lower abdominal core encouraged, knee stays near full extension.

Parameters: 8 to 12 repetitions, 1 to 3 sets, 1 time per day or every other day

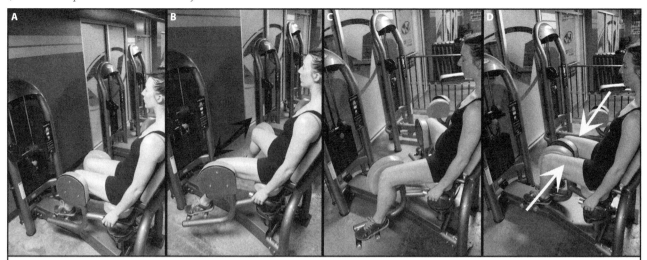

6.04.42 STRENGTHEN: HIP ABDUCTOR AND ADDUCTOR ON WEIGHT MACHINES

<u>POSITION</u>: Seated

<u>TARGETS</u>: Strengthening of hip adductors (adductor brevis, adductor longus, adductor magnus, adductor minimus, pectineus, gracilis, slight obturator externus) and abductors (TFL, gluteus medius and minimus)

<u>INSTRUCTION</u>: *Abductor machine:* Place thighs so that pads are on outer thigh and adjust starting position so that thighs are fully adducted. Patient sits tall and engages the core muscles to stabilize pelvis. Knees are bent 90 degrees with feet on platforms if available. Patient slowly presses thighs away from each other, opening the hips, keeping knees straight and aligned with toes pointed forward. Hold squeeze 2 to 3 seconds and slowly return, stopping just before the weights touch down and repeat (A and B). *Adductor machine:* Place thighs so that pads are on inner thigh and adjust starting position so that there is a slight stretch on the adductors. Patient sits tall and engages the core muscles to stabilize pelvis. Knees are bent 90 degrees with feet on platforms if available. Patient slowly squeezes thighs together, keeping knees straight and aligned with toes pointed forward. Hold squeeze 2 to 3 seconds and slowly return stopping just before the weights touch down and repeat (C and D).

<u>SUBSTITUTIONS</u>: Maintain neutral pelvis; active lower abdominal core encouraged, knee stays near full extension.

<u>PARAMETERS</u>: 8 to 12 repetitions, 1 to 3 sets, 1 time per day or every other day

Where's the Evidence?

Critics argue that although these machines do strengthen these muscles, they are dangerous because the body isn't designed for those movements (abduction and adduction) with the hips flexed (Presto, n.d.). They do not mimic real life movements. The abduction machine also tightens the iliotibial band. A tight iliotibial band can factor into poor patellar alignment with knee movements (Charles, n.d.). Several websites have the hip abductor and adductor machines listed as the top machines to avoid at the gym (Behnken, n.d.; Doll, 2010; Perrine, 2011).

6.04.43 FUNCTIONAL: GAIT PRACTICE

Discussion: There are many activities to increase patients' balance, proprioception, and strength in the LEs with standing. Refer to knee and ankle sections for additional ideas to challenge these areas in the LE. In addition, the hip has specific demands to achieve a normal smooth gait.

The hip demands and compensations during gait:

- The *hip flexors* eccentrically control hip extension at the end of the stance phase and concentrically initiate the swing phase. With loss of flexor function, swing will be initiated by a compensatory posterior lurch of the trunk. Tightness of the hip flexors will prevent full extension into the last half of stance phase, resulting in a shortened stride. This may cause an increase in lumbar lordosis or forward trunk flexion when walking.
- The *hip extensors* eccentrically slow the advancing leg at terminal swing to initial heel contact. Once the foot begins to bear weight in foot flat, the hip extensors concentrically begin to initiate hip extension. A loss of hip extensor function can result in the trunk lurching posteriorly at foot contact. Tightness of the hip extensors can result in a reduced range in the final stage of the swing phase. The patient may compensate by rotating the pelvis to bring the leg through. A tight gluteus maximus may cause greater tension on the ITB, which can result in irritation to the lateral knee.
- The *hip abductors* control lateral pelvic tilt when the opposite leg is swinging through. Poor gluteus medius function can cause a hip drop during swing phase or a compensatory lateral bending of the trunk over the stance side when the opposite leg swings through. Lateral shifting may also occur when a patient has painful hip to lessen the amount or weight and torque that the hip has to endure. The TFL is also an abductor and may alter gait if tight.

REFERENCES

Behnken, M. (n.d.). Top 5 worst weight machines. *Ask the Trainer.* Retrieved from http://www.askthetrainer.com/top-5-worst-weight-Machines/

Boren, K., Conrey, C., Le Coguic, J., Paprocki, L., Voight, M., & Robinson, T. K. (2011). Electromyographic analysis of gluteus medius and gluteus maximus during rehabilitation exercises. *International Journal of Sports Physical Therapy, 6*(3), 206-223.

Brandt, M., Jakobsen, M. D., Thorborg, K., Sundstrup, E., Jay, K., & Andersen, L. L. (2013). Perceived loading and muscle activity during hip strengthening exercises: Comparison of elastic resistance and machine exercises. *International Journal of Sports Physical Therapy, 8*(6), 811-819.

Charles, K. (n.d.). The effectiveness of a hip abduction and adduction exercise machine. *Healthy Living.* Retrieved from http://healthy-living.azcentral.com/effectiveness-hip-abduction-adduction-exercise-machine-20730.html

Distefano, L. J., Blackburn, J. T., Marshall, S. W., & Padua, D. A. (2009). Gluteal muscle activation during common therapeutic exercises. *Journal of Orthopedic and Sports Physical Therapy, 39*(7), 532-540.

Doll, S. (2010). Top 5 machines to avoid in a health club. *Shaping Concepts.* Retrieved from http://www.shapingconcepts.com/blog/health-club-machines-to-avoid/

Lee, J. H., Cynn, H. S., Kwon, O. Y., Yi, C. H., Yoon, T. L., Choi, W. J., & Choi, S. A. (2014). Different hip rotations influence hip abductor muscles activity during isometric side-Lying hip abduction in subjects with gluteus medius weakness. *Journal of Electromyography and Kinesiology, 24*(2), 318-324.

McBeth, J. M., Earl-Boehm, J. E., Cobb, S. C., & Huddleston, W. E. (2012). Hip muscle activity during 3 side-lying hip-strengthening exercises in distance runners. *Journal of Athletic Training, 47*(1), 15-23.

Perrine, S. (2011). Train better: 10 exercise machines to avoid. *Women's Health.* Retrieved from http://www.womenshealthmag.com/fitness/gym-Exercise-Machines?slide=1

Presto, G. (n.d.). Shape fitness/workouts. *Shape.* Retrieved from http://www.shape.com/fitness/workouts/7-Exercises-and-Gym-Machines-skip

Section 6.05

HIP PROTOCOLS AND TREATMENT IDEAS

6.05.1 HIP ARTHROSCOPY DISCUSSION

Hip arthroscopy is a minimally invasive procedure in which the surgeon inserts a small camera into the hip joint. The surgeon uses these images to guide miniature surgical instruments. Generally, this procedure is done for labral tears, femoroacetabular impingement (meaning too much friction in the joint usually due to alterations in femoral heal or acetabular shape), articular cartilage damage, or loose bodies. It is usually performed in an outpatient surgery center, meaning no overnight stay is required. Arthroscopy currently represents the gold standard in both the diagnosis and treatment of labral tears. Initial treatment consisting of PWB may respond if initiated early (Schmerl, Pollard, & Hoskins, 2005). Rehabilitation starts before surgery with a preoperative educational visit for instruction, explanation, and demonstration of the post-operative rehab program. After surgery, post-operative weightbearing status will be determined by the physician as surgery can entail different aspects and each patient will differ in this. Weightbearing restrictions are applied to allow for healing to occur, and also because there often is a significant amount of reflex inhibition and poor muscle firing due to the penetration of the hip with the arthroscopic instruments and the large amount of traction applied to the hip during the arthroscopy. AAROM exercises are begun early, staying within pain-free ranges as avoidance of excessive stretching or end-range pushing. Muscle strengthening exercises begin the first week after surgery, progressing gradually as patient tolerates. Patients should avoid exercises that engage the iliopsoas during the first several weeks after surgery. Iliopsoas tendonitis is a known side effect of hip arthroscopy but can be avoided with appropriate post-operative care, including avoiding exercises that have high activity of the iliopsoas (such as SLRs, resisted hip flexion, abductor strengthening that incorporates significant co-contraction). If the patient had an abductor repair, abductor strengthening will be limited early in the rehabilitation process to allow the tendon to heal back to the bone (University of Wisconsin Sports Rehabilitation, 2013). Micro-fracturing may be done to address small cartilage effects. Micro-fracture is a marrow-stimulation technique in which damaged cartilage is drilled or punched, perforating the subchondral bone and generating a blood clot within the defect that matures into fibro cartilage. Microfracture for the treatment of small cartilage defects of the hip has shown good results (Chandrasekaran et al., 2015).

6.05.2 Hip Arthroscopy Labral Repair With or Without Femoro-Acetabular Impingement Protocol

Protocol adapted from combination of protocols from Bryan T. Kelly, MD, Center for Hip Preservation, Hospital for Special Surgery—Hip Arthroscopy Rehabilitation Labral Debridement with or without FAI post-operative Hip Arthroscopy Rehabilitation Protocol (Kelly, n.d.); Dr. David Hergan's Labral Repair with or without FAI Component (Hergan, n.d.); and University of Wisconsin Sports Rehabilitation—Rehabilitation Guidelines for Hip Arthroscopy Procedures (University of Wisconsin Sports Rehabilitation, 2013).

Phase I: 0 to 4 Weeks Post-Operation: Joint Protection

1. Physical therapy includes bed mobility, transfers and education on donning/doffing brace if applicable, gait with appropriate assistive device if necessary, and discuss increasing walking tolerance. Reinforce sitting, standing, and ADLs modifications with neutral spine postures and proper body mechanics.

2. No active lifting or flexing and rotating hip for 2 to 3 weeks

3. Assistance from a family member/care taker is important for transitioning positions for the first week after surgery

4. No sitting with hip flexed to 90 degrees or more for greater than 30 minutes for first 2 weeks to avoid tightness in the front of the hip

5. Lay on stomach for 2 to 3 hours per day to decrease tightness in the front of the hip (patients with LBP may have to modify position)

6. Weightbearing restrictions without micro-fracturing: 0 to 3 weeks flat foot weightbearing, meaning no weight can be transmitted through the foot, but it is encouraged for the foot to be flat as it makes contact with the ground for balance.

7. Weightbearing restrictions with micro-fracturing: 0 to 3 weeks flat foot weightbearing, then 20 lbs (9kg) weightbearing for another 3 weeks (6 weeks total)

8. Brace:
   a. Set at 0 to 90 degrees extension/flexion for walking
   b. Locked at 0 degrees extension for sleeping, must sleep in brace
   c. Worn at all times the patient is up; must sleep in brace

9. Scar massage: 5 minutes daily at incision portals; begin post-operation day 2 through week 3.

10. Manual therapy: soft tissue to address complaints of soft tissue stiffness, especially for pinching in anterior hip
    a. Consider hip flexors (psoas, iliacus, TFL/ITB, rectus femoris, inguinal ligament, sartorius), gluteus maximus/medius/minimus, quadratus lumborum, adductor group, hamstrings, piriformis, external rotators (gemellus, quadratus femoris, and obturator internus), and erector spinae

11. PROM/AAROM/AROM/ROM; *do not push ROM in any plane 0 to 4 weeks.*
    a. 0 to 2 weeks: Flexion limited to 90 degrees
    b. 0 to 2 weeks: Abduction limited to 30 degrees
    c. 0 to 3 weeks: Internal rotation at 90 degrees flexion limited to 20 degrees
    d. 0 to 3 weeks: External rotation at 90 degrees flexion limited to 30 degrees
    e. 0 to 3 weeks: Prone internal rotation and log roll internal rotation; no limits.
    f. 0 to 3 weeks: Prone external rotation limited to 20 degrees
    g. 0 to 3 weeks: Prone hip extension limited to 0 degrees
    h. 0 to 4 weeks: No active hip flexion past 90 degrees
    i. Joint mobilizations (3 to 12 weeks)
       i. May begin with gentle oscillations for pain grade 1 to 2
       ii. Caudal glide during flexion may begin week 3 and assist with minimizing pinching during ROM
       iii. Begin posterior glides/inferior glides at week 4 to decrease posterior capsule tightness (may use belt mobilizations in supine and side-lying)
       iv. Do not stress anterior capsule for 6 weeks post-operation with joint mobilizations

12. 6.11.3 ROM: Ankle/Foot, Long-Sitting and Ankle Pumps, 4-Way, Active; *supine ankle pumps only AROM (start at week 3).*
    a. 4.02.1 Stretch: Single Knee to Chest; *Passive only, no active hip flexion until 4 weeks.*
    b. 6.01.8 Hip Flexion and Extension, Heel Slide, Active
    c. 6.01.10 ROM: Hip Abduction and Adduction, Heel Slide, Active

13. AROM (start at week 4)
    a. 4.01.7 ROM: Lower Trunk Rotation, Active
    b. 6.01.14 ROM: Hip Internal Rotation and External Rotation, Active; *supine variation only.*
    c. 6.01.4 ROM: Hip Extension, Standing, Active Assistive

14. Isometrics
    a. Hip (start week 1 to 2)
       i. 6.04.2 Strengthen: Isometric; Hip Extension/Gluteus Sets

    ii.   6.04.3 Strengthen: Isometric; Hip Abduction

    iii.   6.04.4 Strengthen: Isometric; Hip Adduction

    iv.   6.04.6 Strengthen: Isometric; Hip External Rotation

    v.   6.04.5 Strengthen: Isometric; Hip Internal Rotation

  b.   Knee (start week 1 to 2)

    i.   6.09.3 Strengthen: Isometric; Knee Flexion, Hamstring Set

    ii.   6.09.2 Strengthen: Isometric; Knee Extension, Quadriceps Set With Ball Squeeze (Vastus Medialis Oblique)

Phase II: 5 to 12 Week Post-Operation: Progressive Strengthening

1.   Stretching

  a.   4.01.2 ROM: Lumbar Extension, Prone on Elbows, Progress to Press Up on Hands, Passive

  b.   3.02.2 Stretch: Thoracic Flexion, "Child's Pose" or "Prayer Stretch," Add Side-Bend or Rotation

  c.   4.02.2 Stretch: Double Knee to Chest, 3-Way

  d.   6.03.3 Stretch: Hip Flexor, Standing Lunge

  e.   6.03.2 Stretch: Hip Flexor, Kneeling Lunge

  f.   6.03.7 Stretch: Hip Adductors, Frog

  g.   6.03.11 Stretch: Hip Adductors on Wall

  h.   6.03.22 Stretch: Piriformis, Figure 4 and Variations

  i.   6.08.1 Stretch: Quadriceps

    i.   Side-lying hand assist

    ii.   Prone belt assist

  j.   6.08.3 Stretch: Hamstrings (try different variations listed below)

    i.   Supine

    ii.   Long-sitting

    iii.   Seated

    iv.   Standing foot on stool

2.   Strengthening

  a.   4.03.1 Strengthen: Isometric; Posterior Pelvic Tilt, Lumbar Spine, With or Without Blood Pressure Cuff for Biofeedback

  b.   4.03.7 Strengthen: Lumbar Spine, Bent-Knee Fall-Outs

  c.   4.03.9 Strengthen: Lumbar Spine, Bent-Knee Lift

  d.   4.01.6 ROM: Pelvic Clocks

  e.   4.03.26 Strengthen: Lumbar Spine, Rocking

  f.   6.04.13 Strengthen: Isotonic; Hip Extension, Mini-Bridge on Towel/Bolster

  g.   6.04.14 Strengthen: Isotonic; Hip Extension, Bridge and Variations (listed below)

    i.   Bridge

    ii.   Bridge with isometric adduction ball squeeze

    iii.   Bridge with isometric hip abduction

    iv.   Bridge in/outs

    v.   Single leg bridge

    vi.   Bridge with knee extension

  h.   6.04.16 Strengthen: Isotonic; Hip Abduction and External Rotation, "Clam" and Variations; *only variations below.*

    i.   Phase I

    ii.   Phase II

  i.   4.03.14 Strengthen: Lumbar Spine, Alternating Arm Lift, Leg Lift, and Combined

  j.   6.04.8 Strengthen: Isotonic; Hip, Straight Leg Raise, 4-Way; *only variations below.*

    i.   Extension

    ii.   Isolate gluteus maximus

3.   Cardiovascular program

  a.   Stationary bike, start at 5 minutes week 3 and increase 3 to 5 minutes each week until at 20 minutes.

  b.   Aquatic physical therapy program; can start after incision healed at 3 weeks.

  c.   Elliptical trainer; week 6, start with 10 minutes increase 3 to 5 minutes; can alternate with bike to achieve 30 minutes continuous activity total between bike and elliptical.

Phase III: Advanced Strengthening: 12 to 16 Weeks Post-Operation

1.   Hip strengthening

  a.   6.04.22 Strengthen: Resistance Band, Hip, Sidestepping

  b.   6.04.15 Strengthen: Hip Extension, Forearm Plank

  c.   6.04.17 Strengthen: Isotonic; Hip Abduction, "Fire Hydrants"

  d.   6.04.23 Strengthen: Resistance Band, Hip, "Clam"

  e.   6.04.24 Strengthen: Resistance Band, Hip Internal Rotation and Variations

  f.   6.04.25 Strengthen: Resistance Band, Hip External Rotation and Variations

  g.   6.04.26 Functional: Hip, Wall Squat

  h.   6.04.28 Functional: Hip, Free-Standing Squat

  i.   6.04.27 Functional: Hip, Wall Sit

  j.   6.04.29 Functional: Hip, Single-Limb Squat

  k.   6.04.33 Functional: Hip, Step-Ups

  l.   6.04.34 Functional: Hip, Lunge and Variations

2.   Core strengthening

  a.   4.03.24 Strengthen: Lumbar Spine, Alternating Hip and Knee Extension, Quadruped

  b.   4.03.23 Strengthen: Lumbar Spine, Alternating Arm Lift, Quadruped

  c.   4.03.24 Strengthen: Lumbar Spine, Alternating Hip and Knee Extension, Quadruped

  d.   4.03.25 Strengthen: Lumbar Spine, Opposite Arm and Leg Lift, Quadruped

   e. 4.03.27 Strengthen: Lumbar Spine, Hold Neutral Spine, Tall-Kneeling

   f. 4.03.28 Strengthen: Lumbar Spine, Arm Lift, Tall-Kneeling

   g. 4.03.29 Strengthen: Lumbar Spine, Reach Toward Floor, Tall-Kneeling

   h. 4.03.30 Strengthen: Lumbar Spine, Reach Toward Floor, Half-Kneeling

   i. 4.03.39 Strengthen: Abdominal, Side Plank and Variations
- i. A: Standing wall (beginner)
- ii. B: Standing chair (beginner)
- iii. C: On elbow and knee (beginner)
- iv. D: On elbow and feet
- v. E: On hand and knee
- vi. F: On hand and feet
- vii. H: With leg lift
- viii. J: Hip dip

   j. 4.03.38 Strengthen: Abdominal, Plank and Variations
- i. A: Standing wall (beginner)
- ii. B: Standing chair (beginner)
- iii. C: Quadruped
- iv. D: Forearm
- v. E: Hands
- vi. F: Forearms to hands
- vii. I: Cheek dips
- viii. J: Tap outs

   k. 4.03.42 Strengthen: Abdominal, Pulsing Crunch, 3-Way (Advanced)

   l. 6.04.37 Functional: Pelvic Drop/Hip Hike

   m. 6.04.38 Functional: Hip, Sidestepping With Mini-Squat

   n. 6.04.39 Functional: Hip, Step-Overs

   o. 6.04.40 Functional: Hip, Backward Walking

   p. 6.04.43 Functional: Gait Practice

   q. 6.14.16 Functional: Ankle/Foot, Rhomberg and Variations

   r. 6.14.18 Functional: Ankle/Foot, Opposite Hip, 4-Way Balance Challenge

3. Plyometrics

   a. 6.09.33 Plyometrics and Variations, Knee below
- i. A: Quiet jumps double leg
- ii. B: Quiet jumps single leg
- iii. C: Box jumps forward

   b. 6.09.34 Reactive Neuromuscular Training and Variations
- i. Uniplanar anterior shift
- ii. Uniplanar lateral shift
- iii. Multiplanar weight shifts
- iv. Squat posterior weight shifts
- v. Squat anterior weight shifts
- vi. Squat posterior medial shifts
- vii. Lunge medial weight shifts
- viii. Single leg squat medial shifts band at knee

4. Sport specific agility drills; adding later in rehabilitation 12 to 16 weeks; clear with physician first.
- i. 6.09.30 Agility: Knee, Speed Ladder Drills and Variations
- ii. 6.09.31 Agility: Knee, Dot Drills and Variations
- iii. 6.09.32 Agility: Knee, Mini-Hurdle Drills and Variations
- iv. 8.01.4 Running Progressions
- v. 8.01.7 Cutting Sequence-Figure 8 Progression
- vi. 8.01.6 Jump-Hop Sequence
- vii. 8.01.5 Sprint Sequence

5. Cardiovascular program

   a. Running, elliptical, bike, swimming, Stairmaster

6. Criteria for discharge; return to sport (clear with physician)

   a. Pain-free or at least a manageable level of discomfort

   b. Manual muscle test within 10% of uninvolved LE

   c. Biodex test of quadriceps and hamstrings peak torque within 15% of uninvolved

   d. Single-leg cross-over triple hop for distance: Score of less than 85% are considered abnormal for male and female

   e. Step Down Test

   f. Y Balance Test for distance

6.05.3 HIP ARTHROPLASTY DISCUSSION

Patients with severe degeneration of the hip joint may opt to undergo a THA. THA replaces damaged bone and cartilage prosthetic components. The damaged femoral head is replaced with a metal stem with a metal or ceramic ball on one end. The stem is placed into the hollow center of the femur. The damaged cartilage surface of the acetabulum is removed and replaced with a metal socket. A plastic, ceramic, or metal spacer is inserted between the new ball and the socket to allow for smooth joint articulation.

THA is one of the most successful and cost-effective of surgical procedures with the primary goals of pain relief and restoration of function. Since THAs were introduced, there has been steady improvement in the technology associated with it, leading to better functional outcome and implant survivorship (Abdulkarim, Ellanti, Motterlini, Fahey, & O'Byrne, 2013). THA can be either cemented or non-cemented. Cemented prosthesis use a fast-drying bone cement to help affix the bone. Over time, the cement may breakdown causing the prosthesis to loosen and requiring a second THA called a *total hip revision* (THR). Noncemented is specially textured to allow the bone to grow into the prosthesis adhering it over time. Cementless bonds tend to last for longer periods of time.

Where's the Evidence?

A recent meta-analysis of randomized controlled trials found no significant difference between cemented and cementless THA patients in terms of implant survival as measured by the revision rate, mortality, or the complication rate. Additionally, they found better short-term clinical outcomes, mainly improved pain score, obtained from cemented fixation (Abdulkarim et al., 2013).

Furthermore, the minimally invasive approach which minimized soft tissue disruption was found to have an even more rapid recovery.

Where's the Evidence?

Berger et al. (2004) evaluated 100 consecutive patients who underwent the minimally invasive THA and found astonishing results. 97% of patients met all the inpatient physical therapy goals required for discharge to home on the day of surgery. 100% of patients achieved these goals within 23 hours of surgery. Outpatient therapy was initiated in 9% of patients immediately, 62% of patients by 1 week, and all patients by 2 weeks. The mean time to discontinued use of crutches, discontinued use of narcotic pain medications, and resumed driving was 6 days postoperatively. The mean time to return to work was 8 days, discontinued use of any assistive device was 9 days, and resumption of all ADL was 10 days. The mean time to walk one-half mile was 16 days. There were no readmissions, no dislocations, and no reoperations.

Physiotherapy rehabilitation after total hip replacement is accepted as a standard and essential treatment. Its aim is to maximize functionality and independence and to minimize complications such as wound infection, DVT, pulmonary embolism, and hip dislocation. The incidence of hip dislocation in the first 3 months after surgery ranges from 3% to 8% and is highest between the fourth and twelfth week post-operatively. The incidence of deep wound infection is 0.2% to 1% in the first 3 months after total joint replacement surgery. The prevalence of DVT after hip replacement surgery, including asymptomatic cases detected by venography, is between 45% and 57%. The prevalence of pulmonary embolism after THR surgery ranges from 0.7% to 30% and 0.34% to 6% for fatal pulmonary embolism.

Where's the Evidence?

Early ambulation is associated with a lower incidence of symptomatic thromboembolism after hip replacement surgery and does not increase the risk of embolization in those patients diagnosed with DVT (Health Quality Ontario, 2005).

Customized preoperative exercise programs are well tolerated by patients with end-stage hip arthritis and are effective in improving early recovery of physical function after THA (Gilbey et al., 2003). Exercise program focusing on hip external rotator muscle may lead to significant improvement of hip abductor muscle strength and gait ability in the acute post-THA stage (Nankaku et al., 2016).

Where's the Evidence?

Di Monaco, Vallero, Tappero, and Cavanna (2009) found convincing evidence in a 2009 and again in a 2013 systematic review of controlled trials to support the effectiveness in the early post-operative phase for treadmill training with partial body-weight support, unilateral resistance training of the quadriceps muscle on the operated side and arm-interval exercises with an arm ergometer. In the late post-operative phase, they found weightbearing exercises with hip abductor eccentric strengthening to be the crucial component and recommended late post-operative programs should include weightbearing exercises with hip abductor eccentric strengthening (Di Monaco & Castiglioni, 2013).

Where's the Evidence?

Recent reviews have found there was no difference in pain, functional outcomes, or patient satisfaction between patients that receive home-based rehabilitation and groups that have inpatient rehabilitation, recommending the use of a home-based rehabilitation protocol following elective primary total hip replacement as the more cost-effective strategy (Mahomed et al., 2008; Okoro, Lemmey, Maddison, & Andrew, 2012).

Physical therapy protocols are based on the surgical approach; anterior/anterolateral, posterior, or global; and whether cemented or cementless, with or without trochanteric osteotomy, and based on other operative complications that may have occurred. The following protocol will guide the therapist in treatment of the THA patient and provide general precautions for each common surgical procedure variance. Precautions are designed to maintain the placement of the prosthesis and prevent dislocation while the stabilizing soft tissues are healing.

6.05.4 HIP ARTHROPLASTY PROTOCOL

Protocol adapted from combination of protocols from the Brigham and Women's Hospital, Inc., Department of Rehabilitation Services THA/Hemiarthroplasty Protocol (Beagan, 2011).

Precautions: Follow for at Least 3 Months; Clear With Surgeon Before Discontinuing

1. All approaches
   a. No hip flexion greater than 90 degrees
   b. No hip internal rotation beyond neutral
   c. No hip adduction beyond neutral
2. Anterior approach and global approach additional precautions
   a. No hip extension or hip external rotation beyond neutral
   b. No bridging, no prone-lying
   c. When the patient is supine, keep the hip flexed to approximately 30 degrees by placing a pillow under the patient's knee or raise the head of the bed.
   d. Patients may perform a step-through gait pattern, but should avoid end-range hip extension ROM.
3. With trochanteric osteotomy
   a. Active hip abduction restricted due to the force of the contraction of the gluteus medius musculature on the reattached greater trochanter. In the post-operative order set, this will present as "Trochanter removed" or "Troch off precautions."
   b. Passive abduction only
   c. Functional abduction only; the patient should not perform hip abduction exercises but may contract the hip abductors for functional mobility such as getting out of bed or ambulating.
4. Weightbearing:
   a. Cemented THA is usually WBAT immediately post-operation
   b. Non-cemented mat be FWB/WBAT or PWB. FWB has been shown to be safe and effective after uncemented THA (Markmiller, Weiss, Kreuz, Rüter, & Konrad, 2011). However, some surgeons may restrict weightbearing post-operatively. Always follow surgeon's orders if they differ from this protocol. Surgeon's orders supersede any discrepancies with this protocol.

Phase IA: Immediate Postsurgical (Day 1 to 4):

Patient may be using a hip abduction pillow, or have the operative extremity in traction suspension based on surgeon preference. The patient may be removed from either device unless specific orders were written to remain in them. The patient does not need to return to use of the traction suspension or the hip abduction pillow unless additional orders specify. A pillow should be placed between the patient's LEs when in bed. Patients with anterior precautions may have but do not require traction suspension or a hip abduction pillow.

1. Goals:
   a. Patient education regarding dislocation precautions; *patient verbalizes understanding.*
   b. Physical therapy includes bed mobility, transfers, and gait with appropriate assistive device if necessary, and discusses increasing walking tolerance.
   c. Reinforce sitting, standing, and ADLs modifications with neutral spine postures and proper body mechanics while following precautions.
   d. Ambulate with an assistive device and ascend/descend stairs if patient must use stairs at home to allow for independence with household activities while maintaining appropriate WB.
   e. Transfer into and out of a vehicle with minimal assistance.
   f. Observe for any signs of DVT: increased swelling, redness, calf pain.
   g. Observe for signs of hip dislocation: uncontrolled pain, obvious leg length discrepancy, leg appears rotated as compared to the nonoperative extremity.
   h. Observe the patient's hip dressing and wound. If a large amount of drainage is present or blistering or frail skin around the hip joint, discuss with the nurse to decide if notifying the surgical team is indicated.
   i. Monitor for signs of pulmonary embolism and loss of peripheral nerve integrity. Notify the medical doctor immediately.
   j. Sleeping positions: a towel roll placed next to thigh just proximal to the knee should be used as needed to maintain neutral hip rotation when supine. Nothing should be placed behind the knee of the operative leg for posterior precautions. If the patient has anterior precautions, a pillow may be placed behind the operative knee to maintain slight hip flexion.
2. PROM/AAROM/ROM within ROM restrictions/postsurgical precautions

3. AROM
    a. 6.11.3 ROM: Ankle/Foot, Long-Sitting and Ankle Pumps, 4-Way, Active; *supine ankle pumps only.*
    b. 6.01.8 ROM: Hip Flexion and Extension, Heel Slide, Active
    c. 6.01.10 ROM: Hip Abduction and Adduction, Heel Slide, Active; *except if trochanteric osteotomy.*
4. Isometrics
    a. Hip
        i. 6.04.2 Strengthen: Isometric; Hip Extension/Gluteus Sets
        ii. 6.04.3 Strengthen: Isometric; Hip Abduction; *except if trochanteric osteotomy.*
        iii. 6.04.4 Strengthen: Isometric; Hip Adduction
        iv. 6.04.6 Strengthen: Isometric; Hip External Rotation
        v. 6.04.5 Strengthen: Isometric; Hip Internal Rotation
    b. Knee
        i. 6.09.3 Strengthen: Isometric; Knee Flexion, Hamstring Set
        ii. 6.09.2 Strengthen: Isometric; Knee Extension, Quadriceps Set With Ball Squeeze (Vastus Medialis Oblique)
5. Isotonics
    a. 6.09.8 Strengthen: Isotonic; Short-Arc Extension (Quadriceps)
    b. 6.09.9 Strengthen: Isotonic; Long-Arc Extension (Quadriceps)
    c. 6.09.10 Strengthen: Isotonic; Hamstring Curl (standing variation)

Phase I: Week 1 to 4

1. Continue previous exercises; progress reps and sets.
2. Gait train
    a. Wean off their assistive device between weeks 4 to 6
3. Closed kinetic chain
    a. 6.09.21 Functional: Knee, Weight Shifts
4. Cardiovascular program
    a. Recumbent bike start at 5 minutes week 3 and increase 3 to 5 minutes each week. Start to add light resistance in week 3 to 4.

Phase II: Week 4 to 6

1. Continue previous exercises
2. Strengthening
    a. 6.04.8 Strengthen: Isotonic; Hip, Straight Leg Raise, 4-Way; *avoid extension with anterior*

approach and abduction with trochanteric osteotomy.
    b. 6.04.34 Functional: Hip, Lunge and Variations; beginner variation only for forward lunge.
    c. 7.03.2 Global Functioning: Treatment Ideas; only variation below.
        i. Sit to stand
3. Closed kinetic chain
    a. 6.09.24 Functional: Knee, Step-Ups; variations listed below.
        i. Beginner
        ii. Forward
        iii. Diagonal
        iv. Lateral
4. Functional standing and gait activities
    a. 6.04.38 Functional: Hip, Sidestepping With Mini-Squat
    b. 6.04.39 Functional: Hip, Step-Overs
    c. 6.04.40 Functional: Hip, Backward Walking
    d. 6.04.43 Functional: Gait Practice
    e. Ambulation on uneven surfaces

Phase III: 5 to 12 Week Post-Operation: Progressive Strengthening:

1. Continue exercises in Phase II; progress resistance, repetitions and sets.
2. Stretching
    a. 6.01.4 ROM: Hip Extension, Standing, Active Assistive; *avoid extension with anterior approach.*
    b. 4.01.2 ROM: Lumbar Extension, Prone on Elbows, Progress to Press Up on Hands, Passive; *avoid extension with anterior approach and abduction with trochanteric osteotomy.*
    c. 6.03.3 Stretch: Hip Flexor, Standing Lunge
    d. 6.03.2 Stretch: Hip Flexor, Kneeling Lunge
    e. 6.03.7 Stretch: Hip Adductors, Frog
    f. 6.03.11 Stretch: Hip Adductors on Wall
    g. 6.03.22 Stretch: Piriformis, Figure 4 and Variations; *careful to avoid flexion > 90 degrees.*
    h. 6.08.1 Stretch: Quadriceps; *avoid extension with anterior approach.*
        i. Side-lying hand assist
        ii. Prone belt assist
    i. 6.08.3 Stretch: Hamstrings (try different variations listed below); *careful to avoid flexion > 90 degrees.*
        i. Supine
        ii. Standing foot on stool
    j. 6.13.7 Stretch: Calf on Step
3. Strengthening
    a. 6.14.7 Strengthen: Isotonic; Heel Raises

b. 4.03.1 Strengthen: Isometric; Posterior Pelvic Tilt, Lumbar Spine, With or Without Blood Pressure Cuff for Biofeedback

c. 4.03.7 Strengthen: Lumbar Spine, Bent-Knee Fall-Outs

d. 4.03.9 Strengthen: Lumbar Spine, Bent-Knee Lift

e. 6.04.13 Strengthen: Isotonic; Hip Extension, Mini-Bridge on Towel/Bolster

f. 6.04.14 Strengthen: Isotonic; Hip Extension, Bridge and Variations (listed below); *avoid extension and bridging with anterior approach.*
    i.   Bridge
    ii. Bridge with isometric adduction ball squeeze
    iii. Bridge with isometric hip abduction
    iv. Bridge in/outs

g. 6.04.16 Strengthen: Isotonic; Hip Abduction and External Rotation, "Clam" and Variations; only variations below; *caution with abduction with trochanteric osteotomy.*
    i.   Phase I

h. 6.04.23 Resistance Band, Hip, "Clam"; *caution with abduction with trochanteric osteotomy.*

i. 4.03.14 Strengthen: Lumbar Spine, Alternating Arm Lift, Leg Lift, and Combined; *avoid extension beyond 90 degrees at hip with anterior approach.*

j. 6.04.22 Strengthen: Resistance Band, Hip, Sidestepping; *caution with abduction with trochanteric osteotomy.*

4. Cardiovascular program
    a. Recumbent bike with resistance working up to 20 minutes
    b. Progressive walking/treadmill program

Phase IV: Advanced Strengthening: 12 to 16 Weeks Post-Operation

1. Balance/coordination/proprioception
    a. 7.03.2 Global Functioning: Treatment Ideas
        i.   A: Vibratory training
        ii.   B: Reaching forward (standing)
        iii. C: Dual-task: Treadmill
        iv.   H: Carrying laundry basket
        v.   I: Carrying a grocery bag
        vi.   J: Pushing grocery cart
        vii. K: Walking, turning on uneven surfaces
        viii. M: Perturbation training

2. Strengthening
    a. 6.04.26 Functional: Hip, Wall Squat
    b. 6.04.28 Functional: Hip, Free-Standing Squat
    c. 6.04.27 Functional: Hip, Wall Sit
    d. 6.14.16 Functional: Ankle/Foot, Rhomberg and Variations; *caution with sharpened Rhomberg due to hip adduction.*

e. 6.04.17 Strengthen: Isotonic; Hip Abduction, "Fire Hydrants"

f. 6.04.33 Functional: Hip, Step-Ups

g. 4.03.39 Strengthen: Abdominal, Side Plank and Variations below
    i.   A: Standing wall (beginner)
    ii. B: Standing chair (beginner)
    iii. C: On elbow and knee (beginner)
    iv. D: On elbow and feet

h. 6.04.15 Strengthen: Hip Extension, Forearm Plank

i. 4.03.24 Strengthen: Lumbar Spine, Alternating Hip and Knee Extension, Quadruped; *cautious with extension with anterior approach.*

j. 4.03.23 Strengthen: Lumbar Spine, Alternating Arm Lift, Quadruped

k. 4.03.25 Strengthen: Lumbar Spine, Opposite Arm and Leg Lift, Quadruped; *cautious with extension with anterior approach.*

l. 4.03.24 Strengthen: Lumbar Spine, Alternating Hip and Knee Extension, Quadruped

m. 4.03.27 Strengthen: Lumbar Spine, Hold Neutral Spine, Tall-Kneeling

n. 4.03.28 Strengthen: Lumbar Spine, Arm Lift, Tall-Kneeling

o. 4.03.30 Strengthen: Lumbar Spine, Reach Toward Floor, Half Kneeling

p. 4.03.29 Strengthen: Lumbar Spine, Reach Toward Floor, Tall-Kneeling

q. 4.03.38 Strengthen: Abdominal, Plank and Variations below
    i.   A: Standing wall (beginner)
    ii. B: Standing chair (beginner)
    iii. C: Quadruped
    iv. D: Forearm
    v.   E: Hands

r. 4.03.42 Strengthen: Abdominal, Pulsing Crunch, 3-Way (Advanced)

s. 6.04.37 Functional: Pelvic Drop/Hip Hike; *cautious with hip adduction.*

t. 6.14.18 Functional: Ankle/Foot, Opposite Hip, 4-Way Balance Challenge

u. 6.14.19 Functional: Ankle/Foot, Single-Leg Mini-Squat and Reach, All Directions

v. 6.14.21 Functional: Ankle/Foot, Nintendo Wii
    i.   For exercise that enhances balance
    ii. For muscle strengthening exercise

3. Criteria for discharge; clear with physician.
    a. Non-antalgic gait
    b. Manual muscle test (MMT) 4+/5 or better
    c. Normal balance
    d. Independent stairs
    e. Independent home program

References

Abdulkarim, A., Ellanti, P., Motterlini, N., Fahey, T., & O'Byrne, J. M. (2013). Cemented versus uncemented fixation in total hip replacement: A systematic review and meta-analysis of randomized controlled trials. *Orthopedic Reviews, 5*(1), e8.

Beagan, C. (2011). Total hip arthroplasty/hemiarthroplasty protocol. *Brigham and Women's Hospital*. Retrieved from http://www.brighamandwomens.org/Patients_Visitors/pcs/RehabilitationServices/Physical-Therapy-Standards-of-Care-and-Protocols/Hip-Total%20Hip%20Arthroplasty.pdf

Berger, R. A., Jacobs, J. J., Meneghini, R. M., Della Valle, C., Paprosky, W., & Rosenberg, A. G. (2004). Rapid rehabilitation and recovery with minimally invasive total hip arthroplasty. *Clinical Orthopedics and Related Research*, (429), 239-247.

Chandrasekaran, S., Lindner, D., Martin, T. J., Lodhia, P., Suarez-Ahedo, C., & Domb, B. G. (2015). Technique of arthroscopically assisted transtrochanteric drilling for femoral head chondral defects. *Arthroscopy Techniques, 4*(4), 287-291.

Di Monaco, M., & Castiglioni, C. (2013). Which type of exercise therapy is effective after hip arthroplasty? A systematic review of randomized controlled trials. *European Journal of Physical Rehabilitation and Medicine, 49*(6), 893-907.

Di Monaco, M., Vallero, F., Tappero, R., & Cavanna, A. (2009). Rehabilitation after total hip arthroplasty: A systematic review of controlled trials on physical exercise programs. *European Journal of Physical and Rehabilitation Medicine, 45*(3), 303-317.

Gilbey, H. J., Ackland, T. R., Wang, A. W., Morton, A. R., Trouchet, T., & Tapper, J. (2003). Exercise improves early functional recovery after total hip arthroplasty. Clinical Orthopedics and Related Research, (408), 193-200.

Health Quality Ontario. (2005). Physiotherapy rehabilitation after total knee or hip replacement. *Ontario Health Technology Assessement Series, 5*(8), 1-91.

Hergan, D. (n.d.). Post-operative hip arthroscopy rehabilitation Protocol: Labral repair with or without FAI component. *David J. Hergan, MD, MS.* Retrieved from http://www.davidherganmd.com/pdf/post-operative-hip-arthroscopy-rehabilitation-protocol-for-dr-hergan.pdf

Kelly, B. T. (n.d.). Hip arthroscopy rehabilitation labral debridement with or without FAI component. *Dr Bryan T Kelly.* Retrieved from http://www.bryankellymd.com/pdf/labral-debridement-fai-component.pdf

Mahomed, N. N., Davis, A. M., Hawker, G., Badley, E., Davey, J. R., Syed, K. A., . . . Wright, J. G. (2008). Inpatient compared with home-Based rehabilitation following primary unilateral total hip or knee replacement: A randomized controlled trial. *Journal of Bone and Joint Surgery, 90*(8), 1673-1680.

Markmiller, M., Weiss, T., Kreuz, P., Rüter, A., & Konrad, G. (2011). Partial weightbearing is not necessary after cementless total hip arthroplasty: A two-year prospective randomized study on 100 patients. *International Orthopedics, 35*(8), 1139-1143.

Nankaku, M., Ikeguchi, R., Goto, K., So, K., Kuroda, Y., & Matsuda, S. (2016). Hip external rotator exercise contributes to improving physical functions in the early stage after total hip arthroplasty using an anterolateral approach: A randomized controlled trial. *Disability and Rehabilitation, 38*(22), 2178-2183.

Okoro, T., Lemmey, A. B., Maddison, P., & Andrew, J. G. (2012). An appraisal of rehabilitation regimes used for improving functional outcome after total hip replacement surgery. *Sports Medicine, Arthroscopy, Rehabilitation, Therapy and Technology, 4*(1), 5.

Schmerl, M., Pollard, H., & Hoskins, W. (2005). Labral injuries of the hip: A review of diagnosis and management. *Journal of Manipulative and Physiological Therapeutics, 28*(8), 632.

University of Wisconsin Sports Rehabilitation. (2013). Rehabilitation guidelines for hip. *UW Health Sports Rehabilitation.* Retrieved from http://www.uwhealth.org/files/uwhealth/docs/pdf2/Rehab_Hip_Arthroscopy.pdf

Section 6.06

KNEE RANGE OF MOTION

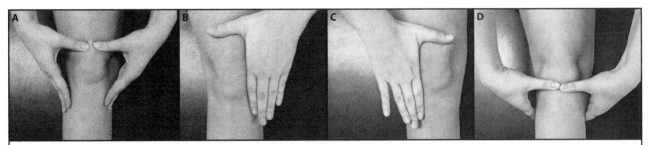

6.06.1 ROM: PATELLAR MOBILIZATION, ACTIVE ASSISTIVE

POSITION: Long-sitting

TARGETS: Mobility of the patella

INSTRUCTION: Patient long sits with knee extended or on a small towel roll for open packed position of the patellofemoral joint. *Inferior glide*: Patient places thumbs on upper edge of patella and slides patella inferiorly (A). *Lateral glide*: Patient places contralateral thumb web space and lateral surface of index finger along medial border of patella and slides patella laterally (B). *Medial glide*: Patient places ipsilateral thumb web space and lateral surface of index finger along lateral border of patella and slides patella medially (C). *Superior glide*: Patient places thumbs on lower edge of patella and slides patella superior (D).

SUBSTITUTIONS: Leg should be stable

PARAMETERS: Hold for 5 seconds, 10 repetitions, repeat 1 to 3 times per day

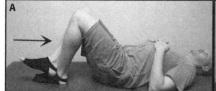
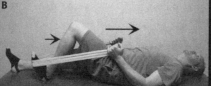
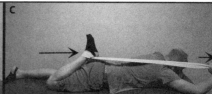

6.06.2 ROM: Knee Flexion, Active Assistive

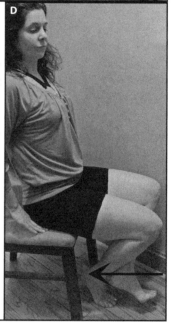

Position: Supine, seated

Targets: Mobility of the knee into flexion

Instruction: *Supine*: Patient slides target heel toward ipsilateral buttock while other ankle is hooked in front of shin, assisting to pull heel closer to buttock. To return, patient hooks behind the ankle with unaffected foot and assists to bring knee back into extension (A). *Supine with belt*: Patient loops strap around foot and pulls with both arms to bring heel closer to buttock as heel slides along mat. To return, patient hooks behind the ankle with unaffected foot and assists to bring knee back into extension (B). *Prone*: Patient bends target knee, bringing heel toward buttock while other ankle is hooked in front of shin, assisting to pull heel further toward the buttock. To return, patient hooks behind the ankle with unaffected foot and assists to bring knee back into extension (C). *Seated*: Patient sits on front half of chair and slides target heel underneath the chair while other ankle is hooked in front of shin, assisting to pull heel further underneath. To return, patient hooks behind the ankle with unaffected foot and assists to bring knee back into extension (D).

Substitutions: Pelvis movements; in chair, patient stays fully seated and trunk upright.

Parameters: Hold for 10 to 15 seconds, 10 repetitions, repeat 1 to 3 times per day

6.06.3 ROM: Knee Flexion, Wall Slide, Active Assistive

Position: Supine

Targets: Mobility of the knee into flexion

Instruction: *Supine*: Patient scoot buttocks toward the wall as therapist assist with legs to place heels on wall. Buttocks are 15 to 25 cm from wall. Patient begins to slide target heel toward ipsilateral buttock while other ankle is hooked in front of shin, assisting to pull heel closer to buttock. To return, patient hooks behind the ankle with unaffected foot and assists to bring knee back into extension (A and B).

Substitutions: Knee stays in line with hip

Parameters: Hold for 10 to 15 seconds, 10 repetitions, repeat 1 to 3 times per day

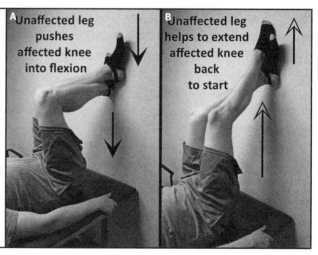

6.06.4 ROM: Knee Flexion, Rocking Chair, Active Assistive

Position: Seated in a rocking chair

Targets: Mobility of the knee into flexion

Instruction: A rocking chair is a great way to increase knee flexion. Patient scoots to edge of rocking chair and brings target foot back as far as possible. Patient then rocks gently forward to increase knee flexion and holds. Patient then rocks back for a rest, attempts to bring heel even further back, and repeats, each time going a little further to increase ROM (not shown).

Substitutions: Pelvic movements; in chair, patient stays fully seated and trunk upright.

Parameters: Hold for 5 to 10 seconds, 10 to 20 repetitions, repeat 1 to 3 times per day

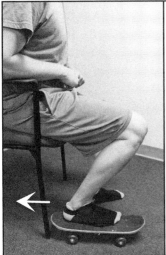

6.06.5 ROM: KNEE FLEXION, SKATEBOARD, ACTIVE ASSISTIVE

POSITION: Seated

TARGETS: Mobility of the knee into flexion

INSTRUCTION: A skateboard is a great way to increase knee flexion. Patient sits in front half of chair and places target foot on skateboard. Patient rolls target foot back underneath as far as possible and then, placing other foot in front, pushes the skateboard further back to assist further knee flexion. Hold and then assist to allow skateboard to come forward and repeat.

SUBSTITUTIONS: Pelvic movements; in chair, patient stays fully seated and trunk upright.

PARAMETERS: Hold for 5 to 10 seconds, 10 to 20 repetitions, repeat 1 to 3 times per day

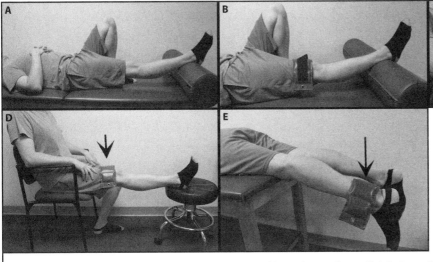

6.06.6 ROM: KNEE EXTENSION, PASSIVE

POSITION: Supine, seated, prone

TARGETS: Mobility of the hip into extension using gravity and weight assist

INSTRUCTION: *Supine:* Prop patient's ankle/foot on a bolster, allowing gravity to pull knee down into extension (A). Add weight to increase the stretch; a cuff weight works well (B). *Seated patient presses:* Patient in long-sitting or slightly reclined, if hamstring tightness is an issue, place leg in same position as described for supine. Patient then presses downward with both hands just above the knee; hold 20 to 30 seconds for 3 to 5 repetitions (C). *Seated:* Prop target ankle onto chair in front of patient and add weight to stretch knee into extension (D). *Prone:* Patient scoots to the edge of the table and allows knee to drop off end. Edge of the table should cross just above the knee. Patient relaxes leg muscles to allow gravity to straighten the knee. Encourage PPT to protect the lumbar spine. Add cuff weight to increase the stretch (E).

SUBSTITUTIONS: Pelvic or trunk movement; hip, knee, and ankle stay in alignment in sagittal plane.

PARAMETERS: Allow end stretch to last 5 to 10 minutes, repeat 1 to 3 times per day

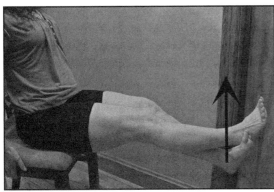

6.06.7 ROM: KNEE EXTENSION, ACTIVE ASSISTIVE

POSITION: Supine, seated

TARGETS: Mobility of the knee into extension

INSTRUCTION: Patient sits in chair and hooks behind the ankle with unaffected foot and assists to bring knee into extension.

SUBSTITUTIONS: Pelvic movements; in chair. patient stays fully seated and trunk upright.

PARAMETERS: Hold for 5 to 10 seconds, 10 repetitions, repeat 1 to 3 times per day

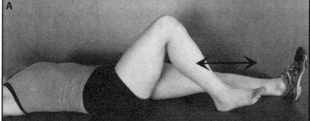

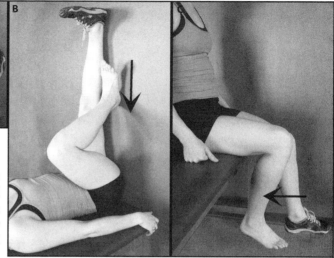

6.06.8 ROM: Knee, Heel Slides, Active

POSITION: Supine, seated

TARGETS: Mobility of the hip into flexion and extension

INSTRUCTION: *Supine*: Patient slides the affected heel toward buttocks as he or she bends the knee. Hold a gentle stretch in this position and then return to fully extended (A). *Supine wall*: Patient scoots buttocks toward the wall as therapist assist with legs to place heels on wall. Buttocks are 15 to 25 cm from wall. Patient slides target heel toward ipsilateral buttock bending the knee, holds for a gentle stretch, and returns to fully extend the knee (B). *Seated*: Patient sits on front half of chair and slides target side heel back under chair to bend knee as far as possible, holds for gentle stretch, and then extends knee fully, keeping heel on floor. Repeat (C).

SUBSTITUTIONS: Pelvic or trunk movement; hip, knee, and ankle stay in alignment in sagittal plane.

PARAMETERS: Hold for 5 to 10 seconds, 10 to 20 repetitions, repeat 1 to 3 times per day

6.06.9 ROM: Knee Flexion and Extension Against Gravity, Active

POSITION: Seated, standing

TARGETS: Mobility of the hip into flexion and extension

INSTRUCTION: *Seated extension*: Patient sitting upright and buttocks back in chair extends the knee, bringing the toes up toward the ceiling (A). *Standing flexion*: Patient holds on to stable object for balance and bends knee, bringing heel toward the buttock (B).

SUBSTITUTIONS: Slow movement encouraged to limit momentum of a kicking action. Limit pelvic or trunk movement; hip, knee, and ankle stay in alignment in sagittal plane.

PARAMETERS: Hold for 2 to 3 seconds, 10 to 20 repetitions, repeat 1 to 3 times per day

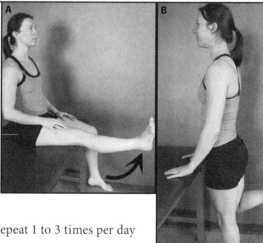

Section 6.07

KNEE JOINT SELF-MOBILIZATION

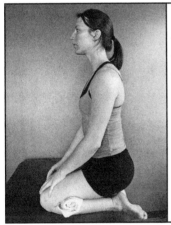

6.07.1 SELF-JOINT MOBILIZATION: KNEE FLEXION

POSITION: Tall-kneeling

TARGETS: Mobility of the tibiofemoral joint into flexion and posterior capsule stretch

INSTRUCTION: Patient kneels with towel roll just below the knee at the level of the tibial tuberosity and sits back until a slight stretch is felt. Patient applies a downward push on top of distal thigh to push further into flexion.

SUBSTITUTIONS: Shifting pelvis or trunk to one side or the other; keep hip, knee and ankle aligned in sagittal plane.

PARAMETERS: Hold 3 to 5 seconds, repeat 10 to 20 times, 1 to 3 times per day

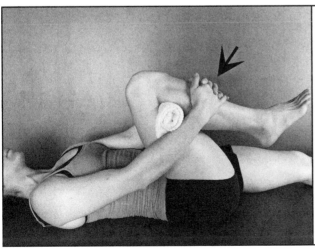

6.07.2 SELF-JOINT MOBILIZATION: ANTERIOR TIBIAL GLIDE

POSITION: Supine

TARGETS: Mobility of the tibiofemoral joint to increase extension and anterior capsule stretch

INSTRUCTION: Place towel roll in popliteal crease of knee and have patient bring knee to chest with hands clasped around anterior tibial plateau while squeezing knee into flexion. Towel roll presses anteriorly on the proximal tibia to assist in anterior gliding.

SUBSTITUTIONS: Encourage stabilization of core and gluteals muscles to avoid pelvic tilting posteriorly.

PARAMETERS: Hold 3 to 5 seconds, repeat 10 to 20 times, 1 to 3 times per day

Section 6.08

KNEE STRETCHING

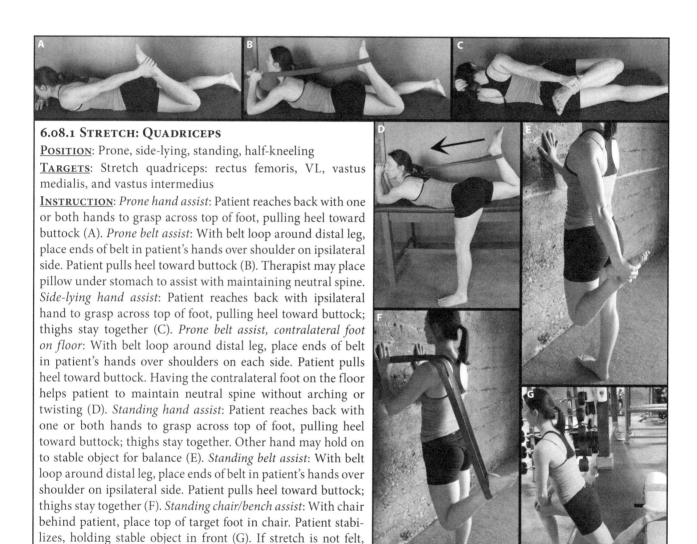

6.08.1 STRETCH: QUADRICEPS

POSITION: Prone, side-lying, standing, half-kneeling

TARGETS: Stretch quadriceps: rectus femoris, VL, vastus medialis, and vastus intermedius

INSTRUCTION: *Prone hand assist*: Patient reaches back with one or both hands to grasp across top of foot, pulling heel toward buttock (A). *Prone belt assist*: With belt loop around distal leg, place ends of belt in patient's hands over shoulder on ipsilateral side. Patient pulls heel toward buttock (B). Therapist may place pillow under stomach to assist with maintaining neutral spine. *Side-lying hand assist*: Patient reaches back with ipsilateral hand to grasp across top of foot, pulling heel toward buttock; thighs stay together (C). *Prone belt assist, contralateral foot on floor*: With belt loop around distal leg, place ends of belt in patient's hands over shoulders on each side. Patient pulls heel toward buttock. Having the contralateral foot on the floor helps patient to maintain neutral spine without arching or twisting (D). *Standing hand assist*: Patient reaches back with one or both hands to grasp across top of foot, pulling heel toward buttock; thighs stay together. Other hand may hold on to stable object for balance (E). *Standing belt assist*: With belt loop around distal leg, place ends of belt in patient's hands over shoulder on ipsilateral side. Patient pulls heel toward buttock; thighs stay together (F). *Standing chair/bench assist*: With chair behind patient, place top of target foot in chair. Patient stabilizes, holding stable object in front (G). If stretch is not felt, patient may lunge on stance leg to deepen stretch. Make sure stance knee does not come more anterior than toes. For even further stretch in chair, patient places top of foot at chair back and stands to the side of the chair. *(continued)*

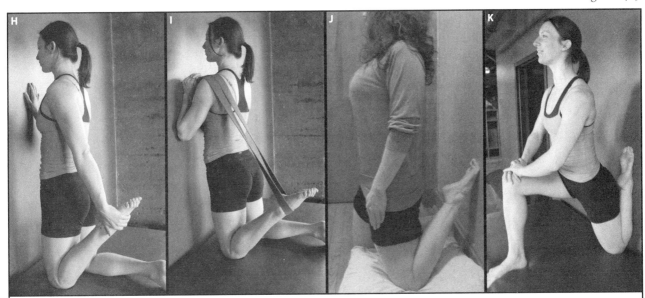

6.08.1 STRETCH: QUADRICEPS (CONTINUED)

Half-kneeling hand assist: Patient half-kneels in front of wall to stabilize balance. With target leg in back, knee directly under hip, patient reaches back with ipsilateral hand to pull heel toward buttock (H). This can also be done with a belt (I). *Tall- and half-kneeling against a wall*: Patient kneels, facing away from wall with feet against wall. Patient leans forward and places target knee side against wall with top of foot lying against wall. Patient then brings trunk back to upright as stretch is felt in anterior thigh (J). This can also be done in half-kneeling with other leg lunged in front of the patient (K).

SUBSTITUTIONS: Quadriceps will pull the pelvis into an anterior tilt; patient should strongly engage lower abdominals to posteriorly pelvic tilt and avoid lumbar extension and any trunk twist during any of the above. Also watch shoulders encouraging scapular retraction when reaching behind and avoid shrugging.

PARAMETERS: Hold for 15 to 30 seconds, 3 to 5 repetitions, 1 to 3 times per day

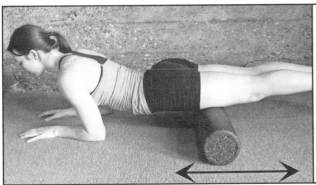

6.08.2 FOAM ROLLER: QUADRICEPS

POSITION: Prone

TARGETS: Soft tissue release, self-massage quadriceps

INSTRUCTION: Patient positions thighs on foam roller and comes into a forearm plank position. Patient rolls body over the foam roller from pelvis to knee and back, slowly holding over sore spots as tolerated.

SUBSTITUTIONS: Avoid pressures that are excessively painful; watch that patient is not shrugging shoulders.

PARAMETERS: Massage 2 to 5 minutes, 1 to 3 times per day

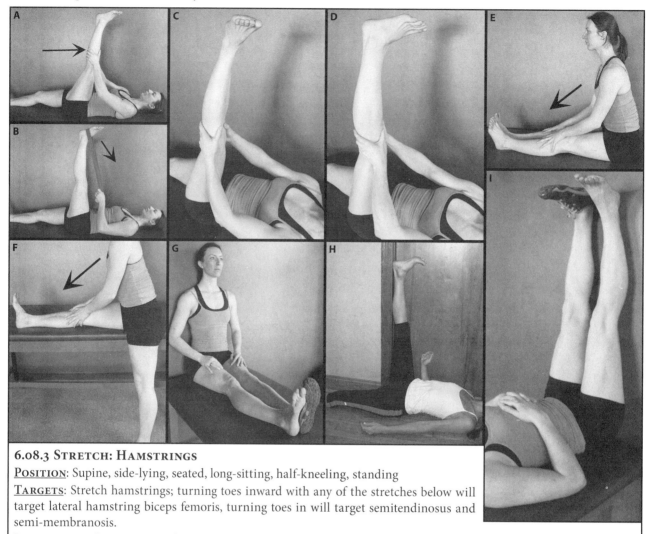

6.08.3 STRETCH: HAMSTRINGS

<u>POSITION</u>: Supine, side-lying, seated, long-sitting, half-kneeling, standing

<u>TARGETS</u>: Stretch hamstrings; turning toes inward with any of the stretches below will target lateral hamstring biceps femoris, turning toes in will target semitendinosus and semi-membranosis.

<u>INSTRUCTION</u>: *Supine*: Patient brings one knee up as other leg stays extended on mat. Patient grasps behind the knee as hip flexes to 90 degrees. Patient then extends the knee as far as possible and pulls the leg toward the chest (A). This can also be done by looping a belt or towel around the arch of the foot and pulling leg toward chest (B). To target medial hamstrings, turn the toes laterally (C). To target lateral hamstrings, turn the toes medially (D.) This modification can be done with any of the hamstring exercises when wanting to target medial or lateral hamstrings. *Long-sitting*: Patient bends non-target knee and tucks foot next to medial thigh of target leg. With back straight, patient bends chest toward extended leg until stretch is felt in back of thigh (E). If patient is on a table, dropping one leg off mat as shown is also effective (F). *Long-sitting against a wall*: Patient sits upright against a wall with hips at 90 degrees and knees extended, patient should feel stretch in bilateral posterior thigh. If not, advance to deeper stretches (G). *Supine doorway/corner*: Patient lies in doorway, along corner with doorjamb, or facing wall on target side. Patient places heel on doorjamb and slides buttock toward wall with knee extended until stretch is felt in posterior thigh. Opposite leg lies extended on floor (H). *Supine wall*: Patient slides buttocks to wall and places heels on wall with knees extended until stretch is felt in posterior thigh (I). *(continued)*

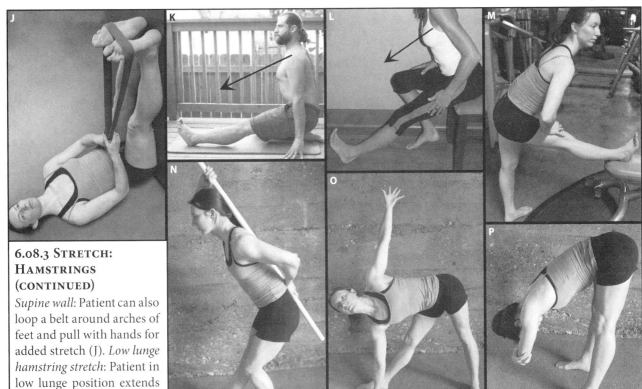

6.08.3 STRETCH: HAMSTRINGS (CONTINUED)

Supine wall: Patient can also loop a belt around arches of feet and pull with hands for added stretch (J). *Low lunge hamstring stretch*: Patient in low lunge position extends front knee and flexes back knee as patient sits back into hips with trunk forward. Patient keeps spine straight as hip hinge forward occurs. Stretch is felt in posterior thigh of extended leg (K). *Seated*: Patient extends one knee and places heel on floor. Patient straightens spine and hinges forward at the hips, leading with the chest, and brings trunk forward over knee until a stretch is felt in back of thigh (L). *Standing foot on bench*: Patient rests target foot on bench or chair and, keeping back straight, leans forward with chest leading the way until stretch is felt in back of thigh (M). *Hip hinge with dowel*: Patient uses the dowel to give feedback and assist with keeping back straight. Patient places the dowel along the spine and attempts to keep contact at the sacrum, lower back, and upper back while placing one foot in front with extended knee. Opposite knee is flexed to 45 degrees. Patient hinges forward at the hips leading with the chest and maintaining all points of contact with dowel rod until stretch is felt in the posterior thigh of the extended leg. This can be done without the dowel rod if patient can maintain a straight spine (N). *Extended triangle pose advanced (yoga)*: Patient stands with wide stance and points target side toes out. Non-target leg toes are pointed forward. Patient abducts shoulders to 90 degrees and stands tall. Patient then reaches laterally with fingertips over target leg and bends at the hips, bringing fingertips to target leg's ankle but pushing hip posteriorly over back leg. Pelvis stays in straight plane directly in line with legs and opposite arm extends fingertips toward ceiling. Patient should feel a stretching posterior thigh of front leg (O). *Forward fold advanced (yoga)*: Patient exhales as patient bends forward at the hips, lengthening the front of the torso. Patient bends elbows and holds onto each elbow with the opposite hand, letting the crown of the head hang down. Patient presses heels to floor as patient lifts the hips toward the ceiling. Knees can be slightly flexed to extended but not locked out (P).

SUBSTITUTIONS: Hamstrings will pull the pelvis into a posterior tilt and flex the lumbar spine; patient should strongly engage lower abdominals and lumbar extensors to maintain neutral spine and pelvis, avoiding lumbar flexion and any trunk twist during any of the above; also watch shoulders, encouraging scapular retraction when reaching and avoid shrugging.

PARAMETERS: Hold for 15 to 30 seconds, 3 to 5 repetitions, 1 to 3 times per day

Where's the Evidence?

Fasen et al. (2009) compared four different hamstring-stretching techniques: two basic types of active stretching, in which ROM is increased through voluntary contraction, and passive stretching, in which ROM is increased through external assistance. The two types of active stretching include neuromobilization and PNF. One hundred subjects between the ages of 21 and 57 were enrolled in the study. Outcome measures included hamstring length and perceived level of hamstring tightness. After 4 weeks of stretching, there was a statistically significant improvement in hamstring length using active stretches as compared with passive stretches. From weeks 4 through 8, hamstring length for the active stretching groups decreased. After 8 weeks of stretching, the SLR passive stretch group had the greatest improvement in hamstring length. Improvement in hamstring flexibility was greatest for the SLR passive stretch.

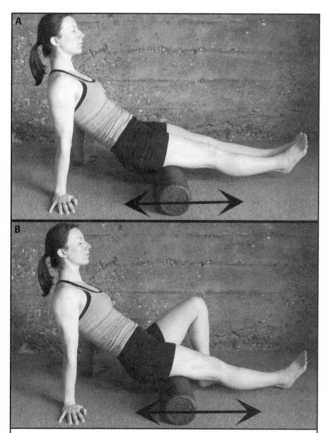

6.08.4 FOAM ROLLER: HAMSTRINGS

POSITION: Long-sitting

TARGETS: Soft tissue release/self-massage hamstrings

INSTRUCTION: Patient positions thighs on foam roller as patient supports weight with arms. Patient rolls body over the foam roller from ischial tuberosities to knee and back, slowly holding over sore spots as tolerated (A). Added pressure to one side is done by bending the other hip and knee (B).

SUBSTITUTIONS: Avoid pressures that are excessively painful; watch that patient is not shrugging shoulders.

PARAMETERS: Massage 2 to 5 minutes, 1 to 3 times per day

6.08.5 STRETCH: OTHER IMPORTANT MUSCLES THAT CROSS KNEE

There are other muscles not listed here that cross the knee as well as the hip or ankle. These muscles are also important to consider when designing a flexibility program for the knee. The stretches can be found under the other joints that they cross in addition to the knee. Listed below are some of these other muscles and where to find in this text:

1. Gracilis (hip adductor, knee flexor)
    a. 6.03.11 Stretch: Hip Adductors on Wall
    b. 6.03.9 Stretch: Hip Adductors With Belt
2. Sartorius (hip flexor, abductor, external rotator, knee flexor)
    a. 6.03.26 Stretch: Sartorius
3. ITB/TFL (hip abductor, knee flexor)
    a. 6.03.18 Stretch: Iliotibial Band With Belt
    b. 6.03.19 Stretch: Iliotibial Band, Leg Hang
    c. 6.03.20 Stretch: Iliotibial Band, Standing Variations
4. Gastrocnemius (ankle plantarflexor, knee flexor)
    a. 6.13.6 Stretch: Soleus Using Strap
    b. 6.13.5 Stretch: Gastrocnemius Using Strap
    c. 6.13.7 Stretch: Calf on Step
    d. 6.13.8 Stretch: Calf on Ramp

REFERENCE

Fasen, J. M., O'Connor, A. M., Schwartz, S. L., Watson, J. O., Plastaras, C. T., Garvan, C. W., . . . Akuthota, V. (2009). A randomized controlled trial of hamstring stretching: comparison of four techniques. *Journal of Strength and Conditioning Research, 23*(2), 660-667.

Section 6.09

KNEE STRENGTHENING

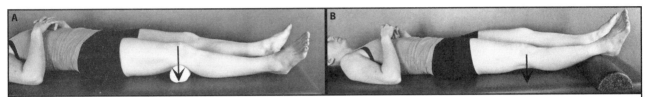

6.09.1 Strengthen: Isometric; Knee Extension, Quadriceps Set

POSITION: Supine, long-sitting

TARGETS: Beginner facilitation and strengthening of quadriceps; rectus femoris, VL, vastus medialis, and vastus intermedius.

INSTRUCTION: Start with small towel roll under knee and progress to no towel roll. Patient presses knee down into towel or mat while tightening top thigh muscles and extending the knee as heel lifts off bed (A). To assist in achieving full extension, place a towel roll under ankle (B). Patient can be supine or long-sitting.

SUBSTITUTIONS: Toes should point straight up to ceiling

PARAMETERS: Hold for 6 to 10 seconds with 1- to 2-second ramp up and down, 8 to 12 repetitions, 1 to 3 sets, 1 time per day or every other day

---

Where's the Evidence?

A study that looked at limb position and ROM to identify muscle activation of VL and vastus medialis found the optimal ROM for VMO is the final 1 degree of extension (Signorile et al., 2014).

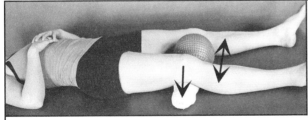

6.09.2 Strengthen: Isometric; Knee Extension, Quadriceps Set With Ball Squeeze (Vastus Medialis Oblique)

POSITION: Supine, long-sitting

TARGETS: Beginner facilitation and strengthening of quadriceps; rectus femoris, VL, VMO, and vastus intermedius, with primary focus on VMO.

INSTRUCTION: Start with small towel roll under knees and progressing to no towel roll. Patient presses squeeze a 15- to 20-cm ball between knees as patient presses knees down into towel or mat while tightening top thigh muscles and extending the knee as heels lift off bed. To assist in achieving full extension, place a towel roll under ankle. Patient can be supine or long-sitting.

SUBSTITUTIONS: Toes should point straight up to ceiling or slightly outward; watch for best activation of VMO.

PARAMETERS: Hold for 6 to 10 seconds with 1- to 2-second ramp up and down, 8 to 12 repetitions, 1 to 3 sets, 1 time per day or every other day

Where's the Evidence?

A randomized, single-blind controlled study found a large number of patellofemoral pain syndrome patients can experience significant improvements in pain, function, and quality of life, at least in the short-term, with quadriceps femoris rehabilitation, with or without emphasis on selective activation of the VMO component. Both approaches would seem acceptable for rehabilitating patients with patellofemoral pain syndrome (Syme, Rowe, Martin, & Daly, 2009).

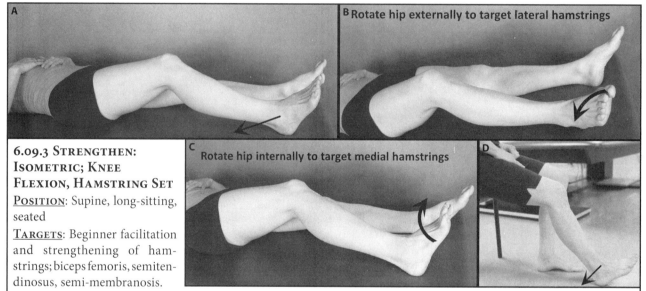

A

B Rotate hip externally to target lateral hamstrings

C Rotate hip internally to target medial hamstrings

D

6.09.3 STRENGTHEN: ISOMETRIC; KNEE FLEXION, HAMSTRING SET

POSITION: Supine, long-sitting, seated

TARGETS: Beginner facilitation and strengthening of hamstrings; biceps femoris, semitendinosus, semi-membranosis.

INSTRUCTION: *Supine, long-sitting*: Start with slight bend in target knee. Patient digs heel into mat while attempting to flex the knee with mat resisting (A). Patient may turn hip outward, externally rotating 45 degrees to target lateral hamstring (bicep femoris) or inward internally rotating 45 degrees to target medial hamstrings (semitendinosus, semi-membranosis) with any of the above exercises (B and C). *Sitting*: Patient slides to front half of chair and brings target heel out to allow slight bend in knee, with other foot planted on floor in 90/90. Patient digs heel into floor while attempting to flex the knee with floor resisting (D).

SUBSTITUTIONS: Patient may substitute with just pressing heel into mat/floor, which will target more gluteus with hamstring assist; to isolate hamstring, patient must focus on attempting to bend knee.

PARAMETERS: Hold for 6 to 10 seconds with 1- to 2-second ramp up and down, 8 to 12 repetitions, 1 to 3 sets, 1 time per day or every other day

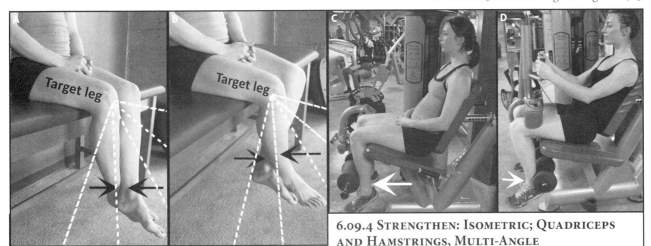

6.09.4 Strengthen: Isometric; Quadriceps and Hamstrings, Multi-Angle

POSITION: Seated

TARGETS: Beginner facilitation and strengthening of quadriceps; rectus femoris, VL, vastus medialis, vastus intermedius, and hamstrings; biceps femoris, semitendinosus, semi-membranosis.

INSTRUCTION: *Quadriceps*: Patient sits with both legs hanging down. Patient places non-target ankle over the top of the target ankle. Patient attempts to lift the target foot up toward ceiling while attempting to extend the knee as the non-target leg resists. This can be done at multiple knee flexion angles (usually 30, 45, 60, 90, and 120 degrees) (A). *Hamstrings*: Patient sits with both legs hanging down. Patient places non-target ankle under the target ankle. Patient attempts to bring the target down and back toward buttock while attempting to flex the knee as the non-target leg resists. This can be done at multiple knee flexion angles (usually 30, 45, 60, 90, and 120 degrees) (B). Multi-angle isometrics can also be done using gym equipment hamstring curl machine (C) and knee extension machines (D). *Weight is set at maximum so that it applies enough force to resist any movement.* Use the machine setting to adjust the angle.

SUBSTITUTIONS: Patient may substitute with just pressing heel into mat/floor, which will target more gluteus with hamstring assist; to isolate hamstring, patient must focus on attempting to bend knee.

PARAMETERS: Hold for 6 to 10 seconds with 1- to 2-second ramp up and down, 8 to 12 repetitions, 1 to 3 sets, 1 time per day or every other day

6.09.5 Strengthen: Isometric; Knee, Straight Leg Raise, 4-Way

This exercise targets the hip and knee. See instructions under hip strengthening **6.04.8**; add cuff weights to increase resistance.

6.09.6 STRENGTHEN: ISOTONIC; STRAIGHT LEG RAISE AND MUNCIE METHOD, (VASTUS MEDIALIS OBLIQUE)

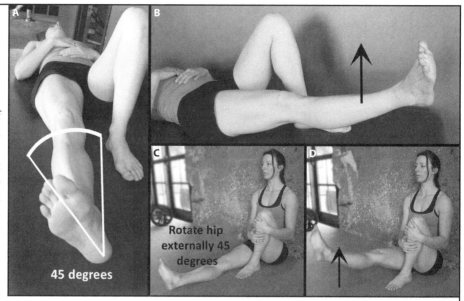

POSITION: Supine, long-sitting

TARGETS: Strengthening of quadriceps and hip flexors with primary focus on VMO

INSTRUCTION: *Supine*: Patient lies supine with unaffected knee bent and foot planted. Patient externally rotates the target hip outward 45 degrees then tightens quadriceps muscle, focusing on "teardrop" VMO medial distal thigh on extended leg. Keeping knee straight, patient lifts foot straight up toward ceiling with toes pointed diagonally outward at a 45-degree angle until heel is 15 cm off mat (A and B). *Muncie method long-sitting taps (advanced)*: Patient sits with buttock scooted up to wall and back straight. Non-target knee is hugged to chest. Patient externally rotates the target hip outward 45 degrees then tightens quadriceps muscle focusing on "teardrop" VMO medial distal thigh on extended leg. Keeping knee straight, patient lifts foot straight up toward ceiling with toes pointed diagonally outward at a 45-degree angle until heel is 15 cm off mat. Patient then lowers leg to "tap" heel on mat and immediately lifts again, repeating until fatigued. Many patients can only do one or two to start (C and D). Add cuff weights to increase resistance.

SUBSTITUTIONS: Maintain neutral pelvis; active lower abdominal core encouraged, knee stays fully extended; do not allow extensor lag (bending of knee); strong active VMO contraction encouraged throughout movements.

PARAMETERS: 8 to 12 repetitions, 1 to 3 sets, 1 time per day or every other day

Where's the Evidence?

In a study comparing traditional therapy in clinic, home therapy, and home therapy with the Muncie method, patients using the Muncie method at home demonstrated improved clinical outcome at a lower cost than traditional home and physical therapy and improved VMO/quadriceps muscle balance. The study suggests patients with anterior knee pain may benefit from applying the Muncie method in a home therapy program (Rousch et al., 2000).

6.09.7 STRENGTHEN: ISOTONIC; STRAIGHT LEG RAISE, ADDUCTION (VASTUS MEDIALIS OBLIQUE)

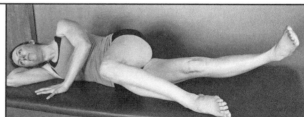

POSITION: Side-lying

TARGETS: Strengthening of hip adductors and quadriceps with primary focus on VMO

INSTRUCTION: Patient side-lying on affected side with top leg placed in front and allowing bent knee to rest on table or with foot planted, patient internally rotates bottom hip so that toes are oriented toward the ceiling, tightens quadriceps muscle on top, and, keeping knee straight, lifts leg up as toes stay pointed toward the ceiling with hip internally rotated. Add cuff weights to increase resistance.

SUBSTITUTIONS: Maintain neutral pelvis; active lower abdominal core encouraged, knee stays fully extended; do not allow bending of knee; strong active VMO contraction encouraged throughout movements.

PARAMETERS: 8 to 12 repetitions, 1 to 3 sets, 1 time per day or every other day

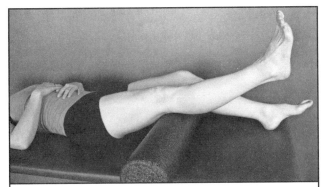

6.09.8 STRENGTHEN: ISOTONIC; SHORT-ARC EXTENSION (QUADRICEPS)

POSITION: Supine, long-sitting

TARGETS: Strengthening of quadriceps; rectus femoris, VL, vastus medialis, and vastus intermedius.

INSTRUCTION: Place a medium bolster or coffee can under the knee. Patient lifts the toes toward the ceiling, keeping the back of the knee in contact with the bolster/can. For VMO focus, rotate the hip to 45 degrees toe out. Add cuff weights to increase resistance.

SUBSTITUTIONS: Lifting knee off bolster or can

PARAMETERS: 8 to 12 repetitions, 1 to 3 sets, 1 time per day or every other day

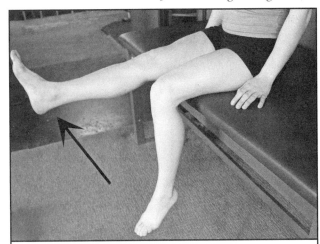

6.09.9 STRENGTHEN: ISOTONIC; LONG-ARC EXTENSION (QUADRICEPS)

POSITION: Seated

TARGETS: Strengthening of quadriceps; rectus femoris, VL, vastus medialis, and vastus intermedius.

INSTRUCTION: Patient lifts the toes toward the ceiling. Add cuff weights to increase resistance.

SUBSTITUTIONS: Maintain neutral pelvis; active lower abdominal core encouraged, knee stays fully extended; do not allow bending of knee; strong active VMO contraction encouraged throughout movements.

PARAMETERS: 8 to 12 repetitions, 1 to 3 sets, 1 time per day or every other day

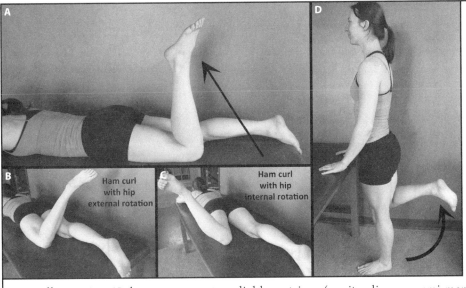

6.09.10 STRENGTHEN: ISOTONIC; HAMSTRING CURL

POSITION: Prone, standing

TARGETS: Strengthening of hamstrings; biceps femoris, semitendinosus, semi-membranosis. Add cuff weights to increase resistance.

INSTRUCTION: *Prone*: Patient lies flat on stomach and brings heel toward buttock, keeping neutral hip rotation (A). Patient may turn hip outward, externally rotating 45 degrees to target lateral hamstring (bicep femoris) (B) or inward, internally rotating 45 degrees to target medial hamstrings (semitendinosus, semi-membranosis) (C). Patient can also do this while squeezing a weighted ball between the ankles to add resistance and hip work. *Standing*: Patient holds onto stable object in front and brings heel toward buttocks keeping neutral hip rotation (D).

SUBSTITUTIONS: Maintain neutral pelvis; active lower abdominal core encouraged, thighs stay in alignment with each other.

PARAMETERS: 8 to 12 repetitions, 1 to 3 sets, 1 time per day or every other day

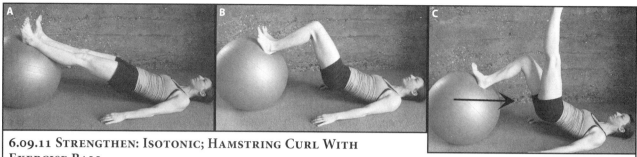

6.09.11 STRENGTHEN: ISOTONIC; HAMSTRING CURL WITH EXERCISE BALL

POSITION: Supine

TARGETS: Strengthening of hamstrings; biceps femoris, semitendinosus, semi-membranosis.

INSTRUCTION: *Bilateral*: Patient places feet on ball with knees near full extension. Patient uses gluteal muscles to lift hips off mat and then, pulling with hamstrings, curls heels toward buttocks, rolling ball toward him or her (A and B). For extra challenge, do this *unilaterally*: Patient lifts non-target leg straight into air as patient curls with target leg as described above (C). This can also be done with a medium-sized foam roll or bolster.

SUBSTITUTIONS: Maintain neutral pelvis; active lower abdominal core encouraged, thighs stay in alignment with each other and hip, knee, and foot stay in straight sagittal plane. Buttocks stay elevated off the mat for entire sequence.

PARAMETERS: 8 to 12 repetitions, 1 to 3 sets, 1 time per day or every other day

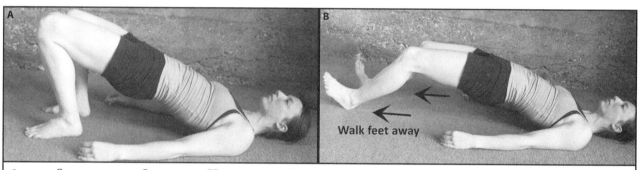

6.09.12 STRENGTHEN: ISOTONIC; HAMSTRING, BRIDGE WALK-OUTS

POSITION: Hook-lying

TARGETS: Strengthening of hamstrings; biceps femoris, semitendinosus, semi-membranosis.

INSTRUCTION: Patient starts with feet close to buttocks, lift hips 15 to 20 cm above mat, and walks each foot out 10 to 15 cm at a time, holding each position for 1 to 2 seconds. Patient walks out as far as possible with hips elevated and knees slightly bent, then slowly steps each foot back to starting position and repeats (A and B).

SUBSTITUTIONS: Maintain neutral pelvis; active lower abdominal core encouraged; hip and knee stay in straight sagittal plane.

PARAMETERS: 8 to 12 repetitions, 1 to 3 sets, 1 time per day or every other day

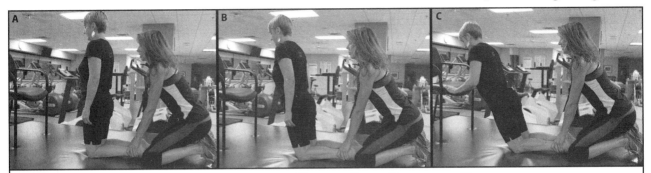

6.09.13 STRENGTHEN: ISOTONIC; HAMSTRING, NORDIC CURL, ECCENTRIC FOCUS

POSITION: Tall-kneeling

TARGETS: Strengthening of hamstrings; biceps femoris, semitendinosus, semi-membranosis with eccentric focus.

INSTRUCTION: Therapist holds patient's ankles as patient straightens spine in tall-kneeling and begins to lean forward, keeping spine straight. The further the patient moves forward, the greater the gravitational pull on trunk. The hamstrings actively control the forward movement of the body by contracting eccentrically. Patient should go as far as possible with slow, controlled movement and return to start (A, B, and C). Placing a chair in front allows the patient to be able to control the body once hamstrings reach maximum tension.

SUBSTITUTIONS: Maintain neutral pelvis; active lower abdominal core encouraged; hip and knee stay in straight sagittal plane.

PARAMETERS: 8 to 12 repetitions, 1 to 3 sets, 1 time per day or every other day

Where's the Evidence?

A 2015 study of over 500 soccer players found that incorporating the Nordic hamstring exercise in regular amateur training significantly reduced hamstring injury incidence, but for those injured, it did not reduce hamstring injury severity (Van der Horst, Smits, Petersen, Goedhart, & Backx, 2015). Anason, Andersen, Holme, Engebretsen, and Bahr (2008) found that eccentric strength training with Nordic hamstring lowers, combined with warm up stretching, appears to reduce the risk of hamstring strains, while no effect was detected from flexibility training alone. Iga, Fruer, Deighan, Croix, and James (2012) found that the greatest recruitment of hamstring muscle fibers was highest during the middle phase of the Nordic hamstring exercise between 31 to 60 degrees of knee flexion and that both hamstrings were engaged to a similar intensity during the exercise regardless of dominance. Tyler, Schmitt, Nicholas, and McHugh (2015) looked at 50 athletes with hamstring injuries who followed a three-phase rehabilitation protocol emphasizing eccentric strengthening with the hamstrings in a lengthened position. They found that none of the 42 compliant patients sustained re-injury within the next 1 to 3 years after return to sport, while four of the eight noncompliant patients sustained re-injury between 3 and 12 months after return to sport. They concluded that compliance with rehabilitation emphasizing eccentric strengthening with the hamstrings in a lengthened position resulted in no re-injuries.

6.09.14 STRENGTHEN: HAMSTRING, BRIDGE AND DEADLIFT DISCUSSION

Bridges and dead lifts work the gluteus maximus and hamstring effectively and can be found under hip strengthening **6.04.12** and **6.04.13** for bridge and **6.04.3** for dead lift.

6.09.15 STRENGTHEN: RESISTANCE BAND, LONG-ARC EXTENSION (KNEE)

<u>POSITION</u>: Seated

<u>TARGETS</u>: Strengthening of quadriceps; rectus femoris, VL, vastus medialis, and vastus intermedius.

<u>INSTRUCTION</u>: Loop band around target ankle and place under non-target foot. Patient brings toes toward ceiling as band resists. Band can also be anchored to back chair leg.

<u>SUBSTITUTIONS</u>: Maintain neutral pelvis; active lower abdominal core encouraged, avoid leaning back with trunk.

<u>PARAMETERS</u>: 8 to 12 repetitions, 1 to 3 sets, 1 time per day or every other day

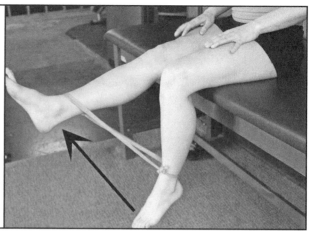

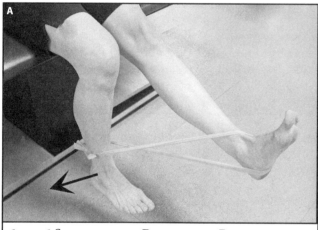

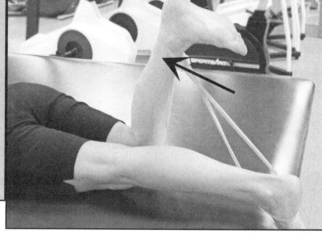

6.09.16 STRENGTHEN: RESISTANCE BAND, FLEXION, HAMSTRING CURL

<u>POSITION</u>: Seated, prone

<u>TARGETS</u>: Strengthening of hamstrings; biceps femoris, semitendinosus, semi-membranosis.

<u>INSTRUCTION</u>: *Seated*: Loop band around non-target ankle and place foot in chair as shown. Place band under non-target foot. Patient brings foot down and underneath as band resists (A). Band can also be anchored in front at knee height. *Prone*: This can also be done prone with anchor below ankle as patient curls heel toward buttocks (B). *Eccentric focus*: Therapist has patient flex the knee and then, with band looped around ankle, therapist applies downward pull with band. Patient slowly lowers foot to mat, resisting and decreasing the speed at which the band and gravity are pulling.

<u>SUBSTITUTIONS</u>: Maintain neutral pelvis; active lower abdominal core encouraged, avoid lifting hip on target side.

<u>PARAMETERS</u>: 8 to 12 repetitions, 1 to 3 sets, 1 time per day or every other day

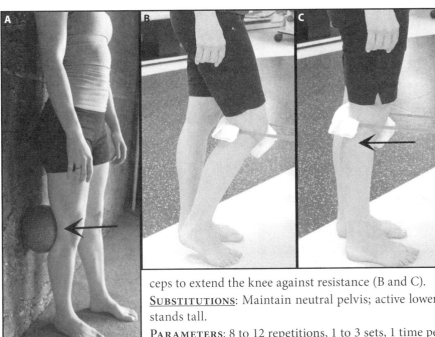

6.09.17 STRENGTHEN: RESISTANCE BAND AND BALL, TERMINAL KNEE EXTENSION

POSITION: Standing

TARGETS: Strengthening of quadriceps primarily VMO

INSTRUCTION: *Ball*: Patient stands with heel against wall and places 10- to 15-cm ball behind knee. Patient extends knee and presses into ball (A). *Resistance band*: Anchor band in front of patient at knee height. Patient steps backward until tension pulls knee into flexion. Patient contracts quadriceps to extend the knee against resistance (B and C).

SUBSTITUTIONS: Maintain neutral pelvis; active lower abdominal core encouraged, patient stands tall.

PARAMETERS: 8 to 12 repetitions, 1 to 3 sets, 1 time per day or every other day

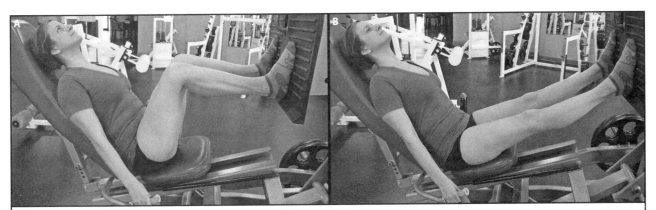

6.09.18 STRENGTHEN: KNEE, LEG PRESS ON WEIGHT MACHINE

POSITION: Seated, reclined

TARGETS: Strengthening hip extensors; gluteus maximus, hamstring, and knee extensors quadriceps.

INSTRUCTION: Patient places feet on platform, hip-width apart and anterior to hips. Adjust seat and back to accommodate full ROM without excessive flexing at the hips > 90 degrees. Patient buttocks should be scooted back into seat with a straight spine. Some machines have handles for the patient to grasp. Patient pushes with the legs to slowly extend the knees to 0 degrees without hyperextending or locking knees out. Patient slowly releases back to start just prior to setting weight down and repeat. Feet remain flat on platform for entire sequence. Depth of squat depends on goals of treatment. Goal is to flex knee to 90 degrees and hip to 90 degrees with knees staying behind the toes (A and B). It is recommended to add an isometric hip adduction ball squeeze with this activity to increase VMO activity.

SUBSTITUTIONS: Maintain neutral pelvis; active lower abdominal core encouraged, patient sits tall and engages core to prevent anterior tilting of pelvis.

PARAMETERS: 8 to 12 repetitions, 1 to 3 sets, 1 time per day or every other day

---

Where's the Evidence?

Peng, Kernozek, and Song (2013) investigated the effects of combining isometric hip adduction with the leg press to assess if VMO activation increased and found that targeted training using the leg press exercise to the last 45 degrees of knee extension/flexion with vigorous hip adduction may be useful in promoting a greater VMO/VL ratio.

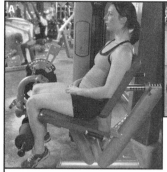
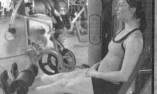
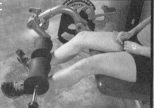
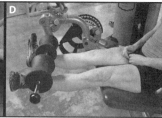

6.09.19 Strengthen: Knee Extension on Weight Machine

Position: Seated

Targets: Strengthening knee extensors, quadriceps

Instruction: Patient places shins behind the leg pads and scoots back into seat with a straight spine. Adjust seat and back to align knee joint with axis of rotation on machine. Some machines have handles for the patient to grasp. Patient lifts the toes slowly, extending the knees to 0 degrees without hyperextending or locking knees out (A and B). *VMO focus*: Set weight to start resisting at 30 degrees of knee flexion by raising shin pad to desired height and placing weight lock in. Patient then lifts shins to meet pad and extends from 30 to 0 degrees with toes pointed outward 45 degrees, holds 2 to 3 seconds, and slowly releases back to start just prior to setting weight down, and repeats. This will target the medial quadriceps, and patient should feel the fatigue at the "teardrop" oblique portion of the muscle (C and D).

Substitutions: Maintain neutral pelvis; active lower abdominal core encouraged, patient sits tall and engages core to prevent anterior tilting of pelvis and raising buttock off seat.

Parameters: 8 to 12 repetitions, 1 to 3 sets, 1 time per day or every other day

6.09.20 Strengthen: Knee Flexion on Weight Machine

Position: Seated, prone

Targets: Strengthening knee flexors, hamstrings with assist from gastrocnemius

Instruction: *Prone*: Patient hooks ankles behind roller pad as hips lie over angled portion of bench. Roller pad should be adjusted to sit just behind the ankles. Patient grasps handles and lays upper body down. Patient then contracts hamstrings to flex the knee while core muscles keep trunk and pelvis against the bench. Squeeze curl at end 2 to 3 seconds and then slowly

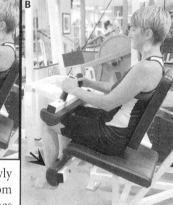

lower (A). *Seated*: Patient places shins under top roller pad and ankles in front of bottom roller pad. Patient scoots all the way back into seat. Adjust setting so that knee joint lines up with rotational axis of machine; shin pad is just below the knee and ankle pad is just posterior to the ankle. Patient engages core to maintain neutral spine and pelvis while bringing the heel down and underneath, flexing the knees slowly. Squeeze at end of bend for 2 to 3 seconds and slowly release back to start just prior to setting weight down and repeat (B).

Substitutions: Maintain neutral pelvis; active lower abdominal core encouraged, patient sits tall and engages core to prevent anterior tilting of pelvis and raising pelvis off seat.

Parameters: 8 to 12 repetitions, 1 to 3 sets, 1 time per day or every other day

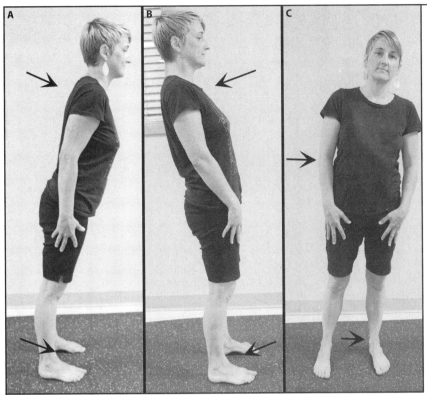

6.09.21 FUNCTIONAL: KNEE, WEIGHT SHIFTS

POSITION: Standing

TARGETS: Strengthening of LEs; working toward accepting weight in different directions.

INSTRUCTION: Patient slightly bends hips and knees with feet placed hip-width apart and toes pointing directly forward, knees in line with second toe on each side. Patient engages core and shifts weight and trunk forward and back to center. Repeat (A). Patient also does this backward by leaning trunk back (B). Lateral weight shifts are done by patient shifting weight and trunk to one side and then the other (C). Diagonal weight shifts involve the patient placing one foot forward and one foot back in a staggered stance and then shifting weight over the front foot and then back foot. Switch feet after doing a full set (not shown).

SUBSTITUTIONS: Maintain neutral pelvis; active lower abdominal core encouraged, knee on target side stays directly behind toes, focus on keeping hips and knee as controlled as possible.

PARAMETERS: 8 to 12 repetitions, 1 to 3 sets, 1 time per day or every other day

6.09.22 KNEE, SQUATS DISCUSSION

Squats and variations work gluteus maximus, hamstring, and quadriceps effectively and can be found under hip strengthening **6.04.26-29, 31, 32**.

Where's the Evidence?

One study identified the effects of performing squat exercises with visual feedback on the activation of the VMO and VL muscles in young adults with an increased quadriceps angle (Q-angle). Both groups performed squat to 90 degrees; one group with visual feedback and one without. The visual feedback group exhibited statistically significant increases in activation of the VMO compared to non-visual group and confirmed that squat exercises with visual feedback are effective in activation of the VMO and VL muscles (Hwangbo, 2015). Another study showed that if patients with patellofemoral pain are trained in eccentric exercises of the quadriceps, pain decreases; thus, isotonic eccentric quadriceps exercises should form a part of treatment in the rehabilitation protocol for the patients with patellofemoral pain syndrome (Eapen, Nayak, & Zulfeequer, 2011). Another study aimed to investigate the effect of altering knee movement and squat depth on the ratio of VMO and VL during squat exercises. They found increased VMO to VL ratio with deeper squats to 50 and 80 degrees as compared to 20 degrees, indicating deeper squats will target VMO most effectively (Jaberzadeh, Yeo, & Zoghi, 2015). Felício, Dias, Silva, Oliveira, and Bevilqauq-Grossi (2011) studied the effects of isometric hip adduction on EMG-monitored VMO recruitment with squat exercises and found squat exercises associated with hip adduction increased VMO muscle activity as well as the activity of gluteus medius. Irish, Millward, Wride, Haas, and Shum (2010) also found that the double-leg squat with isometric hip adduction exercise would be useful in maintaining correct patella tracking and selectively strengthening VMO.

6.09.23 FUNCTIONAL: KNEE, LUNGE AND VARIATIONS

POSITION: Standing

TARGETS: Strengthening of hip extensors (gluteus maximus, hamstrings) and abductors (TFL, gluteus medius and minimus) stabilization of hip internal and external rotators to keep leg aligned and quadriceps extending the knee

INSTRUCTION: *Beginner*: Patient may start with large steps and only mini-lunging. Follow instructions for each, but decrease knee flexion to <90 degrees based on patient tolerances and form.

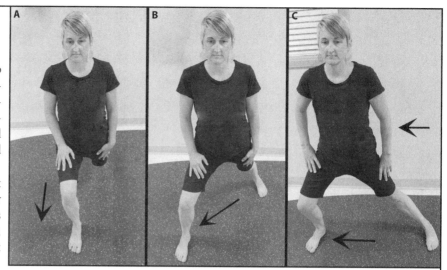

Forward: Patient takes a large step with leg forward and bends both knees to 90 degrees. Keep front knee in straight forward alignment with hip and toes pointed forward. Most of body weight is transferred to front leg. Push off of front leg to return to standing (A). *Diagonal*: Patient takes a large step with leg diagonally halfway between forward and to the side. Lunging, knee bends to 90 degrees and stance leg stays extended. Keep bent knee in straight forward alignment with toes pointed forward. Most of body weight is transferred to laterally placed leg. Push off of front leg to return to standing (B). *Lateral*: Patient takes a large step with leg lateral and slightly forward. Lunging, knee bends to 90 degrees and stance leg stays extended. Keep bent knee in straight forward alignment with toes pointed forward. Most of body weight is transferred to laterally placed leg. Push off of front leg to return to standing (C). *Lunge clocks*: Patient performs lunge forward, diagonal, and lateral in a sequence and repeats (not shown).

SUBSTITUTIONS: Maintain neutral pelvis; active lower abdominal core encouraged, knee on target side stays directly behind toes, focus on keeping hips and knee as controlled as possible.

PARAMETERS: 8 to 12 repetitions, 1 to 3 sets, 1 time per day or every other day

Where's the Evidence?

Irish et al. (2010) studied the effect of closed kinetic chain exercises and open kinetic chain exercise on the muscle activity of VMO and VL and found that the open kinetic chain knee extension exercises produced significantly greater activation of VL than the lunge exercise. They also found the lunge exercise produced the VMO to VL ratio closest to the idealized ratio of 1:1 and recommended the lunge exercise as a key tool in early rehabilitation when restoring preferential VMO to VL ratio is essential.

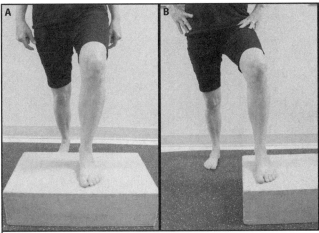
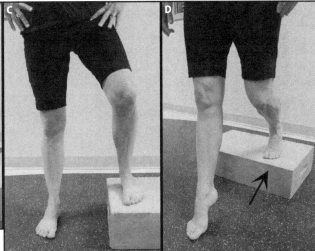

6.09.24 FUNCTIONAL: KNEE, STEP-UPS

POSITION: Standing

TARGETS: Strengthening of hip extensors (gluteus maximus, hamstrings) and abductors (TFL, gluteus medius and minimus), stabilization of hip internal and external rotators to keep leg aligned and quadriceps extending the knee.

INSTRUCTION: A mirror in front provides good feedback on knee position. *Beginner*: Patient may start with small steps and work up to higher steps. Follow instructions for each, but decrease knee flexion based on patient tolerances and form. *Forward*: Patient starts facing step, holding onto stable object to begin. Place one foot on the step and, without pulling up using the railing, step up onto step. Use the leg on the step to lift the remaining body weight, bringing the other foot onto the step. Patient keeps knee over second toes entire sequence (A). *Diagonal*: Patient stands near corner of step and steps, leg diagonally, halfway between forward and to the side. Use the leg on the step to lift the remaining body weight, bringing the other foot onto the step. Patient keeps knee over second toes entire sequence (B). *Lateral*: Patient stands to side of step and steps with leg laterally in sidestep onto step. Use the leg on the step to lift the remaining body weight, bringing the other foot onto the step. Patient keeps knee over second toes entire sequence (C). *Backward*: Patient stands in front of step and steps leg behind onto the step then lifts the remaining body weight with leg on step, bringing the other foot onto the step. Patient keeps knee over second toes entire sequence (D). Patient may also do any of these with just lifting the body to foot level with other foot, and then release back down.

SUBSTITUTIONS: Maintain neutral pelvis; active lower abdominal core encouraged, knee on target side stays directly behind toes, focus on keeping hips and knee as controlled as possible and knee over second toe, knee tends to deviate medially; this must be corrected or can aggravate knee condition.

PARAMETERS: 8 to 12 repetitions, 1 to 3 sets, 1 time per day or every other day

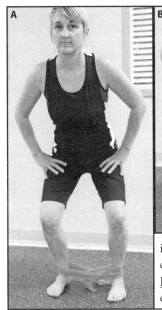
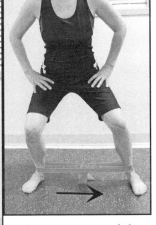

6.09.25 FUNCTIONAL: RESISTANCE BAND, KNEE, SIDE SHUFFLE

POSITION: Standing

TARGETS: Strengthening of hip extensors (gluteus maximus, hamstrings) and abductors (TFL, gluteus medius and minimus), stabilization of hip internal and external rotators to keep leg aligned and quadriceps extending the knee.

INSTRUCTION: Loop band around ankles. Patient squats as far as possible, keeping knees behind toes and engaged abdominal muscles to limit lumbar extension. Patient steps to the side while band resists and then follows, bringing other foot closer to leading foot, and repeat. Perform for desired distance and repeat other direction (A and B).

SUBSTITUTIONS: Maintain neutral pelvis; active lower abdominal core encouraged, knees stay directly behind toes, focus on keeping hips and knee as controlled as possible and knee over second toe, keep trunk upright.

PARAMETERS: Perform for distance to fatigue each direction, 1 to 3 sets, 1 time per day or every other day

6.09.26 FUNCTIONAL: RESISTANCE BAND, KNEE, MONSTER WALK

POSITION: Standing

TARGETS: Strengthening of hip (extensors gluteus maximus, hamstrings) and abductors (TFL, gluteus medius and minimus), stabilization of hip internal and external rotators to keep leg aligned and quadriceps extending the knee

INSTRUCTION: Loop band around ankles. Patient squats as far as possible, keeping knees behind toes and engaged abdominal muscles to limit lumbar extension. Patient walks forward, keeping knees and ankle apart with squat maintained entire sequence (A and B).

SUBSTITUTIONS: Maintain neutral pelvis; active lower abdominal core encouraged, knees stay directly behind toes, focus on keeping hips and knee as controlled as possible and knee over second toe, keep trunk upright.

PARAMETERS: Perform for distance to fatigue each direction, 1 to 3 sets, 1 time per day or every other day

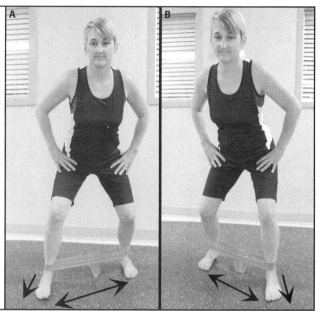

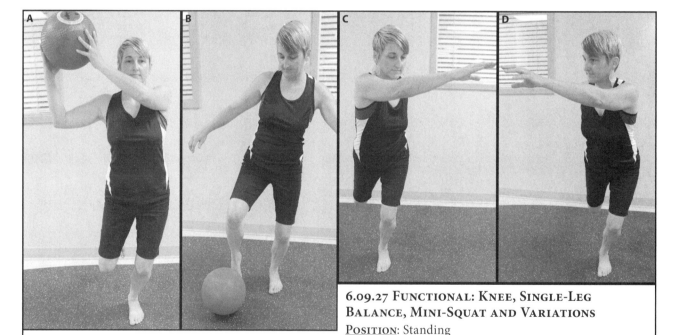

6.09.27 FUNCTIONAL: KNEE, SINGLE-LEG BALANCE, MINI-SQUAT AND VARIATIONS

POSITION: Standing

TARGETS: Strengthening of hip extensors (gluteus maximus, hamstrings) and abductors (TFL, gluteus medius and minimus), stabilization of hip internal and external rotators to keep leg aligned and quadriceps extending the knee

INSTRUCTION: Patient performs single-leg mini-squat with trunk upright. Other knee and hip are flexed to bring foot off floor. In this static position, patient maintains control of the stance knee directly over the second toe and hip in neutral rotation; lower abdominals are engaged and trunk is upright. The following activities can be added to challenge the patient in holding this alignment. *Ball toss*: Throw the ball to the patient, targeting all quadrants (above, overhead right, right side, lower right, lower, lower left, left side, overhead left, and center) (A). *Ball kick*: Roll ball to patient at differing locations as patient kicks the ball back with non-stance leg (B). *Reach twists*: Patient reaches forward across body as far as possible, keeping knee aligned (C). You can further challenge this with reaching for a dumbbell on a table and placing at location on other side then repeating with other arm (D). *(continued)*

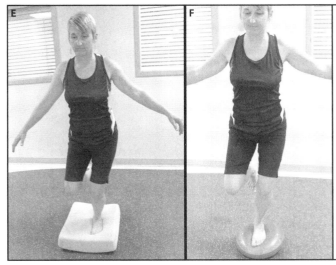

6.09.27 FUNCTIONAL: KNEE, SINGLE-LEG BALANCE, MINI-SQUAT AND VARIATIONS (CONTINUED)

All of these can be done on an unstable surface for further challenge; foam square, mini-trampoline, pillow (E and F).

<u>SUBSTITUTIONS</u>: Maintain neutral pelvis; active lower abdominal core encouraged, knees stay directly behind toes. Focus on keeping hips and knee as controlled as possible and knee over second toe; keep trunk upright.

<u>PARAMETERS</u>: Perform 30 to 60 seconds of each, 1 to 3 sets, 1 time per day or every other day

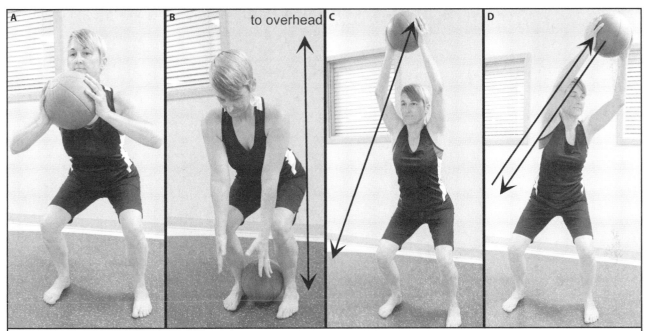

to overhead

6.09.28 FUNCTIONAL: KNEE, SQUAT, BALL VARIATIONS

<u>POSITION</u>: Standing

<u>TARGETS</u>: Strengthening of hip extensors (gluteus maximus, hamstrings) and abductors (TFL, gluteus medius and minimus), stabilization of hip internal and external rotators to keep leg aligned and quadriceps extending the knee.

<u>INSTRUCTION</u>: *Squat chest pass:* Patient starts in the squat position, holding a medicine ball directly in front with shoulder flexed to 90 degrees and elbows extended. Patient stands and brings the ball to the chest. Patient lowers back down to squat and extends ball out in front to repeat sequence (A). *Squat lifts:* Patient starts in the squat position, holding a medicine ball between the ankles. Patient brings ball overhead as patient stands. Patient lowers back down to squat with ball down as well to repeat sequence (B). *Squat slams:* Patient starts in the squat position, holding a medicine ball overhead. Patient slams the ball down as patient stands, catching the ball as it bounces upward. Patient brings ball back overhead and squats to repeat sequence (C). *Squat chop:* Patient starts in the squat position, holding a medicine ball lateral to knee. Patient brings ball over opposite shoulder above head height as patient stands. Patient lowers back down to squat with ball down across lateral knee and repeats sequence. Do full set and then repeat to other side (D).

<u>SUBSTITUTIONS</u>: Maintain neutral pelvis; active lower abdominal core encouraged, knees stay directly behind toes. Focus on keeping hips and knee as controlled as possible and knee over second toe; keep trunk upright.

<u>PARAMETERS</u>: 8 to 12 repetitions, 1 to 3 sets, 1 time per day or every other day

6.09.29 FUNCTIONAL: KNEE, WHOLE BODY VIBRATION MACHINE

<u>POSITION</u>: Standing

<u>TARGETS</u>: Strengthening LE and trunk muscles as a result of a spinal reflex, activates the stretch-reflex to assist training the muscles for good hip-dominant squat and lunge patterns.

<u>INSTRUCTION</u>: *Squat*: Both feet are placed on the whole body vibration platform and squat is performed as described in **6.04.29**. *Lunge*: Both feet are placed in front of machine at a distance at which a large step will place foot onto platform. Patient places one foot on one platform and performs lunge as described in on the whole body vibration platform, and squat is performed as described in **6.09.28** (not shown).

<u>SUBSTITUTIONS</u>: Maintain neutral pelvis; active lower abdominal core encouraged, knees stay directly behind toes. Focus on keeping hips and knee as controlled as possible and knee over second toe; keep trunk upright.

<u>PARAMETERS</u>: 8 to 12 repetitions, 1 to 3 sets, 1 time per day or every other day

Where's the Evidence?

The inclusion of whole body vibration to dynamic resistance exercise can be an added modality to increase strength. Whole body vibration can have varied effects in altering muscle strength in untrained individuals according to the type of resistance training performed. As a dynamic squat with whole body vibration seems to immediately potentiate neuromuscular functioning, the combination of dynamic exercises and whole body vibration could be used as a potential warm-up procedure before resistance exercise (Bush, Blog, Kang, Faigenbaum, & Ratamess, 2015). We concluded that 8 weeks whole body vibration training in 30 hertz (Hz) was more effective than 50 Hz to increase the isometric contraction and dynamic strength of knee extensors as measured using peak concentric torque and equally effective with 50 Hz in improving eccentric torque of knee extensors in healthy young untrained women (Esmaeilzadeh, Akpinar, Polat, Yildiz, & Oral, 2015). Roelants, Delecluse, and Verschueren (2004) investigated the effects of 24 weeks of whole body vibration training on knee-extension strength and speed of movement and on countermovement jump performance in older women. Eighty-nine women aged 58 to 74 were assigned to whole body vibration group, resistance training group, or control group. The whole body vibration group and the resistance training group trained 3 times per week for 24 weeks. The whole body vibration group performed unloaded static and dynamic knee extensor exercises on a vibration platform. The resistance training group trained knee extensors by performing dynamic leg press and leg extension exercises increasing from low to high resistance. The control group did not participate in any training. Isometric and dynamic knee extensor strength increased significantly in the whole body vibration group and the resistance training group after 24 weeks of training, with the training effects not significantly different between the groups. Speed of movement of knee extension and countermovement jump height significantly increased with no significant differences in training effect between the whole body vibration and the resistance training group groups. Most of the gain in knee extension strength and speed of movement and in countermovement jump performance had been realized after 12 weeks of training. They concluded whole body vibration is a suitable training method and is as efficient as conventional resistance training group training to improve knee extension strength and speed of movement and countermovement jump performance in older women. It is suggested that the strength gain in older women is mainly due to the vibration stimulus and not only to the unloaded exercises performed on the whole body vibration platform.

6.09.30 AGILITY: KNEE, SPEED LADDER DRILLS AND VARIATIONS

<u>POSITION</u>: Standing

<u>TARGETS</u>: Strengthening LE, quick muscular responses to improve muscle control and agility while targeting LE neuromuscular control, joint stability, proprioception and facilitating co-contraction of LE muscles.

<u>INSTRUCTION</u>: These drills are started slow as patient works on sequencing and control. Speed is increased as patient can control form. Patients should not be allowed to go too fast as injury can occur if patient is not in control of movements throughout. Allow patient to use arms in alternating swing fashion as with running when applicable. Patient should stay on the balls of the feet for many of the drills; some of the lateral maneuvers will involve placement of the heel down.

A. *One step*: Start with feet hip-width apart facing beginning of ladder. Patient steps in first box on toes with one foot then brings other foot to meet. Repeat entire sequence for distance of ladder. Upon turning around, lead this time with other foot.

B. *Sidestep*: Start with feet hip-width apart facing lateral to beginning of ladder. Patient steps in first box on toes with one foot then brings other foot to meet. Repeat entire sequence for distance of ladder. Return back down ladder, leading this time with other foot.

C. *Alternating tip toes forward*: Start with feet hip-width apart at beginning of ladder. Patient steps in first box with one foot then brings back foot to step in second box. Foot in first box then steps on toes in third box. Patient stays on toes and continues sequence to end of ladder. *(continued)*

6.09.30 Agility: Knee, Speed Ladder Drills and Variations (continued)

D. *High knees forward*: Start with feet hip-width apart facing beginning of ladder. Patient marches hip and knee into >90 degrees flexion and lands in first box on toes with one foot then brings other foot to meet. Repeat entire sequence for distance of ladder. Upon turning around, lead this time with other foot.

E. *High knees lateral*: Start with feet hip-width apart facing lateral to beginning of ladder. Patient marches hip and knee into >90 degrees flexion and lands in first box on toes with one foot, then brings other foot to meet. Repeat entire sequence for distance of ladder. Return back down ladder, leading this time with other foot.

F. *Rabbit hop forward, single box, double box, triple box, lateral*: Start with feet hip-width apart facing beginning of ladder. Patient hops with both feet into first box and continues with quick hops the length of the ladder. Distance of hops can be increased to clear 2 or 3 boxes. This can be done laterally as well.

G. *Skips*: Start with feet hip-width apart facing beginning of ladder. Patient skips, landing each foot in alternating boxes.

H. *Scissor skips*: Start with feet hip-width apart facing beginning of ladder. Patient with one foot in box 1 hops up on both feet and places left foot in box 2. Patient hops with both feet again and brings right foot to box 3. Repeat entire sequence for distance of ladder.

I. *Hop scotch*: Start with feet hip-width apart facing beginning of ladder. Patient hops, landing on left foot into first square then immediately pushing off to land with both feet in next square. Patient then hops to land on right foot and quickly hops to land on both feet again. Repeat entire sequence for distance of ladder.

J. *Ickey shuffle*: Start with feet hip-width apart facing beginning of ladder and left of the ladder. Right foot in box 1 joined by left foot, right foot to right of box 1 joined by left foot. Left foot to box 2 joined by right foot repeating sequence to other side. Repeat entire sequence for distance of ladder. Ickey shuffle can also be done with exaggerated movements lifting knees high and widening lateral steps.

K. *Crossovers*: Start with feet hip-width apart facing lateral to beginning of ladder. Patient steps in first box with a sidestep and then steps across with trailing foot in front of lead foot to next box and repeats entire sequence for distance of ladder.

L. *5 hops and run*: Start with feet hip-width apart facing beginning of ladder. Hop 5 boxes and one landing in fifth hop begins with one step remainder of ladder. This is good for transition training.

M. *Tango*: Start with feet hip-width apart facing beginning of ladder and left of the ladder. Left foot crosses over to land in box 1. Right foot lands to right of box 1 and left foot joins. Right foot now crosses over to land in box 2 as left foot crosses behind to land left of box 2 and then right foot joins. Repeat entire sequence for distance of ladder.

N. *5-count drill*: Start with feet hip-width apart facing beginning of ladder. (1) Right foot steps lateral to box 1; (2) left foot comes forward to inside of box 1; (3) right foot moves to box 1 next to left foot; (4) left foot steps forward into box 2; (5) followed by right foot. Left foot steps to lateral aspect of box three. Sequence repeats. Repeat entire sequence for distance of ladder.

O. *Riverdance*: Start with feet hip-width apart facing beginning of ladder and left of the ladder. Right foot steps into box 1 and left foot crosses behind to land on the other side of the ladder. Right foot steps out to right side of ladder as left foot steps into to ladder box 2, and repeat. "In, behind, out" is a good way to instruct. Repeat entire sequence for distance of ladder.

P. *Side-straddle hop*: Start with feet hip-width apart facing beginning of ladder. Jump into first box and then hop, bringing both feet outside of box 2 then hop again to come inside of box 2. "In, out" is a good way to instruct. Repeat entire sequence for distance of ladder.

Q. *Carioca*: Start with feet hip-width apart facing lateral to beginning of ladder. Bring foot closest to ladder into box 1, cross other foot over to box 2, cross trailing foot behind to box three and repeat. "Over, under, over, under" is a good way to instruct. Repeat entire sequence for distance of ladder.

R. *In and out*: Start with feet hip-width apart facing lateral right side of box 1. Step into box 1 with right foot and follow with left foot, then step back with right foot and follow with left foot. Right foot then steps into box 2 and left foot follows, repeating entire sequence for distance of ladder.

S. *Centipede*: Start with feet hip-width apart facing lateral right side of box 1. Step into box 1 with right foot and follow with left foot, step to box 2 right foot and follow with left foot, right foot then back out of box and left foot follows; right foot then begins sequence again, stepping into third box. Instruct as "two in, two over, two out," repeating entire sequence for distance of ladder.

T. *Slalom double side*: Start with feet hip-width apart facing lateral right side of box 1. Hop laterally into box 1 and then across to other side, repeat into box 2, repeating entire sequence for distance of ladder.

U. *Single side jump cuts*: Start with feet hip-width apart facing lateral right side of box 1. Hop laterally into box 1 and then out back to starting side, repeat into box 2, repeating entire sequence for distance of ladder. Repeat to other side.

Substitutions: Maintain neutral pelvis; active lower abdominal core encouraged, knees stay directly behind toes, focus on keeping hips slightly bent and knee as controlled as possible and knee over second toe, keep trunk upright.

Parameters: 4 to 8 lengths, 1 to 3 sets, 1 time per day or every other day

6.09.31 AGILITY: KNEE, DOT DRILLS AND VARIATIONS

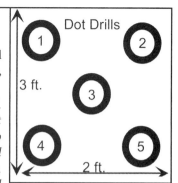

POSITION: Standing

TARGETS: Strengthening LE, quick muscular responses to improve muscle control and agility, strengthening lower while targeting LE neuromuscular control, joint stability, proprioception and facilitating co-contraction of LE muscles.

INSTRUCTION: *These drills are started slow as patient works on sequencing and control. Speed is increased as patient can control form. Patient should not be allowed to go too fast as injury can occur if patient is not in control of movements throughout. Allow patient to use arms in alternating swing fashion as with running when applicable. Patients should stay on the balls of the feet. Exercise for box drills are listed mostly as double-foot hopping, but any of the double-foot hop sequences can be done single foot if patient has good control of stance leg. Dot drill is set up as shown in* **6.09.31**, *using tape usually on the floor to mark the numbers.*

Butterfly: Starting position: Left foot: dot 1, Right foot: dot 2. Both feet jump to dot 3. Both feet jump again, left landing on dot 4 and right on dot 5. Repeat backward.

Butterfly 180 degrees: Starting position: Left foot: dot 1, Right foot: dot 2. Both feet jump to dot 3. Both feet jump again, left landing on dot 4 and right on dot 5. Patient jumps to make a 180-degree turn, landing left foot on dot 5 and right foot on dot 4. Repeat other direction, making 180-degree turns at end of each butterfly.

Figure 8s: Starting position: Both feet follow this sequence of dots: 1, 3, 5, 4, 3, 2, and back to dot 1

Hour glass: Starting position: Both feet follow this sequence of dots: 1, 3, 4, 5, 3, 2, 1

Box 4 corners: Starting position: Both feet follow this sequence of dots: 1, 2, 5, 4 and 1, 4, 5, 2

Bottom triangle: Starting position: Both feet follow this sequence of dots: 1, 2, 3, 1 and 2, 1, 3, 2

Wide triangle: Starting position: Both feet follow this sequence of dots: 3, 4, 1, 3 and 3, 1, 4, 3

Double X: Starting position: Both feet follow this sequence of dots: 1, 3, 4, 3, 5, 3, 2, 3, and back to 1

SUBSTITUTIONS: Maintain neutral pelvis; active lower abdominal core encouraged, knees stay directly behind toes, focus on keeping hips slightly bent, knee as controlled as possible and knee over second toe, keep trunk upright.

PARAMETERS: 8 to 12 each of chosen drill(s), 1 to 3 sets, 1 time per day or every other day

6.09.32 AGILITY: KNEE, MINI-HURDLE DRILLS AND VARIATIONS

POSITION: Standing

TARGETS: Strengthening LE quick muscular responses to improve muscle control and agility

INSTRUCTION: *These drills are started slow as patient works on sequencing and control. Speed is increased as patient can control form. Patients should not be allowed to go too fast as injury can occur if patient is not in control of movements throughout. Allow patient to use arms in alternating swing fashion as with running when applicable. Patients should stay on the balls of the feet. Hurdle spacing is another way to add challenge and variation to these exercises.*

One step: Step over hurdles alternating feet.

One steps: Step over hurdles, bringing feet together in between each hurdle.

Hops: Hop over each hurdle with both feet together.

Sidesteps: Sidestep over hurdle.

Crossovers: Sidestep over hurdles, bringing each foot across to clear next hurdle, with one foot touching between each hurdle.

3 steps forward: Step over hurdles, touching leading leg down, trailing leg, and leading leg again before stepping over hurdle with trailing leg. There are three steps between each hurdle.

3 steps lateral: Stepping laterally over hurdles touch leading leg down, trailing leg, and leading leg again before stepping over hurdle with trailing leg. There are three steps between each hurdle.

SUBSTITUTIONS: Maintain neutral pelvis; active lower abdominal core encouraged, knees stay directly behind toes, focus on keeping hips slightly bent and knee as controlled as possible and knee over second toe, keep trunk upright.

PARAMETERS: 4 to 8 lengths of 10 to 12 hurdles, 1 to 3 sets, 1 time per day or every other day

6.09.33 PLYOMETRICS AND VARIATIONS, KNEE

POSITION: Standing

TARGETS: Strengthening LE, utilizing muscle spindle activity while targeting LE neuromuscular control, joint stability, proprioception and facilitating co-contraction of LE muscles.

INSTRUCTION: *In plyometric exercise, there are three phases: the eccentric phase, the amortization phase, and the concentric phase. The key to plyometrics is an eccentric phase with stretch on the target muscle(s) followed by an immediate concentric contraction of the target muscle(s) with the amortization phase between kept to as minimum length of time as possible. This utilizes the muscle spindle reaction to increase the fiber recruitment and force generation of the target muscle in the concentric phase. There should be no pause between phases of eccentric to concentric phases. Plyometrics should begin once patient demonstrates good strength and control of the LE, as well as good landing mechanics controlling the knees from deviating inward. Always start with low-intensity plyometric drills first before progressing to medium- and high-intensity plyometric drills. Box height should start low and progress in height as proper mechanics are maintained.*

A. *Quiet jumps double leg*: This is a good beginner plyometric exercise utilizing a lower box. Patient squats in front of box and jumps onto box as quietly as possible with knees being flexed to absorb force.

B. *Quiet jumps single leg*: This is a good beginner plyometric exercise utilizing a lower box for single leg control. Patient performs a single leg squat in front of box and jumps onto box as quietly as possible with knees being flexed to absorb force.

C. *Box jumps forward*: Patient starts in a squat position and, keeping knees over heels, jumps onto a box. Patient either steps or jumps back down.

D. *Multiple box jumps forward*: Patient starts in a squat position and, keeping knees over heels, jumps onto a box, then immediately jumps back down and repeats sequence.

E. *Box jumps unilateral*: Patient starts in a squat position and, keeping knees over heels, jumps laterally onto a box. Patient immediately jumps back down and then back up onto box.

F. *Box jumps bilateral*: Patient starts in a squat position and, keeping knees over heels, jumps laterally onto a box. Patient immediately jumps back down and then up onto box on the other side and repeats.

G. *Platform depth jumps forward*: Patient starts in a squat position on a lower box and, keeping knees over heels, jumps forward to land on the ground and immediately jumps onto next box, which can be higher.

H. *Platform depth jumps lateral*: Patient starts in a squat position on a lower box and, keeping knees over heels, jumps laterally to land on the ground and immediately jumps onto next box laterally, which can be higher.

I. *Vertical depth jumps*: Patient starts in a squat position on a box and, keeping knees over heels, jumps off box to land on the ground and immediately jumps straight vertically up in the air as high as possible.

J. *Multiple vertical jumps*: Patient starts in a squat position and jumps as high as possible, lands in a squat, and immediately repeats sequence.

K. *Staircase depth jumps*: Patient starts in a squat position on a box facing a staircase and, keeping knees over heels, jumps off box to land on the ground and immediately jumps to the highest step patient can land on.

L. *Staircase depth jumps*: Patient starts in a squat position on a box facing a staircase and jumps to land on highest step patient can land on in squat position and repeats.

M. *Long depth jumps*: Patient starts in a squat position on a box and, keeping knees over heels, jumps off box to land on the ground and immediately jumps as far forward as patient can land.

N. *Multiple long jumps*: Patient starts in a squat position and jumps as far forward as patient can land and, in squat position, immediately repeats sequence.

O. *Leap frog*: Patient starts in a squat position and jumps forward, landing in squat position, and then immediately jumps backward to start position and repeats sequence.

P. *Around the world leap frog*: Patient starts in a squat position and jumps forward to the right, landing in squat position, and then immediately jumps backward and to the right, then backward and to the left, then forward to the left and forward to the right to start position, and repeats sequence.

Q. *Zig-zag leap frog*: Patient starts in a squat position and jumps forward to the right, landing in squat position, and then immediately jumps forward and to the left, repeating sequence. Once patient finishes, patient jumps backward and to the left, then backward to the right, repeating sequence until patient returns to starting position.

R. *Multiple hurdle jumps*: Patient starts in a squat position and jumps over hurdle, landing in squat position, and immediately repeats sequence.

S. *Box jump march*: Patient starts with one foot on box and one on floor. Patient jumps vertically as patient switches foot positions and immediately repeats sequence. *(continued)*

6.09.33 PLYOMETRICS AND VARIATIONS, KNEE (CONTINUED)

T. *Split jump (also called* jump lunges): Patient starts in lunge position, front knee behind toes. Patient jumps vertically as patient quickly switches foot positions and lunge. Patient immediately repeats sequence.

U. *Split jump with medicine ball*: Patient starts in lunge position, front knee behind toes. Patient holds medicine ball at chest level. Patient jumps vertically, bringing medicine ball overhead as patient quickly switches foot positions and lunges. Patient immediately repeats sequence.

V. *Barrier lateral jumps*: Patient starts in a squat position and, keeping knees over heels, jumps over step, landing in squat, and immediately jumps back over, repeating sequence.

W. *Box lateral shuffle*: Patient starts in a squat position with one foot on step. Patient jumps laterally so that trailing leg lands on step and leading leg on floor. Immediately repeat to other side and repeat sequence.

X. *Bosu lateral shuffle*: Patient starts in a squat position with one foot on Bosu. Patient jumps laterally so that trailing leg lands on Bosu and leading leg on floor. Immediately repeat to other side and repeat sequence.

Y. *Lateral bound "skaters"*: Patient starts in a squat position with weight on outer leg and bounds laterally to land on other leg and immediately repeats back to start position and repeats sequence.

Z. *Lateral bound with medicine ball*: Patient holds medicine ball with extended arms at chest level and starts in a squat position with weight on outer leg. Patient bounds laterally, bringing ball to chest as patient bounds and back to extended arms while landing on other leg and immediately repeats back to start position and repeats sequence.

AA. *Butt kickers*: Patient jogs in place, kicking heels toward buttocks as high as possible and landing soft knees.

BB. *Sprinters*: Patient jogs in place, kicking heels toward buttocks as high as possible and landing soft knees and goes double speed.

CC. *High knees*: Patient marches in place at jogging pace and brings knees as high as possible with each march.

DD. *Front kicks*: Patient kicks one leg out to hip flexion with knee near extended and jumps with stance leg to switch, bringing other leg out and opposite leg lands.

EE. *Tuck jumps*: Patient jumps, bringing both knees to chest and lands, one small hop in between and repeats.

FF. *Superstar jumps*: Patient jumps, bringing both heels to butt and repeats.

GG. *Jump rope*: Patient jogs or hops in place while using jump rope or mimicking jump rope motion.

HH. *One leg side-to-side jump rope*: Patient hops side-to-side on one leg while using jump rope or mimicking jump rope motion.

II. *One leg front-to-back jump rope*: Patient hops front-to-back on one leg while using jump rope or mimicking jump rope motion.

JJ. *Jumping jacks*: Patient jumps, bringing feet out to the side and immediately jumps again to bring feet together. Arms may be added with shoulder abducting when feet hop out wide.

KK. *X jumps*: Patient jumps, bringing feet out and abducting shoulders quickly and bringing back to feet together and arms down for landing.

LL. *Foot switch squat*: Patient in squat, trunk forward, and hands clasped in front of chest slides one foot to side then quickly hops, bringing foot in and sliding other foot out to the side.

MM. *180-degree jumps*: Patient in squat jumps into the air turning body 180 degrees to land and repeats.

NN. *Burpees*: Requires good arm strength; patient jumps vertically in the air and, upon landing, places hands on floor in front and moves into plank position. Patient does a small push up and presses back to standing and jumps vertically again, repeating sequence.

OO. *Quick feet*: Patient in squat, trunk forward, and hands clasped in front of chest quickly brings each foot up off floor, alternating as quickly as possible.

PP. *Donkey kicks alternating*: Requires good arm strength; patient with toes and hands on floor kicks, extends one hip with knee flexion, bringing foot off floor and immediately switches feet so that other hip extends and knee flexes. Repeat sequence.

QQ. *Donkey kicks bilateral*: Requires good arm strength; patient with toes and hands on floor kicks both legs up and out with hip extension and knee flexion, bringing feet off floor and immediately returns to landing. Repeat sequence.

SUBSTITUTIONS: Knees should stay over ankles throughout jumps, attempting to land with knees over ankles and keeping knees lining up with second toe one each foot. Do not allow knees to deviate inward. Encourage engagement of core trunk muscles with activities to maintain neutral spine.

PARAMETERS: 8 to 12 repetitions, 1 to 3 sets, 1 time per day or every other day

Where's the Evidence?

Marcovic's (2007) meta-analytical review confirmed plyometric training provided a statistically significant and practically relevant improvement in vertical jump height. Miller, Herniman, Ricard, Cheatham, and Michael (2006) performed a study to determine if 6 weeks of plyometric training can improve an athlete's agility. Subjects were divided into two groups: a plyometric training and a control group. The plyometric training group performed in a 6-week plyometric training program and the control group did not perform any plyometric training techniques. The plyometric training group had quicker post-test times and reduced time on the ground compared to the control group for the agility tests. The results showed that plyometric training can be an effective training technique to improve agility.

Patellar tendinopathies are a common injury in sports that comprise jump actions. A 2014 systematic review of the literature examined the relation between patellar tendinopathy and take-off and landing kinematics to uncover risk factors and potential prevention strategies. Most differences were found during horizontal landing after forward acceleration, suggesting that horizontal landing poses the greatest threat for developing patellar tendinopathy. A stiff movement pattern with a small post-touchdown ROM and short landing time was associated with the onset of patellar tendinopathy. A flexible landing pattern was the strategy for reducing the risk for developing and redeveloping patellar tendinopathy. Their findings indicated that improving kinetic chain functioning, performing eccentric exercises, and changing landing patterns are potential tools for preventive and therapeutic purposes (Van der Worp, de Poel, Diercks, van den Akker-Scheek, & Zwerver, 2014).

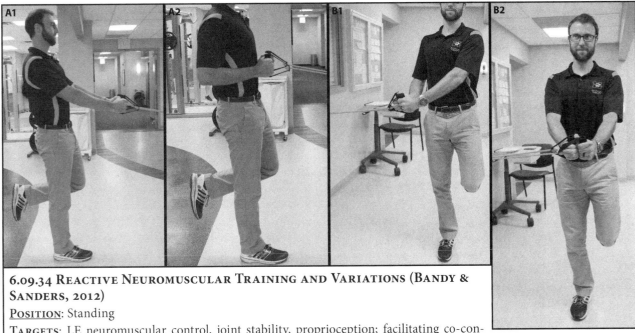

6.09.34 REACTIVE NEUROMUSCULAR TRAINING AND VARIATIONS (BANDY & SANDERS, 2012)

POSITION: Standing

TARGETS: LE neuromuscular control, joint stability, proprioception; facilitating co-contraction of LE muscles.

INSTRUCTION: *RNT uses outside resistance to neurologically turn on an automatic response. It is often seen as a quick fix to faulty movement patterns and designed to improve functional stability and enhance motor control skills with an automatic response. As the body reacts to the applied force, instinct to correct the flawed movements is activated. Clinicians can use these techniques to target specific levels of the central nervous system to stimulate appropriate reflex responses promoting functional static and dynamic stability. These techniques are helpful when verbal cueing is not effective for proper lLE mechanics. If therapist is observing knee "caving in" or excessive trunk movements with squat mechanics these exercises can be useful in correction of the faulty mechanics.*

A. *Uniplanar anterior shift*: Anchor resistance band in front of the patient at waist height, leaving two tails or handles. Patient holds ends of band in each hand. Patient stands on the target extremity, making sure knee is not locked out, and lifts the other foot by bending the knee. Patient balances on the extremity while pulling the band in toward the waist as hands come to outsides of pelvis (A1 and A2).

B. *Uniplanar lateral shift*: Anchor resistance band on the patient's target side at waist height, leaving two tails or handles. Patient holds ends of band in each hand. Patient stands on the target extremity, making sure knee is not locked out, and lifts the other foot by bending the knee. Patient balances on the extremity while pulling the band in front of and behind the body (B1 and B2). *(continued)*

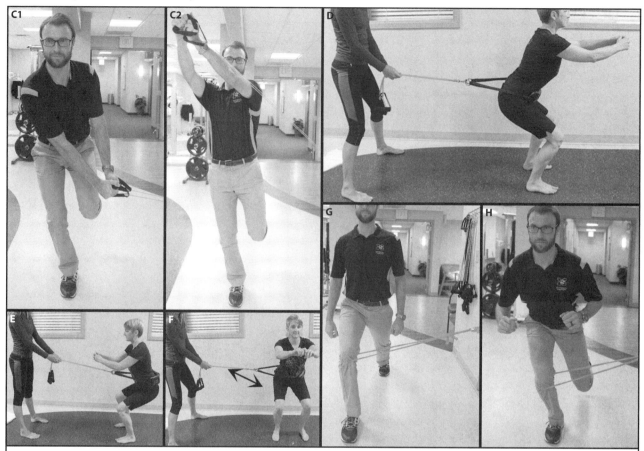

6.09.34 REACTIVE NEUROMUSCULAR TRAINING AND VARIATIONS (CONTINUED)

C. *Mulitplanar weight shifts*: Anchor resistance band on the patient's non-target side at low height, leaving two tails or handles. Patient holds ends of band in each hand. Patient stands on the target extremity, making sure knee is not locked out, and lifts the other foot by bending the knee. Patient balances on the extremity while pulling the band from low on target side to high target side in a diagonal chop pattern (C1 and C2).

D. *Squat, posterior weight shifts*: Anchor resistance band behind the patient so that a loop is formed. Patient places body inside the loop and brings to waist height. A chair is placed behind the patient. Patient squats to almost sit in the chair, keeping feet and knees hip-width apart and knees behind toes, then stands again (D).

E. *Squat, anterior weight shifts*: Anchor resistance band low and in front of the patient so that a loop is formed. Patient places body inside the loop and brings to chest height under the arms or across the shoulder's height. Patient squats to almost sit in a chair, keeping feet and knees hip-width apart and knees behind toes, then stands again (E).

F. *Squat, posterior medial shifts*: Anchor resistance on the non-target side of the patient so that a loop is formed. Patient places body inside the loop and brings to waist height. A chair is placed behind the patient. Patient squats to almost sit in the chair, keeping feet and knees hip-width apart and knees behind toes, then stands again. Band can also be anchored at the knee for variation when trying to correct medial movement of the knee with squat (F).

G. *Lunge, medial weight shifts*: Anchor resistance on the non-target side of the patient so that a loop is formed at knee height. Patient places target leg inside the loop and brings to knee height. Patient steps back so that when lunging with the target leg, the band is in line with knee. Patient steps outward for tension on the knee and performs a slow lunge, leading with the target leg and back to start. Target hip, knee, and ankle stay in alignment with knees behind toes on target leg, then stands again. The band is pulling the knee inward with reactive correction by the patient to bring the knee back into alignment (G).

H. *Single-leg squat, medial shifts band at knee*: Anchor resistance on the non-target side of the patient so that a loop is formed at knee height. Patient places target leg inside the loop and brings to knee height. Patient lifts the non-target leg and single-leg squats, keeping hip, knee, and ankle in alignment and knees behind toes on target leg, then stands again. The band is pulling the knee inward with reactive correction by the patient to bring the knee back into alignment (H).

(continued)

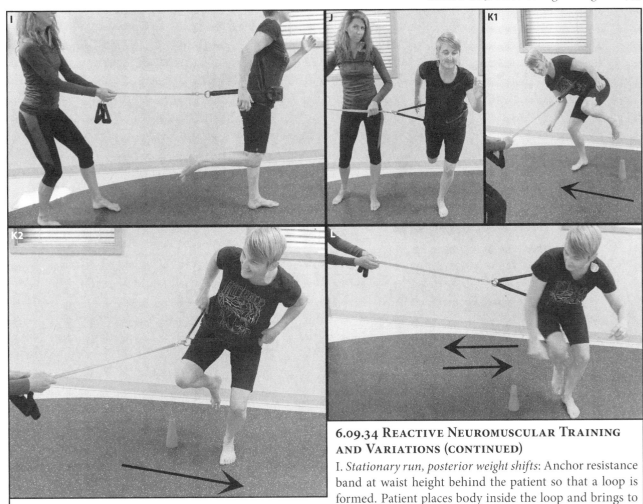

6.09.34 REACTIVE NEUROMUSCULAR TRAINING AND VARIATIONS (CONTINUED)

I. *Stationary run, posterior weight shifts*: Anchor resistance band at waist height behind the patient so that a loop is formed. Patient places body inside the loop and brings to waist height. Patient steps out until there is tension on the band. Patient starts jogging in place, progressing to running pace. The exercise can be advanced to high-knee running (I).

J. *Stationary run, medial weight shifts*: Anchor resistance band at waist height to one side of patient so that a loop is formed. Patient places body inside the loop and brings to waist height. Patient sidesteps out until there is tension on the band. Patient starts jogging in place, progressing to running pace. The exercise can be advanced to high-knee running (J).

K. *Bounding anterior weight shifts*: Anchor resistance band at waist height in front of patient so that a loop is formed. Patient places body inside the loop and brings to waist height. Patient steps back until there is tension on the band. Place a cone to one side of the patient. Patient leaps lateral over the cone and lands, then leaps back over the cone and repeats (K1 and K2).

L. *Bounding medial and lateral weight shifts*: Anchor resistance band at waist height to one side of patient so that a loop is formed. Patient places body inside the loop and brings to waist height. Patient sidesteps out until there is tension on the band. Place a cone to one side of the patient. Patient leaps lateral over the cone and lands one foot at a time, then leaps back over the cone and repeats (L).

SUBSTITUTIONS: Maintain neutral pelvis; active lower abdominal core encouraged, knees stay directly behind toes, focus on keeping hips and knee as controlled as possible and knee over second toe; keep trunk upright or only hinging at hips when activity requires.

PARAMETERS: 8 to 12 repetitions, 1 to 3 sets, 1 time per day or every other day

Where's the Evidence?

A few case studies are available to support RNT. One study utilized RNT to address hamstring tightness. Patient was treated using an RNT technique in which the patient resisted a manual anterior-to-posterior force at the abdomen, sternum, and across the hips while simultaneously bending forward at the hips in an attempt to touch toes. Following one RNT training treatment session, the patient tested negative for hamstring inflexibility and maintained those results at a 5-week follow-up. The authors concluded RNT training was effective for treating hamstring tightness and recommended clinicians should consider using RNT to treat patients with a chief complaint of hamstring tightness (Loutsch, Baker, May & Nasypany, 2015). Another study looked at RNT with a female basketball player with a recent ACL injury of a partial or complete tear of the ACL. They found that 1 week of RNT resulted in dramatic decreases in muscle imbalances at the hip, knee, and ankle and derived this significant gain in strength over such a short period of time was due to increase in neuromuscular control and not strictly strength (Cook, Burton, & Fields, 1999).

REFERENCES

Arnason, A., Andersen, T. E., Holme, I., Engebretsen, L., & Bahr, R. (2008). Prevention of hamstring strains in elite soccer: An intervention study. *Scandanavian Journal of Medicine and Science in Sports, 18*(1), 40-48.

Bandy, W. D., & Sanders, B. (2012). *Therapeutic exercise for physical therapist assistants* (3rd ed.). New York, NY: Lippincott, Williams and Wilkins.

Bush, J. A., Blog, G. L., Kang, J., Faigenbaum, A. D., & Ratamess, N. A. (2015). Effects of quadriceps strength after static and dynamic whole-body vibration exercise. *Journal of Strength and Conditioning, 29*(5), 1367-1377.

Cook, G., Burton, L., & Fields, K. (1999). Reactive neuromuscular training for the anterior cruciate ligament-deficient knee: A case report. *Journal of Athletic Training, 34*(2), 194-201.

Eapen, C., Nayak, C., & Zulfeequer, C. P. (2011). Effect of eccentric isotonic quadriceps muscle exercises on patellofemoral pain syndrome: An exploratory pilot study. *Asian Journal of Sports Medicine, 2*(4), 227-234.

Esmaeilzadeh, S., Akpinar, M., Polat, S., Yildiz, A., & Oral, A. (2015). The effects of two different frequencies of whole-Body vibration on knee extensors strength in healthy young volunteers: A randomized trial. *Journal of Musculoskeletal and Neuronal Interactions, 15*(4), 333-340.

Felício, L. R., Dias, L. A., Silva, A. P., Oliveira, A. S., & Bevilaqua-Grossi, D. (2011). Muscular activity of patella and hip stabilizers of healthy subjects during squat exercises. *Revista Brasileira de Fisioterapia, 15*(3), 206-211.

Hwangbo, P. (2015). The effects of squatting with visual feedback on the muscle activation of the vastus medialis oblique and the vastus lateralis in young adults with an increased quadriceps angle. *Journal of Physical Therapy Science, 27*(5), 1507-1510.

Iga, J., Fruer, C. S., Deighan, M., Croix, M. D., & James, D. V. (2012). 'Nordic' hamstrings exercise—engagement characteristics and training responses. *International Journal of Sports Medicine, 33*(12), 1000-1004.

Irish, S. E., Millward, A. J., Wride, J., Haas, B. M., & Shum, G. L. (2010). The effect of closed-kinetic chain exercises and open-kinetic chain exercise on the muscle activity of vastus medialis oblique and vastus lateralis. *Journal of Strength and Conditioning Research, 24*(5), 1256-1262.

Jaberzadeh, S., Yeo, D., & Zoghi, M. (2015). The effect of altering knee position and squat depth on VMO:VL EMG ratio during squat exercises. *Physiotherapy Research International, 21*(3), 164-173.

Loutsch, R. A., Baker, R. T., May, J. M., & Nasypany, A. M. (2015). Reactive neuromuscular training results in immediate and long term improvements in measures of hamstring flexibility: A case report. *International Journal of Sports Physical Therapy, 10*(3), 371-377.

Marcovic, G. (2007). Does plyometric training improve vertical jump height? A meta-analytical review. *British Journal of Sports Medicine, 41*, 349-355.

Miller, M. G., Herniman, J. J., Ricard, M. D., Cheatham, C. C., & Michael, T. J. (2006). The effects of a 6-week plyometric training program on agility. *Journal of Sports Science and Medicine, 5*(3), 459-465.

Peng, H. T., Kernozek, T. W., & Song, C. Y. (2013). Muscle activation of vastus medialis obliquus and vastus lateralis during a dynamic leg press exercise with and without isometric hip adduction. *Physical Therapy in Sport, 14*(1), 44-49.

Roelants, M., Delecluse, C., & Verschueren, S. M. (2004). Whole-body-vibration training increases knee-extension strength and speed of movement in older women. *Journal of the American Geriatrics Society, 52*(6), 901-908.

Roush, M. B., Sevier, T. L., Wilson, J. K., Jenkinson, D. M., Helfst, R. H., Gehlsen, G. M., & Basey, A. L. (2000). Anterior knee pain: A clinical comparison of rehabilitation methods. *Clinical Journal of Sports Medicine, 10*(1), 22-28.

Signorile, J. F., Lew, K., Stoutenberg, M., Pluchino, A., Lewis, J. E., & Gao, J. (2014). Range of motion and leg rotation affect electromyography activation levels of the superficial quadriceps muscles during leg extension. *Journal of Strength and Conditioning.* [Epub ahead of print].

Syme, G., Rowe, P., Martin, D., & Daly, G. (2009). Disability in patients with chronic patellofemoral pain syndrome: A randomised controlled trial of VMO selective training versus general quadriceps strengthening. *Manual Therapy, 14*(3), 252-263.

Tyler, T. F., Schmitt, B. M., Nicholas, S. J., & McHugh, M. (2015). Rehabilitation after hamstring strain injury emphasizing eccentric strengthening at long muscle lengths: Results of long-term follow-up. *Journal of Sports Rehabilitation, 26*(2), 131-140.

Van der Horst, N., Smits, D. W., Petersen, J., Goedhart, E. A., Backx, F. J. (2015). The preventive effect of the Nordic hamstring exercise on hamstring injuries in amateur soccer players: A randomized controlled trial. *American Journal of Sports Medicine, 43*(6), 1316-1323.

Van der Worp, H., de Poel, H. J., Diercks, R. L., van den Akker-Scheek, I., & Zwerver, J. (2014). Jumper's knee or lander's knee? A systematic review of the relation between jump biomechanics and patellar tendinopathy. *International Journal of Sports Medicine, 35*(8), 714-722.

Section 6.10

KNEE PROTOCOLS AND TREATMENT IDEAS

6.10.1 HAMSTRING INJURIES

Hamstring strains are among the most frequent injuries in sports, especially in events requiring sprinting and running (Lempainen, Sarimo, Mattila, Heikkilä, & Orava, 2007). Injuries to the hamstring muscles can be devastating to the athlete because they can heal slowly and recur with a re-injury risk of 12% to 31% (Ahmad et al., 2013). It is thought that many of the recurrent injuries to the hamstrings are the result of inadequate rehabilitation following the initial injury. The severity of hamstring injuries is usually of first or second degree (partial tears), but occasionally third-degree injuries (complete tear) do occur. Most hamstring strain injuries occur while running or sprinting. Several causative factors have been proposed, including poor flexibility, inadequate strength and/or endurance,

improper synergistic muscle patterns during running, lack of proper warm-up and pre-activity stretching, awkward running style, and a return to activity too soon after previous injury (Agre, 1985). General treatments after first- and second-degree hamstring injuries are rest and immobilization with a gradually increasing program of flexibility, strengthening, and activity. Third-degree hamstring ruptures in the adult are rare and require surgical treatment consisting of reattachment of the hamstring tendon(s) to the origin. Return to athletic competition should only occur once full rehabilitation has been achieved with recovery of full muscle strength, endurance, flexibility, coordination, and athletic agility. Failure to achieve full rehabilitation will only predispose the athlete to recurrent injury.

6.10.2 HAMSTRING STRAIN PROTOCOL

Protocol adapted from AAOS (Hartman, 2004b) and information contained in Valle et al.'s 2015 article proposing a rehabilitation protocol for hamstring muscle injuries based on current basic science and research.

Phase I: Acute 0 to 6 Weeks (Depending on Severity):

1. Rest, ice, compression, elevation, immobilization (usually less than 1 week for even the most severe strain), and mobilization is begun to properly align the regenerating muscle fibers and limit the extent of connective tissue fibrosis (Clanton & Coupe, 1998).

2. No knee extension with hip flexion into pain (stretches hamstring)

3. No active isolated knee flexion or hip extension (contracts hamstring)

4. Gait training to normalize gait pattern (pain-free)
   a. 6.04.43 Functional: Gait Practice

5. AROM
   a. 6.01.8 ROM: Hip Flexion and Extension, Heel Slide, Active
   b. 6.01.10 ROM: Hip Abduction and Adduction, Heel Slide, Active
   c. 4.01.7 ROM: Lower Trunk Rotation, Active

6. Stretching
   a. 6.03.3 Stretch: Hip Flexor, Standing Lunge
   b. 6.03.2 Stretch: Hip Flexor, Kneeling Lunge
   c. 6.03.7 Stretch: Hip Adductors, Frog
   d. 6.08.1 Stretch: Quadriceps
      i. Side-lying hand assist
      ii. Prone belt assist
   e. 6.08.3 Stretch: Hamstrings; initiate once pain decreased; do not do any aggressive stretching, only gentle, gradual and pain-free.
      i. Supine (hip flexed to 90 degrees and allow knee to extend to 45 degrees of flexion)
   f. Calf stretch
      i. 6.13.6 Stretch: Soleus Using Strap
      ii. 6.13.5 Stretch: Gastrocnemius Using Strap
7. Strengthening
   a. Isometrics
      i. 6.04.2 Strengthen: Isometric; Hip Extension/ Gluteus Sets; 50% to 70% sub-maximal contraction.
      ii. 6.09.3 Strengthen: Isometric; Knee Flexion, Hamstring Set (supine)
      iii. 6.09.5 Strengthen: Isometric; Knee, Straight Leg Raise, 4-Way at 45 degrees knee flexion only; 50% to 70% sub-maximal contraction B).
      iv. 6.09.1 Strengthen: Isometric; Knee Extension, Quadriceps Set (use electrical stimulation for increased muscle recruitment as needed)
      v. 6.09.2 Strengthen: Isometric; Knee Extension, Quadriceps Set With Ball Squeeze (Vastus Medialis Oblique)
      vi. 6.04.3 Strengthen: Isometric; Hip Abduction
      vii. 6.04.4 Strengthen: Isometric; Hip Adduction
      viii. 6.04.6 Strengthen: Isometric; Hip External Rotation
      ix. 6.04.5 Strengthen: Isometric; Hip Internal Rotation
   b. Isotonics
      i. 6.04.8 Strengthen: Isotonic; Hip, Straight Leg Raise, 4-Way; *flexion, abduction and adduction only, no extension.*
      ii. 6.14.7 Strengthen: Isotonic; Heel Raises
8. Balance/Coordination
   a. 6.14.16 Functional: Ankle/Foot, Rhomberg and Variations
9. Conditioning
   a. Start light recumbent or upright cycling (no resistance) as long as pain-free

Phase II: Subacute Up to 8 Weeks

1. Modalities and manual therapy: soft tissue to address complaints of soft tissue stiffness; consider psoas, iliacus, TFL/ITB, rectus femoris, sartorius, gluteus maximus/ medius/minimus, quadratus lumborum, adductor group, piriformis, hip external rotators, and erector spinae.
2. Warm-up
   a. Bike
3. Stretching ideas
   a. 6.08.3 Stretch: Hamstrings; *no aggressive stretching,* only gentle, gradual and pain-free.
      i. Supine (hip flexed to 90 degrees and allow knee to extend to 30 degrees of flexion) (C).
   b. 6.03.22 Stretch: Piriformis, Figure 4 and Variations
   c. Advance Calf Stretch (choose one)
      i. 6.13.7 Stretch: Calf on Step
      ii. 6.13.8 Stretch: Calf on Ramp
4. Strengthening ideas
   a. 6.09.5 Strengthen: Isometric; Knee, Straight Leg Raise, 4-Way; progress to 90 degrees knee flexion 50% to 70% sub-maximal contraction (B).
   b. 6.09.10 Strengthen: Isotonic; Hamstring Curl; gentle, start with active, progress to gradual increase in resistance.
   c. 6.09.18 Strengthen: Knee, Leg Press on Weight Machine 0 to 45 degrees
   d. 6.04.26 Functional: Hip, Wall Squat 0 to 45 degrees
   e. 6.04.28 Functional: Hip, Free-Standing Squat 0 to 45 degrees
   f. 6.04.27 Functional: Hip, Wall Sit 0 to 45 degrees
   g. 6.04.34 Functional: Hip, Lunge and Variations 0 to 45 degrees
   h. 6.04.33 Functional: Hip, Step-Ups 4 to 6 inch step
   i. 6.04.14 Strengthen: Isotonic; Hip Extension, Bridge and Variations (listed below)
      i. Bridge
      ii. Bridge with isometric adduction ball squeeze
      iii. Bridge with isometric hip abduction
      iv. Bridge in/outs
   j. 6.04.20 Strengthen: Resistance Band, Hip, 4-Way
   k. 6.04.22 Strengthen: Resistance Band, Hip, Sidestepping
   l. 6.04.17 Strengthen: Isotonic; Hip Abduction, "Fire Hydrants"
   m. 6.04.23 Strengthen: Resistance Band, Hip, "Clam"
   n. 6.04.24 Strengthen: Resistance Band, Hip Internal Rotation and Variations
   o. 6.04.25 Strengthen: Resistance Band, Hip External Rotation and Variations
   p. 6.04.38 Functional: Hip, Sidestepping With Mini-Squat
   q. 6.04.39 Functional: Hip, Step-Overs
   r. 6.04.40 Functional: Hip, Backward Walking
   s. 6.04.8 Strengthen: Isotonic; Hip, Straight Leg Raise, 4-Way; *add variations below as patient tolerates.*
      i. Extension
      ii. Isolate gluteus maximus

5. Core stabilization
   a. 4.03.7 Strengthen: Lumbar Spine, Bent-Knee Fall-Outs
   b. 4.03.9 Strengthen: Lumbar Spine, Bent-Knee Lift
   c. 4.03.23 Strengthen: Lumbar Spine, Alternating Arm Lift, Quadruped
   d. 4.03.24 Strengthen: Lumbar Spine, Alternating Hip and Knee Extension, Quadruped
   e. 4.03.25 Strengthen: Lumbar Spine, Opposite Arm and Leg Lift, Quadruped
   f. 4.03.27 Strengthen: Lumbar Spine, Hold Neutral Spine, Tall-Kneeling
   g. 4.03.28 Strengthen: Lumbar Spine, Arm Lift, Tall-Kneeling
   h. 4.03.29 Strengthen: Lumbar Spine, Reach Toward Floor, Tall-Kneeling
   i. 4.03.30 Strengthen: Lumbar Spine, Reach Toward Floor, Half-Kneeling
   j. 4.03.42 Strengthen: Abdominal, Pulsing Crunch, 3-Way (Advanced)
   k. 4.03.38 Strengthen: Abdominal, Plank and Variations below (progression)
      i. A: Standing wall (beginner)
      ii. B: Standing chair (beginner)
      iii. C: Quadruped
      iv. D: Forearm
      v. E: Hands
   l. 4.03.39 Strengthen: Abdominal, Side Plank and Variations (progression)
      i. A: Standing wall (beginner)
      ii. B: Standing chair (beginner)
      iii. C: On elbow and knee (beginner)
      iv. D: On elbow and feet
      v. E: On hand and knee
      vi. F: On hand and feet

6. Balance/Coordination
   a. 6.14.18 Functional: Ankle/Foot, Opposite Hip, 4-Way Balance Challenge

7. Cardiovascular program
   a. Stationary bike; start at 5 minutes week 3 and increase 3 to 5 minutes each week until at 20 minutes.
   b. Stairmaster initiate slowly; progress gradually as tolerated.
   c. Aquatic; may initiate pool exercise and pool running.
   d. Elliptical trainer; can alternate with bike to work up to 30 minutes continuous activity total between bike and elliptical.

Phase III: Dynamic Strengthening 6 to 16 Weeks

1. Stretching
   a. 6.08.3 Stretch: Hamstrings (try different variations listed below)
      i. Long-sitting
      ii. Seated
      iii. Standing foot on stool
      iv. Hip hinge with dowel
      v. Supine doorway/corner
      vi. Long-sitting against a wall

2. Strengthening
   a. 6.09.16 Strengthen: Resistance Band, Flexion, Hamstring Curl
   b. 6.09.12 Strengthen: Isotonic; Hamstring, Bridge Walk-Outs
   c. 6.09.11 Strengthen: Isotonic; Hamstring Curl With Exercise Ball
   d. 6.09.13 Strengthen: Isotonic; Hamstring, Nordic Curl, Eccentric Focus
   e. 6.09.29 Functional: Knee, Whole Body Vibration Machine (with squat and lunges)
   f. 6.09.18 Strengthen: Knee, Leg Press on Weight Machine 0 to 90 degrees
   g. 6.04.26 Functional: Hip, Wall Squat 0 to 90 degrees
   h. 6.04.28 Functional: Hip, Free-Standing Squat 0 to 90 degrees
   i. 6.04.27 Functional: Hip, Wall Sit 0 to 90 degrees
   j. 6.04.34 Functional: Hip, Lunge and Variations 0 to 90 degrees
   k. 6.04.33 Functional: Hip, Step-Ups 8 to 12 inch step
   l. 6.04.14 Strengthen: Isotonic; Hip Extension, Bridge and Variations (listed below)
      i. Single leg bridge
      ii. Bridge with knee extension
   m. 6.04.15 Strengthen: Hip Extension, Forearm Plank
   n. 6.04.29 Functional: Hip, Single-Limb Squat
   o. 6.04.37 Functional: Pelvic Drop/Hip Hike
   p. 6.09.28 Functional: Knee, Squat, Ball Variations

3. Core stabilization
   a. 4.03.38 Strengthen: Abdominal, Plank and Variations below
      i. I: Cheek dips
      ii. J: Tap outs
   b. 4.03.39 Strengthen: Abdominal, Side Plank and Variations below
      i. H: With leg lift
      ii. J: Hip dip

4. Balance/Coordination ideas; *consider neoprene sleeve during intense dynamic training.*
   a. 6.09.33 Plyometrics and Variations, Knee below
      i. A: Quiet jumps double leg
      ii. B: Quiet jumps single leg
      iii. C: Box jumps forward
      iv. *Consider progressing to other variations per tolerance*
   b. 6.09.34 Reactive Neuromuscular Training and Variations below
      i. Uniplanar anterior shift

    ii. Uniplanar lateral shift

    iii. Multiplanar weight shifts

    iv. Squat, posterior weight shifts

    v. Squat, anterior weight shifts

    vi. Squat, posterior medial shifts

    vii. Lunge medial weight shifts

    viii. Single leg squat medial shifts band at knee

5. Sport specific agility drills; clear with physician first.

    a. 6.09.30 Agility: Knee, Speed Ladder Drills and Variations

    b. 6.09.31 Agility: Knee, Dot Drills and Variations

    c. 6.09.32 Agility: Knee, Mini-Hurdle Drills and Variations

    d. 8.01.4 Running Progressions; gradually increase intensity of running jog to run to sprints.

    e. 8.01.7 Cutting Sequence-Figure 8 Progression

    f. 8.01.6 Jump-Hop Sequence

    g. 8.01.5 Sprint Sequence

6. Cardiovascular program

    a. Running, elliptical, bike, swimming, Stairmaster

7. Criteria for discharge; return to sport (clear with physician).

    a. Isokinetic testing to confirm that muscle-strength imbalances have been corrected, the hamstring-quadriceps ratio is 50% to 60%, and the strength of the injured leg has been restored to within 10% of that of the unaffected leg (Clanton & Coupe, 1998).

    b. Dynamic neuromuscular control with multi-plane activities at high velocity without pain or swelling

    c. Less than 10% deficit on functional testing profile

6.10.3 Hamstring Surgical Repair Protocol

Protocol adapted from guidelines developed collaboratively between Marc Sherry, PT, DPT, LAT, CSCS and the University of Wisconsin Health Sports Medicine Physician Group (2011).

Phase I: Acute 0 to 6 Weeks Post-Operation (Depending on Severity):

1. Weightbearing

    a. Week 0 to 2: Flat foot weightbearing; meaning no weight can be transmitted through the foot, but it is encouraged for the foot to be flat as it makes contact with the ground for balance.

    b. Weeks 3 to 4: 15% to 40% PWB progression

    c. Weeks 5 to 6: WBAT with weaning from crutches

2. Brace

    a. The use of a brace is determined by the surgeon at the time of surgery

3. Precautions

    a. No knee extension with hip flexion into pain (stretches hamstring)

    b. No active isolated knee flexion or hip extension (contracts hamstring)

4. PROM

    a. PROM knee with no hip flexion during knee extension

5. AROM

    a. 6.11.3 ROM: Ankle/Foot, Long-Sitting and Ankle Pumps, 4-Way, Active; *supine ankle pumps only.*

6. Isometrics

    a. 6.09.1 Strengthen: Isometric; Knee Extension, Quadriceps Set; use electrical stimulation for increased muscle recruitment as needed.

    b. 6.09.2 Strengthen: Isometric; Knee Extension, Quadriceps Set With Ball Squeeze (Vastus Medialis Oblique)

    c. 4.03.1 Strengthen: Isometric; Posterior Pelvic Tilt, Lumbar Spine, With or Without Blood Pressure Cuff for Biofeedback

7. Conditioning

    a. 5.04.1 ROM: Shoulder, Warm-Up, Upper Body Ergometer, Active Assistive

8. Aquatics: start weeks 3 to 4

    a. Pool-walking without hip flexion coupled with knee extension, hip abduction, hip extension, and balance exercises

Phase II: 6 to 12 Weeks Post-Operation:

1. Precautions

    a. No dynamic stretching of hamstring

    b. Avoid loading hip at deeper than 45 degrees flexion

    c. No running or impact activities

2. Modalities and manual therapy: soft tissue to address complaints of soft tissue stiffness; consider psoas, iliacus, TFL/ITB, rectus femoris, sartorius, gluteus maximus/medius/minimus, quadratus lumborum, adductor group, piriformis, hip external rotators, and erector spinae.

3. Gait training to normalize gait pattern, pain-free

    a. 6.04.43 Functional: Gait Practice

4. ROM

    a. 6.01.8 ROM: Hip Flexion and Extension, Heel Slide, Active

    b. 6.01.10 ROM: Hip Abduction and Adduction, Heel Slide, Active

c. 4.01.7 ROM: Lower Trunk Rotation, Active

5. Stretching: 6 to 10 weeks

    a. 6.08.3 Stretch: Hamstrings; initiate once pain decreased, *do not do any aggressive stretching,* only gentle, gradual and pain-free.

        i. Supine (hip flexed to 90 degrees and allow knee to extend to 45 degrees of flexion) (A)

        ii. *Progress slowly* to supine (hip flexed to 90 degrees and allow knee to extend to 30 degrees of flexion) (C). **6.03.3**

    b. 6.03.7 Stretch: Hip Adductors, Frog

    c. 6.08.1 Stretch: Quadriceps

        i. Side-lying hand assist

        ii. Prone belt assist

    d. Calf Stretch (choose one)

        i. 6.13.7 Stretch: Calf on Step

        ii. 6.13.9 Stretch: Calf Step on Wall

        iii. 6.13.8 Stretch: Calf on Ramp

6. Stretching: 10 to 12 weeks and beyond

    a. 6.08.3 Stretch: Hamstrings (try different variations listed below)

        i. Long-sitting

        ii. Seated

        iii. Standing foot on stool

        iv. Hip hinge with dowel

        v. Supine doorway/corner

        vi. Long-sitting against a wall

7. Strengthening

    a. Isometrics

        i. 6.04.2 Strengthen: Isometric; Hip Extension/ Gluteus Sets; 50% to 70% sub-maximal contraction

        ii. 6.09.3 Strengthen: Isometric; Knee Flexion, Hamstring Set (supine)

        iii. 6.09.5 Strengthen: Isometric; Knee, Straight Leg Raise, 4-Way; *at 45 degrees knee flexion only,* 50% to 70% sub-maximal contraction (B).

        iv. 6.04.3 Strengthen: Isometric; Hip Abduction

        v. 6.04.4 Strengthen: Isometric; Hip Adduction

        vi. 6.04.6 Strengthen: Isometric; Hip External Rotation

        vii. 6.04.5 Strengthen: Isometric; Hip Internal Rotation

    b. 6.09.11 Strengthen: Isotonic; Hamstring Curl With Exercise Ball

    c. 6.04.14 Strengthen: Isotonic; Hip Extension, Bridge and Variations (listed below)

        i. Bridge

        ii. Bridge with isometric adduction ball squeeze

        iii. Bridge with isometric hip abduction

    d. Isotonics

        i. 6.04.8 Strengthen: Isotonic; Hip, Straight Leg Raise, 4-Way; *flexion, abduction and adduction only, no extension.*

        ii. 6.14.7 Strengthen: Isotonic; Heel Raises

8. Core stabilization

    a. 4.03.7 Strengthen: Lumbar Spine, Bent-Knee Fall-Outs

    b. 4.03.9 Strengthen: Lumbar Spine, Bent-Knee Lift

    c. 4.03.23 Strengthen: Lumbar Spine, Alternating Arm Lift, Quadruped

    d. 4.03.24 Strengthen: Lumbar Spine, Alternating Hip and Knee Extension, Quadruped

    e. 4.03.25 Strengthen: Lumbar Spine, Opposite Arm and Leg Lift, Quadruped

    f. 4.03.27 Strengthen: Lumbar Spine, Hold Neutral Spine, Tall-Kneeling

    g. 4.03.28 Strengthen: Lumbar Spine, Arm Lift, Tall-Kneeling

    h. 4.03.29 Strengthen: Lumbar Spine, Reach Toward Floor, Tall-Kneeling

    i. 4.03.30 Strengthen: Lumbar Spine, Reach Toward Floor, Half-Kneeling

    j. 4.03.42 Strengthen: Abdominal, Pulsing Crunch, 3-Way (Advanced)

    k. 4.03.38 Strengthen: Abdominal, Plank and Variations below (progression)

        i. A: Standing wall (beginner)

        ii. B: Standing chair (beginner)

        iii. C: Quadruped

        iv. D: Forearm

        v. E: Hands

    l. 4.03.39 Strengthen: Abdominal, Side Plank and Variations below (progression)

        i. A: Standing wall (beginner)

        ii. B: Standing chair (beginner)

        iii. C: On elbow and knee (beginner)

        iv. D: On elbow and feet

        v. E: On hand and knee

        vi. F: On hand and feet

9. Balance/Coordination

    a. 6.14.16 Functional: Ankle/Foot, Rhomberg and Variations

    b. 6.09.27 Functional: Knee, Single-Leg Balance, Mini-Squat and Variations

10. Conditioning

    a. Start light recumbent or upright cycling (no resistance) as long as pain-free

Phase III: 12 to 16 Weeks Post-Operation:

1. Warm-up

    a. Bike

2. Strengthening ideas

    a. 6.04.20 Strengthen: Resistance Band, Hip, 4-Way

    b. 6.09.18 Strengthen: Knee, Leg Press on Weight Machine 0 to 45 degrees

    c. 6.04.26 Functional: Hip, Wall Squat 0 to 45 degrees

d. 6.04.28 Functional: Hip, Free-Standing Squat 0 to 45 degrees

e. 6.04.27 Functional: Hip, Wall Sit 0 to 45 degrees

f. 6.04.34 Functional: Hip, Lunge and Variations 0 to 45 degrees

g. 6.04.33 Functional: Hip, Step-Ups 4 to 6 inch step

h. 6.04.22 Strengthen: Resistance Band, Hip, Sidestepping

i. 6.04.17 Strengthen: Isotonic; Hip Abduction, "Fire Hydrants"

j. 6.04.23 Strengthen: Resistance Band, Hip, "Clam"

k. 6.04.24 Strengthen: Resistance Band, Hip Internal Rotation and Variations

l. 6.04.25 Strengthen: Resistance Band, Hip External Rotation and Variations

m. 6.09.16 Strengthen: Resistance Band, Flexion, Hamstring Curl

n. 6.04.38 Functional: Hip, Sidestepping With Mini-Squat

o. 6.04.39 Functional: Hip, Step-Overs

p. 6.04.40 Functional: Hip, Backward Walking

q. 6.09.12 Strengthen: Isotonic; Hamstring, Bridge Walk-Outs

r. 6.04.8 Strengthen: Isotonic; Hip, Straight Leg Raise, 4-Way; *add variations below as patient tolerates.*
   i. Extension
   ii. Isolate gluteus maximus

s. 6.09.13 Strengthen: Isotonic; Hamstring, Nordic Curl, Eccentric Focus

t. 6.04.14 Strengthen: Isotonic; Hip Extension, Bridge and Variations (listed below)
   i. Bridge in/outs
   ii. Single leg bridge
   iii. Bridge with knee extension

3. Core stabilization

a. 4.03.7 Strengthen: Lumbar Spine, Bent-Knee Fall-Outs

b. 4.03.9 Strengthen: Lumbar Spine, Bent-Knee Lift

c. 4.03.23 Strengthen: Lumbar Spine, Alternating Arm Lift, Quadruped

d. 4.03.24 Strengthen: Lumbar Spine, Alternating Hip and Knee Extension, Quadruped

e. 4.03.25 Strengthen: Lumbar Spine, Opposite Arm and Leg Lift, Quadruped

f. 4.03.27 Strengthen: Lumbar Spine, Hold Neutral Spine, Tall-Kneeling

g. 4.03.28 Strengthen: Lumbar Spine, Arm Lift, Tall-Kneeling

h. 4.03.29 Strengthen: Lumbar Spine, Reach Toward Floor, Tall-Kneeling

i. 4.03.30 Strengthen: Lumbar Spine, Reach Toward Floor, Half-Kneeling

j. 4.03.42 Strengthen: Abdominal, Pulsing Crunch, 3-Way (Advanced)

k. 4.03.38 Strengthen: Abdominal, Plank and Variations below (progression)
   i. A: Standing wall (beginner)
   ii. B: Standing chair (beginner)
   iii. C: Quadruped
   iv. D: Forearm
   v. E: Hands

l. 4.03.39 Strengthen: Abdominal, Side Plank and Variations below (progression)
   i. A: Standing wall (beginner)
   ii. B: Standing chair (beginner)
   iii. C: On elbow and knee (beginner)
   iv. D: On elbow and feet
   v. E: On hand and knee
   vi. F: On hand and feet

4. Balance/Coordination

a. 6.14.18 Functional: Ankle/Foot, Opposite Hip, 4-Way Balance Challenge

5. Cardiovascular program

a. Stationary bike; start at 5 minutes week 3 and increase 3 to 5 minutes each week until at 20 minutes.

b. Stairmaster initiate slowly; progress gradually as tolerated.

c. Aquatic; may initiate pool exercise and pool running.

d. Elliptical trainer; can alternate with bike to work up to 30 minutes continuous activity total between bike and elliptical.

Phase IV: Dynamic Strengthening 16 Weeks Post-Operation

1. Criteria to enter this phase

a. Dynamic neuromuscular control with multi-plane activities at low to medium velocity without pain or swelling

b. Less than 25% deficit for side to side hamstring comparison on Biodex testing at 60 degrees and 240 degrees per second

2. Strengthening

a. 6.09.29 Functional: Knee, Whole Body Vibration Machine (with squat and lunges)

b. 6.09.18 Strengthen: Knee, Leg Press on Weight Machine 0 to 90 degrees

c. 6.04.26 Functional: Hip, Wall Squat 0 to 90 degrees

d. 6.04.28 Functional: Hip, Free-Standing Squat 0 to 90 degrees

e. 6.04.27 Functional: Hip, Wall Sit 0 to 90 degrees

f. 6.04.34 Functional: Hip, Lunge and Variations 0 to 90 degrees

g. 6.04.33 Functional: Hip, Step-Ups 8 to 12 inch step

h. 6.04.15 Strengthen: Hip Extension, Forearm Plank

   i. 6.04.29 Functional: Hip, Single-Limb Squat
   j. 6.04.37 Functional: Pelvic Drop/Hip Hike
   k. 6.09.28 Functional: Knee, Squat, Ball Variations
3. Core stabilization
   a. 4.03.38 Strengthen: Abdominal, Plank and Variations below
      i. I: Cheek dips
      ii. J: Tap outs
   b. 4.03.39 Strengthen: Abdominal, Side Plank and Variations below
      i. H: With leg lift
      ii. J: Hip dip
4. Balance/Coordination ideas; consider neoprene sleeve during intense dynamic training.
   a. 6.09.33 Plyometrics and Variations, Knee below
      i.   A: Quiet jumps double leg
      ii. B: Quiet jumps single leg
      iii. C: Box jumps forward
      iv. Consider progressing to other variations per tolerance
   b. 6.09.34 Reactive Neuromuscular Training and Variations below
      i.   Uniplanar anterior shift
      ii. Uniplanar lateral shift
      iii. Multiplanar weight shifts
      iv. Squat posterior weight shifts
      v.   Squat anterior weight shifts
      vi. Squat posterior medial shifts
      vii. Lunge medial weight shifts
      viii. Single leg squat medial shifts band at knee
5. Sport specific agility drills; clear with physician first.
   a. 6.09.30 Agility: Knee, Speed Ladder Drills and Variations
   b. 6.09.31 Agility: Knee, Dot Drills and Variations
   c. 6.09.32 Agility: Knee, Mini-Hurdle Drills and Variations
   d. 8.01.4 Running Progressions; gradually increase intensity of running jog to run to sprints.
   e. 8.01.7 Cutting Sequence-Figure 8 Progression
   f. 8.01.6 Jump-Hop Sequence
   g. 8.01.5 Sprint Sequence
6. Cardiovascular Program
   a. Running, elliptical, bike, swimming, Stairmaster
7. Criteria for discharge; return to sport, clear with physician.
   a. Isokinetic testing to confirm that muscle-strength imbalances have been corrected, the hamstring-quadriceps ratio is 50% to 60%, and the strength of the injured leg has been restored to within 10% of that of the unaffected leg (Clanton & Coupe, 1998).
   b. Dynamic neuromuscular control with multi-plane activities at high velocity without pain or swelling
   c. Less than 10% deficit on functional testing profile

6.10.4 Anterior Cruciate Ligament Tear Discussion

The ACL provides stability to the knee preventing the tibia from translating anteriorly on the femur. It is commonly injured among athletic individuals. Both nonoperative and operative treatment options exist. The optimal treatment of an adult with an ACL tear depends on several factors, including age, occupation, and activity level. In less active patients, physical therapy, bracing, and activity modification can yield successful results. In active patients who want to resume participation in sports or have physically demanding occupations, ACL reconstruction is recommended. Techniques using autograft tissue (patellar and hamstring tendons generally) is preferred over allograft, especially in the younger athlete. Allograft tissue is a reasonable option in the older, less active adult (Bogunovic & Matava, 2013). Partial tearing of the ACL can also occur. There are debates of whether it is advantageous to preserve the ACL remnant and augment it with a graft, or to remove it and proceed with a standard ACL reconstruction. Clinical outcomes of bundle-preserving surgery are promising. An increasingly large body of scientific evidence suggests that augmenting the intact bundle is beneficial in terms of vascularity, proprioception, and kinematics. A number of surgeons have developed techniques to augment the intact bundle of the ACL in partial tears (Sonnery-Cottet & Colombet, 2016). Nonetheless, ACL reconstruction ensures structural ligament repair, whereas rehabilitation protects and maintains the ligament repair and the physical and psychological state and performance capabilities of the athlete (Saka, 2014). Different rehabilitation protocols post-ACL reconstruction exist all over the world, lacking a consensus between practitioners, which leads to uncertainties resulting in aggressive and non-aggressive approaches. Studies in the literature have tried to determine the earliest optimal time to start rehabilitation and how long it should take with new studies surfacing with modifications and development of new protocols (Saka, 2014). Functional bracing after ACL is also highly debated. It has been shown to be useful with high-demand patients, such as skiers, in preventing subsequent knee injury (Sterett, Briggs, Farley, & Steadman, 2006).

Where's the Evidence?

Risberg, Holm, Steen, Eriksson, and Ekeland (1999) evaluated the effect of knee bracing after ACL reconstruction in 60 patients randomized into one of two groups: the braced group wore rehabilitative braces for 2 weeks, followed by functional braces for 10 weeks, and patients in the non-braced group did not wear braces. At all follow-up times, there were no significant differences between the two groups with regard to knee joint laxity, ROM, muscle strength, functional knee tests, or pain. However, patients in the braced group had significantly improved knee function compared with patients in the non-braced group at the 3-month follow-up, even though the braced group showed significantly increased thigh atrophy compared with the non-braced group at 3 months. However, McDevitt et al. (2004) studied 100 volunteers from the three US service academies with acute ACL tears who were randomized into braced or non-braced groups. Only those subjects with ACL tears treated with identical surgical procedures within the first 8 weeks of injury were included. Post-operative physical therapy protocols were also identical for both groups. The braced group was instructed to wear an off-the-shelf functional knee brace for all cutting, pivoting, or jumping activities for the first year after surgery. At 2-year follow-up, 95 subjects were available and results indicated no statistical significant differences between groups in knee stability, functional testing, ROM, or strength testing. Two braced subjects and three non-braced subjects had re-injuries. Birmingham et al. (2008) had similar results in a rather large study of 150 patients after ACL repair comparing neoprene sleeve to functional bracing, with no significant difference found between the two groups with regard to outcomes.

ACL protocols are designed to protect the graft as it undergoes physiological changes as the patellar or hamstring tendon graft becomes more ligamentous. The graft is weakest between 6 and 12 weeks post-operatively and protocols are designed to protect the graft during this period. Additionally, progressive, controlled loading stimulates healing and can improve the quality of graft incorporation.

Early immobilization also can assist to maintain nutrition to articular cartilage nutrition and prevent loss of bone density. Kinematic research shows open-chain contraction of the quadriceps between 10 and 45 degrees of flexion causes the greatest tension on the ACL graft and should be avoided the first 12 weeks post-operation (Cross, 1998).

6.10.5 ANTERIOR CRUCIATE LIGAMENT REPAIR PROTOCOL (HAMSTRING GRAFT AND PATELLAR TENDON GRAFT)

ACL protocol adapted from Tolga Saka's 2014 article in *The World Journal of Orthopedics* and Dr. Michael Hartman's (2004a) ACL protocols following BPTB and hamstring autograft protocols. Saka (2014) attempts to summarize the ACL rehabilitation objectives without indicating a precise timeline, stating the times may overlap and modifications might have to be made on the basis of the criteria associated with the time schedules. He states the basic approach in ACL rehabilitation is to ensure a return to sports activities 6 months post-operatively and that today's post-operative ACL rehabilitation guidelines are time-focused, and while this approach makes implementation of the program easier, it does not cover all cases.

Phase I: Acute 0 to 4 Weeks:

1. Goals
   a. Patient education
   b. Pain control
   c. Decrease edema
   d. Increase ROM
2. Gait
   a. WBAT; crutches 0 to 2 weeks, wean by 2 weeks post-operation.
   b. In brace locked at 0 degrees extension usually; remove brace for treatment and 4 to 5 times per day for self ROM
   c. 6.04.43 Functional: Gait Practice
3. ROM
   a. PROM to achieve full extension in the 1st week
   b. PROM to near full flexion by end of week 3
   c. 6.11.3 ROM: Ankle/Foot, Long-Sitting and Ankle Pumps, 4-Way, Active; supine ankle pumps only.
   d. 6.06.1 ROM: Patellar Mobilization, Active Assistive

   e. 6.01.8 ROM: Hip Flexion and Extension, Heel Slide, Active
   f. 6.01.10 ROM: Hip Abduction and Adduction, Heel Slide, Active
   g. 6.06.2 ROM: Knee Flexion, Active Assistive
   h. 6.06.3 ROM: Knee Flexion, Wall Slide, Active Assistive
4. Stretching
   a. 6.08.3 Stretch: Hamstrings
   b. Calf stretch
      i. 6.13.6 Stretch: Soleus Using Strap
      ii. 6.13.5 Stretch: Gastrocnemius Using Strap
5. Lower extremity strengthening
   a. 6.09.1 Strengthen: Isometric; Knee Extension, Quadriceps Set; use electrical stimulation for increased muscle recruitment as needed.
   b. 6.09.2 Strengthen: Isometric; Knee Extension, Quadriceps Set With Ball Squeeze (Vastus Medialis Oblique)

c. 6.09.3 Strengthen: Isometric; Knee Flexion, Hamstring Set

d. 6.04.2 Strengthen: Isometric; Hip Extension/ Gluteus Sets

e. 6.04.3 Strengthen: Isometric; Hip Abduction

f. 6.04.4 Strengthen: Isometric; Hip Adduction

g. 6.04.6 Strengthen: Isometric; Hip External Rotation

h. 6.04.5 Strengthen: Isometric; Hip Internal Rotation

i. 6.09.9 Strengthen: Isotonic; Long-Arc Extension (Quadriceps); start at 90 degrees flexion and extend to 40 degrees flexion only.

j. 6.09.5 Strengthen: Isometric; Knee, Straight Leg Raise, 4-Way; 90 degrees, 60 degrees and 30 degrees.

k. 6.04.8 Strengthen: Isotonic; Hip, Straight Leg Raise, 4-Way; in brace until no extensor lag.

l. 6.09.21 Functional: Knee, Weight Shifts

m. 6.04.28 Functional: Hip, Free-Standing Squat 0 to 40 degrees

n. 6.09.18 Strengthen: Knee, Leg Press on Weight Machine 0 to 60 degrees

6. Core strengthening:

a. 4.03.1 Strengthen: Isometric; Posterior Pelvic Tilt, Lumbar Spine, With or Without Blood Pressure Cuff for Biofeedback

b. 4.03.33 Strengthen: Abdominal, Partial Sit-Up, 5-Way

c. 4.03.34 Strengthen: Abdominal, Partial Diagonal Sit-Up, 4-Way

7. Aquatics once sutures removed

a. Pool walking

8. Consider upper body and contralateral leg strengthening

a. 5.04.1 ROM: Shoulder, Warm-Up, Upper Body Ergometer, Active Assistive

b. Bicycling knee flexion 90 to 100 degrees; use contralateral leg more than affected side.

Phase II: Week 4 to 7:

1. Gait

a. Brace may be discharged at this time, unless otherwise indicated by physician.

b. FWB; normalize gait.

2. ROM

a. Achieve and maintain full ROM

3. Stretching

a. 6.08.1 Stretch: Quadriceps

i. Side-lying hand assist

ii. Prone belt assist

b. 6.08.3 Stretch: Hamstrings (try different variations listed below)

i. Supine

ii. Long-sitting

iii. Seated

iv. Standing foot on stool

c. 6.03.3 Stretch: Hip Flexor, Standing Lunge or 6.03.2 Stretch: Hip Flexor, Kneeling Lunge

d. 6.03.7 Stretch: Hip Adductors, Frog or **6.03.11** Stretch: Hip Adductors on Wall

e. 6.03.22 Stretch: Piriformis, Figure 4 and Variations

4. Lower extremity strengthening

a. 6.09.24 Functional: Knee, Step-Ups; variations listed below start with 2 inch step.

i. Beginner

ii. Forward

b. 6.04.26 Functional: Hip, Wall Squat 0 to 60 degrees

c. 6.04.27 Functional: Hip, Wall Sit 0 to 60 degrees

d. 6.04.28 Functional: Hip, Free-Standing Squat 0 to 60 degrees

e. 6.04.14 Strengthen: Isotonic; Hip Extension, Bridge and Variations (listed below)

i. Bridge

ii. Bridge with isometric adduction ball squeeze

iii. Bridge with isometric hip abduction

f. 6.09.17 Strengthen: Resistance Band and Ball, Terminal Knee Extension

g. 6.09.18 Strengthen: Knee, Leg Press on Weight Machine 0 to 45 degrees

h. 6.04.23 Strengthen: Resistance Band, Hip, "Clam"

i. 6.04.24 Strengthen: Resistance Band, Hip Internal Rotation and Variations

j. 6.04.25 Strengthen: Resistance Band, Hip External Rotation and Variations

k. 6.09.29 Functional: Knee, Whole Body Vibration Machine (with mini-squat)

5. Balance/Coordination

a. 6.14.16 Functional: Ankle/Foot, Rhomberg and Variations

6. Core strengthening

a. 4.03.42 Strengthen: Abdominal, Pulsing Crunch, 3-Way (Advanced)

b. 4.03.38 Strengthen: Abdominal, Plank and Variations below (progression)

i. A: Standing wall (beginner)

ii. B: Standing chair (beginner)

c. 4.03.39 Strengthen: Abdominal, Side Plank and Variations below (progression)

i. A: Standing wall (beginner)

ii. B: Standing chair (beginner)

iii. D: On elbow and feet

7. Aquatics

a. Swimming; use extended knee flutter kick.

Phase III: 7 to 12 Weeks Post-Operation:

Phase II and III overlap during week 7, depending on patient tolerances may start some of Phase III in Week 7 at therapist's discretion.

1. Stretching

a. Continue stretches as needed

2. Lower extremity strengthening

a. 6.09.24 Functional: Knee, Step-Ups; add variations listed below start with 2 inch step.
   i. Diagonal
   ii. Lateral
b. 6.14.7 Strengthen: Isotonic; Heel Raises
c. 6.09.10 Strengthen: Isotonic; Hamstring Curl
d. 6.09.16 Strengthen: Resistance Band, Flexion, Hamstring Curl
   i. Bridge in/outs
e. 6.09.12 Strengthen: Isotonic; Hamstring, Bridge Walk-Outs
f. 6.09.11 Strengthen: Isotonic; Hamstring Curl With Exercise Ball
g. 6.04.20 Strengthen: Resistance Band, Hip, 4-Way
h. 6.04.22 Strengthen: Resistance Band, Hip, Sidestepping
i. 6.04.38 Functional: Hip, Sidestepping With Mini-Squat
j. 6.09.26 Functional: Resistance Band, Knee, Monster Walk
k. 6.04.17 Strengthen: Isotonic; Hip Abduction, "Fire Hydrants"
l. 6.04.39 Functional: Hip, Step-Overs
m. 6.04.40 Functional: Hip, Backward Walking
n. 6.04.29 Functional: Hip, Single-Limb Squat
o. 6.04.37 Functional: Pelvic Drop/Hip Hike
p. 6.09.13 Strengthen: Isotonic; Hamstring, Nordic Curl, Eccentric Focus
q. 6.09.18 Strengthen: Knee, Leg Press on Weight Machine 0 to 90 degrees
r. 6.04.26 Functional: Hip, Wall Squat 0 to 90 degrees
s. 6.04.28 Functional: Hip, Free-Standing Squat 0 to 90 degrees
t. 6.04.27 Functional: Hip, Wall Sit 0 to 90 degrees
u. 6.04.34 Functional: Hip, Lunge and Variations
   i. Forward: 0 to 45 degrees progress to 60 degrees slowly; work up to 90 degrees by week 12.
v. 6.09.29 Functional: Knee, Whole Body Vibration Machine; already doing with squat, add lunges.
w. 6.04.14 Strengthen: Isotonic; Hip Extension, Bridge and Variations; add variations listed below.
   i. Single leg bridge
   ii. Bridge with knee extension
x. 6.04.15 Strengthen: Hip Extension, Forearm Plank
y. 6.09.20 Strengthen: Knee Flexion on Weight Machine
z. Isokinetic strengthening 100 to 40 degrees
aa. 6.04.29 Functional: Hip, Single-Limb Squat; starting weeks 10 to 12.
ab. Weeks 10 to 12
   i. Chair variation
   ii. Variation using poles
3. Balance/Coordination
   a. 6.14.18 Functional: Ankle/Foot, Opposite Hip, 4-Way Balance Challenge

b. 6.09.27 Functional: Knee, Single-Leg Balance, Mini-Squat and Variations
4. Core strengthening
   a. 4.03.42 Strengthen: Abdominal, Pulsing Crunch, 3-Way (Advanced)
   b. 4.03.38 Strengthen: Abdominal, Plank and Variations below (progression)
      i. D: Forearm
      ii. E: Hands
   c. 4.03.39 Strengthen: Abdominal, Side Plank and Variations below (progression)
      i. F: On hand and feet
5. Cardiovascular program
   a. Stationary bike; start at 5 minutes week 3 and increase 3 to 5 minutes each week until at 20 minutes.
   b. Stairmaster initiate slowly; progress gradually as tolerated.
   c. Elliptical trainer; can alternate with bike to work up to 30 minutes continuous activity total between bike and elliptical.
   d. Walking program
   e. Nordic Track
6. Aquatics
   a. Deep water running
   b. Progress to running backwards
   c. Swimming; use extended knee flutter kick.

Phase IV: 12 to 16 Weeks Post-Operation (3 to 4 Months)

1. Strengthening
   a. 6.04.29 Functional: Hip, Single-Limb Squat
      i. Exercise ball variation
      ii. Progress to bench and free-standing variations as tolerated
   b. 6.09.28 Functional: Knee, Squat, Ball Variations
   c. 6.04.41 Strengthen: "Multi-Hip" 4-Way on Weight Machines
   d. 6.04.30 Functional: Hip, Single-Limb Squat, Circumduction
   e. 6.04.32 Functional: Hip, Single-Limb Squat, Skaters
   f. 6.04.31 Functional: Hip, Single-Limb Squat, Cone Taps
   g. 6.04.35 Functional: Hip, Dynamic Leg Swing, "Running Man"
   h. 6.04.36 Functional: Hip, Deadlift and Variations
2. Core stabilization
   a. 4.03.38 Strengthen: Abdominal, Plank and Variations
      i. I: Cheek dips
      ii. J: Tap outs
   b. 4.03.39 Strengthen: Abdominal, Side Plank and Variations
      i. H: With leg lift
      ii. J: Hip dip

3. Balance/Coordination
   a. 6.09.33 Plyometrics and Variations, Knee below
      i. Quiet jumps double leg
      ii. Quiet jumps single leg
      iii. Box jumps forward
      iv. Consider progressing to other variations as tolerated

Where's the Evidence?

Chmielewski et al. (2016) compared the immediate effect of low- and high-intensity plyometric exercise during rehabilitation after ACL reconstruction on knee function, articular cartilage metabolism, and other clinically relevant measures in 24 patients who underwent unilateral ACL reconstruction. Patients were assigned to 8 weeks (2 per week) of low- or high-intensity plyometric exercise consisting of running, jumping, and agility activities starting at an average of 14 weeks post-operation. Primary outcomes were self-reported knee function and a biomarker of articular cartilage degradation. Secondary outcomes included additional biomarkers of articular cartilage metabolism, serum concentrations of newly formed type II collagen and inflammation, functional performance (maximal vertical jump and single-legged hop), knee impairments (anterior knee laxity, average knee pain intensity, normalized quadriceps strength, quadriceps symmetry index), and psychosocial status. The groups did not significantly differ in the change of any primary or secondary outcome measure. Across groups, significant changes after the intervention were increased in the international knee documentation committee score, vertical jump height, normalized quadriceps strength, quadriceps symmetry index, and knee activity self-efficacy and decreased average knee pain intensity. No significant differences were detected between the low- and high-intensity plyometric exercise groups. The authors concluded that across both groups, plyometric exercise induced positive changes in knee function, knee impairments, and psychosocial status that would support the return to sports participation after ACL reconstruction.

   b. 6.09.34 Reactive Neuromuscular Training and Variations below
      i. Uniplanar anterior shift
      ii. Uniplanar lateral shift
      iii. Multiplanar weight shifts
      iv. Squat posterior weight shifts
      v. Squat anterior weight shifts
      vi. Squat posterior medial shifts
      vii. Lunge medial weight shifts
      viii. Single leg squat medial shifts band at knee
4. Sport specific agility drills; clear with physician first.
   a. 6.09.30 Agility: Knee, Speed Ladder Drills and Variations
   b. 6.09.31 Agility: Knee, Dot Drills and Variations

   c. 6.09.32 Agility: Knee, Mini-Hurdle Drills and Variations
   d. 8.01.4 Running Progressions; gradually increase intensity of running jog to run to sprints.
   e. 8.01.7 Cutting Sequence-Figure 8 Progression
   f. 8.01.6 Jump-Hop Sequence
   g. 8.01.5 Sprint Sequence
5. Cardiovascular program
   a. Running, elliptical, bike, swimming, Stairmaster
6. Criteria for discharge; return to sport, clear with physician.
   a. Good results of functional tests:
      i. Single Leg Hop Test is the most common functional test
      ii. Single leg squat (Hall, Paik, Ware, Mohr, & Limpisvasti, 2015)
      iii. Y-Balance Test (Garrison, Bothwell, Wolf, Aryal, & Thigpen 2015)
   b. Hamstring and quadriceps strength at least 85% of the unaffected leg

Where's the Evidence?

Abrams et al. (2014) systematically reviewed 88 studies and found that, at 6 months post-operatively, a number of isokinetic strength measurements failed to reach 80% Limb Symmetry Index, most commonly isokinetic knee extension testing in both BPTB graft and hamstring autograft groups. They also found the knee flexion strength deficit was significantly less in the BTPB autograft group as compared with those having hamstring autograft at 1 year post-operatively, while no significant differences were found in isokinetic extension strength between the two groups. The results of these functional tests, as reported in the Limb Symmetry Index, improved with increasing time, with nearly all results greater than 90% at 1 year following primary ACL reconstruction.

   c. Flawless running
   d. No swelling, laxity or fear of re-injury by patient

Where's the Evidence?

Ardern, Webster, Taylor, and Feller (2011) looked at 48 studies evaluating 5770 participants at a mean follow-up of 41.5 months. Overall, 82% of participants had returned to some kind of sports participation, 63% had returned to their pre-injury level of participation, and 44% had returned to competitive sport at final follow-up. Approximately 90% of participants achieved normal or nearly normal knee function when assessed post-operatively using impairment-based outcomes such as laxity and strength, and 85% when using activity-based outcomes such as the International Knee Documentation Committee knee evaluation form. Fear of re-injury was the most common reason cited for a post-operative reduction in or cessation of sports participation.

6.10.6 MENISCUS REPAIR DISCUSSION

The meniscus cartilage in the knee includes a medial and a lateral meniscus. The primary function of the menisci is to improve load transmission, shock absorption, lubrication and joint stability. There are two categories of meniscal tears: acute traumatic tears and degenerative tears. Degenerative tears most commonly occur in middle-aged people via repetitive stresses that severely weaken the tissue. Most degenerative tears are surgically removed or conservatively managed with rehabilitation. Acute traumatic tears occur most often in athletes resulting from a twisting injury to the knee with the foot planted (Sherry, 2013a). Meniscal repair is considered for patients with clinically symptomatic meniscal tears who have large, unstable, peripheral, bucket-handle meniscal tears at arthroscopy. Successful repair relieves symptoms and allows the patient to return to full function. Patients with adequate repair of the meniscal tears followed a rehabilitation program that allows immediate ROM and WBAT achieve a clinical result comparable to patients who follow a restrictive rehabilitation program. By using a less-restrictive rehabilitation program, patients may have a shorter interval between the surgical procedure and full return to the ADLs and athletics than offered by previous regimens without compromising the clinical results (Shelbourne, Patel, Adsit, & Porter, 1996).

Where's the Evidence?

Vanderhave, Perkins, and Le (2015) reviewed the current literature on weightbearing status after meniscal repairs to provide evidence-based recommendations for postoperative rehabilitation. They found successful clinical outcomes after both conservative (restricted weightbearing) protocols and accelerated rehabilitation (immediate weightbearing) yielded similar good to excellent results.

Generally, after surgery there will be a period of restricted knee flexion, particularly during weightbearing, to protect the repair. Specific time frames, restrictions, and precautions are given to protect healing tissues and repair. The patient's age, associated injuries, health status, compliance, and injury severity may also affect the rate or progression of the rehabilitation program (Sherry, 2013a). Progressive weightbearing and joint stress are necessary to enhance the functionality of the meniscal repair; however, care should be taken as excessive shear forces may be disruptive (Brindle, Nyland, & Johnson, 2001).

General guidelines are provided here but as with all postsurgical protocols; follow specific physician orders above any guidelines listed here.

6.10.7 MENISCUS REPAIR PROTOCOL

Meniscus repair protocol adapted from Dr. Michael Hartman's Meniscus Protocol (2004c) and Brindle, Nyland and Johnson's 2001 article, "The Meniscus: Review of Basic Principles With Application to Surgery and Rehabilitation."

Phase I: Acute 0 to 2 Weeks:

1. Rest, ice, compression, elevation
2. Brace locked at 0 degrees usually for ambulation and sleeping only
3. Usually PWB 25% to 50%; crutches or walker, some physicians will allow WBAT, follow specific physician orders.
4. ROM
   a. PROM 0 to 90 degrees
   b. 6.11.3 ROM: Ankle/Foot, Long-Sitting and Ankle Pumps, 4-Way, Active; *supine ankle pumps only.*
   c. 6.06.1 ROM: Patellar Mobilization, Active Assistive
   d. 6.01.8 ROM: Hip Flexion and Extension, Heel Slide, Active 60 degrees to 0 degrees (avoid active knee flexion past 60 degrees for first 7 days post-operation)
   e. 6.01.10 ROM: Hip Abduction and Adduction, Heel Slide, Active
5. Stretching
   a. 6.08.3 Stretch: Hamstrings
   b. Calf stretch
      i. 6.13.6 Stretch: Soleus Using Strap
      ii. 6.13.5 Stretch: Gastrocnemius Using Strap

Phase I: Acute 2 to 4 Weeks:

1. Gait
   a. Progress to FWB by week 3; normalize gait.
   b. 6.04.43 Functional: Gait Practice
2. ROM
   a. Gradually increase PROM
      i. Week 2: 0 to 100 degrees
      ii. Week 3: 0 to 120 degrees
      iii. Week 4: 0 to 135 degrees (full)
      iv. 6.06.2 ROM: Knee Flexion, Active Assistive
   b. 6.01.8 ROM: Hip Flexion and Extension, Heel Slide, Active
   c. 6.06.3 ROM: Knee Flexion, Wall Slide, Active Assistive
3. Lower extremity strengthening
   a. 6.09.1 Strengthen: Isometric; Knee Extension, Quadriceps Set; use electrical stimulation for increased muscle recruitment as needed.
   b. 6.09.2 Strengthen: Isometric; Knee Extension, Quadriceps Set With Ball Squeeze (Vastus Medialis Oblique)

c. 6.09.3 Strengthen: Isometric; Knee Flexion, Hamstring Set

d. 6.04.2 Strengthen: Isometric; Hip Extension/ Gluteus Sets

e. 6.04.3 Strengthen: Isometric; Hip Abduction

f. 6.04.4 Strengthen: Isometric; Hip Adduction

g. 6.04.6 Strengthen: Isometric; Hip External Rotation

h. 6.04.5 Strengthen: Isometric; Hip Internal Rotation

i. 6.09.9 Strengthen: Isotonic; Long-Arc Extension (Quadriceps)

j. 6.09.4 Strengthen: Isometric; Quadriceps and Hamstrings, Multi-Angle; 90 degrees, 60 degrees and 30 degrees.

k. 6.04.8 Strengthen: Isotonic; Hip, Straight Leg Raise, 4-Way (no extensor lag)

l. 6.09.21 Functional: Knee, Weight Shifts

m. 6.04.28 Functional: Hip, Free-Standing Squat 0 to 40 degrees

n. 6.04.26 Functional: Hip, Wall Squat 0 to 60 degrees

o. 6.09.18 Strengthen: Knee, Leg Press on Weight Machine 0 to 40 degrees

4. Core strengthening

a. 4.03.1 Strengthen: Isometric; Posterior Pelvic Tilt, Lumbar Spine, With or Without Blood Pressure Cuff for Biofeedback

b. 4.03.33 Strengthen: Abdominal, Partial Sit-Up, 5-Way

c. 4.03.34 Strengthen: Abdominal, Partial Diagonal Sit-Up, 4-Way

5. Conditioning

a. 5.04.1 ROM: Shoulder, Warm-Up, Upper Body Ergometer, Active Assistive

Phase III: 5 to 8 Weeks Post-Operation

1. Brace

a. Usually discontinued by weeks 4 to 5 (physician specific)

2. ROM

a. Full ROM

3. Stretching

a. 6.08.1 Stretch: Quadriceps

i. Side-lying hand assist

ii. Prone belt assist

b. 6.08.3 Stretch: Hamstrings (try different variations listed below)

i. Supine

ii. Long-sitting

iii. Seated

iv. Standing foot on stool

c. 6.03.3 Stretch: Hip Flexor, Standing Lunge or 6.03.2 Stretch: Hip Flexor, Kneeling Lunge

d. 6.03.7 Stretch: Hip Adductors, Frog or **6.03.11** Stretch: Hip Adductors on Wall

e. 6.03.22 Stretch: Piriformis, Figure 4 and Variations

4. Lower extremity strengthening

a. Begin isokinetic strengthening for stability

b. 6.09.24 Functional: Knee, Step-Ups; variations listed below start with 2-inch step

i. Beginner

ii. Forward

iii. Lateral

c. 6.04.20 Resistance Band, Hip, 2-Way

i. Abduction

ii. Adduction

d. 6.04.26 Functional: Hip, Wall Squat 0 to 70 degrees

e. 6.04.27 Functional: Hip, Wall Sit 0 to 70 degrees

f. 6.04.28 Functional: Hip, Free-Standing Squat 0 to 60 degrees

g. 6.04.23 Strengthen: Resistance Band, Hip, "Clam"

h. 6.04.24 Strengthen: Resistance Band, Hip Internal Rotation and Variations

i. 6.04.25 Strengthen: Resistance Band, Hip External Rotation and Variations

j. 6.04.14 Strengthen: Isotonic; Hip Extension, Bridge and Variations

i. Bridge

ii. Bridge with isometric adduction ball squeeze

iii. Bridge with isometric hip abduction

k. 6.09.17 Strengthen: Resistance Band and Ball, Terminal Knee Extension

l. 6.04.22 Strengthen: Resistance Band, Hip, Sidestepping

m. 6.04.39 Functional: Hip, Step-Overs

5. Balance/Coordination

a. 6.14.16 Functional: Ankle/Foot, Rhomberg and Variations

6. Core strengthening:

a. 4.03.42 Strengthen: Abdominal, Pulsing Crunch, 3-Way (Advanced)

7. Cardiovascular program

a. Stationary bike; start at 5 minutes week 3 and increase 3 to 5 minutes each week until at 20 minutes.

8. Aquatics

a. May initiate pool exercise and walking

Phase III: 9 to 16 Weeks Post-Operation

1. Lower extremity strengthening

a. 6.09.24 Functional: Knee, Step-Ups; increased step heights for lateral and forward.

i. Diagonal start at 2-inch step and increase gradually

b. 6.04.26 Functional: Hip, Wall Squat increase to 0 to 90 degrees

c. 6.04.27 Functional: Hip, Wall Sit increase to 0 to 90 degrees

d. 6.04.28 Functional: Hip, Free-Standing Squat increase to 0 to 90 degrees

 e. 6.09.18 Strengthen: Knee, Leg Press on Weight Machine 0 to 90 degrees

 f. 6.14.7 Strengthen: Isotonic; Heel Raises

 g. 6.04.34 Functional: Hip, Lunge and Variations
  i. Forward: 0 to 45 degrees progress to 60 degrees slowly

 h. 6.04.14 Strengthen: Isotonic; Hip Extension, Bridge and Variations (add variation listed below)
  i. Bridge in/outs

 i. 6.04.20 Strengthen: Resistance Band, Hip, 4-Way

 j. 6.09.16 Strengthen: Resistance Band, Flexion, Hamstring Curl

 k. 6.09.12 Strengthen: Isotonic; Hamstring, Bridge Walk-Outs

 l. 6.09.11 Strengthen: Isotonic; Hamstring Curl With Exercise Ball

 m. 6.09.26 Functional: Resistance Band, Knee, Monster Walk

 n. 6.04.17 Strengthen: Isotonic; Hip Abduction, "Fire Hydrants"

 o. 6.04.38 Functional: Hip, Sidestepping With Mini-Squat

 p. 6.04.40 Functional: Hip, Backward Walking

 q. 6.04.37 Functional: Pelvic Drop/Hip Hike

 r. 6.09.29 Functional: Knee, Whole Body Vibration Machine (with squat)

2. Advanced LE strengthening at later stages (weeks 12 to 16)

 a. 6.09.20 Strengthen: Knee Flexion on Weight Machine

 b. 6.04.29 Functional: Hip, Single-Limb Squat

 c. 6.09.13 Strengthen: Isotonic; Hamstring, Nordic Curl, Eccentric Focus

 d. 6.04.34 Functional: Hip, Lunge and Variations; start 0 to 60 degrees and gradually progress to 90 degrees.

 e. 6.04.14 Strengthen: Isotonic; Hip Extension, Bridge and Variations (listed below)
  i. Single leg bridge
  ii. Bridge with knee extension

 f. 6.04.15 Strengthen: Hip Extension, Forearm Plank

 g. 6.04.29 Functional: Hip, Single-Limb Squat

 h. 6.09.29 Functional: Knee, Whole Body Vibration Machine (add lunges)

3. Balance/Coordination

 a. 6.14.18 Functional: Ankle/Foot, Opposite Hip, 4-Way Balance Challenge

 b. 6.09.27 Functional: Knee, Single-Leg Balance, Mini-Squat and Variations

4. Core strengthening

 a. 4.03.38 Strengthen: Abdominal, Plank and Variations (progression)
  i. A: Standing wall (beginner)
  ii. B: Standing chair (beginner)
  iii. C: Quadruped
  iv. D: Forearm
  v. E: Hands

 b. 4.03.39 Strengthen: Abdominal, Side Plank and Variations (progression)
  i. A: Standing wall (beginner)
  ii. B: Standing chair (beginner)
  iii. C: On elbow and knee (beginner)
  iv. D: On elbow and feet
  v. E: On hand and knee
  vi. F: On hand and feet

5. Cardiovascular program

 a. Stairmaster initiate slowly; progress gradually as tolerated.

 b. Elliptical trainer; can alternate with bike to work up to 30 minutes continuous activity total between bike and elliptical.

6. Aquatics

 a. Week 12; may initiate pool running
  i. Deep water running
  ii. Progress to running backwards
  iii. Swimming; *use extended knee flutter kick.*

7. Conditioning

 a. Walking program

Phase IV: 4 to 6 Months:

Continue and progress all strengthening exercises and stretching drills.

1. Strengthening

 a. Deeper squat permitted at 5 months

 b. 6.09.28 Functional: Knee, Squat, Ball Variations

2. Core stabilization

 a. 4.03.38 Strengthen: Abdominal, Plank and Variations
  i. I: Cheek dips
  ii. J: Tap outs

 b. 4.03.39 Strengthen: Abdominal, Side Plank and Variations
  i. H: With leg lift
  ii. J: Hip dip

3. Balance/Coordination

 a. 6.09.33 Plyometrics and Variations, Knee
  i. A: Quiet jumps double leg
  ii. B: Quiet jumps single leg
  iii. C: Box jumps forward
  iv. Consider progressing to other variations per tolerance

 b. 6.09.34 Reactive Neuromuscular Training and Variations
  i. Uniplanar anterior shift
  ii. Uniplanar lateral shift
  iii. Multiplanar weight shifts
  iv. Squat posterior weight shifts

v. Squat anterior weight shifts

vi. Squat posterior medial shifts

vii. Lunge medial weight shifts

viii. Single leg squat medial shifts band at knee

4. Sport-specific agility drills; clear with physician first.

 a. 4 months start straight line running

  i. 8.01.4 Running Progressions; gradually increase intensity of running from jog to run.

 b. 5 months start sprints

  i. 8.01.5 Sprint Sequence

 c. 5 months start pivoting and cutting

  i. 8.01.7 Cutting Sequence-Figure 8 Progression

 d. 5 months start agility training

 i. 6.09.30 Agility: Knee, Speed Ladder Drills and Variations

 ii. 6.09.31 Agility: Knee, Dot Drills and Variations

 iii. 6.09.32 Agility: Knee, Mini-Hurdle Drills and Variations

 iv. 8.01.6 Jump-Hop Sequence

5. Cardiovascular program

 a. Running, elliptical, bike, swimming, Stairmaster

6. Criteria for discharge; return to sport, clear with physician.

 a. Hamstring and quadriceps strength at least 85% of the unaffected leg

 b. Flawless running

 c. No swelling, laxity or fear of re-injury by patient

 d. Good results of functional tests

6.10.8 POSTERIOR CRUCIATE LIGAMENT DISCUSSION

The PCL is approximately twice as strong as the ACL and, therefore, less commonly injured. The PCL functions to limit posterior translation of the tibia in relation to the femur. The PCL also provides support for the collateral ligaments during valgus or varus stresses of the knee. Isolated PCL ruptures are rare and usually a result of a direct blow to the proximal anterior tibia when the knee is flexed. In other PCL injury mechanisms, other knee structures may also be damaged. In isolated, complete tears of the PCL, the majority of studies recommend conservative treatment even in athletes. The outcome seems to depend more on the quadriceps status than on the amount of residual posterior laxity. Conservative treatment protocols focus on intensive quadriceps exercises, with a 2-week immobilization period followed by early controlled activities and early weightbearing (Kannus et al., 1991). If the PCL is repaired surgically, outcomes have historically been inferior to outcomes after ACL reconstruction. This leads some surgeons to be reluctant to recommend reconstruction. However, recent technologic advances have substantially improved PCL reconstructive surgical outcomes. Today, PCL reconstructive surgery often results in excellent function with a return to the patient's pre-injury level of activity. In contrast

to accelerated rehabilitation after ACL reconstructive surgery, slow and deliberate post-operative rehabilitation is recommended to allow early healing to occur after PCL reconstructive surgery (Fanelli, 2008). Post-operation, posterior translation of the tibia in flexion of the knee, especially active flexion, should be avoided. The tendon graft becomes weak by post-operation week 6 and it is recommended during weeks 2 and 3 post-operation, the knee should be immobilized in an extended position. Quadriceps muscle strengthening and straight-leg raising are started immediately after surgery. Passive flexion exercise is performed slight anterior pull on the proximal tibia to 90 degrees of flexion by post-operation weeks 4 to 6. For isolated PCL injuries, weightbearing may begin earlier; however, for combined PCL injuries, PWB is allowed soon after surgery and progressed to FWB at 6 to 12 weeks post-operatively. In addition, PROM should be gradually increased to 140 degrees of flexion avoiding active contraction of the hamstrings. From 12 weeks post-operatively when collagen fibers become organized, flexion exercise is permitted, light jogging is allowed 3 to 6 months after surgery, and sports activities are allowed 6 months after surgery (Lee & Nam, 2011).

6.10.9 POSTERIOR CRUCIATE LIGAMENT REPAIR PROTOCOL

Adapted from University of Wisconsin Sports Rehabilitation protocol (Sherry, 2013b) and Dr. Michael Hartman's Single Tunnel CL-PTG reconstruction protocol (Hartman,2004d).

Phase I: Acute 0 to 2 Weeks:

1. Goals:

 a. Patient education

 b. Pain control

 c. Decrease edema

 d. Increase ROM

 e. *No active flexion*

2. Gait

 a. Partial (>75%) to WBAT; crutches 0 to 2 weeks, wean by 2 weeks post-operation.

 b. In brace locked at 0 degrees extension usually; remove brace for treatment and 4 to 5 times per day for self ROM.

3. ROM
    a. PROM
        i. Day 1 to 3: 0 to 60 degrees
        ii. Day 4 to 7: 0 to 75 degrees
        iii. Week 1 to 2: 0 to 90 degrees
    b. 6.11.3 ROM: Ankle/Foot, Long-Sitting and Ankle Pumps, 4-Way, Active; *supine ankle pumps.*
    c. 6.06.1 ROM: Patellar Mobilization, Active Assistive
    d. 6.01.10 ROM: Hip Abduction and Adduction, Heel Slide, Active
4. Lower extremity strengthening
    a. 6.09.1 Strengthen: Isometric; Knee Extension, Quadriceps Set; use electrical stimulation for increased muscle recruitment as needed.
    b. 6.09.2 Strengthen: Isometric; Knee Extension, Quadriceps Set With Ball Squeeze (Vastus Medialis Oblique)
    c. 6.04.2 Strengthen: Isometric; Hip Extension/Gluteus Sets
    d. 6.04.3 Strengthen: Isometric; Hip Abduction
    e. 6.04.4 Strengthen: Isometric; Hip Adduction
    f. 6.04.6 Strengthen: Isometric; Hip External Rotation
    g. 6.04.5 Strengthen: Isometric; Hip Internal Rotation
    h. 6.09.8 Strengthen: Isotonic; Short-Arc Extension (Quadriceps)
    i. 6.09.9 Strengthen: Isotonic; Long-Arc Extension (Quadriceps); *start at 60 degrees flexion and extend to 0 degrees only.*
    j. 6.04.8 Strengthen: Isotonic; Hip, Straight Leg Raise, 4-Way; in brace until no extensor lag, flexion, abduction and adduction only.
    k. 6.09.21 Functional: Knee, Weight Shifts
    l. 6.04.28 Functional: Hip, Free-Standing Squat 0 to 40 degrees
    m. 6.09.18 Strengthen: Knee, Leg Press on Weight Machine 0 to 60 degrees
5. Core strengthening
    a. 4.03.1 Strengthen: Isometric; Posterior Pelvic Tilt, Lumbar Spine, With or Without Blood Pressure Cuff for Biofeedback
    b. 4.03.33 Strengthen: Abdominal, Partial Sit-Up, 5-Way
    c. 4.03.34 Strengthen: Abdominal, Partial Diagonal Sit-Up, 4-Way
6. Consider conditioning
    a. 5.04.1 ROM: Shoulder, Warm-Up, Upper Body Ergometer, Active Assistive
    b. Bicycling use contralateral leg

Phase II: Week 2 to 6

1. Gait
    a. Brace locked at 0 degrees
    b. 75% or greater WBAT
2. ROM
    a. 0 to 90 degrees

3. Lower Extremity Strengthening:
    a. Week 2
        i. 6.09.4 Strengthen: Isometric; Quadriceps and Hamstrings, Multi-Angle; quadriceps, 60 degrees, 40 degrees and 20 degrees, no hamstring
        ii. 6.04.26 Functional: Hip, Wall Squat 0 to 45 degrees
        iii. 6.09.18 Strengthen: Knee, Leg Press on Weight Machine 0 to 60 degrees
    b. Week 4
        i. 6.04.26 Functional: Hip, Wall Squat 0 to 60 degrees
        ii. 6.04.28 Functional: Hip, Free-Standing Squat 0 to 60 degrees
4. Balance/Coordination
    a. Week 5: 6.14.16 Functional: Ankle/Foot, Rhomberg and Variations
5. Aquatics
    a. Week 4: Pool walking
    b. Week 5: Pool exercises (within restrictions)
6. Conditioning:
    a. 5.04.1 ROM: Shoulder, Warm-Up, Upper Body Ergometer, Active Assistive

Phase III: 7 to 12 Weeks Post-Operation:

1. Gait
    a. Brace unlocked at 0 to 125 degrees
    b. 75% or greater WBAT
    c. Week 12: Discontinue brace
2. ROM
    a. Limit ROM to 0 to 90 degrees; some protocols may allow full ROM at this time, clear with physician first.
    b. 6.01.8 ROM: Hip Flexion and Extension, Heel Slide, Active 0 to 90 degrees
3. Stretching
    a. Calf stretch
        i. 6.13.6 Stretch: Soleus Using Strap
        ii. 6.13.5 Stretch: Gastrocnemius Using Strap
    b. 6.08.1 Stretch: Quadriceps; 0 to 125 degrees only, if no stretch felt at 125 degrees wait until next phase to initiate further.
        i. Side-lying hand assist
        ii. Prone belt assist
    c. 6.08.3 Stretch: Hamstrings; try different variations
        i. Supine
        ii. Long-sitting
    d. 6.03.3 Stretch: Hip Flexor, Standing Lunge or 6.03.2 Stretch: Hip Flexor, Kneeling Lunge
    e. 6.03.7 Stretch: Hip Adductors, Frog or **6.03.11** Stretch: Hip Adductors on Wall
    f. 6.03.22 Stretch: Piriformis, Figure 4 and Variations

4. Lower extremity strengthening
   a. 6.09.3 Strengthen: Isometric; Knee Flexion, Hamstring Set
   b. 6.04.23 Strengthen: Resistance Band, Hip, "Clam"
   c. Week 12: Start isokinetic 0 to 60 degrees (extension/flexion)
   d. Week 12: 6.09.24 Functional: Knee, Step-Ups; add variations start with 2-inch step.
      i.   Beginner
      ii. Forward
      iii. Lateral
   e. Week 12: 6.04.27 Functional: Hip, Wall Sit 0 to 60 degrees
   f. Week 12: 6.09.29 Functional: Knee, Whole Body Vibration Machine (with mini squat)
   g. Week 12: 6.09.17 Strengthen: Resistance Band and Ball, Terminal Knee Extension
   h. Week 12: 6.09.18 Strengthen: Knee, Leg Press on Weight Machine 0 to 45 degrees
   i. Week 12: 6.14.7 Strengthen: Isotonic; Heel Raises
   j. Week 12: 6.09.10 Strengthen: Isotonic; Hamstring Curl (light weight)
5. Balance/Coordination
6. Core strengthening
   a. 4.03.42 Strengthen: Abdominal, Pulsing Crunch, 3-Way (Advanced)
   b. 4.03.38 Strengthen: Abdominal, Plank and Variations (progression)
      i. A: Standing wall (beginner)
      ii. B: Standing chair (beginner)
   c. 4.03.39 Strengthen: Abdominal, Side Plank and Variations (progression)
      i.   A: Standing wall (beginner)
      ii. B: Standing chair (beginner)
      iii. D: On elbow and feet
7. Aquatics
   a. Swimming; use extended knee flutter kick.
   b. Week 12: Initiate pool running

Phase IV: 12 to 16 Weeks Post-Operation (3 to 4 Months)

1. Precautions
   a. No open chain hamstring strengthening or isolated hamstring exercises.
2. ROM
   a. Full ROM
3. Strengthening
   a. 6.04.20 Strengthen: Resistance Band, Hip, 4-Way
   b. 6.04.22 Strengthen: Resistance Band, Hip, Sidestepping
   c. 6.04.38 Functional: Hip, Sidestepping With Mini-Squat
   d. 6.09.26 Functional: Resistance Band, Knee, Monster Walk

   e. 6.04.17 Strengthen: Isotonic; Hip Abduction, "Fire Hydrants"
   f. 6.04.39 Functional: Hip, Step-Overs
   g. 6.04.40 Functional: Hip, Backward Walking
   h. 6.04.29 Functional: Hip, Single-Limb Squat
      i. Chair variation
      ii. Variation using poles
   i. 6.04.37 Functional: Pelvic Drop/Hip Hike
   j. 6.09.18 Strengthen: Knee, Leg Press on Weight Machine 0 to 90 degrees
   k. 6.04.26 Functional: Hip, Wall Squat 0 to 90 degrees
   l. 6.04.28 Functional: Hip, Free-Standing Squat 0 to 90 degrees
   m. 6.04.27 Functional: Hip, Wall Sit 0 to 90 degrees
   n. 6.04.34 Functional: Hip, Lunge and Variations
      i. Forward: 0 to 45 degrees progress to 60 degrees slowly; work up to 90 degrees by week 16.
   o. 6.09.29 Functional: Knee, Whole Body Vibration Machine; with squat and lunges.
4. Balance/Coordination
   a. 6.14.18 Functional: Ankle/Foot, Opposite Hip, 4-Way Balance Challenge
   b. 6.09.27 Functional: Knee, Single-Leg Balance, Mini-Squat and Variations
5. Core strengthening
   a. 4.03.38 Strengthen: Abdominal, Plank and Variations below (progression)
      i. D: Forearm
      ii. E: Hands
   b. 4.03.39 Strengthen: Abdominal, Side Plank and Variations (progression)
      i. F: On hand and feet
6. Cardiovascular program
   a. Stationary bike start at 5 minutes week 3 and increase 3 to 5 minutes each week until at 20 minutes.
   b. Stairmaster initiate slowly with small steps; progress gradually as tolerated.
   c. Walking program

Phase V: 16 to 24 Weeks Post-Operation (5 to 6 Months)

1. Precautions
   a. Avoid post activity swelling
2. ROM
   a. Maintain full ROM
3. Strengthening
   a. 6.09.16 Strengthen: Resistance Band, Flexion, Hamstring Curl
      i. Bridge in/outs
   b. 6.09.12 Strengthen: Isotonic; Hamstring, Bridge Walk-Outs
   c. 6.09.11 Strengthen: Isotonic; Hamstring Curl With Exercise Ball
   d. 6.09.28 Functional: Knee, Squat, Ball Variations

e. 6.04.41 Strengthen: "Multi-Hip" 4-Way on Weight Machines

f. 6.04.30 Functional: Hip, Single-Limb Squat, Circumduction

g. 6.04.32 Functional: Hip, Single-Limb Squat, Skaters

h. 6.04.31 Functional: Hip, Single-Limb Squat, Cone Taps

i. 6.04.35 Functional: Hip, Dynamic Leg Swing, "Running Man"

j. 6.04.36 Functional: Hip, Deadlift and Variations

k. 6.04.29 Functional: Hip, Single-Limb Squat (progression)
   i. Chair variation
   ii. Variation using poles
   iii. Exercise ball variation
   iv. Progress to bench and free-standing variations as tolerated

l. 6.09.13 Strengthen: Isotonic; Hamstring, Nordic Curl, Eccentric Focus

m. 6.04.14 Strengthen: Isotonic; Hip Extension, Bridge and Variations (add variations)
   i. Bridge
   ii. Bridge with isometric adduction ball squeeze
   iii. Bridge with isometric hip abduction
   iv. Progress to Single leg bridge
   v. Progress to Bridge with knee extension

n. 6.04.15 Strengthen: Hip Extension, Forearm Plank

o. 6.09.20 Strengthen: Knee Flexion on Weight Machine

4. Core strengthening
   a. 4.03.38 Strengthen: Abdominal, Plank and Variations
      i. I: Cheek dips
      ii. J: Tap outs
   b. 4.03.39 Strengthen: Abdominal, Side Plank and Variations

   i. H: With leg lift
   ii. J: Hip dip

5. Balance/Coordination
   a. 6.09.33 Plyometrics and Variations, Knee below
      i. A: Quiet jumps double leg
      ii. B: Quiet jumps single leg
      iii. C: Box jumps forward
      iv. Consider progressing to other variations per tolerance
   b. 6.09.34 Reactive Neuromuscular Training and Variations
      i. Uniplanar anterior shift
      ii. Uniplanar lateral shift
      iii. Multiplanar weight shifts
      iv. Squat posterior weight shifts
      v. Squat anterior weight shifts
      vi. Squat posterior medial shifts
      vii. Lunge medial weight shifts
      viii. Single leg squat medial shifts band at knee

6. Sport specific agility drills; clear with physician first.
   a. 6.09.30 Agility: Knee, Speed Ladder Drills and Variations
   b. 6.09.31 Agility: Knee, Dot Drills and Variations
   c. 6.09.32 Agility: Knee, Mini-Hurdle Drills and Variations
   d. 8.01.4 Running Progressions; gradually increase intensity of running jog to run to sprints.
   e. 8.01.7 Cutting Sequence-Figure 8 Progression
   f. 8.01.6 Jump-Hop Sequence
   g. 8.01.5 Sprint Sequence

7. Cardiovascular program
   a. Running, elliptical, bike, swimming, Stairmaster

8. Criteria for discharge; return to sport, clear with physician.
   a. Dynamic neuromuscular control with multi-plane activities, without instability, pain or swelling

6.10.10 Total Knee Arthroplasty Discussion

TKA involves surgical replacement of the knee joint and has become the gold standard treatment for end-stage knee osteoarthritis (Pozzi, Snyder-Mackler, & Zeni, 2013). The goal of TKA is to decrease pain and improve function. DVT is a common concern after TKA and patients typically wear compression stockings and take anticoagulant medication to prevent this. Infection is another major concern and, generally, patients are given a prophylactic antibiotic after surgery for up to 24 hours. While implementing a TKA protocol, the therapist should be aware of these possible complications and alert the physician if observing any signs or symptoms of either. It is important to get the patient moving his or her extremity after surgery to prevent DVT, stiffness, and scarring. CPM machines are often used after surgery.

Where's the Evidence?

A large systematic review in 2014 found minimal evidence to support the use of CPM after TKA (Harvey, Brosseau, & Herbert, 2014). However, Liao et al. in 2015 found evidence that, when clinical performance instrument is applied early with initial high flexion and rapid progress, it can benefit knee function up to 6 months after TKA.

Treatment generally begins post-operation day 1 to begin light strengthening, ROM, gait training, transfer training, and bed mobility. Patients are usually discharged from the hospital fairly quickly and begin home health physical therapy for the first 8 to 10 days before transitioning to an outpatient setting. Other patients with comorbidities, functional limitations, or of increased age may transfer to a skilled nursing facility for a few days to several weeks before transitioning to home. Average TKA is intended to last 10 to 20 years when implants may begin to loosen. Optimal outpatient physical therapy protocols should include strengthening and intensive functional exercises given through land-based or aquatic programs, the intensity of which is increased based on patient progress. Due to the highly individualized characteristics of these types of exercises, outpatient physical therapy performed in a clinic under the supervision of a trained physical therapist may provide the best long-term outcomes after the surgery (Pozzi et al., 2013).

6.10.11 Total Knee Arthroplasty Protocol

Adapted from University of Wisconsin Health Orthopedics and Rehabilitation (The Specialty Team for Arthroplasty Rehabilitation [STAR] Team, 2014) and Vanderbilt Orthopedic Institute Postsurgical TKA protocols (Vanderbilt Orthopaedic Institute, 2011).

Phase I: Acute 0 to 2 Weeks

1. Ice, elevation
2. CPM high flexion and rapid progress (Liao et al., 2015)
3. Bed mobility, transfers
4. Gait training to normalize gait pattern, pain-free (assistive device as needed)
   a. WBAT usually (follow specific physician orders if different)
   b. 6.04.43 Functional: Gait Practice
5. AROM
   a. 6.11.3 ROM: Ankle/Foot, Long-Sitting and Ankle Pumps, 4-Way, Active; *supine ankle pumps only.*
   b. 6.01.8 ROM: Hip Flexion and Extension, Heel Slide, Active
   c. 6.06.1 ROM: Patellar Mobilization, Active Assistive
   d. 6.06.2 ROM: Knee Flexion, Active Assistive
   e. 6.01.10 ROM: Hip Abduction and Adduction, Heel Slide, Active
6. Stretching
   a. 6.08.3 Stretch: Hamstrings
   b. Calf stretch
      i. 6.13.6 Stretch: Soleus Using Strap
      ii. 6.13.5 Stretch: Gastrocnemius Using Strap
7. Strengthening
   a. Isometrics
      i. 6.04.2 Strengthen: Isometric; Hip Extension/ Gluteus Sets
      ii. 6.09.3 Strengthen: Isometric; Knee Flexion, Hamstring Set (supine)
      iii. 6.09.1 Strengthen: Isometric; Knee Extension, Quadriceps Set; use electrical stimulation for increased muscle recruitment as needed.
      iv. 6.09.2 Strengthen: Isometric; Knee Extension, Quadriceps Set With Ball Squeeze (Vastus Medialis Oblique)
      v. 6.04.3 Strengthen: Isometric; Hip Abduction
      vi. 6.04.4 Strengthen: Isometric; Hip Adduction
      vii. 6.04.6 Strengthen: Isometric; Hip External Rotation
      viii. 6.04.5 Strengthen: Isometric; Hip Internal Rotation
   b. Isotonics
      i. 6.04.8 Strengthen: Isotonic; Hip, Straight Leg Raise, 4-Way (may not be able to tolerate extension due to pressure on knee in prone)
      ii. 6.09.8 Strengthen: Isotonic; Short-Arc Extension (Quadriceps)
      iii. 6.09.9 Strengthen: Isotonic; Long-Arc Extension (Quadriceps)
8. Conditioning
   a. 5.04.1 ROM: Shoulder, Warm-Up, Upper Body Ergometer, Active Assistive

Phase II: 3 to 6 Weeks Post-Operation:

1. Gait
   a. Normalize gait pattern; wean assistive device if able.
2. ROM
   a. PROM to increase to 0 to 120 degrees or plateau (may be less due to pre-surgical status)
   b. Consider increasing frequency of visits if ROM not progressing
3. Stretching
   a. 6.08.3 Stretch: Hamstrings
      i. Long-sitting
      ii. Seated
   b. 6.03.22 Stretch: Piriformis, Figure 4 and Variations
   c. Advance Stretch (choose one)
      i. 6.13.7 Stretch: Calf on Step
      ii. 6.13.8 Stretch: Calf on Ramp
4. Nerve glides
   a. 6.15.1 Nerve Glide: Sciatic Nerve, Flossing and Variations
5. Strengthening
   a. 6.14.7 Strengthen: Isotonic; Heel Raises
   b. 6.09.17 Strengthen: Resistance Band and Ball, Terminal Knee Extension
   c. 6.09.10 Strengthen: Isotonic; Hamstring Curl
   d. 6.04.9 Strengthen: Isotonic; Hip Flexion, Marching

e. 6.09.18 Strengthen: Knee, Leg Press on Weight Machine 0 to 45 degrees

f. 6.04.26 Functional: Hip, Wall Squat 0 to 45 degrees

g. 6.04.28 Functional: Hip, Free-Standing Squat 0 to 45 degrees

h. 6.04.27 Functional: Hip, Wall Sit 0 to 45 degrees

i. 6.04.33 Functional: Hip, Step-Ups 2 to 6 inches step

j. 6.04.13 Strengthen: Isotonic; Hip Extension, Mini-Bridge on Towel/Bolster

k. 6.04.22 Strengthen: Resistance Band, Hip, Sidestepping

l. 6.04.23 Strengthen: Resistance Band, Hip, "Clam"

m. 6.04.38 Functional: Hip, Sidestepping With Mini-Squat

n. 6.04.39 Functional: Hip, Step-Overs

o. 6.04.40 Functional: Hip, Backward Walking

6. Balance/Coordination

a. 6.14.16 Functional: Ankle/Foot, Rhomberg and Variations

7. Conditioning

a. Start light recumbent cycling (no resistance) as long as pain-free; can do partial revolutions until ROM allows full revolution.

8. Aquatics, start weeks 3 to 4

a. Pool-walking without hip flexion coupled with knee extension, hip abduction, hip extension, and balance exercises

Phase III: 6 to 12 Weeks Post-Operation

1. Strengthening

a. 6.09.16 Strengthen: Resistance Band, Flexion, Hamstring Curl

b. 6.09.12 Strengthen: Isotonic; Hamstring, Bridge Walk-Outs

c. 6.09.11 Strengthen: Isotonic; Hamstring Curl With Exercise Ball

d. 6.04.14 Strengthen: Isotonic; Hip Extension, Bridge and Variations (listed below)

   i. Bridge

   ii. Bridge with isometric adduction ball squeeze

   iii. Bridge with isometric hip abduction

e. 6.09.29 Functional: Knee, Whole Body Vibration Machine (with squat)

f. 6.04.20 Strengthen: Resistance Band, Hip, 4-Way

g. 6.09.18 Strengthen: Knee, Leg Press on Weight Machine; to tolerance ROM but not beyond 90 degrees.

h. 6.04.26 Functional: Hip, Wall Squat; to tolerance ROM but not beyond 90 degrees.

i. 6.04.28 Functional: Hip, Free-Standing Squat; to tolerance ROM but not beyond 90 degrees.

j. 6.04.27 Functional: Hip, Wall Sit; to tolerance ROM but not beyond 90 degrees.

k. 6.04.34 Functional: Hip, Lunge and Variations start 0 to 45 degrees

l. 6.04.15 Strengthen: Hip Extension, Forearm Plank

m. 6.04.37 Functional: Pelvic Drop/Hip Hike

2. Core stabilization ideas

a. 4.03.42 Strengthen: Abdominal, Pulsing Crunch, 3-Way (Advanced)

b. 4.03.38 Strengthen: Abdominal, Plank and Variations (progression)

   i. A: Standing wall (beginner)

   ii. B: Standing chair (beginner)

c. 4.03.39 Strengthen: Abdominal, Side Plank and Variations (progression)

   i. A: Standing wall (beginner)

   ii. B: Standing chair (beginner)

3. Balance/Coordination

a. 6.14.18 Functional: Ankle/Foot, Opposite Hip, 4-Way Balance Challenge

b. 6.14.17 Functional: Ankle/Foot, Steps-Overs, Step-Behinds, and Carioca/Braiding

c. 7.03.2 Global Functioning: Treatment Ideas

4. Cardiovascular program

a. Walking, cycling, swimming

5. Criteria for discharge; clear with physician.

a. ROM 0 to 125 degrees

b. Normal gait

c. Reciprocal gait on stairs no rails

d. Independent transfers and function

e. No extensor lag

REFERENCES

Abrams, G. D., Harris, J. D., Gupta, A. K., McCormick, F. M., Bush-Joseph, C. A., Verma, N. N., . . . Bach, B. R. Jr. (2014). Functional performance testing after anterior cruciate ligament reconstruction: A systematic review. *Orthopedic Journal of Sports Medicine, 2*(1), 2325967113518305.

Agre, J. C. (1985). Hamstring injuries. Proposed aetiological factors, prevention, and treatment. *Sports Medicine, 2*(1), 21-33.

Ahmad, C. S., Redler, L. H., Ciccotti, M. G., Maffulli, N., Longo, U. G., & Bradley, J. (2013). Evaluation and management of hamstring injuries. *American Journal of Sports Medicine, 41*(12), 2933-2947.

Ardern, C. L., Webster, K. E., Taylor, N. F., & Feller, J. A. (2011). Return to sport following anterior cruciate ligament reconstruction surgery: A systematic review and meta-analysis of the state of play. *British Journal of Sports Medicine, 45*(7), 596-606.

Birmingham, T. B., Bryant, D. M., Giffin, J. R., Litchfield, R. B., Kramer, J. F., Donner, A., & Fowler, P. J. (2008). A randomized controlled trial comparing the effectiveness of functional knee brace and neoprene sleeve use after anterior cruciate ligament reconstruction. *American Journal of Sports Medicine, 36*(4), 648-655.

Bogunovic, L., & Matava, M. J. (2013). Operative and nonoperative treatment options for ACL tears in the adult patient: A conceptual review. *Physician and Sports Medicine, 41*(4), 33-40.

Brindle, T., Nyland, J., & Johnson, D. L. (2001). The meniscus: Review of basic principles with application to surgery and rehabilitation. *Journal of Athletic Training, 36*(2), 160-169.

Chmielewski, T. L., George, S. Z., Tillman, S. M., Moser, M. W., Lentz, T. A., Indelicato, P. A., . . ., Leeuwenburgh, C. (2016). Low- versus high-intensity plyometric exercise during rehabilitation after anterior cruciate ligament reconstruction. *American Journal of Sports Medicine, 44*(3), 609-617.

Clanton, T. O., & Coupe, K. J. (1998). Hamstring strains in athletes: Diagnosis and treatment. *Journal of the American Academy of Orthopedic Surgeons, 6*(4), 237-248.

Cross, M. J. (1998). Anterior cruciate ligament injuries: Treatment and rehabilitation. *Encyclopedia of Sports Medicine and Science.* Retrieved from http://www.sportsci.org/encyc/aclinj/aclinj.html#6

Fanelli, G. C. (2008). Posterior cruciate ligament rehabilitation: How slow should we go? *Arthroscopy, 24*(2), 234-235.

Garrison, J. C., Bothwell, J. M., Wolf, G., Aryal, S., & Thigpen, C. A. (2015). Y balance test™ anterior reach symmetry at three months is related to single leg functional performance at time of return to sports following anterior cruciate ligament reconstruction. *International Journal of Sports Physical Therapy, 10*(5), 602-611.

Hall, M. P., Paik, R. S., Ware, A. J., Mohr, K. J., & Limpisvasti, O. (2015). Neuromuscular evaluation with single-leg squat test at 6 months after anterior cruciate ligament reconstruction. *Orthopedic Journal of Sports Medicine, 3*(3), 2325967115575900.

Hartman, M. (2004a). ACL patellar tendon autograft protocol. *AAOS Health Library.* Retrieved from http://orthodoc.aaos.org/Hartman/ACL%20Regular%20BTB%20Autograft.pdf

Hartman, M. (2004b). Hamstring strain protocol. *AAOS Health Library.* Retrieved from http://orthodoc.aaos.org/Hartman/Hamstring%20Strain.pdf

Hartman, M. (2004c). Meniscus repair rehabilitation (peripheral tears). *AAOS Health Library.* Retrieved from http://orthodoc.aaos.org/Hartman/Meniscus%20Repair%20-%20Peripheral%20Tears.pdf

Hartman, M. (2004d). Rehabilitation protocol following single-tunnel PCL-PTG reconstruction. *AAOS Health Library.* Retrieved from http://orthodoc.aaos.org/Hartman/PCL%20Reconstruction%20Single%20Tunnel.pdf

Harvey, L. A., Brosseau, L., & Herbert, R. D. (2014). Continuous passive motion following total knee arthroplasty in people with arthritis. *Cochrane Database of Systematic Reviews,* (2), CD004260.

Kannus, P., Bergfeld, J., Järvinen, M., Johnson, R. J., Pope, M., Renström, P., & Yasuda, K. (1991). Injuries to the posterior cruciate ligament of the knee. *Sports Medicine, 12*(2), 110-131.

Lee, B. K., & Nam, S. W. (2011). Rupture of posterior cruciate ligament: Diagnosis and treatment principles. *Knee Surgery and Related Research, 23*(3), 135-141.

Lempainen, L., Sarimo, J., Mattila, K., Heikkilä, J., & Orava, S. (2007). Distal tears of the hamstring muscles: review of the literature and our results of surgical treatment. *British Journal of Sports Medicine, 41*(2), 80-83.

Liao, C. D., Huang, Y. C., Lin, L. F., Chiu, Y. S., Tsai, J. C., Chen, C. L., & Liou, T. H. (2016). Continuous passive motion and its effects on knee flexion after total knee arthroplasty in patients with the knee osteoarthritis. *Knee Surgery, Sports Traumatology, Arthroscopy, 24*(8), 2578-2586.

McDevitt, E. R., Taylor, D. C., Miller, M. D., Gerber, J. P., Ziemke, G., Hinkin, D., . . ., Pierre, P. S. (2004). Functional bracing after anterior cruciate ligament reconstruction: A prospective, randomized, multicenter study. *American Journal of Sports Medicine, 32*(8), 1887-1892.

Pozzi, F., Snyder-Mackler, L., & Zeni, J. (2013). Physical exercise after knee arthroplasty: A systematic review of controlled trials. *European Journal of Physical and Rehabilitative Medicine, 49*(6), 877-892.

Risberg, M. A., Holm, I., Steen, H., Eriksson, J., & Ekeland, A. (1999). The effect of knee bracing after anterior cruciate ligament reconstruction. A prospective, randomized study with two years' follow-up. *American Journal of Sports Medicine, 27*(1), 76-83.

Saka, T. (2014). Principles of post-operative anterior cruciate ligament rehabilitation. *World Journal of Orthopedics, 5*(4), 450-459.

Shelbourne, K. D., Patel, D. V., Adsit, W. S., & Porter, D. A. (1996). Rehabilitation after meniscal repair. *Clinics in Sports Medicine, 15*(3), 595-612.

Sherry, M. (2011). Rehabilitation guidelines following proximal hamstring primary repair. *University of Wisconsin Sports Medicine.* Retrieved from http://www.uwhealth.org/files/uwhealth/docs/pdf5/SM-27464_Hamstring_Protocol.pdf

Sherry, M. (2013a). Rehabilitation guidelines for meniscal repair. *University of Wisconsin Sports Medicine.* Retrieved from http://www.uwhealth.org/files/uwhealth/docs/pdf/SM14890_Meniscus_Repair8.pdf

Sherry, M. (2013b). Rehabilitation guidelines for posterior cruciate ligament reconstruction. *University of Wisconsin Sports Medicine.* Retrieved from http://www.uwhealth.org/files/uwhealth/docs/pdf2/SM_PCL.pdf

Sonnery-Cottet, B., & Colombet, P. (2016). Partial tears of the anterior cruciate ligament. *Orthopedics and Traumatology, Surgery and Research, 102*(1 Suppl), S59-67.

Sterett, W. I., Briggs, K. K., Farley, T., & Steadman, J. R. (2006). Effect of functional bracing on knee injury in skiers with anterior cruciate ligament reconstruction: A prospective cohort study. *American Journal of Sports Medicine, 34*(10), 1581-1585.

The Specialty Team for Arthroplasty Rehabilitation (STAR) Team; UW Health Joint Replacement Surgeons. (2014). Outpatient rehabilitation guidelines for total knee arthroplasty. *University of Wisconsin Sports Medicine.* Retrieved from http://www.uwhealth.org/files/uwhealth/docs/sportsmed/RE-38789-14_TKA_OP.pdf

Valle, X., Tol, J. L., Hamilton, B., Rodas, G., Malliaras, P., Malliaropoulos, N., . . ., Jardi, J. (2015). Hamstring muscle injuries, a rehabilitation protocol purpose. *Asian Journal of Sports Medicine, 6*(4), e25411.

Vanderbilt Orthopaedic Institute. (2011). Total knee arthroplasty (TKA) and unicondylar rehabilitation guideline. *Vanderbilt University Medical Center.* Retrieved from http://www.mc.vanderbilt.edu/documents/orthopaedics/files/Total_Knee_Arthropasty_2011.pdf

VanderHave, K. L., Perkins, C., & Le, M. (2015). Weightbearing versus nonweightbearing after meniscus repair. *Sports Health, 7*(5), 399-402.

Section 6.11

ANKLE AND FOOT RANGE OF MOTION

6.11.1 ROM: ANKLE/FOOT, WARM-UP, STATIONARY OR RECUMBENT BIKE

<u>POSITION</u>: Seated

<u>TARGETS</u>: Mobility of the ankle dorsi- and plantarflexion, warm-up for LE

<u>INSTRUCTION</u>: Patient places feet in/on pedals and cycles. Set the seat. The recumbent bike has the pedal oriented in front of the patient with a back rest and offers more back support and thus may be more com-

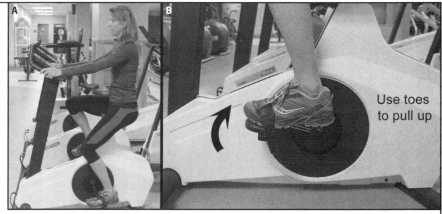

Use toes to pull up

fortable for people with LBP. For patients new to exercise or who are obese, a recumbent bike may be more comfortable. *Upright bike and recumbent*: Adjust the seat height so that at the lowest/furthest position, the leg is almost, but not fully, extended. This prevents the patient from rocking hips to reach the pedal. If patient is using handlebars, handles should be within reach so patient can almost fully extend the elbows. If there are foot straps, adjust them so patient's foot feels snug but not so tight that circulation is impeded. With foot straps, instruct the patient to also pull up on the upstroke (A and B).

<u>SUBSTITUTIONS</u>: Pelvic movements; in chair, patient stays fully seated and trunk upright with chest up and straight spine.

<u>PARAMETERS</u>: Cycle for 5 to 10 minutes for warm-up, increase for cardio training goals, 10 repetitions, repeat 1 to 3 times per day

Where's the Evidence?

An EMG study of 10 non-cyclist males comparing recumbent upright bike found that differences in average peak muscle activity were not statistically significant for any of the four muscles tested: rectus femoris, anterior tibialis, semi-tendinosis, and medial gastrocnemius. Pedaling a recumbent ergometer resulted in greater activity in semitendinosus and tibialis anterior. Rectus femoris muscle demonstrated greater activity during upright pedaling (Lopes, Alouche, Hakansson, & Cohen, 2014).

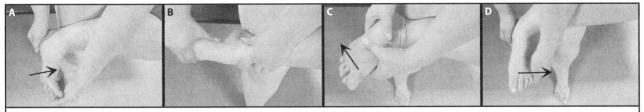

6.11.2 ROM: Ankle/Foot, Self-Assisted, All 4 Ways

POSITION: Seated

TARGETS: Mobility of the talocrural and subtalar joints

INSTRUCTION: *Dorsiflexion*: Patient sits with target leg crossed over non-target thigh. Patient uses opposite hand to assist in pointing the toes while other hand stabilizes the lower leg (A). *Plantarflexion*: Patient sits with target leg crossed over non-target thigh. Patient uses opposite hand to assist in pushing the toes up toward the shin while other hand stabilizes the lower leg (B). *Inversion*: Patient sits with target leg crossed over non-target thigh. Patient uses opposite hand grasping at calcaneus and assists in bringing the sole of the foot toward the ceiling while other hand stabilizes the lower leg (C). *Eversion*: Patient places bend of target leg knee over non-target thigh with foot oriented laterally. Patient grasps calcaneus and assists to bring the sole of the foot up toward the ceiling while other hand stabilizes the lower leg (D).

SUBSTITUTIONS: Leg should be stable

PARAMETERS: Hold for 5 to 10 seconds, 10 repetitions, repeat 1 to 3 times per day

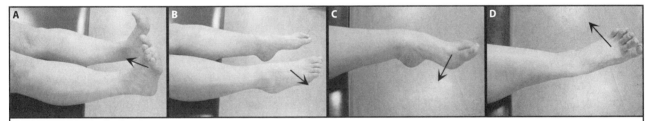

6.11.3 ROM: Ankle/Foot, Long-Sitting and Ankle Pumps, 4-Way, Active

POSITION: Long-sitting, supine

TARGETS: Mobility of the talocrural and subtalar joints

INSTRUCTION: With foot off edge of bed to allow for movement without friction, patient pulls the toes up (dorsiflexion), points the toes (plantarflexion), turns the sole of the foot toward the other foot (inversion), and then outward (eversion). Each activity should be performed multiple repetitions before moving to next movement (A through D). Lower leg may also be propped on pillows as alternative position. *Ankle pumps*: Patient lies supine and pumps ankle into dorsiflexion followed by plantarflexion, holding each 1 to 2 seconds, and repeats.

SUBSTITUTIONS: Leg should be stable; do not allow hip to rotate.

PARAMETERS: 10 to 20 each way, repeat 1 to 3 times per day

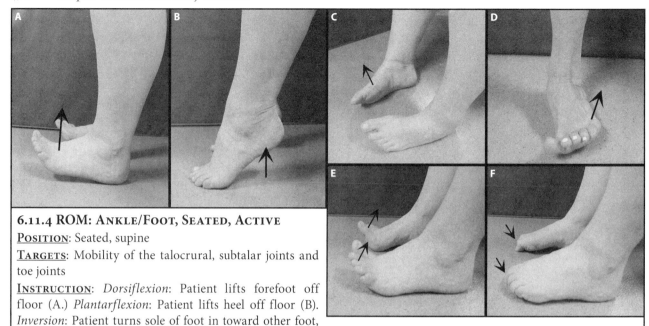

6.11.4 ROM: Ankle/Foot, Seated, Active

Position: Seated, supine

Targets: Mobility of the talocrural, subtalar joints and toe joints

Instruction: *Dorsiflexion*: Patient lifts forefoot off floor (A.) *Plantarflexion*: Patient lifts heel off floor (B). *Inversion*: Patient turns sole of foot in toward other foot, keeping heel on floor (C). *Eversion*: Patient turns sole of foot out away from other foot, keeping heel on floor (D). *Toe extension*: Patient lifts toes off floor, keeping forefoot in contact with floor (E). *Toe flexion*: Patient curls toes to place tips of toes on floor, heel stays in contact with floor (F).

Substitutions: Leg should be stable; do not allow hip to rotate.

Parameters: 10 to 20 each way, repeat 1 to 3 times per day

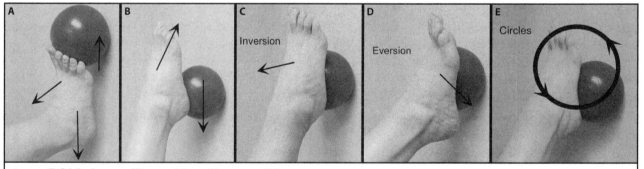

6.11.5 ROM: Ankle/Foot, Mini-Ball on Wall

Position: Supine

Targets: Mobility of the talocrural and subtalar joints

Instruction: Patient lies in 90/90 position with bottom of foot on 15- to 20-cm ball on wall as shown. *Dorsiflexion/Plantarflexion*: Patient rolls the ball up and down, keeping the entire sole of the foot on the ball (A and B). *Inversion/Eversion*: Patient rolls the ball medially and laterally, keeping the entire sole of the foot on the ball (C and D). *Circles*: Patient rolls the ball in circles clockwise, keeping the entire sole of the foot on the ball. Repeat counter-clockwise (E).

Substitutions: Leg should be stable; do not allow hip to rotate.

Parameters: 10 to 20 each way, repeat 1 to 3 times per day

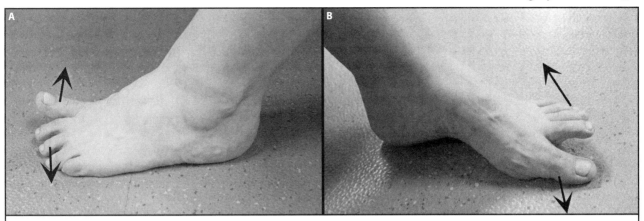

6.11.6 ROM: Toe Yoga, Active

<u>Position</u>: Seated

<u>Targets</u>: Mobility of the toes and early facilitation of toe extensors and flexors and foot intrinsics

<u>Instruction</u>: Patient lifts big toe off the floor as far as possible, keeping toes 2 through 5 on the floor (A). Patient then lifts smaller toes 2 through 5 off the floor as far as possible, keeping big toe on the floor (B).

<u>Substitutions</u>: Minimize movements of the leg

<u>Parameters</u>: 10 to 20 each, repeat 1 to 3 times per day

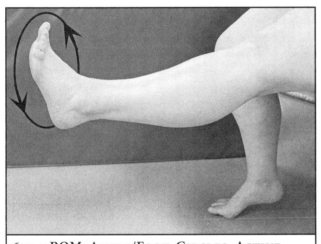

6.11.7 ROM: Ankle/Foot, Circles, Active

<u>Position</u>: Seated

<u>Targets</u>: Mobility of the ankle

<u>Instruction</u>: Patient extends knee to lift foot off floor and, keeping leg still, moves foot around in circles clockwise and then counter-clockwise.

<u>Substitutions</u>: Minimize movements of the leg

<u>Parameters</u>: 10 to 20 circles each way, repeat 1 to 3 times per day

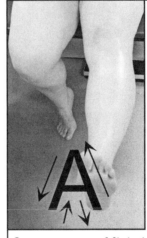

6.11.8 ROM: Ankle/ Foot, Alphabet, Active

<u>Position</u>: Seated

<u>Targets</u>: Mobility of the ankle; also facilitates neuromuscular control and proprioception.

<u>Instruction</u>: Patient extends knee to lift foot off floor and, keeping leg still, moves foot, drawing each letter of the alphabet with tip of toe acting as the end of a pencil.

<u>Substitutions</u>: Minimize movements of the leg

<u>Parameters</u>: A to Z, may also do lower case a to z, repeat 1 to 3 times per day

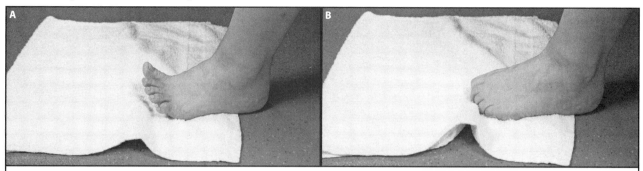

6.11.9 ROM: Toe Scrunches With Towel, Active

Position: Seated

Targets: Mobility of the toes and facilitation of muscles that support the arch of the foot and toe flexors

Instruction: This works best on a smooth surface. Place small towel on floor in front of patient's foot. Patient crunches the towel by curling the toes, keeping the heel on the floor. Patient attempts to continue scrunching while pulling the towel toward him or her (A and B).

Substitutions: Leg movements; in chair, patient stays fully seated and spine straight; patient may lean forward slightly to see foot.

Parameters: 10 to 20 scrunches (4 to 5 hand towel lengths), repeat 1 to 3 times per day

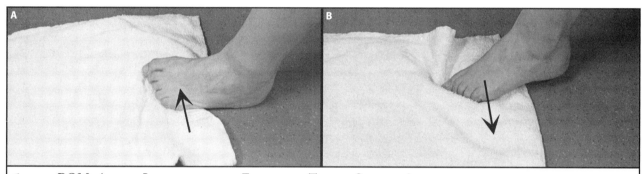

6.11.10 ROM: Ankle Inversion and Eversion, Towel Slides, Active

Position: Seated

Targets: Mobility of the subtalar joint and beginner facilitation of ankle evertors and invertors

Instruction: This works best on a smooth surface. Place small towel on floor in front of patient's foot. Patient places forefoot on towel and, without lifting heel or moving leg, inverts the foot to slide the towel medially and repeats for towel length (A). Patient then reverses and slides towel laterally by everting the foot along the entire towel length. Patient attempts to continue scrunching while pulling the towel laterally (B).

Substitutions: Leg movements; patient may place hands on knee to monitor that knee is stationary; in chair, patient stays fully seated and spine straight; patient may lean forward slightly to see foot.

Parameters: 10 to 20 each way (4 to 5 hand towel lengths), repeat 1 to 3 times per day

6.11.11 ROM: Ankle Dorsiflexion, Chair Slides, Active

Position: Seated

Targets: Mobility of the talocrural joint for dorsiflexion

Instruction: This works best on a smooth surface. Patient slides foot back, keeping sole of foot on floor and toes pointed forward as floor assists dorsiflexion.

Substitutions: Leg movements; patient may place hands on knee to monitor that knee is stationary; in chair, patient stays fully seated and spine straight; patient may lean forward slightly to see foot.

Parameters: 10 to 20 each way (4 to 5 hand towel lengths), repeat 1 to 3 times per day

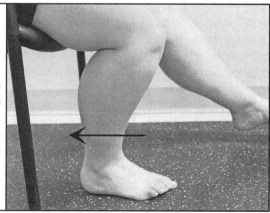

6.11.12 ROM: ANKLE/FOOT, PROSTRETCH, ACTIVE ASSISTIVE

POSITION: Seated, standing

TARGETS: Mobility of the talocrural joints into dorsiflexion and plantarflexion

INSTRUCTION: ProStretch is used for calf stretching and will be listed under stretch as well but is also a nice way to perform controlled ROM into plantarflexion and dorsiflexion. Patient stands on ProStretch and rocks heels down toward floor then forward, bringing toes toward floor. Patient can also do this in sitting. The non-target leg assists in furthering ROM on the target ankle (not shown).

SUBSTITUTIONS: Lower leg stays in neutral alignment; heel and forefoot stay in contact with platform of ProStretch.

PARAMETERS: Hold for 5 to 10 seconds, 10 repetitions, repeat 1 to 3 times per day

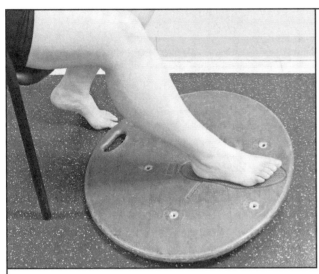

6.11.13 ROM: BIOMECHANICAL ANKLE PLATFORM SYSTEM/WOBBLE BOARD, ACTIVE

POSITION: Seated

TARGETS: Mobility of the talocrural and subtalar joint and beginner facilitation of muscles that control ankle movements, neuromuscular control and proprioception.

INSTRUCTION: The BAPS has one side for each foot. Depending on which foot is desired to mobilize, find correct side and place foot in outlined region. Starting with the smallest ball (beginner), patient balances the BAPS so no edges are touching. *Circles:* Patient touches the front edge down and, without moving the knee, uses the movements of the ankle and touches down the edges in a circle, making sure all sides of the BAPS board touch the floor. This can be done clockwise and counter-clockwise. *Front/back taps:* Patient taps the front edge and then the back edge by dorsiflexing and plantarflexing the ankle. *Side/side taps:* Patient taps the medial edge and then the lateral edge by inverting and everting the ankle. All of these can be done with a wobble board if a BAPS board is unavailable.

SUBSTITUTIONS: Leg movements; patient may place hands on knee to monitor that knee is stationary; in chair, patient stays fully seated and spine straight; patient may lean forward slightly to see foot.

PARAMETERS: 10 to 20 each way repeat 1 to 3 times per day

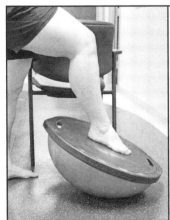

6.11.14 ROM: ANKLE/FOOT, BOSU CIRCLES, ACTIVE

POSITION: Standing

TARGETS: Mobility of the talocrural and subtalar joint and beginner facilitation of muscles that control ankle movements, neuromuscular control and proprioception.

INSTRUCTION: While in the standing position, patient holds onto stable object for balance, places foot in the center of an inverted Bosu, and moves ankle in a circular pattern. Perform in a clockwise then reverse to a counter-clockwise direction.

SUBSTITUTIONS: Leg movements; patient may place hands on knee to monitor that knee is stationary.

PARAMETERS: 10 to 20 each way repeat 1 to 3 times per day

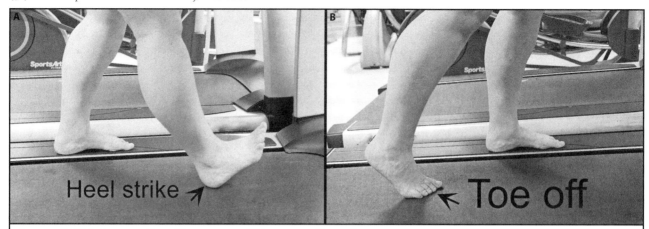

6.11.15 ROM: Single-Leg Treadmill Walking, Gait Simulation

<u>Position</u>: Standing

<u>Targets</u>: Mobility of the talocrural and beginner facilitation of proper ankle movements for gait

<u>Instruction</u>: While in standing, patient places non-target leg to the lateral side of the treadmill walking area but at the same level. Start the treadmill at low speed as patient transfers all weight to non-target leg and uses target leg to make a stride movement forward, contacts in front with heel strike, allowing forefoot to lower into loading response, maintains contact to pass the stance leg, and continues on plantarflexing until toe comes to walking area, then advances to repeat another stride. This activity mimics gait without weightbearing and works on the movements of the ankle necessary for normal gait (A and B).

<u>Substitutions</u>: Stance leg should be keep with good alignment of hip, knee, and ankle; moving leg does not bear weight during entire sequence.

<u>Parameters</u>: 20 to 30 strides, repeat 1 to 3 times per day. Allow rests for stance leg as needed.

Reference

Lopes, A. D., Alouche, S. R., Hakansson, N., & Cohen, M. (2014). Electromyography during pedaling on upright and recumbent ergometer. *International Journal of Sports Physical Therapy, 9*(1), 76-81.

Section *6.12*

ANKLE JOINT SELF-MOBILIZATION

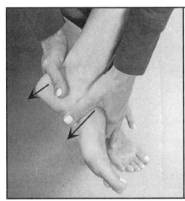

6.12.1 SELF-JOINT MOBILIZATION: ANKLE DISTRACTION

POSITION: Seated

TARGETS: Mobility of the talocrural joint

INSTRUCTION: Patient crosses target leg over non-target thigh in a figure 4 position as shown. Patient uses web spaces between thumb and index fingers to grasp at calcaneus and anterior ankle. Patient elicits a distraction force pulling calcaneus distally from distal tibia.

SUBSTITUTIONS: Target ankle is not relaxed

PARAMETERS: Hold 3 to 5 seconds, repeat 10 to 20 times, 1 to 3 times per day

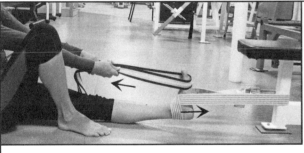

6.12.2 SELF-JOINT MOBILIZATION: BANDED ANKLE DISTRACTION WITH DORSIFLEXION

POSITION: Long-sitting

TARGETS: Mobility of the talocrural joint

INSTRUCTION: Patient loops rigid band around ankle in figure 8 pattern as shown. Band is anchored at floor height. Patient scoots away from band until distraction force occur. Patient then loops another band around forefoot and pulls the foot into dorsiflexion.

SUBSTITUTIONS: Target ankle is not relaxed.

PARAMETERS: Hold 3 to 5 seconds, repeat 10 to 20 times, 1 to 3 times per day

6.12.3 SELF-JOINT MOBILIZATION: WITH MOVEMENT, DORSIFLEXION

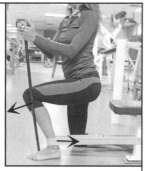

POSITION: Half-kneeling

TARGETS: Mobility of the talocrural joint; posterior glide of tibia to improve dorsiflexion.

INSTRUCTION: Patient kneels on non-target knee with towel roll under the knee for comfort. Rigid strap is looped around stable base behind the stance/target foot at ankle height. Loop band around the ankle just above the malleoli. Patient scoots out until pressure is felt in band around ankle. The foot should be in a position which results in knee flexed 90 degrees. Use a dowel rod or PVC pipe to keep the foot and ankle in a relatively neutral position. Place the dowel vertically, with one end on the ground on the outside of the foot. The knee goes to the inside of the foot so that the dowel crosses in front of the tibia. This keeps the foot in a good biomechanical position. Keep the dowel vertical. Patient then bends target knee bringing tibia forward and dorsiflexing the ankle as the band applies pressure to the distal tibia posteriorly.

SUBSTITUTIONS: Position of band below malleoli; foot arch dropping/pronation.

PARAMETERS: Hold 3 to 5 seconds, repeat 10 to 20 times, 1 to 3 times per day

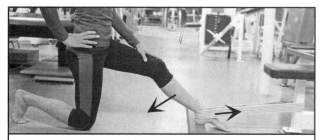

6.12.4 SELF-JOINT MOBILIZATION: WITH MOVEMENT, PLANTARFLEXION

POSITION: Standing

TARGETS: Mobility of the talocrural joint; anterior glide of tibia to improve plantarflexion.

INSTRUCTION: Patient stands with target heel on small block and toes on floor in front, ankle slightly plantarflexed. Rigid strap is looped around stable base in front of the stance/target foot at ankle height. Loop band around the ankle just above the malleoli. Patient scoots back until pressure is felt in band around ankle. Patient then bends opposite knee, keeping target knee straight while sinking down into hips to plantarflex the target foot, bringing tibia posteriorly as the band applies pressure to the distal tibia anteriorly.

SUBSTITUTIONS: Poor control of non-target side with lunge

PARAMETERS: Hold 3 to 5 seconds, repeat 10 to 20 times, 1 to 3 times per day

Where's the Evidence?

Hoch et al. (2012) examined the effect of a 2-week anterior-to-posterior ankle joint mobilization intervention on weightbearing dorsiflexion ROM, dynamic balance, and self-reported function in subjects with chronic ankle instability. The results indicate that dorsiflexion ROM, reach distance in all directions, and the Foot and Ankle Ability Measure all improved following the intervention. At 1 week follow-up, measures remained improved, indicating that the joint mobilization intervention that targeted posterior talar glide was able to improve measures of function in adults for at least 1 week. Vincenzo, Branjerdporn, Teys, and Jordan (2006) evaluated two Mulligan's Mobilization of the Elbow With Movements techniques on 16 patients with recurrent lateral ankle sprains based on recent evidence indicating that a lack of posterior talar glide and weightbearing ankle dorsiflexion was a common physical impairment in individuals with recurrent ankle sprains and found that both the weightbearing and non-weightbearing Mulligan's Mobilization of the Elbow With Movements treatment techniques significantly improved posterior talar glide by 55% and 50% of the pre-application deficit between affected and unaffected sides. The weightbearing and non-weightbearing Mulligan's Mobilization of the Elbow With Movements treatment techniques improved weightbearing dorsiflexion by 26% compared to 9% for the control condition. They concluded suggesting that this technique should be considered in rehabilitation programs following lateral ankle sprain. Collins et al. found similar results in a double-blind, randomized controlled trial of 14 subjects with subacute grade II lateral ankle sprains that measured the initial effects of the Mulligan's Mobilization of the Elbow With Movements treatment on weightbearing dorsiflexion and pressure and thermal pain threshold. Significant improvements in dorsiflexion occurred initially post-Mulligan's Mobilization of the Elbow With Movements; however, no significant changes in pressure or thermal pain threshold were observed after the treatment condition. Results indicate that the Mulligan's Mobilization of the Elbow With Movements treatment for ankle dorsiflexion has a mechanical rather than hypoalgesic effect in subacute ankle sprains (Collins, Teys, & Vincenzino, 2004).

REFERENCES

Collins, N., Teys, P., & Vicenzino, B. (2004). The initial effects of a Mulligan's mobilization with movement technique on dorsiflexion and pain in subacute ankle sprains. *Manual Therapy, 9*(2), 77-82.

Hoch, M. C., Andreatta, R. D., Mullineaux, D. R., English, R. A., McKeon, J. M., Mattacola, C. G., & McKeon, P. O. (2012). Two-week joint mobilization intervention improves self-reported function, range of motion, and dynamic balance in those with chronic ankle instability. *Journal of Orthopedic Research, 30*(11), 1798-1804.

Vicenzino, B., Branjerdporn, M., Teys, P., & Jordan, K. (2006). Initial changes in posterior talar glide and dorsiflexion of the ankle after mobilization with movement in individuals with recurrent ankle sprain. *Journal of Orthopedic Sports Physical Therapy, 36*(7), 464-471.

Section 6.13

ANKLE AND FOOT STRETCHING

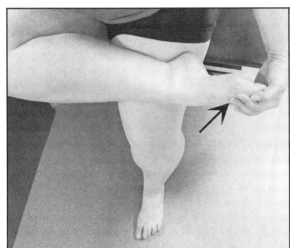

6.13.1 STRETCH: ANTERIOR TIBIALIS (BEGINNER)

POSITION: Seated

TARGETS: Stretch anterior lower leg and ankle/foot structures; anterior tibialis and toe extensors.

INSTRUCTION: Patient sits with target leg crossed over non-target thigh. Patient uses opposite hand to assist in pointing the toes while other hand stabilizes the lower leg.

SUBSTITUTIONS: Quadriceps will pull the pelvis into an anterior tilt; patient should strongly engage lower abdominals to posteriorly pelvic tilt and avoid lumbar extension and any trunk twist during any of the above; also watch shoulders, encouraging scapular retraction when reaching behind and avoid shrugging.

PARAMETERS: Hold for 15 to 30 seconds, 3 to 5 repetitions, 1 to 3 times per day

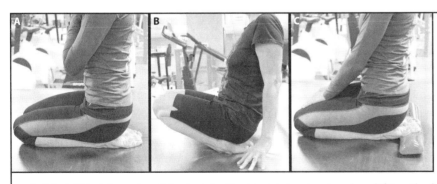

6.13.2 STRETCH: ANTERIOR TIBIALIS, HEEL SIT

POSITION: Tall-kneeling

TARGETS: Stretch anterior lower leg and ankle/foot structures; anterior tibialis and toe extensors.

INSTRUCTION: *Heel-sit*: Patient places dorsum of feet on mat, toes pointing backward while slowly lowering hips to heels. Patient places hands in front or behind (A). Advancing this stretch, if patient tolerates, involves lifting the knee up to further stretch across top of foot (B). A foam roll can be placed under the knee during the stretch to allow shoulder to relax. *Heel-sit with small foam roll*: Place a small foam roll under the toes to increase toe extensors stretch, and perform instructions under heel sit (C).

SUBSTITUTIONS: Quadriceps will pull the pelvis into an anterior tilt; patient should strongly engage lower abdominals to posteriorly pelvic tilt and avoid lumbar extension and any trunk twist during any of the above; also watch shoulders encouraging scapular retraction when reaching behind and avoid shrugging.

PARAMETERS: Hold for 15 to 30 seconds, 3 to 5 repetitions, 1 to 3 times per day

6.13.3 STRETCH: ANTERIOR TIBIALIS, STANDING

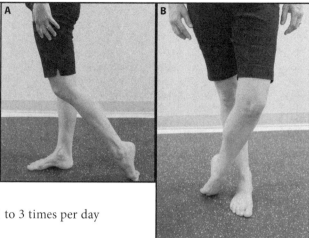

POSITION: Standing

TARGETS: Stretch anterior lower leg and ankle/foot structures; anterior tibialis and toe extensors.

INSTRUCTION: *Behind*: Patient places top of metatarsal heads on floor behind and presses ankle forward to increase plantarflexion and toe curl (A). *Ballet shin stretch*: Patient places top of metatarsal heads on floor lateral to opposite foot and presses ankle down toward the floor to increase plantarflexion and toe curl (B).

SUBSTITUTIONS: Watch that patient is focusing on sagittal plane movement and avoid hyperinverting ankle.

PARAMETERS: Hold for 15 to 30 seconds, 3 to 5 repetitions, 1 to 3 times per day

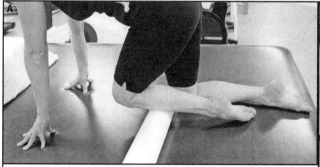
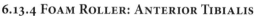
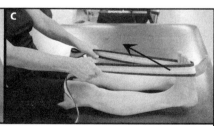

6.13.4 FOAM ROLLER: ANTERIOR TIBIALIS

POSITION: Quadruped

TARGETS: Soft tissue release/self-massage anterior tibialis

INSTRUCTION: Patient positions shins on foam roller while rolling the body over the foam roller from tibial tuberosity to ankle and back slowly holding over sore spots as tolerated (A). For increased pressure, this can be done one leg at a time (B). Patient can also do this with a rolling pin or muscle roller by sitting with knees bent and feet on the floor. Patient rolls along the anterior tibialis muscle from tibial tuberosity to ankle.

SUBSTITUTIONS: Avoid pressures that are excessively painful; watch that patient is not shrugging shoulders.

PARAMETERS: Massage 2 to 5 minutes, 1 to 3 times per day

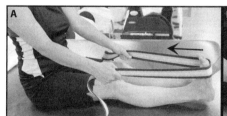
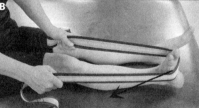

6.13.5 STRETCH: GASTROCNEMIUS USING STRAP

POSITION: Long-sitting, seated

TARGETS: Stretch gastrocnemius

INSTRUCTION: Loop towel, belt, or sheet around forefoot. Patient grasps ends and pulls the toes toward him or her, keeping knee straight but not hyperextended (A). *Medial gastrocnemius*: To target, patient externally rotates hip slightly so that toes are pointed slightly outward (B). *Lateral gastrocnemius*: To target, patient externally rotates hip slightly so that toes are pointed slightly outward (C). All of the above can be done with the patient seated on the edge of a chair or mat with the knee extended.

SUBSTITUTIONS: Knee should never be locked out or hyperextended; monitor shoulders to ensure patient retracts scapula and avoids shrugging; toes should be pointed straight up in sagittal plane unless targeting medial or lateral specifically.

PARAMETERS: Hold for 15 to 30 seconds, 3 to 5 repetitions, 1 to 3 times per day

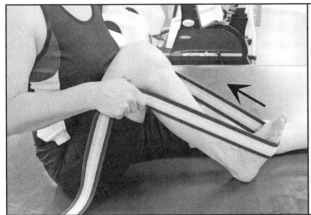

6.13.6 Stretch: Soleus Using Strap

<u>Position</u>: Long-sitting, seated

<u>Targets</u>: Stretch gastrocnemius

<u>Instruction</u>: Loop towel, belt, or sheet around forefoot. Patient grasps ends and bends knee, then pulls the toes toward him or her. This can also be done seated with heel on floor as the patient pulls up with the belt.

<u>Substitutions</u>: Monitor shoulders to ensure patient retracts scapula and avoids shrugging; toes should be pointed straight in sagittal plane.

<u>Parameters</u>: Hold for 15 to 30 seconds, 3 to 5 repetitions, 1 to 3 times per day

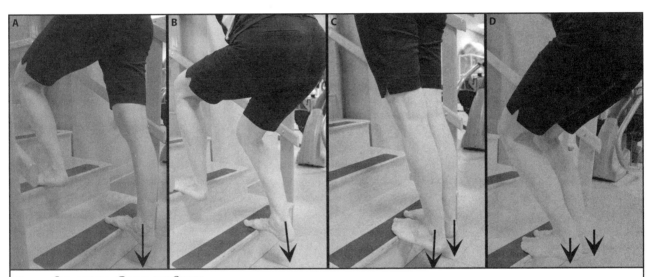

6.13.7 Stretch: Calf on Step

<u>Position</u>: Standing

<u>Targets</u>: Stretch gastrocnemius and soleus

<u>Instruction</u>: *Gastrocnemius focus, unilateral*: Patient stands on step so that target heel is off step while other foot remains planted on step. Patient drops target heel down toward floor, keeping knee extended until stretch felt. Leg remaining on step can flex at the hip and knee (A). *Soleus focus, unilateral*: Patient stands on step so that target heel is off step while other foot remains planted on step. Patient bends target knee, keeping knee aligned with hip and ankle while dropping target heel down toward floor until stretch felt. Leg remaining on step can flex at the hip and knee (B). *Gastrocnemius focus, bilateral*: Patient stands on step so that both heels are off step. Patient drops both heels down toward floor, keeping knees extended until stretch felt (C). *Soleus focus, bilateral*: Patient stands on step so that both heels are off step. Patient flexes both knees and drops both heels down toward floor, keeping knees extended until stretch felt (D).

<u>Substitutions</u>: Monitor shoulders to ensure patient retracts scapula and avoids shrugging; feet should be pointed straight forward in sagittal plane, do not let arch drop inward.

<u>Parameters</u>: Hold for 15 to 30 seconds, 3 to 5 repetitions, 1 to 3 times per day

6.13.8 STRETCH: CALF ON RAMP

POSITION: Standing

TARGETS: Stretch gastrocnemius and soleus

INSTRUCTION: A ramp should be placed so that patient has something stable to hold onto in front of him or her. *Gastrocnemius focus*: Patient stands on ramp, allowing both ankles to dorsiflex. Patient may lean back to begin placement of feet and then lean forward, keeping knees extended until stretch felt (A). *Medial gastrocnemius focus*: Patient turns toes out slightly (B). *Lateral gastrocnemius focus*: Patient turns toes in slightly (C). *Soleus focus, bilateral*: Patient stands on ramp, so that ankles are dorsiflexed. Patient flexes both knees and squats, pushing ankles into more dorsiflexion (D).

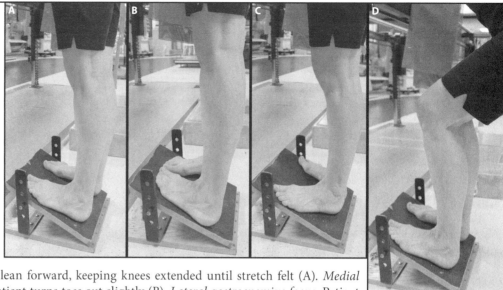

SUBSTITUTIONS: Monitor shoulders to ensure patient retracts scapula and avoids shrugging; feet should be pointed straight forward in sagittal plane, allow patient to hold stable object in front of him or her to assist pulling and depth of stretch, *do not let arch drop inward.*

PARAMETERS: Hold for 15 to 30 seconds, 3 to 5 repetitions, 1 to 3 times per day

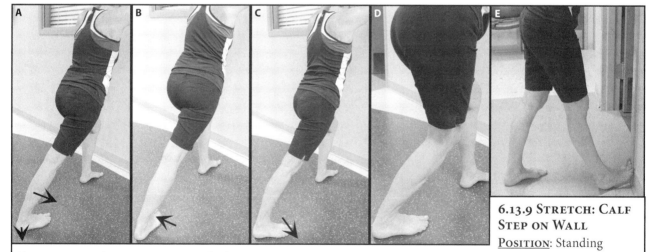

6.13.9 STRETCH: CALF STEP ON WALL

POSITION: Standing

TARGETS: Stretch gastrocnemius and soleus

INSTRUCTION: Patient facing a wall stands 3 to 4 feet away from wall. Patient steps forward with non-target leg. *Gastrocnemius focus*: Back knee is straight as patient leans into wall, bending non-target knee until stretch is felt in back calf. Toes are pointed forward. (A). This can also be done with a table in front. *Medial gastrocnemius focus*: Patient turns toes out slightly (B). *Lateral gastrocnemius focus*: Patient turns toes in slightly (C). *Soleus focus*: Patient stands on ramp so that ankles are dorsiflexed. Patient flexes both knees, squatting while pushing ankles into more dorsiflexion. Knees aligned with hips and ankles (D). This can also be done with a table in front. *Alternate doorway calf stretch*: Patient can also stretch the calf by placing the target forefoot on the doorjamb and hold jamb with hands as shown. Patient then transfers weight, pushing with back leg to forward leg while pressing hips forward, increasing dorsiflexion with the knee straight (E).

SUBSTITUTIONS: Feet should be pointed straight forward in sagittal plane unless working on isolation of medial or lateral gastrocnemius; allow patient to hold stable object in front of them to assist pulling and depth of stretch; *do not let arch drop inward.*

PARAMETERS: Hold for 15 to 30 seconds, 3 to 5 repetitions, 1 to 3 times per day.

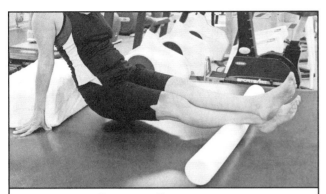

6.13.10 FOAM ROLLER: GASTROCNEMIUS AND SOLEUS

POSITION: Long-sitting

TARGETS: Soft tissue release, self-massage gastrocnemius and soleus

INSTRUCTION: Patient positions target calf on foam roller and crosses other leg on top while rolling the body over the foam roller from back of knee to ankle and back, slowly holding over sore spots as tolerated.

SUBSTITUTIONS: Avoid pressures that are excessively painful; watch that patient is not shrugging shoulders.

PARAMETERS: Massage 2 to 5 minutes, 1 to 3 times per day

6.13.12 STRETCH: PLANTAR FASCIA SOFT TISSUE RELEASE WITH TENNIS BALL

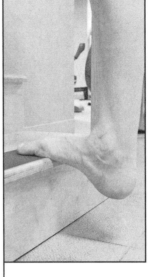

POSITION: Sitting, standing

TARGETS: Soft tissue release, self-massage plantar fascia

INSTRUCTION: Patient positions arch of foot on top of tennis ball and presses down while rolling the arch over the ball from distal portion of calcaneus to metatarsal heads.

SUBSTITUTIONS: Avoid pressures that are excessively painful.

PARAMETERS: Massage 2 to 5 minutes, 1 to 3 times per day

6.13.11 STRETCH: PLANTAR FASCIA ON STEP

POSITION: Standing

TARGETS: Stretch plantar fascia

INSTRUCTION: Patient stands on step so that target heel is off step while other foot remains planted on step. The focus is on planting the forefoot as close to the edge as possible. Patient drops target heel down toward floor, focusing on stretching in the arch of the foot. Leg remaining on step can flex at the hip and knee.

SUBSTITUTIONS: Feet should be pointed straight forward in sagittal plane.

PARAMETERS: Hold for 15 to 30 seconds, 3 to 5 repetitions, 1 to 3 times per day.

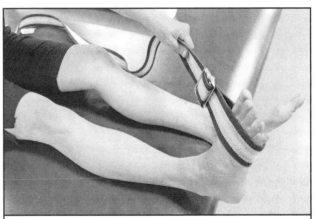

6.13.13 STRETCH: EVERTORS

POSITION: Long-sitting, seated

TARGETS: Stretch ankle evertors: peroneus longus, brevis and tertius; this generally assists to increase ROM into inversion.

INSTRUCTION: Loop towel, belt, or sheet around forefoot. Patient grasps ends and pulls sole of the foot inward while inverting the foot.

SUBSTITUTIONS: Knee should never be locked out or hyperextended; monitor shoulders to ensure patient retracts scapula and avoids shrugging; toes should be pointed straight up in sagittal plane, ankle in 0 degrees of dorsi- and plantarflexion.

PARAMETERS: Hold for 15 to 30 seconds, 3 to 5 repetitions, 1 to 3 times per day

6.13.14 STRETCH: INVERTORS

<u>POSITION</u>: Long-sitting, seated

<u>TARGETS</u>: Stretch ankle invertors anterior and posterior tibialis to a slight degree; this generally assists to increase ROM into eversion.

<u>INSTRUCTION</u>: Loop towel, belt, or sheet around forefoot. Patient grasps ends and pulls sole of the foot outward while everting the foot.

<u>SUBSTITUTIONS</u>: Knee should never be locked out or hyperextended; monitor shoulders to ensure patient retracts scapula and avoids shrugging; toes should be pointed straight up in sagittal plane, ankle in 0 degrees of dorsi- and plantarflexion.

<u>PARAMETERS</u>: Hold for 15 to 30 seconds, 3 to 5 repetitions, 1 to 3 times per day

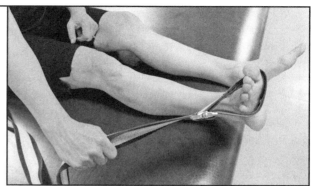

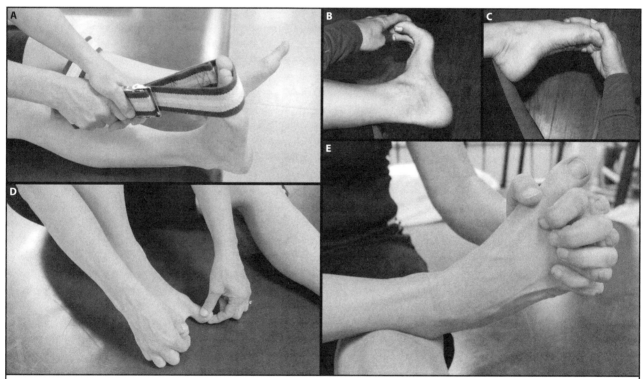

6.13.15 STRETCH: TOES

<u>POSITION</u>: Seated, long-sitting

<u>TARGETS</u>: Stretch toe flexors (flexor digitorum longus and brevis, flexor hallucis longus and brevis, lumbricals and quadratus plantae), toe extensors (extensor digitorum longus and brevis, extensor hallucis longus and brevis) and toe adductors (adductor hallucis, interossei)

<u>INSTRUCTION</u>: *Flexors:* In long-sitting, patient uses towel to loop around bottom of toes and pulls back to stretch toes into extension (A). Patient can also isolate each toe by manually grasping each toe, and pulling into extension (B). *Extensors:* Patient sits with target leg crossed over non-target thigh and curls hand around toes pulling them into flexion (C). Patient can also isolate each toe by manually grasping each toe and curling into flexion. *Adductors:* Patient in long-sitting, target knee bent and foot planted pulls each adjacent toe laterally or medially away from adjacent toes (D). Patient can globally adduct by placing fingers inbetween toes. This is a common technique used in massage (E).

<u>SUBSTITUTIONS</u>: Lower leg is stable during ankle/foot movements

<u>PARAMETERS</u>: Hold for 15 to 30 seconds, 3 to 5 repetitions, 1 to 3 times per day

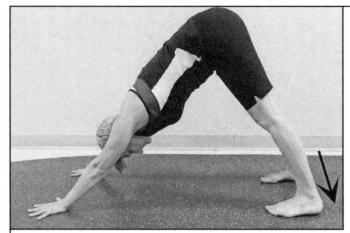

6.13.16 STRETCH: YOGA; CALF STRETCH, DOWNWARD-FACING DOG

POSITION: Quadruped

TARGETS: Stretch gastrocnemius and soleus

INSTRUCTION: Patient is on hands and knees with knees directly below hips and hands slightly forward of shoulders with palms spread and index fingers parallel or slightly turned out. Patient turns toes under and lifts knees away from the floor. At first, patient may keep the knees slightly bent and the heels lifted away from the floor. Patient lengthens tailbone, lifting hips up toward the ceiling. Patient pushes top of thighs back and stretches heels down toward the floor. Patient straightens knees but does not to lock them. To protect the arms, firm the arms and press the bases of the index fingers actively into the floor, lifting along inner arms from the wrists to shoulders. Patient also retracts and depresses scapula toward the tailbone. Patient's head stays between the upper arms and does not hang. Patient may "walk the dog" by allowing one knee to bend while pressing the other heel further toward the floor for a unilateral calf stretch and alternate. Patient may also press both heels down for a bilateral stretch.

SUBSTITUTIONS: Monitor shoulders to ensure patient retracts scapula and avoids shrugging; feet should be pointed straight forward in sagittal plane; do not let arch drop inward.

PARAMETERS: Hold for 15 to 30 seconds, 3 to 5 repetitions, 1 to 3 times per day

Section 6.14

ANKLE AND FOOT STRENGTHENING

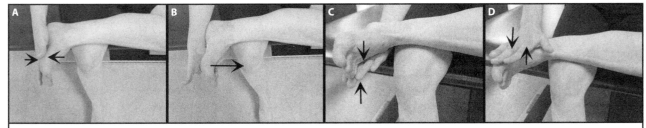

6.14.1 STRENGTHEN: ISOMETRIC; ANKLE, HAND RESIST, 4-WAY

<u>POSITION</u>: Long-sitting

<u>TARGETS</u>: Beginner facilitation and strengthening of ankle muscles: dorsiflexors (anterior tibialis), evertors (peroneus longus, brevis, tertius), plantarflexors (gastrocnemius, soleus, posterior tibialis), invertors (anterior and posterior tibialis).

<u>INSTRUCTION</u>: Cross target leg over non-target thigh in figure 4 position as shown. Patient stabilizes the lower leg with the ipsilateral hand. Ankle is in neutral. *Plantarflexion*: Contralateral hand is placed on plantar surface of metatarsal heads and patient attempts to plantarflex as hand resists (A) *Dorsiflexion*: Contralateral hand is placed over the dorsum (top) of the metatarsal heads and patient attempts to dorsiflex as hand resists (B). *Eversion*: Contralateral hand is placed along the inside of the first metatarsal and patient attempts to invert the foot (cue to attempt to bring sole down toward floor) as hand resists (C). *Inversion*: Contralateral hand is placed along the inside of the first metatarsal and patient attempts to invert the foot (cue to attempt to bring sole up toward ceiling) as hand resists (D).

<u>SUBSTITUTIONS</u>: Ankle stays in neutral; no movement allowed, avoid hip rotations or knee flexion/extension.

<u>PARAMETERS</u>: Hold for 6 to 10 seconds with 1- to 2-second ramp up and down, 8 to 12 repetitions, 1 to 3 sets 1 time per day or every other day

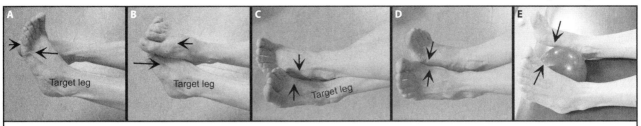

6.14.2 STRENGTHEN: ISOMETRIC; ANKLE, FOOT RESIST, 4-WAY

POSITION: Long-sitting

TARGETS: Beginner facilitation and strengthening of ankle muscles: dorsiflexors (anterior tibialis), evertors (peroneus longus, brevis, tertius), plantarflexors (gastrocnemius, soleus, posterior tibialis), invertors (anterior and posterior tibialis).

INSTRUCTION: *Plantarflexion*: Patient places dorsum (top) of non-target foot under the metatarsal heads of target foot. Patient attempts to plantarflex as other foot resists (A). *Dorsiflexion*: Patient places sole of non-target foot on top of metatarsal heads of target foot. Patient attempts to dorsiflex as other foot resists (B). *Eversion*: Patient crosses ankles while placing lateral non-target foot against lateral target foot. Patient attempts to evert (turn out) target foot as other foot resists (C). *Inversion*: Patient places feet side-by-side with medial feet touching. Patient attempts to invert (turn in) target foot as other foot resists (D). This can also be done with a 10- to 15-cm ball between feet (E).

SUBSTITUTIONS: Ankle stays in neutral; no movement allowed, avoid hip rotations or knee flexion/extension

PARAMETERS: Hold for 6 to 10 seconds with 1- to 2-second ramp up and down, 8 to 12 repetitions, 1 to 3 sets 1 time per day or every other day

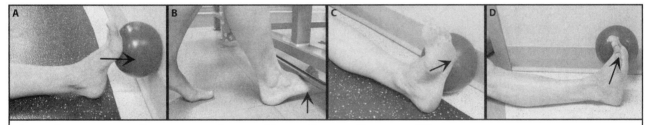

6.14.3 STRENGTHEN: ISOMETRIC; ANKLE, FIXED OBJECT RESIST, 4-WAY

POSITION: Long-sitting, seated

TARGETS: Beginner facilitation and strengthening of ankle muscles: dorsiflexors (anterior tibialis), evertors (peroneus longus, brevis, tertius), plantarflexors (gastrocnemius, soleus, posterior tibialis), invertors (anterior and posterior tibialis).

INSTRUCTION: *Plantarflexion*: Patient places metatarsal heads of target foot against a fixed object. Patient attempts to plantarflex as stable object resists (A). *Dorsiflexion*: Patient places target foot metatarsal heads under stable object such as couch. Patient attempts to dorsiflex as stable object resists (B). *Eversion*: Patient places lateral foot against a stable object. Patient attempts to evert (turn out) target foot as stable object resists. This can also be done against a wall in long-sitting (C). *Inversion*: Patient places medial foot against a stable object. Patient attempts to invert (turn in) target foot as stable object resists. This can also be done against a wall in long-sitting (D).

SUBSTITUTIONS: Ankle stays in neutral; no movement allowed, avoid hip rotations or knee flexion/extension.

PARAMETERS: Hold for 6 to 10 seconds with 1- to 2-second ramp up and down, 8 to 12 repetitions, 1 to 3 sets 1 time per day or every other day

6.14.4 STRENGTHEN: ISOMETRIC; TOE EXTENSION AND FLEXION

<u>POSITION</u>: Standing

<u>TARGETS</u>: Beginner facilitation and strengthening of toe flexors (flexor digitorum longus and brevis, flexor hallucis longus and brevis, lumbricals and quadratus plantae) and toe extensors (extensor digitorum longus and brevis, extensor hallucis longus and brevis).

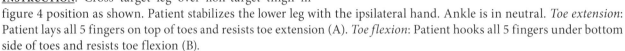

<u>INSTRUCTION</u>: Cross target leg over non-target thigh in figure 4 position as shown. Patient stabilizes the lower leg with the ipsilateral hand. Ankle is in neutral. *Toe extension*: Patient lays all 5 fingers on top of toes and resists toe extension (A). *Toe flexion*: Patient hooks all 5 fingers under bottom side of toes and resists toe flexion (B).

<u>SUBSTITUTIONS</u>: Ankle stays in neutral; no movement allowed.

<u>PARAMETERS</u>: Hold for 6 to 10 seconds with 1- to 2-second ramp up and down, 8 to 12 repetitions, 1 to 3 sets 1 time per day or every other day

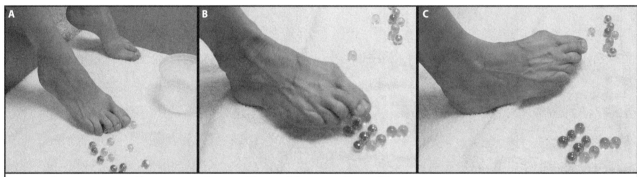

6.14.5 STRENGTHEN: ISOTONIC; ANKLE/FOOT, MARBLE PICK-UPS

<u>POSITION</u>: Seated

<u>TARGETS</u>: Beginner facilitation and strengthening of toe flexors (flexor digitorum longus and brevis, flexor hallucis longus and brevis, lumbricals and quadratus plantae), toe extensors (extensor digitorum longus and brevis, extensor hallucis longus and brevis), and toe adductors (adductor hallucis, interossei); this exercise also utilizes the ankle movements and thus helps early activation of ankle dorsiflexors (anterior tibialis), evertors (peroneus longus, brevis, tertius), plantarflexors (gastrocnemius, soleus, posterior tibialis), invertors (anterior and posterior tibialis), as well as proprioception and neuromuscular control.

<u>INSTRUCTION</u>: Place 15 to 20 marbles on the floor. Patient picks up marbles one at a time using the toes and places them in a bowl (A). *Isolate inversion/eversion*: Patient places heel down and, keeping knee stable, moves marbles from one side of toes to the other and reverse (B and C).

<u>SUBSTITUTIONS</u>: Excessive use of hip and knee; target mainly on ankle foot.

<u>PARAMETERS</u>: 15 to 20 marbles of varying sizes, 1 to 3 sets 1 time per day or every other day

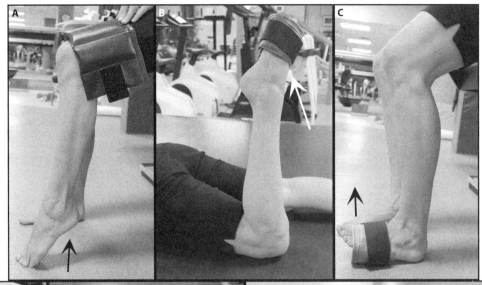

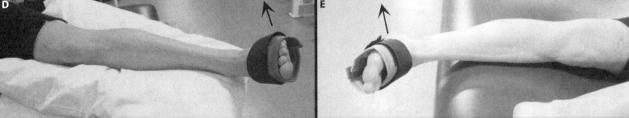

6.14.6 Strengthen: Isotonic; Ankle, Cuff Weights

<u>Position</u>: Seated, prone, side-lying

<u>Targets</u>: Strengthening of plantarflexors (gastrocnemius, soleus, posterior tibialis), dorsiflexors (anterior tibialis), evertors (peroneus longus, brevis, tertius), and invertors (anterior and posterior tibialis).

<u>Instruction</u>: *Plantarflexion*: Place cuff weight over knee with patient seated with ankle directly under. Patient lifts heel, plantarflexing the ankle and bringing weight up (A). This can also be done prone. Both of these will isolate soleus (B). *Dorsiflexion*: Place cuff weight around metatarsal heads. Patient seated with ankle directly under knee attempts to dorsiflex, lifting toes and weight off floor, heel stays in contact with floor (C). *Eversion*: Place cuff weight around metatarsal heads. Patient lies on contralateral side and slides to edge of bed so ankle is hanging off. Patient attempts to evert (turn out) target foot, lifting weight without turning the hip into external rotation (D). *Inversion*: Place cuff weight around metatarsal heads. Patient lies on ipsilateral side and slides to edge of bed so ankle is hanging off. Patient attempts to invert (turn in) target foot, lifting weight without turning the hip into internal rotation (E).

<u>Substitutions</u>: Excessive use of hip and knee; target mainly on ankle foot.

<u>Parameters</u>: 15 to 20 marbles of varying sizes, 1 to 3 sets 1 time per day or every other day

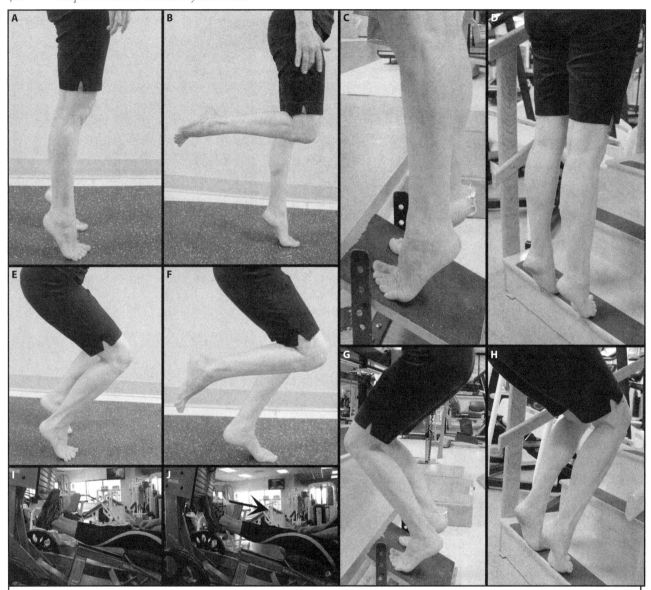

6.14.7 Strengthen: Isotonic; Heel Raises

<u>Position</u>: Standing

<u>Targets</u>: Strengthening of plantarflexors (gastrocnemius, soleus, posterior tibialis)

<u>Instruction</u>: *Standing gastrocnemius focus, phase I*: Patient raises up on toes, lifting heels off ground as far as possible (A). *Standing gastrocnemius focus, phase II*: To advance, have patient bring one foot off of ground and lift heel on stance leg only (B). *Standing gastrocnemius focus, phase III*: Perform on step or ramp, patient drops heels down into dorsiflexion and then raises up on toes, lifting heels off ground as far as possible (C). *Standing gastrocnemius focus, phase IV*: Perform on step or ramp, patient lifts one foot off ramp/step and drops target heel down into dorsiflexion and then raises up on toes, lifting heel off ground as far as possible (shown in picture with both legs) (D). *Standing soleus focus, phase I*: Patient bends both knees and raises up on toes, lifting heels off ground as far as possible (E). *Standing soleus focus, phase II*: To advance, have patient bring one foot off of ground and, with stance knee bent, lift heel on stance leg only (F). *Standing soleus, focus phase III*: Perform on step or ramp, patient drops heel down into dorsiflexion, then bends knee and raises heel (G). *Standing soleus focus, phase IV*: Perform on step or ramp, patient lifts one foot off ramp/step and bends the other knee while dropping target heel down into dorsiflexion and then raises up on toes, lifting heel off ground as far as possible (shown in picture with both legs) (H). *Using leg press machine*: Patient places forefoot on bottom edge of leg press base plate. Patient then allows the heels to drop, bringing the ankles into dorsiflexion. Patient then presses, to plantar flex the ankle, pressing on the base plate at the forefeet. This can be done bilaterally or unilaterally (I and J).

<u>Substitutions</u>: Rolling ankle out; keep calcaneus in alignment and equal weight distribution through metatarsal heads.

<u>Parameters</u>: 8 to 12 repetitions, 1 to 3 sets, 1 time per day or every other day

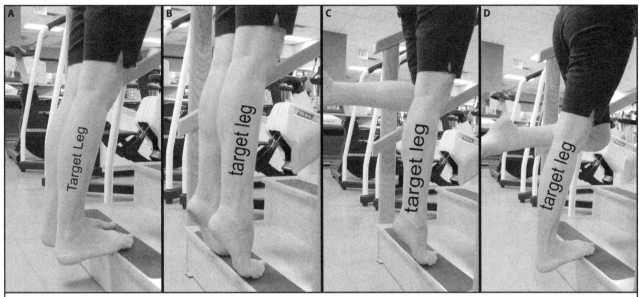

6.14.8 STRENGTHEN: ISOTONIC; HEEL RAISES, ECCENTRIC FOCUS

POSITION: Standing

TARGETS: Eccentric strengthening of plantarflexors (gastrocnemius, soleus, posterior tibialis)

INSTRUCTION: Perform on step or ramp, dropping heels down into dorsiflexion and then raising up on toes using the non-dominant leg only. Patient then transfers weight to target leg and very slowly lowers the target heel to full dorsiflexion (A through D).

SUBSTITUTIONS: Rolling ankle out; keep calcaneus in alignment and equal weight distribution through metatarsal heads.

PARAMETERS: 8 to 12 repetitions, 1 to 3 sets, 1 time per day or every other day

6.14.9 STRENGTHEN: ISOTONIC; TOE RAISES

POSITION: Seated, standing

TARGETS: Strengthening of dorsiflexors (anterior tibialis)

INSTRUCTION: Patient holds stable object for balance and, with target leg, lifts toes off floor, dorsiflexing the ankle. This can also be done seated.

SUBSTITUTIONS: Leaning back

PARAMETERS: 8 to 12 repetitions, 1 to 3 sets, 1 time per day or every other day

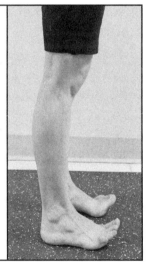

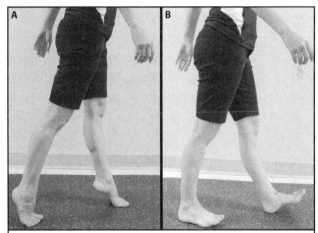

6.14.10 STRENGTHEN: ISOTONIC; HEEL-TOE WALKING

POSITION: Standing

TARGETS: Strengthening of dorsiflexors (anterior tibialis) and plantarflexors (gastrocnemius, soleus, posterior tibialis)

INSTRUCTION: *Toe walking*: Patient lifts heels off the ground and walks forward, keeping heels elevated (A). *Heel walking*: Patient lifts toes off the ground and walks forward, keeping toes elevated (B).

SUBSTITUTIONS: Leaning back, pitching forward, poor ankle control

PARAMETERS: 20 to 50 feet, 1 to 3 sets, 1 time per day or every other day

6.14.11 STRENGTHEN: ISOTONIC; ARCH LIFTS

<u>POSITION</u>: Standing

<u>TARGETS</u>: Strengthening of posterior tibialis, quadratus plantae

<u>INSTRUCTION</u>: Patient raises the arches of the foot, pulling the big toe toward the heel without curling the toes (A and B).

<u>SUBSTITUTIONS</u>: Leaning back, pitching forward, poor ankle control

<u>PARAMETERS</u>: 10 to 50 repetitions (to build endurance), 1 to 3 sets, 1 time per day or every other day

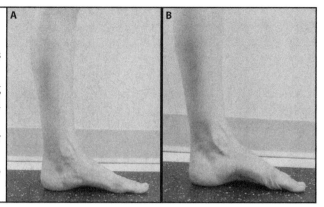

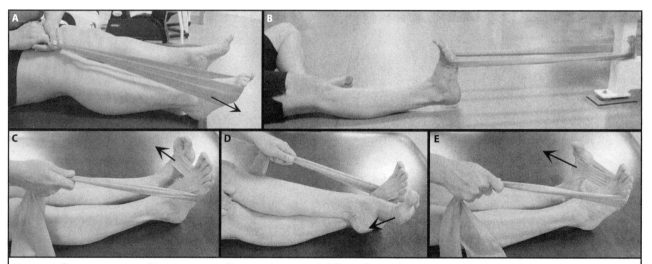

6.14.12 STRENGTHEN: RESISTANCE BAND; ANKLE, 8-WAY, SELF-ASSISTED

<u>POSITION</u>: Long-sitting

<u>TARGETS</u>: Beginner facilitation and strengthening of ankle muscles: dorsiflexors (anterior tibialis, extensor digitorum longus assist from peroneus tertius), evertors (peroneus longus, brevis, tertius), plantarflexors (gastrocnemius, soleus, posterior tibialis), invertors (anterior and posterior tibialis). *Dorsiflexion/eversion*: Targets anterior tibialis primarily. *Dorsiflexion/inversion*: Targets peroneus tertius. *Plantarflexion/eversion*: Targets peroneus longus and brevis. *Plantarflexion/inversion*: Targets posterior tibialis.

<u>INSTRUCTION</u>: *Plantarflexion*: Loop band around metatarsal head and give ends to patient to grasp. Patient applies tension to the band while plantarflexing (A). *Dorsiflexion*: Anchor the band so it is aligned with bottom of foot and loop band around top of foot. Patient scoots back to put resistance on band and pulls toes toward them while dorsiflexing against the band's resistance (B). *Eversion*: Patient places both feet together. Band is looped around target foot and under non-target foot with patient holding other end(s). Patient everts the foot, bringing the foot away from the other foot and turning the sole of the foot outward against the band's resistance (C). *Inversion*: Patient crosses target ankle over non-target ankle. Band is looped around target foot and under non-target foot with patient holding other end(s). Patient inverts the foot, bringing the foot away from the other foot and turning the sole of the foot against the band's resistance (D). All of these can be done sitting with target leg extended. *Dorsiflexion/eversion*: Patient places feet together and places metatarsal heads of non-target foot against band with band looped around target foot. Patient pushes band below the target foot to gain resistance from a downward anchor like pushing down a gas pedal. Patient pulls target toes up and everts the foot, turning the sole of the foot outward against the band's resistance (E). *(continued)*

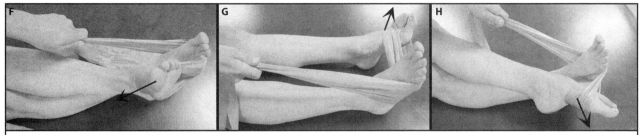

6.14.12 STRENGTHEN: RESISTANCE BAND; ANKLE, 8-WAY, SELF-ASSISTED (CONTINUED)

Dorsiflexion/inversion: Patient crosses target ankle over non-target ankle and places metatarsal heads of non-target foot against band with band looped around target foot. Patient pushes band below the target foot to gain resistance from a downward anchor. Patient pulls target toes up and inverts the foot, turning the sole of the foot inward against the band's resistance (F). *Plantarflexion/eversion*: Patient places feet together and places outside edge metatarsal heads of non-target foot against band with band looped around target foot. Patient presses band outward above target foot to gain resistance from an upward anchor. Patient points and everts the foot, turning the sole of the foot outward against the band's resistance (G). *Plantarflexion/inversion*: Patient crosses non-target ankle over non-target ankle and places metatarsal heads of non-target foot against band with band looped around target foot. Patient presses band outward above target foot to gain resistance from an upward anchor. Patient points and inverts the foot, turning the sole of the foot medially against the band's resistance (H).

<u>SUBSTITUTIONS</u>: Hip stays in neutral; avoid hip rotations or knee flexion/extension; with inversion and eversion, keep ankle in 0 degrees of dorsi/plantarflexion.

<u>PARAMETERS</u>: 8 to 12 repetitions, 1 to 3 sets, 1 time per day or every other day

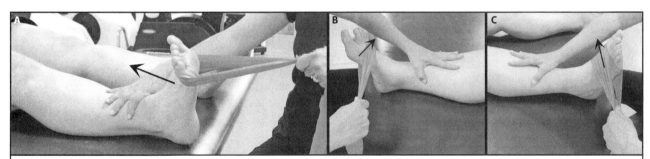

6.14.13 STRENGTHEN: RESISTANCE BAND; ANKLE, 8-WAY, THERAPIST-ASSISTED

<u>POSITION</u>: Long-sitting

<u>TARGETS</u>: Beginner facilitation and strengthening of ankle muscles: dorsiflexors (anterior tibialis, extensor digitorum longus assist from peroneus tertius), evertors (peroneus longus, brevis, tertius), plantarflexors (gastrocnemius, soleus, posterior tibialis), invertors (anterior and posterior tibialis). *Dorsiflexion/eversion*: Targets anterior tibialis primarily. *Dorsiflexion/inversion*: Targets peroneus tertius. *Plantarflexion/eversion*: Targets peroneus longus and brevis. *Plantarflexion/inversion*: Targets posterior tibialis.

<u>INSTRUCTION</u>: *Plantarflexion*: Band is looped around target foot, therapist or patient holds ends and anchors superior to ankle. Patient presses toes down, like pressing a gas pedal, to plantarflex (**6.14.12.A**). *Dorsiflexion*: Band is looped around top of foot; therapist holds ends and anchors inferior to ankle, and patient pulls toes up toward head (A). *Eversion*: Band is looped around target foot, therapist holds ends and anchors medial to metatarsal heads, and patient everts the foot, turning the sole of the foot outward (B). *Inversion*: Band is looped around target foot, therapist holds ends and anchors lateral to metatarsal heads, and patient inverts the foot, turning the sole of the foot inward (C). *(continued)*

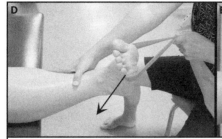

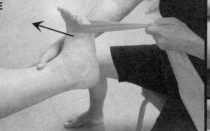

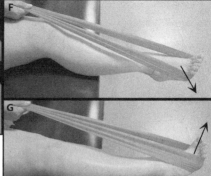

6.14.13 STRENGTHEN: RESISTANCE BAND; ANKLE, 8-WAY, THERAPIST-ASSISTED (CONTINUED)

Dorsiflexion/eversion: Band is looped around target foot; therapist holds ends and anchors inferior and medial to metatarsal heads, and patient pulls toes up and everts the foot, turning the sole of the foot outward (D). *Dorsiflexion/inversion*: Band is looped around target foot, therapist holds ends and anchors inferior and lateral to metatarsal heads, and patient pulls toes up and inverts the foot, turning the sole of the foot inward (E). *Plantarflexion/eversion*: Band is looped around target foot, therapist holds ends and anchors superior and medial to metatarsal head, and patient presses foot down, like pressing a gas pedal, and everts the foot, turning the sole of the foot outward (F). *Plantarflexion/inversion*: Band is looped around target foot, therapist holds ends and anchors superior and lateral to metatarsal heads, and patient presses foot down, like pressing a gas pedal, and inverts the foot, turning the sole of the foot outward (G).

SUBSTITUTIONS: Hip stays in neutral; avoid hip rotations or knee flexion/extension; with inversion and eversion, keep ankle in 0 degrees of dorsi-/plantarflexion; therapist stabilizes lower leg just above malleoli for all exercises.

PARAMETERS: 8 to 12 repetitions, 1 to 3 sets, 1 time per day or every other day

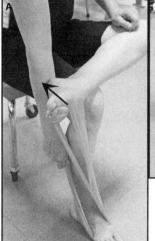

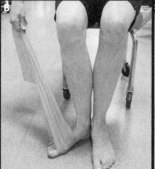

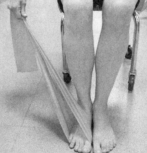

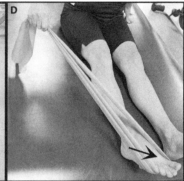

6.14.14 STRENGTHEN: RESISTANCE BAND; POSTERIOR TIBIALIS, VARIATIONS

POSITION: Seated, long-sitting

TARGETS: Strengthening of posterior tibialis

INSTRUCTION: *Seated cross-legged*: Patient crosses target leg over non-target thigh. Band is looped around target foot, therapist brings band under stance foot and holds ends on lateral side of non-target knee so there is tension on the target foot pulling toward the floor. Patient then inverts and plantarflexes the target ankle (A). *Seated "windshield wipers"*: Patient, with both feet flat on floor, loops band around target metatarsal heads and anchor lateral to him or her. Tension so that foot is turned out with hip and knee staying aligned. Patient pulls forefoot inward as the arch rises without letting the foot lift off the floor. Keep toes relaxed (B and C). *Long-sitting*: This can also be done in long-sitting by having the patient loop band around metatarsal heads and pulling band to the lateral side of the hip and up as patient plantarflexes and inverts the foot against resistance (D).

SUBSTITUTIONS: Patient should feel the burn in the lower medial posterior leg and foot arch; if not, make sure inversion and plantarflexion are occurring with seated cross-legged and long-sitting version; avoid hip rotations or knee flexion/extension with long-sitting variation.

PARAMETERS: 8 to 12 repetitions, 1 to 3 sets, 1 time per day or every other day

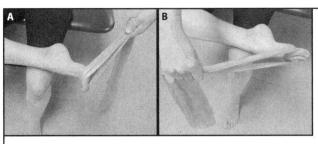

6.14.15 STRENGTHEN: RESISTANCE BAND; TOE EXTENSION AND FLEXION

<u>POSITION</u>: Seated

<u>TARGETS</u>: Strengthening of toe flexors (flexor digitorum longus and brevis, flexor hallucis longus and brevis, lumbricals and quadratus plantae) and toe extensors (extensor digitorum longus and brevis, extensor hallucis longus and brevis).

<u>INSTRUCTION</u>: Cross target leg over non-target thigh in figure 4 position as shown. *Toe extension*: Patient loops band around toes and holds, anchoring ends away from plantar aspect of toes. Patient extends toes without dorsiflexing as band resists (A). *Toe flexion*: Patient loops band around toes and holds anchoring ends away from dorsal aspect of toes. Patient flexed toes without plantarflexing as band resists (B).

<u>SUBSTITUTIONS</u>: Ankle stays in neutral; no movement allowed.

<u>PARAMETERS</u>: 8 to 12 repetitions, 1 to 3 sets, 1 time per day or every other day

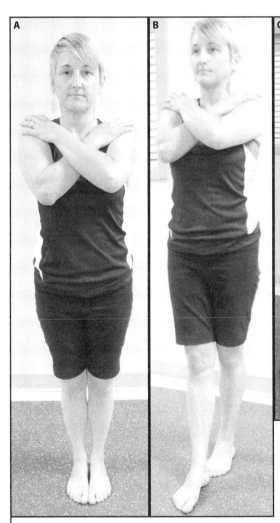

6.14.16 FUNCTIONAL: ANKLE/FOOT, RHOMBERG AND VARIATIONS

<u>POSITION</u>: Standing

<u>TARGETS</u>: Strengthening of ankle and foot, facilitate balance reactions, neuromuscular control and proprioception

<u>INSTRUCTION</u>: *Rhomberg*: Patient stands with feet together, starting with index fingers on a stable surface (for balance only), and eventually without, crossing arms across chest, starting with eyes open and progressing to eyes closed (A). *Sharpened Rhomberg*: Patient stands heel to toe, starting with index fingers on a stable surface (for balance only), and eventually without, crossing arms across chest, starting with eyes open and progressing to eyes closed (B). *Unilateral stance*: Patient stands on one leg. To begin, allow patient to touch down with opposite toe as needed and progress to without. Patient may also start with index fingers on a stable surface (for balance only) and eventually without, crossing arms across chest, starting with eyes open and progress to eyes closed (not shown). *Multi-surface*: To progress both of these variations, change the surface to unstable: foam square, pillow, mini-trampoline, air disc, Bosu (upside or downside), tilt board forward or sideways, wobble board (C). *Ball toss*: Add ball toss in any of the above positions and surfaces to challenge balance. *Perturbations*: Therapist may provide external force to attempt to disturb the patient's center of gravity. These small to medium forces can be applied at the shoulders and pelvis anterior to posterior and reverse, lateral, transverse/rotational. *Weight shifts*: Patient shifts weight forward/backward/left/right with any of the stance positions—*Rhomberg, Sharpened Rhomberg, or Unilateral stance*. May add variations reaching for an object forward, lateral, or diagonal, and high to low.

<u>SUBSTITUTIONS</u>: Patient should bear weight equally in the foot in the triad of medial metatarsal heads, lateral metatarsal heads, and calcaneus. Do not allow arch to drop; as patient moves to unstable surface, this may not be possible.

<u>PARAMETERS</u>: 10 to 60 seconds, 3 to 10 repetitions, 1 time per day or every other day

6.14.17 FUNCTIONAL: ANKLE/FOOT, STEPS-OVERS, STEP-BEHINDS, AND CARIOCA/BRAIDING

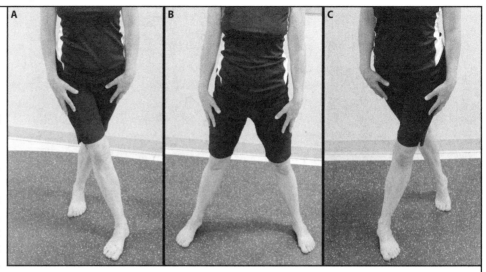

POSITION: Standing

TARGETS: Strengthening of ankle and foot, facilitate balance reactions, neuromuscular control and proprioception

INSTRUCTION: *Step-overs*: Patient steps in front and over right foot with left foot, brings right foot back to right side of left foot, and repeats. This can also be done stepping foot behind and over. Repeat to both sides. *Carioca/braiding*: Patient steps in front and over right foot with left foot, brings right foot back to right side of left foot, followed by stepping behind right foot to land on other side of foot, then brings right foot back to medial side of left foot as if braiding "over, under, over, under" (A through C).

SUBSTITUTIONS: Therapist may allow patient to hold onto the therapist's hands in the beginner phase and progress to no hands.

PARAMETERS: 30 to 50 feet both ways, 3 to 10 repetitions, 1 time per day or every other day

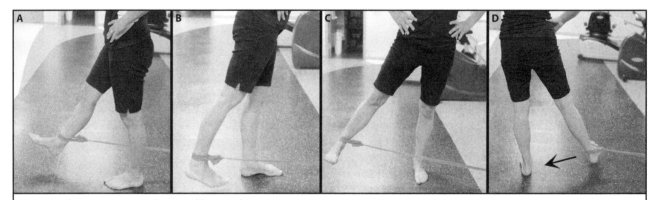

6.14.18 FUNCTIONAL: ANKLE/FOOT, OPPOSITE HIP, 4-WAY BALANCE CHALLENGE

POSITION: Standing

TARGETS: Strengthening of ankle and foot, facilitate balance reactions, neuromuscular control and proprioception

INSTRUCTION: With band anchored at ankle height, loop band around non-target ankle. *Flexion*: Patient faces away from anchor, stands straight up and tightens quadriceps to keep knee fully extended while bringing leg forward against the resistance of the band (A). *Extension*: Patient faces toward anchor, stands straight up, and tightens quadriceps to keep knee fully extended while bringing leg backward against the resistance of the band (B). *Abduction*: Patient stands with target side away from anchor and steps out so that there is tension on the band. Patient stands straight up and tightens quadriceps to keep knee fully extended while bringing leg away from other leg against the resistance of the band (C). *Adduction*: Patient standing with target side toward anchor and steps out so that hip is abducted with tension on the band. Patient stands straight up and tightens quadriceps to keep knee fully extended while bringing leg toward the other leg and crosses in front or behind against the resistance of the band (D). All of these can be done with just the non-target leg movements without the resistance band to begin and then adding resistance band as a progression. By doing this with the unaffected leg as the actively moving leg, it challenges the stance leg all directions. Varying surfaces add an extra challenge.

SUBSTITUTIONS: Maintain neutral pelvis; active lower abdominal core encouraged, moving knees stay fully extended but not locked out or hyperextended, encourage patient to tighten quadriceps on stance leg to lift the patella.

PARAMETERS: 8 to 12 repetitions, 1 to 3 sets, 1 time per day or every other day

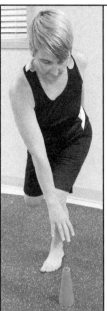

6.14.19 FUNCTIONAL: ANKLE/FOOT, SINGLE-LEG MINI-SQUAT AND REACH, ALL DIRECTIONS

POSITION: Standing

TARGETS: Strengthening of ankle and foot, facilitate balance reactions, neuromuscular control and proprioception with functional movement of reaching

INSTRUCTION: Patient with feet hip-width apart and knees and ankle in good alignment performs a mini-squat and then reaches as far forward as possible, then returns. This may trigger a stepping response, which is a good training technique to encourage these reactions, but ultimately the object of this exercise is to maintain stance. Therapist may have the patient reach toward the therapist's hand or an object. Once forward-reaching repetitions are completed, work on reaching laterally to target side, and reaching diagonally (forward lateral and down combinations and forward, lateral, and up combinations).

SUBSTITUTIONS: Straining shoulder or neck

PARAMETERS: 8 to 12 repetitions each direction, 1 to 3 sets, 1 time per day or every other day

6.14.20 FUNCTIONAL: ANKLE/FOOT, SINGLE-LEG HOPS AND VARIATIONS

POSITION: Standing

TARGETS: Strengthening, facilitating quicker power movements, neuromuscular control and proprioception of the ankle and foot

INSTRUCTION: Patient starts with double leg hops and jumps and progresses to single leg. *Hop in place*: Patient starts by mini-hopping in place. Allow them to hold stable object to star and progress to no hands. *Dot jumps*: Refer to **6.09.31** for full description of a variation of dot drills that can be progressed to single leg.

SUBSTITUTIONS: Hard landings; the hip, knee, and ankle/foot mechanism should be watched carefully to ensure patients are absorbing the landing shock.

PARAMETERS: 8 to 12 repetitions, 1 to 3 sets, 1 time per day or every other day

6.14.21 FUNCTIONAL: ANKLE/FOOT, NINTENDO WII

POSITION: Standing

TARGETS: Strengthening, facilitating balance, reaction times, neuromuscular control and proprioception of the ankle and foot.

INSTRUCTION: *For muscle-strengthening exercise*: Lunges, single-leg extensions, sideways leg lifts, single-leg twists, and rowing squats can be performed. In lunges, players begin with a posture of lacing the fingers behind the head and with front hip and knee at 90 degrees flexion, back foot about two steps behind also at 90 degrees knee flexion and slight hip flexion, keeping the torso straight. The more weight players put on the ankle, the higher the red gauge moves. The gauge has to reach at least above the blue line.

In *single-leg* extensions, players stand on one leg and keep other hip and knee joint slightly flexed, moving the bent leg in anterior to posterior directions. In order to maintain the body's balance, the center of the body needs to not deviate from the yellow part. In order to reinforce the ankle, the patient concentrates on the ankle when applying weight. In *sideways leg lifts*, the patient begins standing on one foot and abducts of opposite shoulder and hip while maintaining the center of the body within the boundary of the yellow part, concentrating on the ankle. In the *single-leg twists*, the patient stands on one foot and maintains flexion opposite hip and knee. At the same time, patient lowers the arms in a diagonal direction and twist the body such that the back of the hand touched the knee. In the *rowing squats*, the patient repeats flexion and extension of both legs concurrently with repetition of flexing the elbows as if trying to touch anterior shoulder while extending the shoulder joint. The center of the body has to stay within the interior of the blue part as the knee avoids advancing before the toe.

For exercise that enhances balance: Patient heads imaginary soccer balls, tightrope walks, table tilts, and slalomes on both snowboards and skis. In *soccer heading*, patients head soccer balls by moving the center of the body left to right. Patients get higher scores in case of continuous headers. The players also avoid any objects that are not soccer balls and are able to think ahead, as the number of soccer balls remaining is displayed on the upper-left part of the screen. In *ski slalom*, the players pass flag marks in sequence by moving left to right and anterior to posterior. The number of missed flags, elapsed time, and current speed are all displayed on the screen. Patients can see how the center of gravity is moving at the current time by looking at the screen. Time is measured upon reaching the arrival point, and final times are calculated by adding the time-converted number of missed flags. *(continued)*

6.14.21 FUNCTIONAL: ANKLE/FOOT, NINTENDO WII (CONTINUED)

In *tightrope walk*, patients control the characters to avoid falling from the single stripe. When the body is tilted toward one side, the player has to immediately balance toward the opposite side in order not to fall. The patient has to do this as quickly as possible since there is a time limit. Obstacles appear frequently in order to interrupt the progress, and the character has to jump adeptly to avoid them, after which balancing is important in the landing process. In *table tilt*, the patient puts a bead in holes by moving the body left-right and anterior-posterior. The number of beads or difficulty level increases in the higher stages. This exercise requires concentration since there is a time limit. The patient can proceed to the next level once clearing one stage. The *snowboard slalom* requires the patient stand on the Wii Balance Board vertically, as if actually snowboarding. The patient maintains body balance by moving forward and backward while standing sideways on the board. The patient has to pass the flag marks in regular sequence in order to obtain a high score. The final score is computed by adding up the times the patient took to pass the flags.

SUBSTITUTIONS: Hip, knee, and ankle/foot mechanisms should be watched carefully to ensure patients are controlling ankle movements.

PARAMETERS: 20 minutes, 1 time per day or every other day

Where's the Evidence?

The Nintendo Wii Fit Plus contains programs that aim to enhance muscle strength as well as those that aim to enhance the sense of balance. Kim, Jun, and Heo (2015) examined the effects of a training program using the Nintendo Wii Fit Plus on the ankle muscle strengths of subjects in their 20s who had functional ankle instability. They were randomized to a Wii strength training group and a Wii balance training group. Both groups demonstrated increased strength in plantar- and dorsiflexion. The balance training group using Wii Fit Plus showed better results in strength of inversion and eversion than the strengthening training group. Consequently, it is recommended to add the balance training program of the Wii Fit Plus to conventional exercise programs to improve ankle muscle strength in functional ankle instability.

REFERENCE

Kim, K. J., Jun, H. J., & Heo, M. (2015). Effects of Nintendo Wii Fit Plus training on ankle strength with functional ankle instability. *Journal of Physical Therapy Science, 27*(11), 3381-3385.

Section 6.15

LOWER EXTREMITY NERVE GLIDES

In the LE, there are two nerves that can be damaged or trapped anywhere along the LE. This could be due to scar tissue, impingement, or tightness. Nerves with poor gliding through the leg become inflamed and painful. Gentle nerve glides, also called *nerve flossing* or *neural glides/flossing*, can relieve this inflammation and nerve pain if done properly.

Nerve glides are still preferred in the acute and subacute phases to avoid further irritation. The two main nerves in the LE are the sciatic and femoral nerves.

Where's the Evidence?

A 2008 study found that gliding techniques were more effective at moving the nerve through the tissue than tensioning the nerve. Nerve sliding works by elongating the nerve bed at one joint while simultaneously shortening it at another (Coppieters & Butler, 2008). This allows the nerve to move without creating a strain on the nerve. Ellis and Hing, in a 2008 systematic review of the literature, found that although neural mobilization is advocated for treatment of neurodynamic dysfunction, the primary justification for using neural mobilization had been based on a few clinical trials and primarily anecdotal evidence. The review found majority of these studies concluded a positive therapeutic benefit from using neural mobilization; however, in consideration of their methodological quality, qualitative analysis of these studies revealed that there is only limited evidence to support the use of neural mobilization.

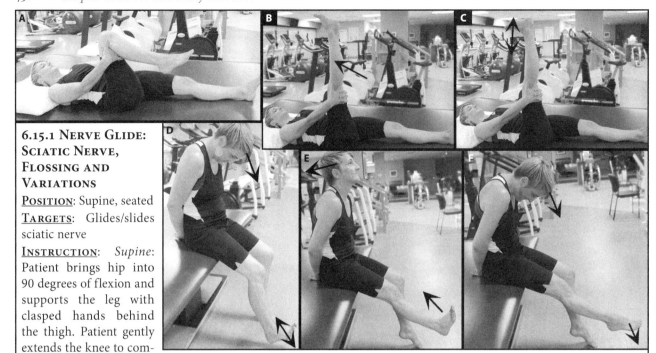

6.15.1 NERVE GLIDE: SCIATIC NERVE, FLOSSING AND VARIATIONS

POSITION: Supine, seated

TARGETS: Glides/slides sciatic nerve

INSTRUCTION: *Supine*: Patient brings hip into 90 degrees of flexion and supports the leg with clasped hands behind the thigh. Patient gently extends the knee to comfortable tension. Once tension felt, bend knee just slightly out of that range and pump the ankle into dorsiflexion and then plantarflexion. Once completed, extend knee into new range, and repeat instructions from beginning (A through C). *Seated slump*: Patient sits with slouched posture with hands behind the back. Patient drops the head down and extends the knee until slight tension is felt. Once tension felt, bend knee just slightly out of that range and pump the ankle into dorsiflexion and then plantarflexion. Once completed, extend knee into new range, and repeat instructions from beginning (D). *Seated with neck movement*: With trunk erect, patient extends knee until slight tension is felt. Patient bends the knee just slightly to remove tension. Patient then extends the neck (not fully, watch neck control) and dorsiflexes the ankle at the same time, followed by then bringing the neck back to neutral as patient plantarflexes 20 repetitions. Once completed, extend knee into new range and repeat instructions from beginning (E and F).

SUBSTITUTIONS: Stretching nerve, nerve pain, excessive tensioning; stop and re-instruct.

PARAMETERS: Each set is done 20 times and then moved into new range, perform sequence 3 times, repeat 1 to 3 times per day as needed.

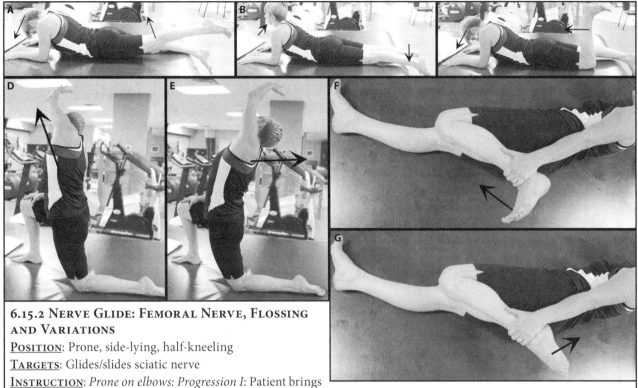

6.15.2 NERVE GLIDE: FEMORAL NERVE, FLOSSING AND VARIATIONS

POSITION: Prone, side-lying, half-kneeling

TARGETS: Glides/slides sciatic nerve

INSTRUCTION: *Prone on elbows: Progression I*: Patient brings hip into extension, keeping knee straight, and flexes the neck. Leg is then lowered back to mat as patient extends the neck back to neutral (A). *Progression II*: Patient bends the knee while bending the neck into flexion. Lower leg back to mat as patient brings neck back to neutral (B and C). *Half-kneeling*: Patient in tall-kneeling with target knee down. Patient reaches overhead with ipsilateral arm and side bends contralaterally. Patient rolls forward and then backward. Use towel under knee for comfort (D and E). *Side-lying*: Lying on unaffected side, bring target heel toward buttock and hold with top hand. Patient then flexes and extends the neck mid-range (F and G).

SUBSTITUTIONS: Stretching nerve, nerve pain, excessive tensioning; stop and re-instruct.

PARAMETERS: Each set is done 20 times, perform sequence 3 times, repeat 1 to 3 times per day as needed

REFERENCES

Coppieters, M. W., & Butler, D. S. (2008). Do 'sliders' slide and 'tensioners' tension? An analysis of neurodynamic techniques and considerations regarding their application. *Manual Therapy, 13*(3), 213-221.

Ellis, R. F., & Hing, W. A. (2008). Neural mobilization: A systematic review of randomized controlled trials with an analysis of therapeutic efficacy. *Journal of Manual and Manipulative Therapy, 16*(1), 8-22.

Section 6.16

ANKLE AND FOOT PROTOCOLS AND TREATMENT IDEAS

6.16.1 ANKLE INSTABILITY

Inversion injuries, primarily sprains of the ankle are one of the most commonly treated injuries. Lateral ankle sprains are classified into three categories: Grade I, II, and III. A Grade I mild sprain is stretching or minor tearing of a few fibers of the ligament with no loss of function and only slight swelling and tenderness and usually involves the ATFL. A Grade II moderate sprain involves extensive tearing of the ligament fibers, resulting in profuse swelling, pain with movement, and significant tenderness with discoloration and usually involves the ATFL and calcaneofibular ligament. A Grade III severe sprain is painful with significant loss of motion, swelling, bruising, and tenderness and involves all three lateral ligaments: ATFL, calcaneofibular ligament, and posterior talofibular ligament. The three main treatments for acute lateral ankle ligament injuries are immobilization, functional treatment consisting of early mobilization and an external support (brace, rigid taping), and surgical reconstruction (Kerkhoffs, Handoll, de Bie, Rowe, & Strujis, 2002). Chronic lateral ankle instability occurs in 10% to 20% of people after an acute ankle sprain. Initial treatment is generally conservative; however, if conservative treatment fails and ligament laxity is present, surgery is indicated.

Where's the Evidence?

Conservative treatment consisting of neuromuscular training alone has been shown to be effective in the short term. If surgical correction is performed, studies also show early rehabilitation is superior to 6 weeks post-operation immobilization (de Vries, Krips, Sierevelt, Blankenvoort, & van Dijk, 2011).

Handoll, Rowe, Quinn, and de Brie (2001) found evidence to suggest that wearing a semi-rigid ankle support such as an air cast may even prevent ankle sprains in high-risk sporting activities such as basketball and soccer.

Seah and Mani-Bubu's review of the evidence in 2011 found that for mild-to-moderate ankle sprains, functional treatment options consisting of elastic bandaging, soft casting, taping, or orthoses with associated coordination training was better than immobilization for multiple outcomes measures. They also found that for severe ankle sprains, a short period of immobilization resulted in a quicker recovery. Other findings included that lace-up supports are a more effective functional treatment than elastic bandaging and result in less swelling in the short-term when compared with semi-rigid ankle supports, elastic bandaging, and tape.

Petersen et al.'s review of available evidence through 2013 also supported these ideas stating that the majority of grades I, II, and III lateral ankle ligament ruptures could be managed without surgery. Their systematic review also supported protocol of a short-term immobilization for grade III injuries followed by a semi-rigid brace.

In a study by Janssen, van Mechelen, and Verhagen (2014) of 384 athletes who had previously sustained a lateral ankle sprain, bracing was found to be somewhat superior to neuromuscular training in reducing the incidence but not the severity of self-reported recurrent ankle sprains after usual care.

One relatively new approach is hyaluronic acid injections into the ankle which may have a role in expediting return to sport after ankle sprain (Seah & Mani-Babu, 2011). Balance and proprioceptive training are effective key approaches for rehabilitation of the unstable ankle (Hupperets, Verhagen, & van Mechelen, 2009). Different approaches to balance training have all shown similar improvement for sprained ankle (Faizullin & Faizullina, 2015). A three-phase protocol is outlined here. Phase I focuses on rest, protecting the stretched and torn ligaments to allow for healing and reducing swelling and usually lasts 1 to 4 weeks depending on the severity. Phase II focuses on restoring ROM, strength, proprioception, and flexibility while continuing to protect healing structures and may last up to 3 to 6 weeks. Phase III gradually returns the patient to activities that do not require turning or twisting and progressing exercises followed eventually by activities that require cutting, agility, plyometrics, running, and sports activities up to 3 to 4 months.

6.16.2 ANKLE SPRAIN/INSTABILITY NON-OPERATIVE PROTOCOL

Adapted from Dr. Lind's (2015a,b) non-operative lateral ankle sprain protocols at Rosenberg Cooley Metcalf Orthopedic Clinic in Park City and Mattacola and Dwyers' (2002) article, "Rehabilitation of the Ankle After Acute Sprain or Chronic Instability."

Advice for patient: Always try to step heel-first, especially when walking on uneven terrain and off steps.

Phase I:

- Grade I and II: 0 to 1 week
- Grade III: 0 to 4 weeks

1. Week 1: Rest, ice, compression, elevation
2. Decreased weightbearing; may use crutches
3. Grade III injuries generally in a splint, boot or cast for up to 6 weeks
4. Gait training to normalize gait pattern, pain-free
   a. 6.04.43 Functional: Gait Practice
5. AROM
   a. 6.11.3 ROM: Ankle/Foot, Long-Sitting and Ankle Pumps, 4-Way, Active; no end range especially plantarflexion (ATFL) and inversion.
6. Strengthening
   a. Ankle Isometrics; choose one strategy, whichever keeps patient in most neutral position.
      i. 6.14.3 Strengthen: Isometric; Ankle, Fixed Object Resist, 4-Way
      ii. 6.14.2 Strengthen: Isometric; Ankle, Foot Resist, 4-Way
      iii. 6.14.1 Strengthen: Isometric; Ankle, Hand Resist, 4-Way
   b. 6.14.4 Strengthen: Isometric; Toe Extension and Flexion
7. Early conditioning
   a. 6.11.1 ROM: Ankle/Foot, Warm-Up, Stationary or Recumbent Bike
   b. 6.11.15 ROM: Single-Leg Treadmill Walking, Gait Simulation
8. Aquatics
   a. Non-impact pool program

Phase II:

- Grade I and II: 1 to 2 weeks
- Grade III: 4 to 6 weeks

1. Continue to address swelling and pain (modalities)
2. Wean crutches
3. AROM
   a. 6.11.3 ROM: Ankle/Foot, Long-Sitting and Ankle Pumps, 4-Way, Active; focus on full AROM, especially dorsiflexion.
   b. 6.11.13 ROM: Biomechanical Ankle Platform System/ Wobble Board, Active (also targets proprioception)
   c. 6.11.8 ROM: Ankle/Foot, Alphabet, Active
   d. 6.11.11 ROM: Ankle Dorsiflexion, Chair Slides, Active
4. Stretching
   a. Calf stretch
      i. 6.11.12 ROM: Ankle/Foot, Prostretch, Active Assistive
      ii. 6.13.6 Stretch: Soleus Using Strap
      iii. 6.13.5 Stretch: Gastrocnemius Using Strap
5. Strengthening
   a. 6.11.10 ROM: Ankle Inversion and Eversion, Towel Slides, Active; focus on eversion primarily and inversion only 50% range.
   b. 6.14.13 Strengthen: Resistance Band; Ankle, 8-Way, Therapist-Assisted
      i. Plantarflexion
      ii. Dorsiflexion
      iii. Eversion
      iv. Inversion; 75% ROM only to start, progress to full inversion slowly.
      v. Dorsiflexion/eversion
      vi. Dorsiflexion/inversion
      vii. Plantarflexion/eversion
      viii. Plantarflexion/inversion (50% range)
   c. *Or* 6.14.12 Strengthen: Resistance Band; Ankle, 8-Way, Self-Assisted
      i. Plantarflexion
      ii. Dorsiflexion
      iii. Eversion
      iv. Inversion; 75% ROM only to start, progress to full inversion slowly.

     v. Dorsiflexion/eversion

     vi. Dorsiflexion/inversion

     vii. Plantarflexion/eversion

     viii. Plantarflexion/inversion (50% range)

  d. 6.14.5 Strengthen: Isotonic; Ankle/Foot, Marble Pick-Ups

  e. 6.14.9 Strengthen: Isotonic; Toe Raises (seated)

  f. 6.14.10 Strengthen: Isotonic; Heel-Toe Walking (heel walking only)

  g. 6.14.11 Strengthen: Isotonic; Arch Lifts

  h. 6.14.7 Strengthen: Isotonic; Heel Raises (avoid extreme end range)

  i. 6.11.9 ROM: Toe Scrunches With Towel, Active (also strengthens intrinsic)

  j. 6.09.18 Strengthen: Knee, Leg Press on Weight Machine

  k. 6.04.26 Functional: Hip, Wall Squat

  l. 6.04.28 Functional: Hip, Free-Standing Squat

  m. 6.04.34 Functional: Hip, Lunge and Variations

     i. Beginner and forward only

  n. 6.04.8 Strengthen: Isotonic; Hip, Straight Leg Raise, 4-Way (hip strengthening)

  o. 6.04.33 Functional: Hip, Step-Ups 4- to 6-inch step

6. Balance/Coordination

  a. 6.14.16 Functional: Ankle/Foot, Rhomberg and Variations

     i. Flat stable surfaces only; eyes open and closed

       1. Rhomberg

       2. Sharpened Rhomberg

       3. Unilateral stance

       4. Ball toss

       5. Weight shifts; with functional reaches.

       6. Perturbations; with stable surface and Rhomberg, sharpened Rhomberg and unilateral stance.

7. Conditioning

  a. Bike, elliptical, treadmill walking

8. Aquatics

  a. Light jogging

Phase III:

- Grade I and II: 2 to 3 weeks
- Grade III: 6 to 8 weeks

1. Balance/Coordination

  a. 6.14.18 Functional: Ankle/Foot, Opposite Hip, 4-Way Balance Challenge

2. Stretching ideas

  a. Advance Calf Stretch (choose one)

     i. 6.13.7 Stretch: Calf on Step

     ii. 6.13.8 Stretch: Calf on Ramp

3. Strengthening ideas

  a. 6.14.10 Strengthen: Isotonic; Heel-Toe Walking (add toe walking)

  b. 6.04.22 Strengthen: Resistance Band, Hip, Sidestepping

  c. 6.04.34 Functional: Hip, Lunge and Variations

     i. Add lateral

     ii. Add diagonal

4. Balance/Coordination

  a. 6.14.16 Functional: Ankle/Foot, Rhomberg and Variations

     i. Progress to multiple surfaces, eyes open and closed

       1. Rhomberg

       2. Sharpened Rhomberg

       3. Unilateral stance

       4. Ball toss

       5. Weight shifts; with functional reaches.

       6. Perturbations; with stable surface and Rhomberg, sharpened Rhomberg and unilateral stance.

  b. 6.14.18 Functional: Ankle/Foot, Opposite Hip, 4-Way Balance Challenge

  c. 6.04.35 Functional: Hip, Dynamic Leg Swing, "Running Man"

     i. Stand on affected leg

  d. 6.14.17 Functional: Ankle/Foot, Steps-Overs, Step-Behinds, and Carioca/Braiding

  e. 6.14.19 Functional: Ankle/Foot, Single-Leg Mini-Squat and Reach, All Directions

  f. 6.09.33 Plyometrics and Variations, Knee

     i. Quiet jumps double leg: box 2 to 6 inch height

  g. 6.09.30 Agility: Knee, Speed Ladder Drills and Variations

     i. One step

     ii. Sidestep

5. Conditioning

  a. Start light jogging

Phase IV:

- Grade I and II: 3 to 6 weeks
- Grade III: 8 to 12 weeks

1. Balance/Coordination ideas; wear brace (lace-up, air cast or rigid taping) for advanced agility, cutting and sprinting drills.

  a. 6.09.33 Plyometrics and Variations, Knee below

     i. B: Quiet jumps single leg

     ii. C: Box jumps forward

     iii. Consider progressing to other variations per tolerance

  b. 6.09.34 Reactive Neuromuscular Training and Variations below

     i. Uniplanar anterior shift

     ii. Uniplanar lateral shift

     iii. Multiplanar weight shifts

     iv. Squat posterior weight shifts

     v. Squat anterior weight shifts

     vi. Squat posterior medial shifts

     vii. Lunge medial weight shifts

viii. Single leg squat medial shifts band at knee

2. Sport specific agility drills; clear with physician first.

    a. 6.09.30 Agility: Knee, Speed Ladder Drills and Variations

    b. 6.09.31 Agility: Knee, Dot Drills and Variations

    c. 6.09.32 Agility: Knee, Mini-Hurdle Drills and Variations

    d. 8.01.4 Running Progressions; gradually increase intensity of running jog to run to sprints

    e. 8.01.7 Cutting Sequence-Figure 8 Progression

    f. 8.01.6 Jump-Hop Sequence

    g. 8.01.5 Sprint Sequence

3. Cardiovascular program

    a. Running, elliptical, bike, swimming, Stairmaster

4. Criteria for discharge; return to sport, physician directed.

    a. Good scoring on strength and agility tests

    b. Negative clinical exam

6.16.3 LATERAL ANKLE LIGAMENT RECONSTRUCTION PROTOCOL

Adapted from Royal National Orthopedic Hospital's (2008), "Rehabilitation Guidelines for Patients Undergoing Surgery for Lateral Ligament Reconstruction of the Ankle."

Advice for patient: Always try to step heel-first, especially when walking on uneven terrain and off steps.

Phase I: 0 to 6 Weeks

1. Weightbearing; depending on surgery may be PWB or WBAT and wearing brace, may use crutches as needed.

    a. Brace (hinged boot/hinged splint)

      i. 0 to 2 weeks: Locked in neutral

      ii. 3 to 4 weeks: 10 degrees dorsiflexion to 20 degrees plantarflexion

      iii. 5 to 6 weeks: 20 degrees dorsiflexion to 40 degrees plantarflexion

2. Start physical therapy:

    a. 3 weeks if anatomic repair; *will start gentle PROM of ankle out of boot* (Karlsson, Rudholm, Bergsten, Faxén, & Styf, 1995).

    b. 6 weeks if secondary extrinsic repair (i.e. peroneal tenodesis)

3. *No active eversion for 6 weeks if peroneal tenodesis technique utilized

4. Elevation after surgery for edema

Circulatory exercises after surgery:

5. AROM

    a. 6.01.8 ROM: Hip Flexion and Extension, Heel Slide, Active

    b. 6.01.10 ROM: Hip Abduction and Adduction, Heel Slide, Active

6. Stretching

    a. 6.08.3 Stretch: Hamstrings

7. Strengthening; muscle pump leg isometrics, *no ankle exercises.*

    a. 6.04.2 Strengthen: Isometric; Hip Extension/ Gluteus Sets

    b. 6.09.3 Strengthen: Isometric; Knee Flexion, Hamstring Set (supine)

    c. 6.09.1 Strengthen: Isometric; Knee Extension, Quadriceps Set

    d. 6.09.2 Strengthen: Isometric; Knee Extension, Quadriceps Set With Ball Squeeze (Vastus Medialis Oblique)

    e. 6.04.3 Strengthen: Isometric; Hip Abduction

    f. 6.04.4 Strengthen: Isometric; Hip Adduction

Phase II: 6 to 12 Weeks

1. Precautions

    a. No stretching into inversion

    b. No impact exercises

    c. No balance exercises until strength 4/5

2. Wean out of boot/splint into normal footwear

3. Wean assistive device

4. Gait training to normalize gait pattern, pain-free

    a. 6.04.43 Functional: Gait Practice

5. AROM

    a. 6.11.3 ROM: Ankle/Foot, Long-Sitting and Ankle Pumps, 4-Way, Active; focus on full AROM, especially dorsiflexion however caution with end range especially plantarflexion and inversion.

    b. 6.11.13 ROM: Biomechanical Ankle Platform System/ Wobble Board, Active (also targets proprioception)

      i. Seated

    c. 6.11.8 ROM: Ankle/Foot, Alphabet, Active

    d. 6.11.11 ROM: Ankle Dorsiflexion, Chair Slides, Active

6. Stretching

    a. Calf stretch

      i. 6.11.12 ROM: Ankle/Foot, Prostretch, Active Assistive

      ii. 6.13.6 Stretch: Soleus Using Strap

      iii. 6.13.5 Stretch: Gastrocnemius Using Strap

7. Strengthening

    a. Ankle Isometrics; choose one strategy, whichever keeps patient in most neutral position.

      i. 6.14.3 Strengthen: Isometric; Ankle, Fixed Object Resist, 4-Way

    ii. 6.14.2 Strengthen: Isometric; Ankle, Foot Resist, 4-Way

    iii. 6.14.1 Strengthen: Isometric; Ankle, Hand Resist, 4-Way

    iv. 6.14.4 Strengthen: Isometric; Toe Extension and Flexion

  b. Progress to isotonics

    i. 6.14.13 Strengthen: Resistance Band; Ankle, 8-Way, Therapist-Assisted

      1. Plantarflexion

      2. Dorsiflexion

      3. Eversion

      4. Inversion; 75% ROM only to start, progress to full inversion slowly.

      5. Dorsiflexion/eversion

      6. Dorsiflexion/inversion

      7. Plantarflexion/eversion

      8. Plantarflexion/inversion (50% range)

    ii. *Or* 6.14.12 Strengthen: Resistance Band; Ankle, 8-Way, Self-Assisted

      1. Plantarflexion

      2. Dorsiflexion

      3. Eversion

      4. Inversion; 75% ROM only to start, progress to full inversion slowly.

      5. Dorsiflexion/eversion

      6. Dorsiflexion/inversion

      7. Plantarflexion/eversion

      8. Plantarflexion/inversion (50% range)

  c. Other strengthening

    i. 6.11.9 ROM: Toe Scrunches With Towel, Active (also strengthens intrinsic)

    ii. 6.14.5 Strengthen: Isotonic; Ankle/Foot, Marble Pick-Ups

    iii. 6.14.9 Strengthen: Isotonic; Toe Raises (seated)

    iv. 6.14.10 Strengthen: Isotonic; Heel-Toe Walking (heel walking only)

    v. 6.14.11 Strengthen: Isotonic; Arch Lifts

    vi. 6.14.7 Strengthen: Isotonic; Heel Raises (avoid extreme end range)

    vii. 6.09.18 Strengthen: Knee, Leg Press on Weight Machine

    viii. 6.04.26 Functional: Hip, Wall Squat

    ix. 6.04.28 Functional: Hip, Free-Standing Squat

    x. 6.04.34 Functional: Hip, Lunge and Variations

      1. Beginner and forward only

    xi. 6.04.8 Strengthen: Isotonic; Hip, Straight Leg Raise, 4-Way (hip strengthening)

    xii. 6.04.33 Functional: Hip, Step-Ups 4 to 6 inch step

8. Balance/Coordination

  a. 6.14.16 Functional: Ankle/Foot, Rhomberg and Variations

    i. Flat stable surfaces only; eyes open and closed

      1. Rhomberg

      2. Sharpened Rhomberg

      3. Unilateral stance

      4. Ball toss

      5. Weight shifts; with functional reaches.

      6. Perturbations; with stable surface and Rhomberg, sharpened Rhomberg and unilateral stance.

9. Conditioning

  a. Bike, treadmill, walking

10. Core strengthening

  a. 4.03.42 Strengthen: Abdominal, Pulsing Crunch, 3-Way (Advanced)

  b. 4.03.38 Strengthen: Abdominal, Plank and Variations below (progression)

    i. C: Quadruped

  c. 4.03.39 Strengthen: Abdominal, Side Plank and Variations below (progression)

    i. C: On elbow and knee (beginner)

    ii. E: On hand and knee

11. Early conditioning

  a. 6.11.1 ROM: Ankle/Foot, Warm-Up, Stationary or Recumbent Bike

  b. 6.11.15 ROM: Single-Leg Treadmill Walking, Gait Simulation

12. Aquatics

  a. Non-impact pool program

Phase III: 12 Weeks to 6 Months

1. Stretching ideas

  a. Advance Calf Stretch (choose one)

    i. 6.13.7 Stretch: Calf on Step

    ii. 6.13.8 Stretch: Calf on Ramp

2. Strengthening ideas

  a. 6.14.10 Strengthen: Isotonic; Heel-Toe Walking (add toe walking)

  b. 6.04.22 Strengthen: Resistance Band, Hip, Sidestepping

  c. 6.04.34 Functional: Hip, Lunge and Variations

    i. Add lateral

    ii. Add diagonal

3. Balance/Coordination

  a. 6.14.18 Functional: Ankle/Foot, Opposite Hip, 4-Way Balance Challenge

  b. 6.14.16 Functional: Ankle/Foot, Rhomberg and Variations

    i. Progress to multi surfaces eyes open and closed

      1. Rhomberg

      2. Sharpened Rhomberg

      3. Unilateral stance

      4. Ball toss

      5. Weight shifts; with functional reaches.

6. Perturbations; with stable surface and Rhomberg, sharpened Rhomberg and unilateral stance.

c. 6.14.18 Functional: Ankle/Foot, Opposite Hip, 4-Way Balance Challenge

d. 6.04.35 Functional: Hip, Dynamic Leg Swing, "Running Man"

   i. Stand on affected leg

e. 6.14.17 Functional: Ankle/Foot, Steps-Overs, Step-Behinds, and Carioca/Braiding

f. 6.14.19 Functional: Ankle/Foot, Single-Leg Mini-Squat and Reach, All Directions

g. 6.09.33 Plyometrics and Variations, Knee

   i. Quiet jumps double leg: box 2 to 6 inches height

h. 6.09.30 Agility: Knee, Speed Ladder Drills and Variations

   i. One step

   ii. Sidestep

4. Conditioning

a. Start light jogging

Advanced Later Stages of Phase IIII—Clear With Physician Before Beginning

1. Balance/Coordination ideas; wear brace (lace-up, air cast or rigid taping) for advanced agility, cutting and sprinting drills.

a. 6.09.33 Plyometrics and Variations, Knee below

   i. B: Quiet jumps single leg

ii. C: Box jumps forward

iii. *Consider progressing to other variations per tolerance*

b. RNT and Variations below

   i. Uniplanar anterior shift

   ii. Uniplanar lateral shift

   iii. Multiplanar weight shifts

   iv. Squat posterior weight shifts

   v. Squat anterior weight shifts

   vi. Squat posterior medial shifts

   vii. Lunge medial weight shifts

   viii. Single leg squat medial shifts band at knee

2. Sport specific agility drills; clear with physician first.

a. 6.09.30 Agility: Knee, Speed Ladder Drills and Variations

b. 6.09.31 Agility: Knee, Dot Drills and Variations

c. 6.09.32 Agility: Knee, Mini-Hurdle Drills and Variations

d. 8.01.4 Running Progressions; gradually increase intensity of running jog to run to sprints.

e. 8.01.7 Cutting Sequence-Figure 8 Progression

f. 8.01.6 Jump-Hop Sequence

g. 8.01.5 Sprint Sequence

3. Cardiovascular program

a. Running, elliptical, bike, swimming, Stairmaster

4. Criteria for discharge; return to sport, physician directed.

a. Good scoring on strength and agility tests

b. Negative clinical exam

6.16.4 ACHILLES TENDON RUPTURE AND REPAIR DISCUSSION

The Achilles tendon is one of the largest and strongest tendons in the human body, but it is also the most frequently ruptured (Jiang, Wang, Chen, Dong, & Yu, 2012). Although Achilles tendon problems are considered frequent in active individuals from overuse or a single acute episode, problems in the Achilles tendon can be a consequence of inflammatory and autoimmune conditions, genetically determined collagen abnormalities, infectious diseases, tumors, and neurological conditions that are not of a primary surgical nature (Ames, Longo, Denaro, & Maffulli, 2008). The acute rupture of the Achilles tendon is a protracted injury generally requiring surgery. The rehabilitation protocol is integral in restoring the patient back to pre-injury activity level. Despite several studies available comparing different treatment regimes, there had been minimal consensus regarding the optimal protocol.

Patient may also recover without surgery, usually being casted for 6 weeks after injury; however, patients managed conservatively have been shown to have a higher risk or re-rupture (Jiang et al., 2012).

Where's the Evidence?

Suchak, Spooner, Reid, and Jomha (2006) found early functional treatment protocols, when compared with post-operative immobilization, led to more excellent rated subjective responses and no difference in re-rupture rate.

This was further supported by Brumann, Baumbach, Mutschler, and Polzer's review of current evidence in 2014. They found the combination of FWB and early ankle mobilization compared to immobilization was most beneficial. They recommended the rehabilitation protocol after Achilles tendon repair should allow immediate FWB and, after the second post-operative week, controlled ankle mobilization by free plantarflexion and limited dorsiflexion at 0 degrees.

Braunstein, Baumbach, Boecker, Carmont, and Polzer (2015) also confirmed this in a systematic review of the literature and recommended immediate weightbearing in a functional brace, together with early mobilization, stating it is safe and has superior outcome following minimally invasive repair of Achilles tendon rupture.

6.16.5 Achilles Tendon Repair Post Surgical Protocol

Adapted from University of Wisconsin Health Sports Medicine Center's (2015) "Rehabilitation Guidelines for Achilles Tendon Repair."

Phase I: 0 to 2 Weeks

1. Weightbearing: Flat foot weightbearing/touchdown/toe touch weightbearing; only putting foot down for balance but no weight through foot, use of assistive device as needed.
   a. Brace (hinged boot/hinged splint); general recommendation, this is physician specific, follow specific orders of physician if differing.
      i. 0 to 2 weeks: Locked in 20 to 30 degrees plantarflexion; may require use of heel lift if non-hinged boot.
   Circulatory exercises after surgery:
2. AROM
   a. 6.01.8 ROM: Hip Flexion and Extension, Heel Slide, Active
   b. 6.01.10 ROM: Hip Abduction and Adduction, Heel Slide, Active
3. Stretching
   a. 6.08.3 Stretch: Hamstrings
4. Strengthening; muscle pump leg isometrics, no ankle exercises:
   a. 6.04.2 Strengthen: Isometric; Hip Extension/Gluteus Sets
   b. 6.09.3 Strengthen: Isometric; Knee Flexion, Hamstring Set (supine)
   c. 6.09.1 Strengthen: Isometric; Knee Extension, Quadriceps Set
   d. 6.09.2 Strengthen: Isometric; Knee Extension, Quadriceps Set With Ball Squeeze (Vastus Medialis Oblique)
   e. 6.04.3 Strengthen: Isometric; Hip Abduction
   f. 6.04.4 Strengthen: Isometric; Hip Adduction

Phase II: 2 to 4 Weeks

1. Weightbearing: WBAT
   a. Brace (hinged boot/hinged splint/boot); general recommendation, this is physician specific, follow specific orders of physician if differing.
      i. 2 to 3 weeks: 10 degrees plantarflexion; may require use of heel lift if non-hinged boot.
      ii. 3 to 4 weeks: 0 degrees plantarflexion; may require use of heel lift if non-hinged boot.
2. Wean assistive device
3. AROM
   a. 6.11.3 ROM: Ankle/Foot, Long-Sitting and Ankle Pumps, 4-Way, Active; *pain-free*, gentle plantarflexion and dorsiflexion.
   b. 6.11.13 ROM: Biomechanical Ankle Platform System/Wobble Board, Active (also targets proprioception)
      i. Seated

c. 6.11.8 ROM: Ankle/Foot, Alphabet, Active
   d. 6.11.10 ROM: Ankle Inversion and Eversion, Towel Slides, Active
4. Ankle strengthening
   a. Ankle Isometrics; choose one strategy, whichever keeps patient in most neutral position; *plantarflexion only 50% contraction to start.*
      i. 6.14.3 Strengthen: Isometric; Ankle, Fixed Object Resist, 4-Way *or*
      ii. 6.14.2 Strengthen: Isometric; Ankle, Foot Resist, 4-Way *or*
      iii. 6.14.1 Strengthen: Isometric; Ankle, Hand Resist, 4-Way *and*
      iv. 6.14.4 Strengthen: Isometric; Toe Extension and Flexion
5. Hip strengthening (open chain only)
   a. 6.04.8 Strengthen: Isotonic; Hip, Straight Leg Raise, 4-Way (hip strengthening)
6. Core strengthening ideas
   a. 4.03.42 Strengthen: Abdominal, Pulsing Crunch, 3-Way (Advanced)
   b. 4.03.38 Strengthen: Abdominal, Plank and Variations below (progression)
      i. C: Quadruped (feet off the table)
   c. 4.03.39 Strengthen: Abdominal, Side Plank and Variations Below (progression)
      i. C: On elbow and knee (beginner)
      ii. E: On hand and knee
7. Conditioning
   a. 5.04.1 ROM: Shoulder, Warm-Up, Upper Body Ergometer, Active Assistive

Phase III: 4 to 8 Weeks

1. Gradually wean out of boot/splint into normal footwear using heel lifts and gradually removing heel lifts during week 5 to 8
2. Gait training to normalize gait pattern, pain-free
   a. 6.04.43 Functional: Gait Practice
3. Stretching
   a. Calf stretch; *no aggressive calf stretching*
      i. 6.11.12 ROM: Ankle/Foot, Prostretch, Active Assistive (*gentle*)
      ii. 6.13.6 Stretch: Soleus Using Strap (*gentle*)
      iii. 6.13.5 Stretch: Gastrocnemius Using Strap (*gentle*)
4. Continue AROM; goal 5 degrees dorsiflexion to 40 degrees plantarflexion and within normal limits inversion/eversion.
5. Strengthening
   a. Progress to isotonics week 6

    i. 6.14.13 Strengthen: Resistance Band; Ankle, 8-Way, Therapist-Assisted
1. Plantarflexion
2. Dorsiflexion
3. Eversion
4. Inversion
5. Dorsiflexion/eversion
6. Dorsiflexion/inversion
7. Plantarflexion/eversion
8. Plantarflexion/inversion

    ii. *Or* 6.14.12 Strengthen: Resistance Band; Ankle, 8-Way, Self-Assisted
1. Plantarflexion
2. Dorsiflexion
3. Eversion
4. Inversion
5. Dorsiflexion/eversion
6. Dorsiflexion/inversion
7. Plantarflexion/eversion
8. Plantarflexion/inversion

b. Other strengthening
    i. 6.11.9 ROM: Toe Scrunches With Towel, Active (also strengthens intrinsic)
    ii. 6.14.5 Strengthen: Isotonic; Ankle/Foot, Marble Pick-Ups
    iii. 6.14.9 Strengthen: Isotonic; Toe Raises (seated)
    iv. 6.14.11 Strengthen: Isotonic; Arch Lifts
    v. 6.09.18 Strengthen: Knee, Leg Press on Weight Machine 0 to 30 degrees
    vi. 6.04.29 Functional: Hip, Free-Standing Squat 0 to 30 degrees
    vii. 6.04.34 Functional: Hip, Lunge and Variations 0 to 30 degrees
        1. Beginner and forward only
    viii. 6.04.33 Functional: Hip, Step-Ups 2 to 4 inch step

6. Balance/Coordination
a. 6.14.16 Functional: Ankle/Foot, Rhomberg and Variations
    i. Flat stable surfaces only; eyes open and closed.
        1. Rhomberg
        2. Sharpened Rhomberg
        3. Unilateral stance (week 7 to 8)
        4. Perturbations: with stable surface and Rhomberg, sharpened Rhomberg and unilateral stance (week 7 to 8)

7. Conditioning
a. Continue UBE

8. Aquatics
a. Non-impact pool program

Phase IV: 8 to 16 Weeks

1. AROM; goal 15 degrees dorsiflexion to 50 degrees plantarflexion.

2. Early conditioning
a. 6.11.1 ROM: Ankle/Foot, Warm-Up, Stationary or Recumbent Bike
b. 6.11.15 ROM: Single-Leg Treadmill Walking, Gait Simulation

3. Stretching ideas
a. May consider advancing calf stretch (choose one); *with caution, pain-free.*
    i. 6.13.7 Stretch: Calf on Step
    ii. 6.13.8 Stretch: Calf on Ramp

4. Strengthening ideas
a. 6.14.7 Strengthen: Isotonic; Heel Raises
b. 6.14.10 Strengthen: Isotonic; Heel-Toe Walking
c. 6.04.22 Strengthen: Resistance Band, Sidestepping
d. 6.09.18 Strengthen: Knee, Leg Press on Weight Machine; progress gradually to 0 to 45 degrees, then 0 to 60 degrees then 0 to 70 degrees.
e. 6.04.28 Functional: Hip, Free-Standing Squat 0 to 30 degrees; progress gradually to 0 to 45 degrees, then 0 to 60 degrees then 0 to 70 degrees.
f. 6.04.34 Functional: Hip, Lunge and Variations 0 to 30 degrees; progress gradually to 0 to 45 degrees, then 0 to 60 degrees then 0 to 70 degrees.
    i. Add lateral
    ii. Add diagonal
g. 6.04.33 Functional: Hip, Step-Ups 4 to 8 inches step

5. Balance/Coordination
a. 6.14.18 Functional: Ankle/Foot, Opposite Hip, 4-Way Balance Challenge
b. 6.14.16 Functional: Ankle/Foot, Rhomberg and Variations
    i. Progress to multi surfaces eyes open and closed
        1. Rhomberg
        2. Sharpened Rhomberg
        3. Unilateral stance
        4. Ball toss; start stable surfaces and progress to multi surface.
        5. Weight shifts: with functional reaches; start stable surfaces and progress to multi surface.
        6. Perturbations: with stable surface and Rhomberg, sharpened Rhomberg and unilateral stance
c. 6.04.35 Functional: Hip, Dynamic Leg Swing, "Running Man"
    i. Stand on affected leg
d. 6.14.17 Functional: Ankle/Foot, Steps-Overs, Step-Behinds, and Carioca/Braiding
e. 6.14.19 Functional: Ankle/Foot, Single-Leg Mini-Squat and Reach, All Directions

6. Conditioning
a. 6.11.1 ROM: Ankle/Foot, Warm-Up, Stationary or Recumbent Bike
b. Stairmaster
c. Swimming

Phase V: Starting 4 Months Post-Operation

1. Balance/Coordination ideas
   a. 6.09.33 Plyometrics and Variations, Knee
   b. 6.09.30 Agility: Knee, Speed Ladder Drills and Variations
      i. One step
      ii. Sidestep
   c. 6.09.33 Plyometrics and Variations, Knee below
      i. Quiet jumps double leg: box 2 to 6 inch height
      ii. Progress to B: Quiet jumps single leg
      iii. C: Box jumps forward
      iv. Consider progressing to other variations per tolerance
   d. 6.09.34 Reactive Neuromuscular Training and Variations below
      i. Uniplanar anterior shift
      ii. Uniplanar lateral shift
      iii. Multiplanar weight shifts
      iv. Squat posterior weight shifts
      v. Squat anterior weight shifts
      vi. Squat posterior medial shifts
      vii. Lunge medial weight shifts
      viii. Single leg squat medial shifts band at knee
2. Sport specific agility drills; clear with physician first.
   a. 6.09.30 Agility: Knee, Speed Ladder Drills and Variations
   b. 6.09.31 Agility: Knee, Dot Drills and Variations
   c. 6.09.32 Agility: Knee, Mini-Hurdle Drills and Variations
   d. 8.01.4 Running Progressions; gradually increase intensity of running jog to run to sprints, no limp with jog or fun.
   e. 8.01.7 Cutting Sequence-Figure 8 Progression
   f. 8.01.6 Jump-Hop Sequence
   g. 8.01.5 Sprint Sequence
3. Cardiovascular program
   a. Running, elliptical, bike, swimming, Stairmaster
4. Criteria for discharge; return to sport (physician directed)
   a. Good scoring on strength and agility tests
   b. Negative clinical exam

REFERENCES

Ames, P. R., Longo, U. G., Denaro, V., & Maffulli, N. (2008). Achilles tendon problems: Not just an orthopaedic issue. *Disability and Rehabilitation, 30*(20-22), 1646-1650.

Braunstein, M., Baumbach, S. F., Boecker, W., Carmont, M. R., & Polzer, H. (2015). Development of an accelerated functional rehabilitation protocol following minimal invasive Achilles tendon repair. *Knee Surgery, Sports Traumatology, Arthroscopy.* [Epub ahead of print]

Brumann, M., Baumbach, S. F., Mutschler, W., & Polzer, H. (2014). Accelerated rehabilitation following Achilles tendon repair after acute rupture—Development of an evidence-based treatment protocol. *Injury, 45*(11), 1782-1790.

de Vries, J. S., Krips, R., Sierevelt, I. N., Blankevoort, L., & van Dijk, C. N. (2011). Interventions for treating chronic ankle instability. *Cochrane Database of Systematic Reviews*, (8), CD004124.

Faizullin, I., & Faizullina, E. (2015). Effects of balance training on post-sprained ankle joint instability. *International Journal of Risk and Safety in Medicine, 27*(Suppl 1), S99-S101.

Handoll, H. H., Rowe, B. H., Quinn, K. M., & de Bie, R. (2001). Interventions for preventing ankle ligament injuries. *Cochrane Database of Systematic Reviews*, (3), CD000018.

Hupperets, M. D., Verhagen, E. A., & van Mechelen, W. (2009). Effect of unsupervised home based proprioceptive training on recurrences of ankle sprain: Randomised controlled trial. *The BMJ, 339*, b2684.

Janssen, K. W., van Mechelen, W., & Verhagen, E. A. (2014). Bracing superior to neuromuscular training for the prevention of self-reported recurrent ankle sprains: A three-arm randomised controlled trial. *British Journal of Sports Medicine.* [Epub ahead of print]

Jiang, N., Wang, B., Chen, A., Dong, F., & Yu, B. (2012). Operative versus nonoperative treatment for acute Achilles tendon rupture: A meta-analysis based on current evidence. *International Orthopedics, 36*(4), 765-773.

Karlsson, J., Rudholm, O., Bergsten, T., Faxén, E., & Styf, J. (1995). Early range of motion training after ligament reconstruction of the ankle joint. *Knee Surgery, Sports Traumatology, Arthroscopy, 3*(3), 173-177.

Kerkhoffs, G. M., Handoll, H. H., de Bie, R., Rowe, B. H., & Struijs, P. A. (2002). Surgical versus conservative treatment for acute injuries of the lateral ligament complex of the ankle in adults. *Cochrane Database of Systematic Reviews*, (2), CD000380.

Lind, C. C. (2015a). Lateral ankle sprain Grade I-II nonoperative protocol. *Rosenburg Cooley Metcalf the Orthopedic Clinic at Park City.* Retrieved from https://www.rcmclinic.com/pdfs/foot-ankle/lateral_ankle_grade_I_II.pdf

Lind, C. C. (2015b). Lateral ankle sprain Grade III nonoperative protocol. *Rosenburg Cooley Metcalf the Orthopedic Clinic at Park City.* Retrieved from https://www.rcmclinic.com/pdfs/foot-ankle/lateral_ankle_grade_III.pdf

Mattacola, C. G., & Dwyer, M. K. (2002). Rehabilitation of the ankle after acute sprain or chronic instability. *Journal of Athletic Training, 37*(4), 413-429.

Petersen, W., Rembitzki, I. V., Koppenburg, A. G., Ellermann, A., Liebau, C., Brüggemann, G. P., & Best, R. (2013). Treatment of acute ankle ligament injuries: A systematic review. *Archives of Orthopedic and Trauma Surgery, 133*(8), 1129-1141.

Royal National Orthopedic Hospital. (2008). Rehabilitation guidelines for patients undergoing surgery for lateral ligament reconstruction of the ankle. Retrieved from https://www.rnoh.nhs.uk/sites/default/files/downloads/physiotherapy_rehabilitation_guidelines_lateral_ligament_reconstruction_of_the_ankle.pdf

Seah, R., & Mani-Babu, S. (2011). Managing ankle sprains in primary care: What is best practice? A systematic review of the last 10 years of evidence. *British Medical Bulletin, 97*, 105-135.

Suchak, A. A., Spooner, C., Reid, D., & Jomha, N. (2006). Post-operative rehabilitation protocols for Achilles tendon ruptures: A meta-analysis. *Clinical Orthopedics and Related Research, 445*, 216-221.

University of Wisconsin Health Sports Medicine Center. (2015). Rehabilitation guidelines for Achilles tendon repair. Retrieved from http://www.uwhealth.org/files/uwhealth/docs/sportsmed/SM-41576_AchillesTendonProtocol.pdf

Chapter 7
SPECIALTY PROGRAMS

Section 7.01

VESTIBULAR EXERCISE

7.01.1 BENIGN PAROXYSMAL POSITIONAL VERTIGO DISCUSSION

BPPV is characterized by brief recurrent episodes of vertigo, triggered by changes in head position. Vertigo represents a subset of dizziness and is defined as an illusion of movement, usually rotational, of the patient or the patient's surroundings. The illusion of motion may be of oneself, subjective vertigo, or of external objects, objective vertigo (Koelliker, Summers, & Hawkins, 2001). BPPV is the most common etiology of recurrent vertigo and is caused by abnormal stimulation of the inner ear organs that sense gravity and linear acceleration. There are free-floating calcium debris and canaliths (also referred to as *otoliths*) in the inner ear that move when the head accelerates and stimulate tiny hairs, giving feedback to the brain about the head's spatial orientation and movement. BPPV is thought to be attributed to this debris collecting in one part of the inner ear (Hain, 2010). Typical symptoms and signs of BPPV are evoked when the head is positioned so that the plane of the affected semicircular canal is spatially vertical and thus aligned with gravity (Lee & Kim, 2010). Movements that may trigger episodes include turning over in bed, getting in and out of bed, bending over and then straightening up, extending the neck to look up (such as reaching for an item from a shelf, top-shelf vertigo), or hanging up washing (Fife et al., 2008).

Vertigo and nystagmus develop after performing the Dix-Hallpike maneuver in posterior-canal BPPV and during the supine roll test in horizontal-canal BPPV (Lee & Kim, 2010).

Positioning the head in the opposite direction usually reverses the direction of the nystagmus. Spontaneous recovery may be expected, even with conservative treatments. However, *canalith repositioning* maneuvers usually provide an immediate resolution of symptoms by clearing the canaliths from the semicircular canal into the bulbous center vestibule (Lee & Kim, 2010). Evidence has shown that canalith repositioning procedure remains the gold standard in the treatment of BPPV except for very occasional intractable cases that might require surgery (Ibekwe & Rogers, 2012).

Technique

Dix-Hallpike Maneuver begins in long-sitting. The patient is instructed to rotate his or her head 45 degrees toward the direction of the ear being tested. With the assistance of the clinician, the patient is then instructed to quickly lie back onto the table so that the neck is extended approximately 30 degrees. If the patient lacks cervical extension, the test position can be modified by positioning a pillow or wedge under the patient's shoulders. The clinician then observes the patient's eyes for approximately 60 seconds. BPPV of the posterior canal is diagnosed if an upward and ipsitorsional nystagmus is observed by the evaluator and the patient reports symptoms of vertigo (Rehabilitation Institute of Chicago, 2012a).

Supine Roll Test begins in supine with neck flexed 20 degrees. Head is quickly rolled to one side for 1 minute, observe presence and direction of nystagmus, and then return to midline, maintaining neck flexion. The procedure is repeated to the other side. Note patient report of vertigo (Rehabilitation Institute of Chicago, 2012b).

Where's the Evidence?

A single study comparing the Dix-Hallpike and side-lying tests. For the Dix-Hallpike test, the estimated sensitivity was 79%, specificity was 75%. For the side-lying test, the estimated sensitivity was 90%, specificity was 75% (Halker, Barrs, Wellik, Winger, & Demaerschalk, 2008).

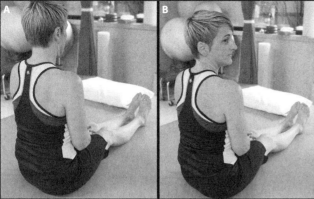

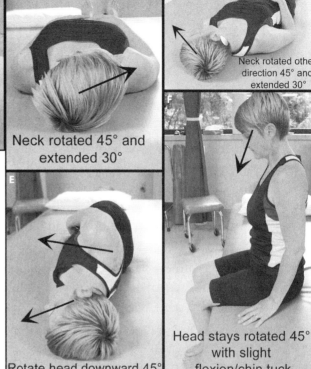

Neck rotated 45° and extended 30°

Neck rotated other direction 45° and extended 30°

Rotate head downward 45°

Head stays rotated 45° with slight flexion/chin tuck

7.01.2 MODIFIED EPLEY CANALITH REPOSTIONING MANEUVER

POSITION: Supine, seated

TARGETS: BPPV posterior and anterior canals; uses gravity to reposition free-floating particles from affected canal back into utricle.

INSTRUCTION: Listed step by step below; follow each step in order, *do not skip any steps*.

1. Patient begins in an upright long-sitting posture (A), and the head rotated 45 degrees toward the side in the same direction that gives a positive Dix–Hallpike test (B).

2. The patient is then quickly and passively forced down backward by the clinician performing the treatment into a supine position with the head held approximately in a 30-degree neck extension (Dix-Hallpike position), and still rotated to the same. The clinician observes the patient's eyes for primary stage nystagmus (C).

3. The patient remains in this position for approximately 1 to 2 minutes.

4. The patient's head is then rotated 90 degrees to the opposite direction so that the opposite ear faces the floor, while maintaining the 30-degree neck extension (D).

5. The patient remains in this position for approximately 1 to 2 minutes.

6. Keeping the head and neck in a fixed position relative to the body, the individual rolls onto the shoulder, rotating the head another 90 degrees in the direction in which facing. The patient is now looking downward at a 45-degree angle (E).

7. The eyes should be immediately observed by the clinician for secondary stage nystagmus, and this secondary stage nystagmus should be in the same direction as the primary stage nystagmus. The patient remains in this position for approximately 1 to 2 minutes.

8. Finally, the patient is slowly brought up to an upright sitting posture, while maintaining the 45 degrees rotation of the head and slight chin tuck. The patient holds sitting position for up to 30 seconds (F).

9. During every step of this procedure, the patient may experience some dizziness.

10. Patient should wait 10 minutes before going home or resuming any activities.

11. Patient should sleep recumbent (lying down no further than at a 45-degree angle) for the following 2 nights. Most patients will sleep in a recliner during this time.

12. During the day, patients should try to keep head vertical; no bending over, drying hair, dentist, shaving face, eye drops, picking things off a high shelf, or activities that would move head out of vertical position.

For 1 week, patient should avoid head positions that might bring BPPV on again. Use two pillows when sleeping and avoid sleeping on the "bad" side. Don't turn head far up or far down. Be careful to avoid head extended position, when lying on the back, especially with head turned toward the affected side.

SUBSTITUTIONS: The patient may be instructed to be cautious of bending over, lying backward, moving the head up and down, or tilting the head to either side.

PARAMETERS: The entire procedure is performed 3 times in 1 sitting.

Where's the Evidence?

Several studies have confirmed the efficacy of the Epley Maneuver. Ruckenstein (2001) studied 86 cases with patients diagnosed with BPPV and then treated with the Epley Maneuver. It was found that 84% of cases that were treated with one or two canalith repositioning maneuvers had a resolution of vertigo as a direct result of the maneuver. Waleem, Malik, Ullah, and ul Hassan (2008) studied 44 patients with positive Dix-Hallpike divided into 2 groups. Fourteen patients of the 22 in the treated group reported to be symptom-free after the maneuver compared to 1 out of 22 for the control group, concluding that Epley Maneuver is a much better form of management for BPPV. A more recent study by Gaur et al. (2015) analyzing the response to the Epley Maneuver in a series of patients with posterior canal BPPV, and comparing the results with those treated exclusively by medical management alone, reinforces the validity of the Epley Maneuver in comparison with the medical management.

7.01.3 MODIFIED EPLEY CANALITH REPOSITIONING MANEUVER, FOR HOME

POSITION: Supine, seated

TARGETS: BPPV posterior and anterior canals; uses gravity to reposition free-floating particles from affected canal back into utricle.

INSTRUCTION: Listed step by step below; follow each step in order, *do not skip any steps.*

If vertigo comes from *right ear* and side, instruct patient:

1. Sit on the edge of the bed.
2. Turn the head 45 degrees to the left.
3. Place a pillow under patient so when lying down, pillow rests between the shoulders rather than under the head.
4. Quickly lie down to the left side, face up, with the head on the bed (still at the 45-degree angle). The pillow should be under the shoulders. Wait 30 seconds for any vertigo to stop.
5. Turn the head half-way (90 degrees) to the right without raising it. Wait 30 seconds.
6. Turn the head and body on its side to the right, looking at the floor. Wait 30 seconds.
7. Slowly sit up to the right side but remain on the bed a few minutes.

If vertigo comes from *left ear*, reverse these instructions.

SUBSTITUTIONS: The patient may be instructed to be cautious of bending over, lying backward, moving the head up and down, or tilting the head to either side.

PARAMETERS: The entire procedure is performed 3 times in one sitting and repeated 1 time per day until free from vertigo for more than 24 hours

---

Where's the Evidence?

Radtke et al. (2004) compared the efficacy of a self-applied modified Semont Maneuver with self-treatment with a modified Epley procedure in 70 patients with posterior canal BPPV. The response rate after 1 week, defined as absence of positional vertigo and nystagmus on positional testing, was 95% in the modified Epley procedure group vs 58% in the modified Semont Maneuver group.

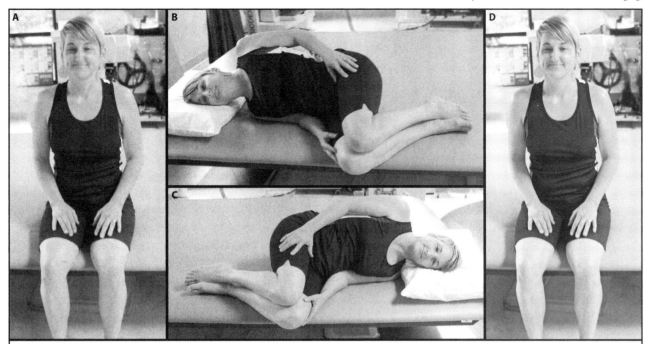

7.01.4 MODIFIED SEMONT MANEUVER, FOR HOME

POSITION: Supine, seated

TARGETS: BPPV posterior and anterior canals; uses gravity to reposition free-floating particles from affected canal back into utricle.

INSTRUCTION: Listed step by step below; follow each step in order, *do not skip any steps.*

If vertigo comes from *right ear* and side, instruct patient:

1. Patient sits upright, turns head to right 45 degrees.
2. Drops quickly to right side, so that head touches the bed behind the right ear. Wait 30 seconds.
3. Move head and trunk in a swift movement toward the other side without stopping, so that head comes to rest on the left side of the forehead. Wait 30 seconds. Sit back to upright position (A through D).

If vertigo comes from *left ear* and side, reverse these instructions.

SUBSTITUTIONS: The patient may be instructed to be cautious of bending over, lying backward, moving the head up and down, or tilting the head to either side. Since this maneuver requires speed, it can be difficult for the elderly.

PARAMETERS: The entire procedure is performed 3 times in one sitting and repeated 1 time per day until free from vertigo for more than 24 hours

Where's the Evidence?

Liu, Wang, Zhang, Bai, and Zhang (2015), using network meta-analysis, aimed to compare the efficacy and safety of the Epley and Semont Maneuvers as treatment options for posterior canal BPPV. Randomized controlled studies that used an Epley or Semont Maneuver in posterior canal BPPV patients were analyzed. Of 589 articles, 12 studies that enrolled 999 posterior canal BPPV patients were selected. The pooled analysis revealed that the Epley Maneuver was as efficacious as the Semont Maneuver, in both the 1-week recovery rate and end of study recovery rate and had a similar recurrence rate. These two techniques were both better than sham-controlled treatment. They concluded the Epley Maneuver was similar to the Semont Maneuver in both efficacy and safety for posterior canal BPPV in short-term effects, and both were superior to the sham-controlled treatment.

Wang et al. (2014) investigated the treatment of BPPV of posterior semicircular canal by Epley Maneuver combined with the Semont Maneuver. One hundred fifty patients with BPPV of posterior semicircular canal were randomly divided into three groups: one group treated with the Epley Maneuver, one group with the Semont Maneuver, and one group treated with the Epley Maneuver combined with the Semont Maneuver. Statistics of treatment effects and follow-up studies with 3 months after the recovery were assessed. They found that the primary cure rate was increased, the numbers of treatments were reduced, and the relapse was decreased by the use of the Epley Maneuver combined with the Semont Maneuver in the treatment of BPPV of posterior semicircular canal and suggested the Epley Maneuver combined with the Semont Maneuver in the clinic.

7.01.5 BRANDT-DAROFF (HABITUATION)

POSITION: Supine, seated

TARGETS: BPPV posterior and anterior canals; uses gravity to reposition free-floating particles from affected canal back into utricle.

INSTRUCTION: Brandt-Daroff is different than Semont in that patient does not stay in positions for more than 1 to 2 seconds, thus speed is increased. Also, number of repetitions and frequency is greater. Listed step by step below; follow each step in order, *do not skip any steps.*

If vertigo comes from *right ear* and side, instruct patient:

1. Patient sits upright, turns head to right 45 degrees.
2. Drops quickly to right side, so that head touches the bed behind the right ear. Wait 1 to 2 seconds.
3. Move head and trunk in a swift movement toward the other side without stopping, so that head comes to rest on the left side of the forehead. Wait 1 to 2 seconds. Sit back to upright position (**7.01.4 A through D**).

If vertigo comes from *left ear* and side, reverse these instructions.

SUBSTITUTIONS: The patient may be instructed to be cautious of bending over, lying backward, moving the head up and down, or tilting the head to either side. Since this maneuver requires speed, it can be difficult for the elderly.

PARAMETERS: Perform entire maneuver 5 times, repeat 3 times per day for up to 2 weeks; stop once symptoms absent more than 24 hours.

Where's the Evidence?

A 2011 study evaluated the efficacy of three physical treatments for BPPV: Brandt-Daroff habituation exercises, the Semont Maneuver, and the Epley Maneuver. A total of 106 BPPV patients were randomly assigned to one of the three treatment groups, and responses were evaluated 1 week, 1 month, and 3 months after the initial treatment. At the 1-week follow-up, similar cure rates were obtained with the Semont and Epley Maneuvers (74% and 71%, respectively), both cure rates being significantly higher than that obtained with Brandt-Daroff exercises (24%). By the 3-month follow-up, the cure rate obtained with the Epley Maneuver was higher (93%) than that obtained with the Semont Maneuver (77%), though both remained higher than that obtained with the Brandt-Daroff Maneuver (62%) (Soto Varela et al., 2001).

7.01.6 OCULOMOTOR: SACCADES

POSITION: Standing, seated

TARGETS: Improved control of eye movements with stationary head

INSTRUCTION: *Horizontal*: Place 2 targets side by side on the wall at the same vertical height, distance variable, larger distance between objects adds difficulty. Patient stands 1 foot away from the wall and looks right and left toward each target without moving the head. Start slowly and progress speed. For additional progression, move patient further from wall to 3 feet.

Vertical: Place two targets above and below on the wall on the same vertical plane, distance variable, larger distance between objects adds difficulty. Patient stands 1 foot away from the wall and looks up and down toward each target without moving the head. Start slowly and progress speed. For additional progression, move patient further from wall to 3 feet.

Diagonal: Place two targets diagonal to each other on the wall, distance variable, larger distance between objects add difficulty. Patient stands 1 foot away from the wall and looks up and down toward each target without moving the head. Start slowly and progress speed. For additional progression, move patient further from wall to 3 feet.

Dice on tongue depressor: A fun way to work on eye movements with head still is to place a tongue depressor between the front teeth; as patient closes teeth, so does tongue depressor in parallel to floor. Patient then attempts to stack dice on the end of the tongue depressor. This is also good for hand-eye coordination.

SUBSTITUTIONS: Do not allow head movements with these exercises, allow patient to sit at first and progress to standing, proper posture/alignment of the spine is encouraged; target to remain in focus; limit distractions to allow patient to concentrate.

PARAMETERS: Each set is done 20 repetitions, perform sequence 1 to 3 times, repeat 1 to 3 times per day as needed

7.01.7 OCULOMOTOR: SMOOTH PURSUITS

POSITION: Standing, seated

TARGETS: Improved control of eye movements with stationary head

INSTRUCTION: Keeping eyes fixed on a target and head still. Patient or therapist moves target slowly up and down, side to side, and diagonally as patient follows with the eyes but not the head.

SUBSTITUTIONS: Do not allow head movements with these exercises, allow patient to sit at first and progress to standing, proper posture/alignment of the spine is encouraged; target to remain in focus; limit distractions to allow patient to concentrate.

PARAMETERS: Each set is done 20 repetitions, perform sequence 3 times, repeat 1 to 3 times per day as needed

7.01.8 GAZE STABILIZATION

POSITION: Standing, seated

TARGETS: Improved gaze stabilization, the ability to focus on an object when movements of the head are occurring

INSTRUCTION: Target is held by patient or therapist. Patient focuses on target while moving the head right to left. Repeat for bringing head up and down and diagonal. Target stays fixed and eyes focused on target entire sequence.

SUBSTITUTIONS: Allow patient to sit at first and progress to standing, proper posture/alignment of the spine is encouraged; target to remain in focus; limit distractions to allow patient to concentrate.

PARAMETERS: Each set is done 20 repetitions, perform sequence 1 to 3 times, repeat 1 to 3 times per day as needed

Where's the Evidence?

Hall, Heusel-Gillig, Tusa, and Herdman (2010) performed a study to determine whether the addition of gaze stability exercises to balance rehabilitation would lead to greater improvements of symptoms and postural stability in older adults with normal vestibular function who reported dizziness. Participants who were referred to outpatient physical therapy for dizziness were randomly assigned to the gaze stabilization group or control group. Dizziness was defined as symptoms of unsteadiness, spinning, a sense of movement, or lightheadedness. Participants were evaluated at baseline and discharged on symptoms, balance confidence, visual acuity during head movement, balance, and gait measures. The gaze stabilization group performed vestibular adaptation and substitution exercises designed to improve gaze stability, and the control group performed placebo eye exercises designed to be vestibular neutral. In addition, both groups performed balance and gait exercises. The gaze stabilization group demonstrated a significantly greater reduction in fall risk compared with the control group, providing evidence that in older adults with symptoms of dizziness and no documented vestibular deficits, the addition of vestibular-specific gaze stability exercises to standard balance rehabilitation results in greater reduction in fall risk. Diehl and Pidcoe (2010) compared gaze stability and stepping responses between young and aging adults. They found young adults were better at maintaining gaze fixation than older adults and made linear correlations demonstrating significant negative relationships between gaze fixation and step latencies. They concluded the ability to maintain gaze fixation of a target may be important in reducing step latency following a perturbation. Whitney, Marchetti, Pritcher, and Furman (2009) attempted to determine if there was a relationship between clinical measures of walking performance and the gaze stability test in patients with vestibular disorders and in healthy subjects. They hypothesized that impairment of the ability to keep objects in focus during active head movement would be correlated with walking performance. They found in older subjects with vestibular disorders gaze stability is associated with reduced test scores on measures of gait performance such as the Timed Get Up and Go test and the Dynamic Gait Index.

7.01.9 VISIO-VESTIBULAR

POSITION: Standing, seated

TARGETS: Improved oculomotor and vestibular functioning

INSTRUCTION:

Same Direction: Target is held by patient or therapist. Patient focuses on target. Target is moved by the patient or therapist, and the patient follows with the eyes *and* head right to left. Repeat for bringing head up and down and diagonally. Target stays fixed and eyes focused on target entire sequence.

Opposite Direction: Target is held by patient or therapist. Patient focuses on target. Target is moved by the patient or therapist and the patient follows with the eyes, but moves the head in the *opposite* direction. For example, the target goes to the right as the eyes follow to the right, but the patient rotates head to left. Repeat for bringing head up and down and diagonally. Target stays fixed and eyes focused on target entire sequence.

SUBSTITUTIONS: Allow patient to sit at first and progress to standing, proper posture/alignment of the spine is encouraged; target to remain in focus; limit distractions to allow patient to concentrate.

PARAMETERS: Each set is done 20 repetitions, perform sequence 1 to 3 times, repeat 1 to 3 times per day as needed

7.01.10 CAWTHORNE COOKSEY

POSITION: Standing, seated

TARGETS: Improved oculomotor and vestibular functioning

INSTRUCTION: (Zanardini, Zeigelboim, Jurkiewicz, Marques, & Martins-Bassetto, 2007)

1. Head and eye movements seated:
    a. Sitting, start with having the patient perform eye movements, at first slow, then quick looking up and down, side to side allowing head to move as well.
    b. Sitting, focusing on finger moving from 3 feet to 1 foot away from face.
    c. Sitting, start head movements at first slow, then quick, eventually progressing to eyes closed. Patient extends and flexes the neck and rotates from right to left. Repeat with eyes closed.
2. Head and body movements seated:
    a. Bending forward and picking up objects from the ground; look at object entire sequence.
    b. Bending forward and move objects from in front of toes to behind heel and repeat; look at object entire sequence.
3. Changing from sitting to standing position with eyes open and shut:
    a. Standing perform 1a and 1c above
4. Dynamic activities:
    a. Patient walks while looking right and left
    b. Patient makes brisk 90-degree turns when walking, progress to eyes closed.
    c. Ascend and descend stairs, eyes open and then closed; walk up and down slope with eyes open and then closed before attempting stairs.
    d. Stand on one foot, eyes open and then closed
    e. Stand on soft surface
    f. Walk on soft surfaces
    g. Baby steps with eyes open and closed
    h. Walk across room with eyes open and then closed
    i. Any game involving stooping and stretching and aiming, such as bowling and basketball throwing a small ball from hand to hand above eye level; try having patient throw a ball from hand to hand and under the knee, and patient circle around therapist as therapist throws patient a ball and patient return throws it.

SUBSTITUTIONS: Allow patient to sit at first and progress to standing; proper posture and alignment of the spine is encouraged.

PARAMETERS: Each set is done 10 to 20 repetitions, perform each activity 1 to 3 sets, repeat 1 to 3 times per day as needed

Where's the Evidence?

Ribeiro and Pereira (2005) attempted to verify whether specific therapeutic approach of the Cawthorne Cooksey exercises can promote motor learning and can contribute to the improvement of balance and to decrease the likelihood of falls. They studied 15 women, aged 60 to 69, 3 times a week for 1 hour for 3 months. They were evaluated with the Berg Balance Scale, whose scores determine the possibility of fall. Significant improvement in Berg scores were noted and they concluded Cawthorne Cooksey exercises were able to promote significant improvement in the balance of this sample, and the exercises can be applied as prevention and treatment in balance disturbances in elderly people. Corna et al. (2003) performed a study to compare Cawthorne Cooksey exercises with instrumented balance training on a moving platform for patients with unilateral vestibular deficits. The authors found that both Cawthorne Cooksey exercises and instrumental rehabilitation are effective for treating balance disorders of vestibular origin, and that improvement affected both control of body balance and performance of ADLs. The larger decrease in body sway and greater improvement of dizziness after instrumental rehabilitation suggested that it is more effective than Cawthorne Cooksey exercises in improving balance control; however, both are effective.

References

Corna, S., Nardone, A., Prestinari, A., Galante, M., Grasso, M., & Schieppati, M. (2003). Comparison of Cawthorne-Cooksey exercises and sinusoidal support surface translations to improve balance in patients with unilateral vestibular deficit. *Archives of Physical Medicine and Rehabilitation, 84*(8), 1173-1184.

Diehl, M. D., & Pidcoe, P. E. (2010). The influence of gaze stabilization and fixation on stepping reactions in younger and older adults. *Journal of Geriatric Physical Therapy, 33*(1), 19-25.

Fife, T. D., Iverson, D. J., Lempert, T., Furman, J. M., Baloh, R. W., Tusa, R. J., . . . Quality Standards Subcommittee, American Academy of Neurology. (2008). Practice parameter: Therapies for benign paroxysmal positional vertigo (an evidence-based review): Report of the Quality Standards Subcommittee of the American Academy of Neurology. *Neurology, 70*(22), 2067-2074.

Gaur, S., Awasthi, S. K., Bhadouriya, S. K., Saxena, R., Pathak, V. K., & Bisht, M. (2015). Efficacy of Epley's maneuver in treating BPPV patients: A prospective observational study. *International Journal of Otolarygology, 2015,* 1-5.

Hain, T. C. (2010). Otoliths. *Dizziness-and-balance.com.* Retrieved from http://www.dizziness-and-balance.com/disorders/bppv/otoliths.html

Halker, R. B., Barrs, D. M., Wellik, K. E., Wingerchuk, D. M., & Demaerschalk, B. M. (2008). Establishing a diagnosis of benign paroxysmal positional vertigo through the Dix-Hallpike and side-lying maneuvers: A critically appraised topic. *Neurologist, 14*(3), 201-204.

Hall, C. D., Heusel-Gillig, L., Tusa, R. J., & Herdman, S. J. (2010). Efficacy of gaze stability exercises in older adults with dizziness. *Journal of Neurologic Physical Therapy, 34*(2), 64-69.

Ibekwe, T. S., & Rogers, C. (2012). Clinical evaluation of posterior canal benign paroxysmal positional vertigo. *Nigerian Medical Journal, 53*(2), 94-101.

Koelliker, P., Summers, R. L., & Hawkins, B. (2001). Benign paroxysmal positional vertigo: Diagnosis and treatment in the emergency department—A review of the literature and discussion of canalith-repositioning maneuvers. *Annals of Emergency Medicine, 37*(4), 392-398.

Lee, S.H. & Kim, J.S. (2010). Benign paroxysmal positional vertigo. *Journal of Clinical Neurology, 6*(2), 51-63.

Liu, Y., Wang, W., Zhang, A. B., Bai, X., & Zhang, S. (2015). Epley and Semont maneuvers for posterior canal benign paroxysmal positional vertigo: A network meta-analysis. *Laryngoscope, 126*(4), 951-955.

Radtke, A., von Brevern, M., Tiel-Wilck, K., Mainz-Perchalla, A., Neuhauser, H., & Lempert, T. (2004). Self-treatment of benign paroxysmal positional vertigo: Semont maneuver vs Epley procedure. *Neurology, 63*(1), 150-152.

Rehabilitation Institute of Chicago, Center for Rehabilitation Outcomes Research, Northwestern University Feinberg School of Medicine Department of Medical Social Sciences Informatics Group. (2012a). Rehab measures: Dix–Hallpike maneuver. *Rehabilitation Measures Database.* Retrieved from http://www.rehabmeasures.org/Lists/RehabMeasures/PrintView.aspx?ID=1010

Rehabilitation Institute of Chicago, Center for Rehabilitation Outcomes Research, Northwestern University Feinberg School of Medicine Department of Medical Social Sciences Informatics Group. (2012b). Rehab measures: Roll test. *Rehabilitation Measures Database.* Retrieved from http://www.rehabmeasures.org/Lists/RehabMeasures/DispForm.aspx?ID=1158

Ribeiro, A. S., & Pereira, J. S. (2005). Balance improvement and reduction of likelihood of falls in older women after Cawthorne and Cooksey exercises. *Brazilian Journal of Otorhinolaryngology, 71*(1), 38-46.

Ruckenstein, M. J. (2001). Therapeutic efficacy of the Epley canalith repositioning maneuver. *Laryngoscope, 111*(6), 940-945.

Soto Varela, A., Bartual Magro, J., Santos Pérez, S., Vélez Regueiro, M., Lechuga García, R., Pérez-Carro Ríos, A., & Caballero, L. (2001). Benign paroxysmal vertigo: A comparative prospective study of the efficacy of Brandt and Daroff exercises, Semont and Epley maneuver. *Revue de Laryngologie, 122*(3), 179-183.

Waleem, S. S., Malik, S. M., Ullah, S., & ul Hassan, Z. (2008). Office management of benign paroxysmal positional vertigo with Epley's maneuver. *Journal of Ayub Medical College, 20*(1), 77-79.

Wang, T., An, F., Xie, C., Chen, J., Zhu, C., & Wang, Y. (2014). [The treatment of benign positional paroxysmal vertigo of posterior semicircular canal by Epley maneuver combined with Semont maneuver] [Article in Chinese]. *Journal of Otorhinolaryngology, Head & Neck Surgery, 28*(19), 1469-1471.

Whitney, S. L., Marchetti, G. F., Pritcher, M., & Furman, J. M. (2009). Gaze stabilization and gait performance in vestibular dysfunction. *Gait & Posture, 29*(2), 194-198.

Zanardini, F. H., Zeigelboim, B. S., Jurkiewicz, A. L., Marques, J. M., & Martins-Bassetto, J. (2007). [Vestibular rehabilitation in elderly patients with dizziness] [Article in Portuguese]. *Jornal da Sociedade Brasileira de Fonoaudiologia, 19*(2), 177-184.

Section 7.02

PELVIC FLOOR

7.02.1 KEGEL

POSITION: Hook-lying

TARGETS: Strengthen pelvic floor muscles: superficial perineal layer (bulbocavernosus, ischiocavernosus, superficial transverse perineal, external anal sphincter), deep urogenital diaphragm layer (compressor urethera, retrovaginal sphincter, deep transverse perineal), and pelvic diaphragm (levator ani: pubococcygeus, iliococcygeus, coccygeus/ischiococcygeus, piriformis, obturator internus); use of electrical stimulation and biofeedback devices is helpful if patient is unable to

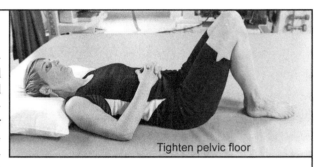

Tighten pelvic floor

understand how to perform the Kegel or has difficulty with contracting the pelvic floor muscles.

INSTRUCTION: Patient tightens the pelvic floor muscles *without* tightening the muscles in the abdomen, thigh, or buttocks.

SUBSTITUTIONS: Do not do Kegel exercises to start and stop urine stream. Doing Kegel exercises while emptying bladder can actually lead to incomplete emptying of the bladder, which can increase the risk of a urinary tract infection.

PARAMETERS: Hold 5 to 10 seconds, relax for 10 seconds between repetitions, 1 to 3 sets of 6 to 10, 2 to 3 times per day

---

Where's the Evidence?

García-Sánchez, Rubio-Arias, Ávila-Gandía, Ramos-Campo, and López-Román (2015) analyzed the content of various published studies related to physical exercise and its effects on urinary incontinence to determine the effectiveness of pelvic floor muscle exercise (pelvic floor muscles) programs. They conducted a thorough search of multiple databases and selected three full-text articles on treating urinary incontinence in female athletes and six full-text articles and one abstract on treating urinary incontinence in women in general. The nine studies included in the review achieved positive results and therefore concluded physical exercise, specifically pelvic floor muscles programs, has positive effects on urinary incontinence, especially urinary incontinence. Chang, Lam, and Patel (2015) studied men post-prostatectomy to determine the effects of pelvic floor muscles on incontinence following the surgery. This systematic review of the literature using 11 studies based on selection criteria found evidence to suggest that preoperative pelvic floor muscles improves early continence rates but not long-term continence rates. *(continued)*

Where's the Evidence? *(continued)*

Lee and Choi (2015) compared pelvic floor muscles with pelvic floor muscles using electrical stimulation and biofeedback, and found that maximum pressure of vaginal contraction in the experimental group showed a statistically significant increase compared to the control group, indicating increased recruitment of pelvic floor muscles using such devices. Another study performed by Ong et al. (2015) compared pelvic floor muscles to pelvic floor muscles training with the Vibrance kegel device, a biofeedback device that creates a vibration when the proper muscles are contracting. Forty patients were recruited and divided into control group and device group and underwent 16 weeks of training. The Vibrance kegel device group reported significantly earlier improvement in urinary incontinence scores. However, there was no significant difference between the groups' urinary incontinence scores at week 16. The subjective cure rate was similar in both groups at week 16. Furthermore, Harvey (2003) studied the evidence-based effectiveness of peripartum pelvic floor exercises in the prevention of pelvic floor problems including urinary and anal incontinence and prolapse. Antepartum pelvic floor exercises, when used with biofeedback and taught by trained health care personnel using a conservative model, did not result in significant short-term (3 months) decrease in postpartum urinary incontinence or pelvic floor strength. However, postpartum pelvic floor exercises, when performed with a vaginal device providing resistance or feedback, appear to decrease postpartum urinary incontinence and to increase strength. Reminder and motivational systems to perform Kegel exercises were not found to be effective in preventing postpartum urinary incontinence. Postpartum pelvic floor exercises did not consistently reduce the incidence of anal incontinence. Overall, Harvey (2003) concluded postpartum pelvic floor exercises appear to be effective in decreasing postpartum urinary incontinence.

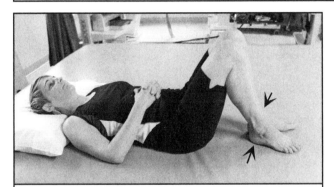

7.02.2 KEGEL, "QUICK FLICKS"

POSITION: Hook-lying

TARGETS: Strengthen pelvic floor muscles: superficial perineal layer (bulbocavernosus, ischiocavernosus, superficial transverse perineal, external anal sphincter), deep urogenital diaphragm layer (compressor urethera, retrovaginal sphincter, deep transverse perineal), and pelvic diaphragm (levator ani: pubococcygeus, iliococcygeus, coccygeus/ischiococcygeus, piriformis, obturator internus)

INSTRUCTION: Patient squeezes heels together with toes out as patient tightens the pelvic floor.

SUBSTITUTIONS: Focus on Kegel and *not* tightening the muscles in the abdomen, thighs, or buttocks.

PARAMETERS: Hold 5 to 10 seconds, relax for 10 seconds between repetitions, 1 to 3 sets of 6 to 10, 2 to 3 times per day; inhale on tightening phase and exhale on relaxation phase.

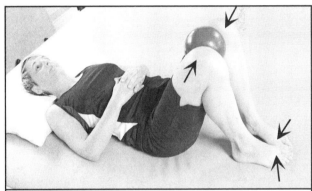

7.02.3 KEGEL, ROLL-IN

POSITION: Hook-lying

TARGETS: Strengthen pelvic floor muscles: superficial perineal layer (bulbocavernosus, ischiocavernosus), superficial transverse perineal, external anal sphincter), deep urogenital diaphragm layer (compressor urethera, retrovaginal sphincter, deep transverse perineal), and pelvic diaphragm (levator ani: pubococcygeus, iliococcygeus, coccygeus/ischiococcygeus, piriformis, obturator internus)

INSTRUCTION: Place a small ball between the knees. Patient squeezes toes and knees together as patient tightens the pelvic floor.

SUBSTITUTIONS: Focus on Kegel and *not* tightening the muscles in the abdomen, thighs, or buttocks.

PARAMETERS: Hold 5 to 10 seconds, relax for 10 seconds between repetitions, 1 to 3 sets of 6 to 10, 2 to 3 times per day; inhale on tightening phase and exhale on relaxation phase.

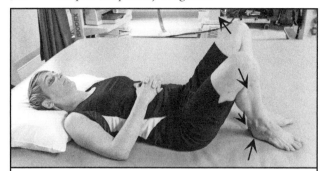

7.02.4 KEGEL, ROLL-OUT

POSITION: Hook-lying

TARGETS: Strengthen pelvic floor muscles: superficial perineal layer (bulbocavernosus, ischiocavernosus, superficial transverse perineal, external anal sphincter), deep urogenital diaphragm layer (compressor urethera, retrovaginal sphincter, deep transverse perineal), and pelvic diaphragm (levator ani: pubococcygeus, iliococcygeus, coccygeus/ischiococcygeus, piriformis, obturator internus)

INSTRUCTION: Patient lets hips roll out to shoulder-width apart, squeezes heels together with toes out as patient tightens the pelvic floor. Add resistance band looped around just above the knees as a modification.

SUBSTITUTIONS: Focus on Kegel and *not* tightening the muscles in the abdomen, thighs, or buttocks.

PARAMETERS: Hold 5 to 10 seconds, relax for 10 seconds between repetitions, 1 to 3 sets of 10, 2 to 3 times per day; inhale on tightening phase and exhale on relaxation phase.

7.02.7 KEGEL, "THE ELEVATOR"

POSITION: Seated

TARGETS: Strengthen pelvic floor muscles: superficial perineal layer (bulbocavernosus, ischiocavernosus, superficial transverse perineal, external anal sphincter), deep urogenital diaphragm layer (compressor urethera, retrovaginal sphincter, deep transverse perineal), and pelvic diaphragm (levator ani: pubococcygeus, iliococcygeus, coccygeus/ischiococcygeus, piriformis, obturator internus)

INSTRUCTION: Patient imagines the pelvic floor region is an elevator going from the first to the fourth floor of a building. The patient contracts the pelvic muscles a little at a time, tightening at each floor, taking the pelvic floor right up to the fourth floor, where muscles are as tight as possible, and holds followed by a gradual release back to the ground floor.

SUBSTITUTIONS: Focus on Kegel and *not* tightening the muscles in the abdomen, thighs, or buttocks.

PARAMETERS: Hold 5 to 10 seconds, relax for 10 seconds between repetitions, 1 to 3 sets of 10, 2 to 3 times per day; inhale on tightening phase and exhale on relaxation phase.

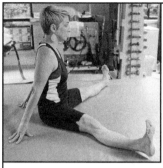

7.02.5 KEGEL, WIDE LEG

POSITION: Supine

TARGETS: Strengthen pelvic floor muscles: superficial perineal layer (bulbocavernosus, ischiocavernosus, superficial transverse perineal, external anal sphincter), deep urogenital diaphragm layer (compressor urethera, retrovaginal sphincter, deep transverse perineal), and pelvic diaphragm (levator ani: pubococcygeus, iliococcygeus, coccygeus/ischiococcygeus, piriformis, obturator internus)

INSTRUCTION: Patient lies with hips abducted and knees extended. Patient tightens pelvic floor and holds. This can be done in long-sitting or cross-legged.

SUBSTITUTIONS: Focus on Kegel and *not* tightening the muscles in the abdomen, thighs, or buttocks.

PARAMETERS: Hold 5 to 10 seconds, relax for 10 seconds between repetitions, 1 to 3 sets of 10, 2 to 3 times per day; inhale on tightening phase and exhale on relaxation phase.

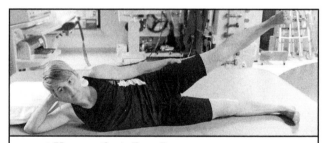

7.02.6 KEGEL, SIDE LEG LIFT

POSITION: Side-lying

TARGETS: Strengthen pelvic floor muscles: superficial perineal layer (bulbocavernosus, ischiocavernosus, superficial transverse perineal, external anal sphincter), deep urogenital diaphragm layer (compressor urethera, retrovaginal sphincter, deep transverse perineal), and pelvic diaphragm (levator ani: pubococcygeus, iliococcygeus, coccygeus/ischiococcygeus, piriformis, obturator internus)

INSTRUCTION: Patient lies on one side and tightens the pelvic floor, tightens quadriceps, and lifts leg into straight plane hip abduction. After completing a set, place the top leg behind the bottom leg and, tightening pelvic floor, lift bottom leg into straight plane hip adduction (not shown).

SUBSTITUTIONS: Focus on Kegel primarily, although other muscles are working to lift the leg. Hips are stacked.

PARAMETERS: Hold 5 to 10 seconds, relax for 10 seconds between repetitions, 1 to 3 sets of 10, 2 to 3 times per day; inhale on tightening phase and exhale on relaxation phase.

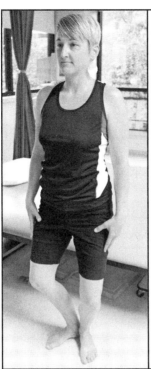

7.02.8 KEGEL, SMALL KNEE BENDS/PLIÉS

<u>POSITION</u>: Standing

<u>TARGETS</u>: Strengthen pelvic floor muscles: superficial perineal layer (bulbocavernosus, ischiocavernosus, superficial transverse perineal, external anal sphincter), deep urogenital diaphragm layer (compressor urethera, retrovaginal sphincter, deep transverse perineal), and pelvic diaphragm (levator ani: pubococcygeus, iliococcygeus, coccygeus/ischiococcygeus, piriformis, obturator internus)

<u>INSTRUCTION</u>: Patient squeezes heels together with toes out as patient tightens the pelvic floor. Patient bends knees, rolling hips outward on the way down, and then rises back as patient rolls hips in.

<u>SUBSTITUTIONS</u>: Focus on Kegel and *not* tightening the muscles in the abdomen, thighs, or buttocks.

<u>PARAMETERS</u>: Hold 5 to 10 seconds, relax for 10 seconds between repetitions, 1 to 3 sets of 10, 2 to 3 times per day; inhale on tightening phase and exhale on relaxation phase.

REFERENCES

Chang, J. I., Lam, V., & Patel, M. I. (2015). Preoperative pelvic floor muscle exercise and postprostatectomy incontinence: A systematic review and meta-analysis. *European Urology, 69*(3), 460-467.

García-Sánchez, E., Rubio-Arias, J. A., Ávila-Gandía, V., Ramos-Campo, D. J., & López-Román, J. (2015). Effectiveness of pelvic floor muscle training in treating urinary incontinence in women: A current review. *Actas Urologicas Espanolas, 40*(5);271-278.

Harvey, M. A. (2003). Pelvic floor exercises during and after pregnancy: A systematic review of their role in preventing pelvic floor dysfunction. *Journal of Obstetrics and Gynaecology Canada, 25*(6), 487-498.

Lee, J. B., & Choi, S. Y. (2015). [Effects of electric stimulation and biofeedback for pelvic floor muscle exercise in women with vaginal rejuvenation women] [Article in Korean]. *Journal of Korean Academic of Nursing, 45*(5), 713-722.

Ong, T. A., Khong, S. Y., Ng, K. L., Ting, J. R., Kamal, N., Yeoh, W. S., . . . Razack, A. H. (2015). Using the Vibrance Kegel device with pelvic floor muscle exercise for stress urinary incontinence: A randomized controlled pilot study. *Urology, 86*(3), 487-491.

Section 7.03

GLOBAL FUNCTIONAL ACTIVITIES FOR ELDERLY

BALANCE AND FALL PREVENTION

7.03.1 FALL RISK IN THE ELDERLY: TREATMENT DISCUSSION

Fall risk in the elderly is a big concern, as elderly patients are more prone to serious injury when falling and commonly incur shoulder and/or hip fractures among other injuries due to fragile bones. Patients can end up moving from independent living to skilled nursing and long-term care facilities.

Where's the Evidence?

Falls can lead to morbidity, immobility. and even death (Jeon, Jeong, Petrofsky, Lee, & Yim, 2014). This can be costly for the families and health care system, and all measures should be utilized to prevent such falls at home or in health care facilities. Furthermore, due to falls in health care settings, nurses' fears about patient falls may lead to unjustified restraint use. Restraint use has been linked to even lower independence scores as the restraints interfere with the patient's abilities to perform ADLs (Dever Fitzgerald et al., 2015). Landers, Oscar, Sasaoka, and Vaughn (2015) found balance confidence was the best predictor of falling, followed by fear of falling avoidance behavior and the Timed Up and Go Test. Fall history, presence of pathology, and physical tests did not predict falling. These findings suggest patients have had a better sense of their fall risk than with a test that provides a snapshot of their balance. Jeon et al. (2014) found subjects enrolled in a 12-week recurrent fall prevention program, comprised of strength training, balance training, and patient education, showed improvement in muscle strength and endurance of the ankles and the LEs, dynamic balance, depression, and compliance with preventive behavior related to falls, fear of falling, and fall self-efficacy, demonstrating a fall prevention program effectively improves muscle strength and endurance, balance, and psychological aspects in elderly women with a fall history. A large systematic of randomized trials by Gillespie et al. (2012) found group and home-based exercise programs and home safety interventions reduce rate of falls and risk of falling. In the elderly population, the requirements to produce rapid movements often occurs when performing other attention-demanding tasks, such as walking while talking or carrying an object. Furthermore, Muir-Hunter and Wittwer (2015) found that fall risk was associated with changes in gait under dual-task testing. Adding dual- and multi-tasks to the 12-week program also has been shown to reduce concerns about falling and improved gait in older adults with osteoporosis and increased fall risk (Halvarsson, Oddsson, Franzén, & Ståhle, 2015). Six weeks of dual-task training on a treadmill demonstrated improved scores on tests of mobility, functional performance tasks, and cognition in elderly fallers. Dual-task training can be readily implemented by therapists as a component of a fall risk reduction training program (Dorfman, Herman, Brozgol, Shema, & Weiss, 2014).

7.03.2 GLOBAL FUNCTIONING: TREATMENT IDEAS

Vibratory training: Patient can perform a multitude of tasks on a vibratory training machine. Basic stance, marching in place, mini squats, heel raises, toe raises, sharpened Rhomberg, and unilateral stance are a few examples.

Where's the Evidence?

A randomized controlled trial of 56 participants with a mean age of near 82 years compared a control group receiving usual care physiotherapy to intervention group receiving vibratory training at a frequency 30 to 50 Hz which occurred 3 times per week until discharge. Amplitude of the Vibratory training progressively increased from 2 to 5 mm to allow the program to be individually tailored to the participant. The study used the following outcome measures: physiological profile assessment and Functional Independence Measure and Modified Falls Efficacy Scale. The study found a statistically significant difference between the two groups in terms of Functional Independence Measure score and Modified Falls Efficacy Scale after treatment, concluding that for older people admitted to an inpatient rehabilitation facility there may be some beneficial effect to the use of vibratory training in conjunction with usual care physiotherapy in terms of improved functional ability. Implications for rehabilitation vibratory training may assist in reducing the risk of falling among at-risk older people (Parsons, Mathieson, Jull, & Parsons, 2015).

Sit-to-stand: Patient performs sit-to-stand from various surfaces: desk chair, recliner, rocking chair, bench, etc., at differing heights and both hands use, one hand use, and no hand use.

Where's the Evidence?

Adding variable standing surfaces may also challenge the patient. For patients with hemiparesis after a stroke, repetitive sit-to-stand training that involves positioning the non-paretic leg on a step during sit-to-stand can be considered a significant form of training that improves their symmetric posture adjustment and balance (Kim, Kim, & Kang, 2015).

Pick item off floor (seated, standing): Therapist places items on the floor at differing distances from the feet forward, lateral, and diagonal, and patient bends to pick them up. Patient may hold stable object to begin and progress to no hands.

Reaching forward (standing): Keeping feet planted, patient reaches for targets as determined by therapist. Progression involves increasing distance and moving from stable to unstable surfaces.

Reaching overhead (standing): Patient takes objects and places them overhead on higher shelf. Patient may also reach for preset targets using a clock pattern. Therapist can alter pattern of reach by calling out clock numbers and patient attempts to touch that number. Progression involves increasing distance and moving from stable to unstable surfaces.

Dual-task: Treadmill (Silsupadol, Siu, Shumway-Cook, & Woollacott, 2006)

a. *Auditory discrimination during gait*: While patient performs walking on treadmill, even surface or variable surface, patient is asked to identify noises or voices from a recording. Examples include discriminating between a woman, man, or child's voice or identifying noises such a car horn, barking dog, meowing cat, snapping fingers, bell, door slam, etc.

b. *Random digit generation*: Therapist gives patient a range of numbers such as 0 to 500 and asks patient to speak random number between the ranges out loud while walking.

c. *Backward verbal task*: Patient recites day of the week/month backward or counts backward from 50, 100, or 200 by 1s or 2s out loud while walking.

d. *Visual spatial matrix task*: Therapist creates a matrix of imaginary headers such as colors, people, places, foods. Therapist shows the patient pictures of items and asks patient to place them verbally in one of the imaginary headers while walking on a treadmill.

e. *Math tasks*: Patients are asked to perform math skills while walking on treadmill. Avoid automated response types of questions such a 1+1, but more complex questions such as 221+131 or a-3=7, solve for a, while walking on the treadmill.

f. *Visual imaginary spatial task*: Patient imagines the route from his or her home to another familiar destination, such as church, grocery store, post office, and verbally describes the routes.

g. *Remembering things*: Therapist give patient a series of numbers, prices, objects, or words to remember and then, after a brief period, asks patient to recite them out loud while walking.

h. *Storytelling*: Therapist asks patient to tell a story such as what patient did this morning, on a vacation, or how patient made a recipe out loud while walking.

i. *Tell opposite direction of action*: Patient says the opposite side of the leg patient is using, so when stepping with left leg patient says" right" out loud while walking. Therapist may ask which arm is swinging now, and patient replies with the opposite answer.

j. *Spelling backward*: Therapist gives patient a word, asks patient to spell it backward out loud while walking.

k. *Stroop task*: Therapist has a set of words written on index cards. Each word is in different colors of ink. Therapist shows word to patient and patient is asked to reply with the color of the word, done while patient walks on treadmill.

l. *Dual-task*: Visual discrimination during balance activities: Show the patient a picture of something (a person, a plant, a building) and ask patient to memorize the photo. The patient then performs the balance activity. After completion, the therapist shows the patient the same or slightly different picture and asks patient if it is the same or different.

Carrying laundry basket: Patient carries laundry basket over various surfaces, up and down ramps, stairs, sets on shelf, sets on floor, any tasks related to home laundry set up.

Carrying a grocery bag: Patient mimics taking groceries out of car, carrying into house over curb, steps, varied surfaces, setting on counter, putting items away. Challenge patient by talking to patient during the activity, asking patient random questions. This should be done with carrying plastic bags to the side and paper bags in front.

Pushing grocery cart: Patient pushes a grocery cart around various objects in an obstacle course format. Challenge the patient by adding weight to the cart and offering distractions.

Walking, turning on uneven surfaces: Challenge gait on multiple surfaces, walk outside, on grass, gravel, carpet.

Stairs and ramp with arm movements: Add bicep curl movements or touching hands to head and back to waist during stair training.

Perturbation training: On multiple challenging surfaces, patient attempts to maintain static balance while therapist gives gentle to moderate pushes from all directions at shoulders and pelvis. Progress to moving toward dynamic activities such as walking or marching in place while perturbations are enacted.

Unilateral stance: Add functional activities to standing on leg such as brushing teeth, combing hair, dishes, etc.

Walking the line: Narrow patient's base of support to walk on a line forward, sideways, backward.

Eye tracking: As described under **7.01.6-8**, there are several eye activities that can be done while having patient do functional tasks, such as marching in place, standing on one leg, walking on treadmill and also with static positions on challenging surfaces such as Rhomberg on a trampoline.

Balancing wand: Using a lightly weighted wand such as a yard stick, an umbrella, or cane, patient sits in an armless chair and attempts to balance the wand vertically in the palm of hand.

Grapevine/Carioca: As described under **6.14.17**, patient performs task with the added challenge of adding a line to follow around objects in an obstacle course fashion.

Steps up forward, lateral, backward: As described under **6.08.24**, patient performs task with the added challenge of adding arm and eye challenges, such as catching/throwing ball, reaching, carrying objects, looking right, left, up, and down.

Walking with distractions: Head moves side to side, up and down during any walking activities.

Stance positioning while reading: Patient reads from a book or a poster while maintaining balance in standing in Rhomberg, sharpened Rhomberg, unilateral stance as described under **6.14.16**.

Getting in/out of car: Patient simulates getting into and out of car. This can be done with sitting first, and then bringing legs in and also with lifting leg to place on car floor before sitting, other leg following. Try with holding back of seat and then no hands.

Shower simulation: Patient simulates getting into and out of shower and performing shower activities, washing one foot is especially challenging.

Stepping over tub: Patient simulates getting into and out of bathtub. Use a tall object for patient to step over. Patient sits as if in tub, then gets up to stand and exits tub. Perform on slicker surfaces such as linoleum. Grab bars can be used if patient has these at home, but progress to without grab bars for practice.

Obstacle course: These are very useful for putting all of the above together. Obstacle course should challenge patient in activities patient may be doing at home like carrying objects, stairs, ramp, curb, uneven surfaces, stepping over and around objects, sitting, standing, turning, etc. Turning lights down low to remove some visual feedback can also further challenge patient.

7.03.3 GLOBAL FUNCTIONING: USE OF NINTENDO WII

<u>POSITION</u>: Standing

<u>TARGETS</u>: Strengthening, facilitating balance, reaction times, neuromuscular control and proprioception; there is a growing interest in the potential of virtual reality-based interventions for balance training in older adults and there is evidence to support it; patients also find it quite fun and enjoyable.

Where's the Evidence?

Laufer, Dar, and Kodesh (2015) performed a systematic review. Seven relevant studies were retrieved. The four studies examining the effect of Wii-based exercise, compared with no exercise, reported positive effects on at least one outcome measure related to balance performance in older adults. Studies comparing Wii-based training with alternative exercise programs generally indicated that the balance improvements achieved by Wii-based training are comparable with those achieved by other exercise programs. The review indicated that Wii-based exercise programs may serve as an alternative to more conventional forms of exercise aimed at improving balance control. Another 2015 study of 42 adult patients with stroke found that Wii training was as effective as Bobath Neurodevelopmental Training on daily living functions and quality of life in subacute stroke patients. The Wii group used five games selected from the Wii Sports and Wii Fit packages for upper limb and balance training, respectively, for 45- to 60-minute treatments, 3 times per week for 10 weeks. The patients in Bobath Neurodevelopmental Training group were applied a therapy program included UE activities, strength, balance, gait, and functional training. They also found the patients in Wii group were more satisfied from the therapy (Şimşek & Çekok, 2015). Roopchand-Martin, McLean, Gordon, and Nelson (2015) looked at the effects of 6 weeks of training, using activities from the Wii Fit Plus disc, on balance in community-dwelling Jamaicans 60 years and older. Participants completed 30-minute training sessions on the Wii Fit twice per week for 6 weeks. Activities used included "Obstacle Course," "Penguin Slide," "Soccer Heading," "River Bubble," "Snow Board," "Tilt Table," "Skate Board," and "Yoga Single Tree Pose." Significant improvement was noted on the Berg Balance Scale, the Multi Directional Reach Test, and the Star Excursion Balance Test, indicating games on the Wii Fit Plus disc can be used as a tool for balance training in community-dwelling persons 60 years of age and older (Roopchand-Martin et al., 2015).

<u>INSTRUCTION</u>: Below is a list of appropriate activities found on the Wii Fit Plus. Follow the instructions as the game dictates.

    a.   Yoga: Tree pose
    b.   Yoga: Warrior
    c.   Yoga: Half moon
    d.   Yoga: Deep breathing
    e.   Yoga: Spine extension
    f.   Yoga: Gate
    g.   Strength training: Single leg extension
    h.   Strength training: Torso twists
    i.   Strength training: Lunge
    j.   Strength training: Side lunge
    k.   Strength training: Single leg reach (for advanced patients)
    l.   Aerobic: Hula hoop
    m.   Aerobic: Basic step
    n.   Balance: Soccer heading
    o.   Balance: Table tilt
    p.   Training plus: Balance: Perfect 10
    q.   Training plus: Balance: Bird's eye bulls eye
    r.   Training plus: Balance: Snowball fight

As the therapist, you should try all of the games so you can properly prescribe exercises. Other games and activities on the Wii may be used. The above list includes the basic suggestions but can certainly be expanded in practice.

<u>SUBSTITUTIONS</u>: Stay close to the patient in the early stages of Wii Fit use, as balance will be challenged varying degrees. Watch for good ankle, knee, hip, and trunk control. Allow use of assistive devices and hand holds when first teaching the Wii Fit as needed.

<u>PARAMETERS</u>: 20 minutes, 1 time per day or every other day

REFERENCES

Dever Fitzgerald, T., Hadjistavropoulos, T., Williams, J., Litimes, L., Zahir, S., Alfano, D., & Scudds, R. (2015, Oct). The impact of fall risk assessment on nurse fears, patient falls, and functional ability in long-term care. *Disability and Rehabilitation*, 1-12.

Dorfman, M., Herman, T., Brozgol, M., Shema, S., Weiss, A., Hausdorff, J. M., & Mirelman, A. Dual-task training on a treadmill to improve gait and cognitive function in elderly idiopathic fallers. (2014, Oct). *Journal of Neurologic Physical Therapy*, 246-53. doi:10.1097/NPT.0000000000000057

Halvarsson A, Oddsson L, Franzén E, Ståhle A. (2015, Sep). Long-term effects of a progressive and specific balance-training programme with multi-task exercises for older adults with osteoporosis: A randomized controlled study. *Clinical Rehabilitation*, EPub ahead of print. doi:0269215515605553

Gillespie, L. D., Robertson, M., Gillespie, W. J., Sherrington, C., Gates, S., Clemson, L.M., & Lamb, S.E. Interventions for preventing falls in older people living in the community. (2012, Sep). *The Chochrane Database of Systematic Reviews*, 9. doi:10.1002/14651858.CD007146. pub3

Jeon, M. Y., Jeong, H., Petrofsky, J., Lee, H., & Yim, J. (2014, Nov). Effects of a randomized controlled recurrent fall prevention program on risk factors for falls in frail elderly living at home in rural communities. *Medical Science Monitor: International Medical Journal of Experiments and Clinical Research*, 2283-2291. doi:10.12659/MSM.890611

Kim, K., Kim, Y. M., Kang, D. Y. (2015, Aug). Repetitive sit-to-stand training with the step-foot position on the non-paretic side, and its effects on the balance and foot pressure of chronic stroke subjects. *Journal of Physical Therapy Science*, 2621-2624. doi:10.1589/jpts.27.2621

Landers, M. R., Oscar, S., Sasaoka, J., & Vaughn, K. (2015, Aug). Balance confidence and fear of falling avoidance behavior are most predictive of falling in older adults: Prospective analysis. *Physical Therapy*, EPub ahead of printing.

Laufer, Y., Dar, G., Kodesh, E. (2015, Oct). Does a Wii-based exercise program enhance balance control of independently functioning older adults? A systematic review. *Clinical Interventions in Aging*, 1803-1813. doi:10.2147/CIA.S69673

Muir-Hunter, S. W., Wittwer, J. E. (2015, Jul). Dual-task testing to predict falls in community-dwelling older adults: a systematic review. *Physiotherapy*, EPub ahead of printing. doi:10.1016/j.physio.2015.04.011

Parsons, J. M. S. (2015, Dec). Does vibration training reduce the fall risk profile of frail older people admitted to a rehabilitation facility? A randomised controlled trial. *Disability and Rehabilitation*, 1-7.

Roopchand-Martin, S., McLean, R., Gordon, C., Nelson, G. (2015, Jun). Balance Training with Wii Fit Plus for community-dwelling persons 60 years and older. *Games for Health Journal*, 247-252. doi:10.1089/g4h.2014.0070

Silsupadol, P., Siu, K. C., Shumway-Cook, A., Woollacott, M. H. (2006, Feb). Training of balance under single- and dual-task conditions in older adults with balance impairment. *Physical Therapy*, 269-281.

Şimşek, T. T., Çekok, K. (2015, Dec). The effects of Nintendo Wii[TM]-based balance and upper extremity training on ADLs and quality of life in patients with sub-acute stroke: a randomized controlled study. *The International Journal of Neuroscience*, 1-10.

Section 7.04

YOGA AND TAI CHI

7.04.1 YOGA: TREATMENT DISCUSSION

Yoga is an ancient practice widely known for its benefits to mind and body. Many of the aspects of yoga are excellent for patients with various musculoskeletal and medical issues. Yoga focuses on core stability, scapular stability, hip flexibility, and deep breathing techniques, among other things. There are seven main types of yoga that will be discussed: Hatha, Vinyasa, Iyengar, Bikram, Kundalini, Ashtanga, and Kripalu. These are briefly described here for reference.

1. *Hatha*: Good for beginners. Hatha combines poses with breathing techniques to develop flexibility, balance, and is generally relaxing and restorative. Hatha yoga encompasses all the various styles of yoga as discussed below.

2. *Vinyasa*: Good for weight loss as it is more fast paced with continuous flow between poses and focuses on strength, flexibility, and balance. Inversion poses (where feet are above the head) are also utilized.

3. *Iyengar*: A form of Hatha yoga that uses props as aids in performing poses. Props include blocks, belts, blankets, cushions, benches, and straps. It helps develop strength, flexibility, and balance while reducing the risks of injury.

4. *Bikram*: Primarily it is designed to increase flexibility and is also known as hot yoga as it is performed in a heated room with sauna-like conditions, usually 105 ° F and 40% humidity.

5. *Kundalini*: Good for a more spiritual experience, this yoga form relaxes the mind and energizes the body through chanting, mantras, and breathing.

6. *Ashtanga*: A more advanced form of yoga, Ashtanga is a fast-paced repetitive transition between poses and requires significant strength and endurance.

7. *Kripalu*: Uses classic poses, breath work, development of a quiet mind, and the practice of relaxation with emphasis on following the flow of prana, or life-force energy, practicing compassionate self-acceptance, observing the activity of the mind without judgment, and taking what is learned into daily life.

Where's the Evidence?

Yoga has been shown to assist in managing hypertension by increasing parasympathetic activity and decreasing sympathetic activity, arguably mainly by increasing gamma-aminobutyric acid activity, thus counteracting excess activity of the sympathetic nervous system, which has been associated with hypertension (Cramer, 2016). Nejati, Zahiroddin, Afrookhteh, Rahmani, and Hoveida's (2015) study showed that the mean scores of lifestyle, emotion-focused coping strategies, problem-focused coping strategies, diastolic blood pressure, and systolic blood pressure were significantly different between the intervention and control group after the intervention of mindfulness-based stress reduction yoga. Posadzki, Cramer, Kuzdzal, Lee, and Ernst's (2014) systematic review of literature on yoga for hypertension also found encouraging evidence to support yoga as a treatment for hypertension, but felt more rigorous trials were warranted.

Cramer et al. (2014) in a systematic review also revealed evidence for clinically important effects of yoga on most biological cardiovascular disease risk factors and deduced that yoga could be considered as an ancillary intervention for the general population and for patients with increased risk of cardiovascular disease.

(continued)

Where's the Evidence? (continued)

Yoga has also demonstrated benefits for patients with Parkinson's syndrome (Ni et al., 2016).

A systematic review by Luu and Hall (2016) found Hatha yoga was also beneficial for increasing *executive function*, such as working memory, reasoning, flexibility, and problem solving as well as planning and execution. Cramer, Lauche, Haller, and Dobos's (2013) systematic review also found strong evidence for short-term effectiveness and moderate evidence for long-term effectiveness of yoga for chronic LBP in the most important patient-centered outcomes and recommended yoga as an additional therapy to chronic LBP patients.

A pilot study by Sharan, Manjula, Urmi, and Ajeesh (2014) assessed the effects of yoga on reducing myofascial pain syndrome of the neck. The study was done among eight physiotherapists with minimum 6 months of experience using a structured yoga protocol designed and implemented for 5 days a week for 4 weeks. The outcome variables—DASH; NDI; VAS; pressure pain threshold for trigger points; CROM, AROM, and PROM; and grip and pinch strengths—improved significantly after intervention.

Amin and Goodman (2014) assessed the effect of Iyengar yoga on hamstring and lumbar flexibility and found a significant increase in flexibility after 6 weeks of single-session yoga training, indicating it may be effective in increasing erector spinae and hamstring flexibility.

Farinatti, Rubini, Silva, and Vanfraechem (2014) compared the flexibility of elderly individuals before and after having practiced Hatha yoga and calisthenics for 1 year at least 3 times a week. This fairly large study of 66 subjects was divided into three groups: control, Hatha yoga and calisthenics. Between-group comparison showed that increases in the Hatha yoga group were greater than in the calisthenics group for most flexibility indexes, particularly the overall flexibility. In conclusion, the practice of Hatha yoga (i.e., slow/passive movements) was more effective in improving flexibility compared to calisthenics (i.e., fast/dynamic movements), but calisthenics was also able to prevent flexibility losses observed in sedentary elderly subjects.

DiBenedetto et al. (2014) studied the effects of and Iyengar and Hatha yoga programs tailored to elderly persons and designed to improve lower body strength and flexibility on 23 healthy adults. Findings of this study suggested that yoga practice may improve hip extension, increase stride length, and decrease APT in healthy elders, and that yoga programs tailored to elderly adults may offer a cost-effective means of preventing or reducing age-related changes in these indices of gait function.

Zettergren, Lubeski, and Viverito (2011) examined the impact of an 8-week therapeutic yoga program on postural control, mobility, rising from the floor, and gait speed in community-living older adults. Eight patients, all women with a mean age of 84, underwent an 8-week, 80-minute, biweekly Kripalu yoga class designed specifically for community-dwelling older adults. Patients were compared to a control group of 5 women and 3 men, mean age 81 years. Post-test differences were found for yoga participants in balance scores and fast-walking speed. Improvements in postural control as measured by the Berg Balance Scale and gait, as measured by fast-gait speed, indicated that research subjects benefited from the yoga intervention. The yoga program designed for this study included activities of standing, sitting, and lying on the floor.

Schmid, Miller, Van Puymbroeck, and DeBaun-Sprague (2014) assessed change in physical functioning (pain, ROM, strength, and endurance) after 8 weeks, twice per week, of therapeutic yoga in people with chronic stroke randomized to therapeutic yoga or wait-list control groups. Yoga was delivered in a standardized and progressive format with postures, breathing and meditation, and relaxation in sitting, standing and supine. Pain, neck ROM, hip PROM, UE strength, and the 6-minute walk scores all significantly improved after 8 weeks of engaging in yoga. No changes occurred in the wait-list control group. They concluded a group therapeutic yoga intervention may improve multiple aspects of physical functioning after stroke, and such an intervention may be complementary to traditional rehabilitation.

It was also shown to positively affect depression and anxiety in post-stroke patients (Chan, Immink, & Hillier, 2012). A large study of 131 subjects compared yoga with relaxation training and the effects on stress and anxiety. Yoga was found to be as effective as relaxation in reducing stress and anxiety and improving health status, and yoga was more effective than relaxation in improving mental health (Smith, Hancock, Blake-Mortimer, & Eckert, 2007).

Furthermore, Patel, Newstead, and Ferrer's (2012) systematic review and meta-analysis of related studies from 1950 to November 2010 suggested that the benefits of yoga may exceed those of conventional physical activity interventions in elderly people for self-rated health status, aerobic fitness, and strength.

The growing body of research supports the practice of yoga as an adjunct to traditional therapies and exercise interventions. Yoga is a powerful tool that can be applied by practitioners to help patients reach established goals. Used in conjunction with manual therapy, modalities, and other procedures, yoga may be applied in some or all of the rehab stages. In addition, the psychological benefits are also helpful side effects.

In implementing yoga into current practice, therapists must incorporate *synchronized breathing* with the postures and movements. Each exercise and pose will list the breathing schedule for the patient and should be the primary focus of the intervention. Secondly, posture and alignment are fundamental to proper yoga. Therapists should continuously monitor and cue the patient as needed.

7.04.2 YOGA: BASIC POSES FOR CLINICIANS

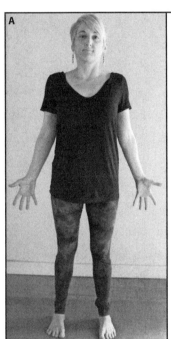

MOUNTAIN POSE (TADASANA):
Mountain pose will help create a good foundation for all additional poses. It is important to understand this pose fully and know the micro-adjustments that can be made for proper alignment and muscle engagement. Patient stands with feet hips-width apart and weight distributed evenly. Patient stands tall, as if a string is pulling the top of the head toward the ceiling. Patient breathes deeply and slowly. Hands are down, with palms forward. Patient lifts the thighs and patella upward. Have the patient lift shoulders to the ears, slightly pulled forward, and then have them pull shoulders down, pulled slightly back, to reset posture. Gaze is forward. Patient may take prayer position with hands to heart. Patient brings scapula back and down to avoid shrugging the shoulders while reaching. Use the phrase, "bring the shoulders down away from the ears" to assist the patient in understanding.
__TARGETS__: Postural control, balance, spine lengthening, core strengthening

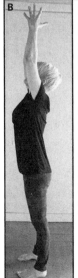

UPWARD SALUTE (URDHVA HASTASANA):
From *Mountain Pose* (A), patient inhales while looking up and bringing arms out to the sides, then patient reaches toward the ceiling, palms facing each other into an "H" position shoulder-width apart. Patient brings scapula back and down to avoid shrugging the shoulders, as patient reaches, kiss the shoulder blades. Patient may then bring the hands together and clasp/weave fingers, leaving the index finger straight and pointed toward the ceiling. Encourage patient to breathe deeply and work on extending spine, pulling shoulders down way from the ears. Extend arms so that upper arm is parallel to ears. Additionally, a block may be placed in between the thighs for spinal support. Using a block between the thighs will help aid in proper alignment as patient squeezes the block and lengthens the tailbone down toward the block. It is important to gently remind patients of the breath. Often, when struggling with any pose, the patient will hold the breath. This creates anxiety in the patient and frustration with the poses. Cue the breath with deep inhales and exhales to aid the patient into full expression of any pose (B).
__TARGETS__: Postural control, balance, spine lengthening, shoulder stretch

"Rag Doll" or Standing Forward Bend (Uttanasana):

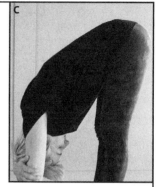

Patient stands tall with a deep inhale, then exhales slowly as patient swan dives down, as if diving into a swimming pool, and bends forward from the hip joints, not from the waist. As patient bends, draw the navel in and away from the groin area to open the space between the pubis and top sternum. The emphasis is on lengthening the front torso as patient moves further into the position. Knees may be slightly bent, eventually working to extend them fully, careful to avoid hyperextension. Once knees are straightened, patient crosses the forearms and holds the elbows. Instruct patient to press the heels firmly into the floor and lift the ischial tuberosities, sitting bones, toward the ceiling, turning the hips slightly inward. Patient inhales deeply and lifts and lengthens the front torso slightly, followed by deep exhale and release more into the forward bend. Patient may put the hands on the floor if possible, but watch that patient is not shrugging the shoulders. Patient's head hangs relaxed with top of head toward the floor. Stay in this pose 30 seconds to 1 minute repeating deep breathing and sinking into the pose further. When coming back up, instruct patient to deeply inhale while gently rolling up one vertebra at a time with the hands on the hips for additional support and alignment. Patient presses tailbone down and into the pelvis. Patient may feel a little dizzy upon standing so remain close.

<u>Targets</u>: Spine decompression and lengthening, stretch spinal extensors and hamstrings, neck stretching and strengthening

Flat Back or "Halfway Lift" (Ardha Uttanasana):

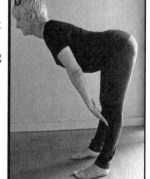

Full *Rag Doll* (C), therapist may have the patient perform a few flat back movements. Patient will place fingertips on floor or shins while inhaling and lifting up, straightening the spine and looking forward at the floor 1 to 2 feet in front of them. Patient will hold briefly, kissing the shoulder blades, and then exhale while folding forward again into rag doll.

<u>Targets</u>: Spine lengthening, activates spinal extensors primarily in thoracic spine

Where's the Evidence?

Half-way lift targets longissimus thoracic per EMG studies (Ni, Mooney, Harriell, Balachandran, & Signorile, 2014).

Downward-Facing Dog (Adho Mukha Svanasana):

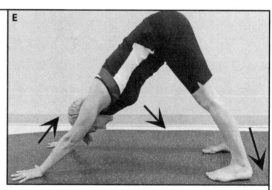

Patient begins in quadruped with wrists directly under the shoulders and the knees directly under hips, fingers are pointed forward. Patient spreads fingers wide and presses firmly through the palms, fingers, and knuckles to distribute weight evenly across the hands. Patient exhales while tucking toes under and lifting knees off floor while reaching the pelvis up toward the ceiling drawing ischial tuberosities, sit bones, toward the wall behind the patient. Patient then gently begins to straighten the knees without locking knees. The patient's body should be in the shape of an "A." Ask the patient to imagine the hips and thighs being pulled backward. Gaze is between the legs. Patient continues to press the floor way from the patient while bringing the shoulders away from the ears in scapular retraction and depression. Patient continues to press the floor away as spine lengthens, patient lifts the sit bones up toward the ceiling while pressing down equally through heels and the palms of hands. Patient continues to draw chest toward the thighs. Heels sink into the floor, stretching the calf muscles. The heels do not have to touch the floor. Patient does not need to walk hands closer to feet to make this happen. Patient holds for at least 5 deep breaths up to 20 breaths. To release, patient exhales while bending knees to come back to quadruped. Weight of the hands in this pose should be in the thumb and forefinger, lifting the palm of the hand off the ground as if cupping a basketball. Inner thighs rotate toward the back and create space between the shoulders and ears to avoid sagging or crunching into the shoulder region. Patients with wrist problems such as carpal tunnel should not do this exercise.

<u>Targets</u>: Spine lengthening, hamstring and gastrocnemius stretching, scapular strengthening, external oblique activation

Where's the Evidence?

Downward-Facing Dog poses are effective for strengthening external obliques per EMG studies (Ni et al., 2014).

LOW LUNGE (ANJANEYASANA):

From *Downward-Facing Dog* (E), extend the right leg toward the sky. Rotate the big toe down to align the hips. Take a deep breath in, and on the exhale, with hands firmly planted on the ground in front, create a slight bend in the knee and bring the right foot slowly forward and

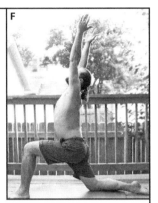

place gently between the two hands, with right knee bent. Use the arms to create balance between both legs and gently draw the right hip back a little to even the spine. Pull the right calf toward the left thigh to also create balance and strengthen these interior muscles. Create a flow when repeating this action on the left side, by bringing right foot back to meet the left into a high-plank and then pushing back up to *Downward-Facing Dog*.

<u>MODIFICATION</u>: Drop left knee down to the ground, and vice versa, when extending the opposite foot forward. Be sure the knee patient is resting on has that resting foot extended straight out without inverting of the foot.

<u>TARGETS</u>: Spine lengthening, activates spinal extensors primarily in thoracic spine, abdominal strengthening, psoas muscle stretch, hamstring stretch

CRESCENT MOON (ALANASANA):

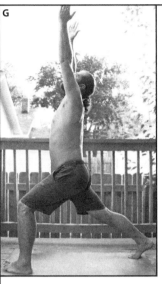

From *Low Lunge* (F), patient gently raises knee back and both hips away from the ground while extending hands firmly in the air. Create space between shoulders and neck and rotate palms to face each other. Create micro-adjustments by slightly rotating the hip of the backward leg forward. Draw the front knee open and engage to avoid strain on that knee. The knee should be directly on top of the ankle, not bending inward. Rotate thigh of the backward extended leg externally and imagine front foot is pulling toward back leg to create inner torso balance with abdominal strength.

Imagine a connection from tailbone to the top of the head, creating one long line of energy. Lightly hug ribs toward the back of the body and draw the tailbone to the earth.

<u>TARGETS</u>: Spine lengthening, activates spinal extensors primarily in thoracic spine, abdominal strengthening, hamstring stretch, psoas muscle stretch

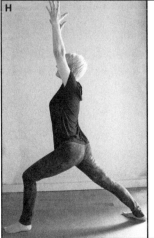

WARRIOR I (VIRABHADRASANA I):

From *Crescent Moon* (G), drop back heel down to the ground and bring front foot back a few inches. Toes should be at a 45-degree angle outward from the heel, with the weight going into the lateral aspect "knife edge" of the foot. Patient may visualize being on a train track with one foot on each track. Increase or decrease the length between the front and back foot and widen or shorten the width of the train track to level of comfort. Gently bring the hip of the back leg forward to square the hips to the front of the room while drawing the front hip back slightly. Placing both hands on hips is a good way to tune into this micro-adjustment. Distribute weight evenly between all four corners of the feet. Patient may extend the arms up or press palms firmly together at the heart with the elbows bent.

<u>TARGETS</u>: Spine lengthening, activates spinal extensors primarily in thoracic spine

Where's the Evidence?

Warrior poses are effective for strengthening gluteus maximus per EMG studies (Ni et al., 2014).

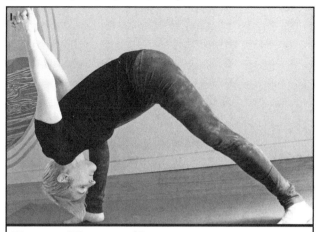

HUMBLE WARRIOR (BADDHA VIRABHADRASANA):

From *Warrior I* (H), patient clasps hands behind back and bends elbows to flatten palms against each other while avoiding overextending elbows. Take a deep breath in, and on the exhale, patient slowly bends forward tucking shoulder on the inside of the extended knee. Tune in to micro-adjustments at hips, gently pulling hip anteriorly on bent leg side and posteriorly on extended knee side. Relax head so the crown reaches toward the ground and slowly straighten arms. By keeping elbows bent, this allows the patient to keep the palms flush with each other until patient is ready to straighten them. Be careful to avoid overextending elbows. Hold this pose for a few breaths and then gently rise up and switch sides.

<u>TARGETS</u>: Spine lengthening, activates spinal extensors primarily in thoracic spine

REVERSE WARRIOR (VIPARITA VIRABHADRASANA):

From *Warrior II* (J), begin to reach the front extended hand toward the sky while creating a slight bend in lower back and reaching back hand toward the back leg or calf. Avoid putting any pressure on the knee. Gaze is up toward the extended hand. Again, be mindful the knee is not

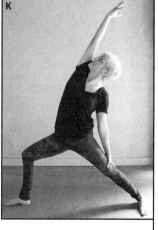

deviating medially. The more the knee is drawing outward or laterally, the more protection the patient has of the lower back and knee. Create a gentle twist in lower abdomen by lightly rotating chest and both shoulders toward the sky.

Use any of these poses to build a sequence leading up to this pose: *Crescent Moon* (G), *Warrior I (H)*, *Warrior II* (J).

<u>TARGETS</u>: Spine lengthening, activates spinal extensors primarily in thoracic spine, neck strengthening

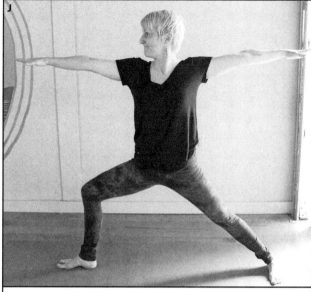

WARRIOR II (VIRABHADRASANA II):

Patient may arrive at this pose from *Crescent Moon* (G) or *Warrior I* (H). With front knee still bent and back leg extended, slowly begin to rotate the back foot so that it is perpendicular to the front heel. Open the front knee to avoid strain, with knee stacked directly over the ankle and thigh parallel to the ground. Extend both arms out with palms face down and gaze out over front middle finger. Notice that torso is not leaning to either side, as shoulders should be stacked directly above hips. The hips are open to the side instead of facing forward. Create more space (distance) between front and back foot while energetically drawing them toward each other, sinking deeper into the hips with every exhale. This creates a strengthening in hip flexors, hamstrings, and gluteals. Remember to drop shoulders down and reach shoulders blades toward each other, chest and chin high. Mindfully rotate the thigh of the back extended leg internally and front thigh externally gently and toward the sky. Weight should be in the outer "knife edge" of the back foot. Inhale to lengthen and exhale to deepen as patient settles into this pose.

<u>TARGETS</u>: Spine lengthening, activates spinal extensors primarily in thoracic spine

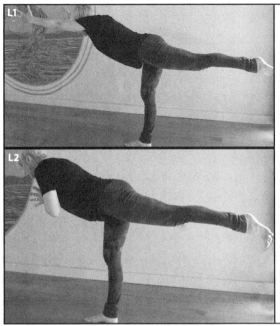

WARRIOR III (VIRABHADRASANA III):

Warrior III can be best achieved from *Mountain Pose* (A) or *Crescent Moon* (G). From *Crescent Moon*, draw both arms behind. It's a good practice to create a Vinyasa, or flow, with this movement, moving from arms extended above to flowing them back behind on inhales and exhales and leaning forward from hips as swinging arms back on the exhale. Chest is pointed down to the ground and neck is long, again, creating one nice long line of energy. On next rotation of the Vinyasa, as arms move backward, softly lift the back leg off of the ground and extend it long behind, then gently lunge forward. Draw pinky toe to the ground to rotate the hips square to the earth. Lift up through the standing leg and extend arms out parallel to the head. Palms face each other as gaze is directed downward. Flex toes of extended leg toward the face to create additional stability (L1). Patient may also bring hands to heart for added balance challenge (L2).

<u>TARGETS</u>: Spine lengthening, activates spinal extensors primarily in thoracic spine

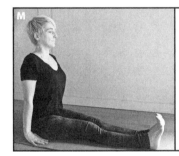

STAFF POSE (DANDASANA):

Start in long-sitting with both hands by the side. Reach up with the head while pulling the shoulder blades down. The patient lengthens from the pubic bone to the sternum with the spine long and tall. Patient presses the knees down by contracting the quadriceps. The pelvis tilts anterior while the patient pulls the toes towards them by dorsi flexing. The patient also presses the hands into the surface they are sitting on while spreading the toes and lengthening through the legs by pushing the heels away.

<u>TARGETS</u>: Spine lengthening, hamstring stretching, postural strengthening

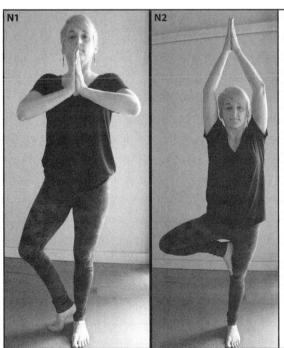

TREE POSE (VRKSASANA):

Start from *Mountain Pose* (A) with both hands by the sides. With feet rooted firmly in the ground, slowly reach for one ankle with the hand and pull the sole of the foot to rest gently on the opposite leg's inner calf (N1) or upper thigh (N2). Always avoid placing the foot inside of the knee as this could cause injury. Engage the inner thigh of the opposite leg to create a shelf for the foot to wedge into. Lift through the arch of the rooted foot. Place both hands on hips and find a focal point (drishti) to help with balance. Open the bent knee wide, externally rotating and abducting the hip while drawing pelvis in and hips down in a posterior tilt. Pull navel to spine to help activate the hips and pelvis alignment. Once patient has a strong hold on balance, gently extend one arm toward the sky. Eventually patient will extend both arms to the sky as patient "grows the tree." Patient may also bring both hands to prayer pose at the chest until patient feels confident enough to extend upwards.

<u>TARGETS</u>: Spine lengthening, activates spinal extensors primarily in thoracic spine

CHAIR POSE (UTKATASANA):

This is another pose that can be accomplished from *Mountain Pose* (A). With both feet planted firmly on the ground, side by side and hip-width apart, arches lifted, extend arms long above the head. Take a deep breath in and, as exhaling, begin to bend the knees and drop the hips down toward the calves as if patient is sitting in an imaginary chair, keeping the thighs parallel to the ground. Knees should be in line with each other. Tail bone is tucked under as patient pulls the belly into the spine and leans forward slightly. Gaze is toward the front of the room. Using a block in between the thighs can aid in strengthening and proper alignment.

TARGETS: Spine lengthening; activates spinal extensors primarily in thoracic spine, ankles, quadriceps, hamstrings, and gluteal strengthening; chair pose can help correct flat feet when arches are correctly lifted.

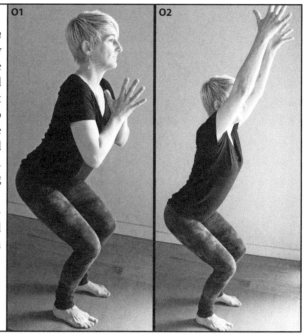

Where's the Evidence?

Chair poses are effective for strengthening gluteus maximus longissimus thoracis per EMG studies (Ni et al., 2014).

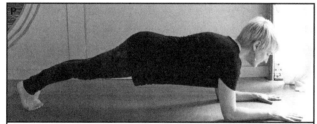

DOLPHIN PLANK POSE (MAKARA ADHO MUKHA SVANASANA):

Beginning in *Downward-Facing Dog* (E), patient slowly pushes self forward so that patient is in a *High-Plank* position with wrists directly under shoulders. Stack the joints: shoulders, elbows, wrists. Begin to lower the body down and place elbows and anterior forearms on the ground. It is very important to have the elbows pulled in under the shoulders to avoid shoulder strain. Draw the heels of the feet to the back of the room to create one flat line from heels to the crown of the head and to avoid sinking into the shoulders. Gaze is downwards. Lift through the shoulders with tail bone tucked under and pull the navel inward to create strength in the back. Be sure to breathe. Beginning practitioners will have a tendency to hold the breath in this pose. This is a great pose for developing the core abdominal muscles.

TARGETS: Spine lengthening, activates spinal extensors primarily in thoracic spine, core strengthening

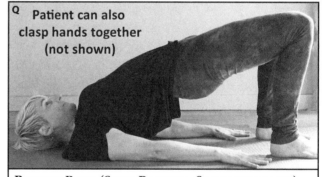

Patient can also clasp hands together (not shown)

BRIDGE POSE (SETU BANDHA SARVANGASANA):

Start by lying supine. Flex the knees, bringing feet toward buttocks with the ankles stacked directly underneath the knees. Lift the pelvis off of the ground and clasp hands underneath the buttocks with shoulders wrapped underneath. Continue to reach pelvis toward the sky on each exhale. Pull the chin away from the chest to reduce any crunching in the neck and protect the spine. Feet should be hip-width apart and knees squeezing toward each other. Placing a block between the thighs will aid in proper alignment.

TARGETS: Spine strengthening, activates spinal extensors primarily in thoracic spine, chest opener

SIDE-SIT TWIST (BHARADVAJASANA I):

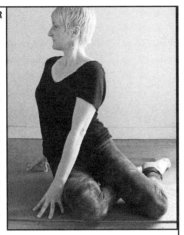

Description is for right spine twist. Reverse directions for left spine twist.

Start in a side-sitting position with both hips and knees flexed. Place the right hand on the ground behind and the left hand in front of the right thigh. Gently pull with the right hand and push against the thigh with the left hand to generate a pleasant twisting affect through the spine. Patient should look over the right shoulder. The patient can get deeper into the twist by taking a deep breath and then applying more pressure with the rooted hands as exhaling.

Please take extra precaution with this exercise with any previous hip or spine problems.

TARGETS: Spine lengthening, spinal rotation

EASY POSE (SUKHASANA):

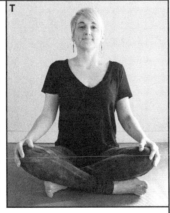

This is a seated pose and is similar to sitting with shins crossed and knees open wide, slowly tuck each foot under the opposite knee. Try to keep feet parallel to each other as this is a little easier on the knees. A great way to get acclimated into this pose is to place a block or a blanket under the buttocks, lifting the posterior pelvis off the ground slightly. This will help to alleviate any pressure on the knees that may be felt. Sit in an upright position and be present to the spine alignment. As the crown of the head lifts toward the ceiling, shoulders drop away from the ears and heart is pushed forward, lifting the chest. Tilt the tailbone down in the seat.

This may also be initially attempted with the back against a wall for added support.

TARGETS: Spine lengthening, activates spinal extensors primarily in thoracic spine

EXTENDED HAND TO BIG TOE POSE (UTTHITA HASTA PADANGUSTASANA):

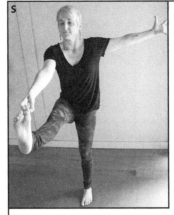

This pose is a more advanced pose and should be attempted *only* if the patient has previous experience or can be assisted. Beginning in standing pose with feet firmly rooted to the ground, place hands on natural waist, not hips. Transfer the weight onto one side and, on the inhale, draw the knee of the opposite leg up toward the belly. Wrap the arms around the calf and breathe. A great way to adjust to the next steps of this pose is to cradle the bent knee in the arms, as if you are rocking a baby. Rotate the knee out and begin to bring the foot to a horizontal position with the knee. Wrap one arm around the thigh and tuck the sole of the foot into the bent elbow part of the other arm to create a cradling effect. Gently rock this cradle until patient is comfortable with balance. Next, remain in the standing position and lower the foot so it is below the knee. Reach down and grab the big toe with the same side of hand of the extended leg and gradually begin to extend the leg out. Patient may keep a slight bend in the leg to help with balance. Patient may find a focal point on the wall to help stay connected to the breath. Once the leg is extended, advancement is to begin to horizontally abduct the hip to the side of the body. For an added challenge and balance definition, try gazing in the opposite direction of the extended leg in this final pose (not shown).

To aid in balance until patient is able to achieve full expression of the pose, patient may place one hand on a wall. A strap or belt can also be used to wrap around the foot to extend reach if patient cannot grasp big toe. This may prevent any injury due to tight hamstrings or weak ankles. Another modification is to keep the knee bent until the body is ready for the full stretch.

TARGETS: Spine lengthening, activates spinal extensors primarily in thoracic spine

LOCUST POSE (SALABHASANA):

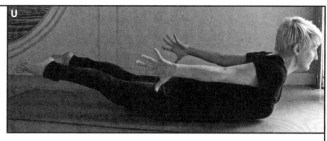

Begin this pose by lying prone. A blanket may be placed under the hip/pelvic area for padding. All 10 toes, forehead, and nose should be touching the ground with the hands by the sides. Big toes are flush with the ground, with hips slightly externally rotated to avoid any sickling of the feet. Take a deep breath in and, as exhaling, begin to lift the forehead, nose, chin, and chest while simultaneously lifting feet, knees, and thighs off of the ground. Broaden through the chest while arms are extended and reaching toward back wall. Engaging buttocks in this pose will help support lower spine.

Modifications for this pose are to clasp hands behind the back. Again, keep the palms flush with each other and a slight bend in the elbows.

TARGETS: Spine lengthening, activates spinal extensors primarily in thoracic spine

TRIANGLE POSE (TRIKONASANA):

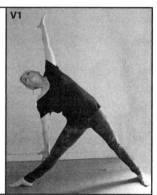

Navigate to triangle pose from *Warrior II* (J). Begin by straightening the front leg. The back leg should be straight with the foot at a 45-degree angle and weight in the outer knife edge. Extend one arm out in front and one behind as is done in *Warrior II* with hips facing the side, not forward. Stack shoulders above hips. Gaze is over the front middle finger. Rotate the front thigh internally and back thigh externally to help square the hips to the side. Check in with the shoulders and spine. Shoulders should be directly over the hips with no hinging of the hips to either side.

TARGETS: Spine lengthening, activates spinal extensors primarily in thoracic spine, hamstring stretch, abdominal strengthening

EXTENDED TRIANGLE POSE (UTTHITA TRIKONASANA):

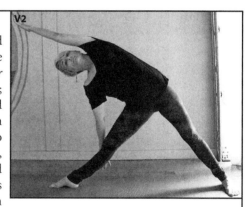

Start in *Warrior II* (J) by straightening the front leg. The back leg should be straight with the foot at a 45-degree angle and weight in the outer knife edge. Extend one arm out in front and one behind as is done in *Warrior II*, with hips facing the side, not forward. Stack shoulders above the hips; gaze is over the front middle finger. Rotate the front thigh internally and the back thigh externally to help square the hips to the side. Check in with the shoulders and spine. Shoulders should be directly over the hips with no hinging of the hips to either side. Take a deep breath and, while exhaling, slowly hinge from hips by reaching the front extended arm forward and draw the back hip in the opposite direction. Once the arm is extended as far as possible, rotate that arm to the ground while extending the other arm toward the sky, stacking the shoulders. The front arm can be placed in front of the calf or, for a deeper stretch, reach behind the front calf. Rotate the front hip so it is in line with the back hip. The patient can pretend to be in between two panes of glass with this pose. Micro-adjustments to the thighs may be needed to ensure the hips are squared to the side while energetically drawing them together to support the lower spine. Roll the rib cage open and toward the ceiling. Gaze may either be toward the ground or (for a challenge) to the sky. Lift up through the side abdominals and rotate the rib cage toward the ceiling (V1). The arm may be brought overhead toward the front foot for an advanced side-body stretch (V2). A block may be used for the front hand that is reaching toward the ground for additional support.

TARGETS: Spine lengthening, activates spinal extensors primarily in thoracic spine

DOLPHIN POSE (ARDHA PINCHA MAYURASANA):
Begin in *Downward-Facing Dog* (E), check in with the alignment. Apply weight in the thumb and index fingers, creating a cup of air under the palms as if cupping a ball. Inner thighs are rotated externally, belly to spine and sacrum reaching toward the sky. The heels do not need to touch the ground unless fully warmed up. Begin to bend the elbows until anterior forearms are flush with the ground and parallel to each other. Elbows should not be open wider than the shoulders and even drawn in tighter if possible. Patient may walk the feet a few inches

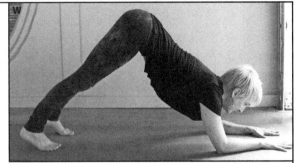

back away from the face to help achieve the pose and as patient becomes more acclimated, begin to take tiny steps toward the face. Use the forearms to carefully push the chest toward the thighs to deepen this stretch. A strap or a belt can be used to aid in proper alignment of the elbows and shoulders. Place the strap around the biceps and tighten to comfort.

TARGETS: Spine lengthening, activates spinal extensors primarily in thoracic spine, shoulder opener, hamstring stretch, calf stretch

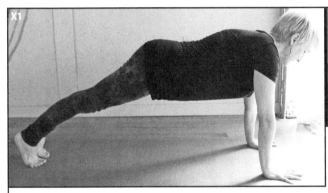

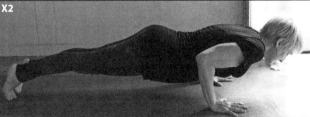

HIGH-TO-LOW PLANK (CHATARANGA DANDASANA):
Start in *High Plank* with hands facing forward, fingers spread wide, and wrists stacked directly below the shoulders. Draw the heels to the back of the room and engage core abdominal muscles and low ribs by pulling belly into spine. Hug the muscles into the midline and point the crown of the head toward the front of the room (X1). On the exhale, begin to shift forward on the toes and slowly lower down so that the elbows are at a 90-degree angle and anterior forearms are resting on mat. It is very important to keep the elbows tucked in toward the body, kissing the ribs. Continue to draw the thighs upward. Avoid drooping in the shoulders and/or raising hips in the air. The body should be one, long straight line from head to toe (X2). Repeat back to *High Plank* when fatigued or lower slowly to the mat.

TARGETS: Spine lengthening, activates spinal extensors primarily in thoracic spine, core and arm strengthening

Where's the Evidence?

Low plank and high plank poses are effective for strengthening external obliques per EMG studies (Ni et al., 2014).

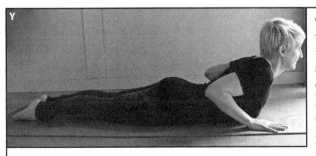

COBRA POSE (BHUJANGASANA): Lying prone, extend the legs long with 10 toes and pelvic bone pressed firmly into the ground. Bring hands directly under shoulders and spread fingers wide. Relax neck and gaze toward the edge of the mat. Contract the hips and thighs to support the lower back and, on the inhale, gradually push the forehead, chin, and chest away from the mat with hands still in place, keeping elbows firmly at the ribs. For extra strengthening, lift the hands off the floor so they float above the ground.

Check in with the body. The shoulders are drawn down and pulled back, tops of the feet and thighs are rooted into the floor, and the chest is lifted. These are all micro-adjustments that can be made in this pose.

TARGETS: Spine lengthening, activates spinal extensors primarily in thoracic spine

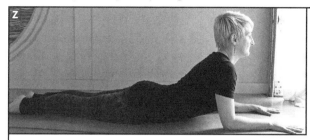

Sphinx Pose (Salamba Bhujangasana):

This pose can be achieved from *Cobra Pose* (Y). Create the alignment as in *Cobra*. Place both forearms on the ground below and slowly push away from the ground using forearms and elbows, with hands directly in front of patient, fingers spread wide, and elbows kissing the ribs. Bring shoulders away from the ears and ground down through the hips, thighs, and tops of the feet. Focus on extending the thoracic spine. Patient may also press up through the elbows to extend them fully (avoid hyperextension) as the thoracic and lumbar spine extend further.

Targets: Spine lengthening, activates spinal extensors primarily in thoracic spine, stretch abdominals with full elbow extension

Bound Angle Pose (Baddha Konasana):

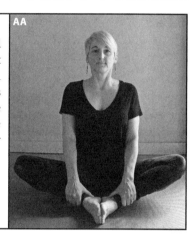

Begin seated in *Staff Pose* (M) with spine straight and legs extended in front. Bend knees, drawing heels in toward the pelvis. Press the soles of the feet together and let knees drop open to both sides, but only as far as possible. Do not press on knees in this pose. Clasp big toes with first two fingers on each side and press the outer edges of the feet firmly together and into the floor. Sit up straight, extending through the length of the entire spine, lifting the crown of the head. Gaze straight ahead. Hold the pose for up to 5 minutes. To release, first release the clasp from the toes, then gently lift knees, and extend the legs once again along back to *Staff Pose*.

Targets: Hip opener

Half Lord of the Fishes Pose (Ardha Matsyendrasana):

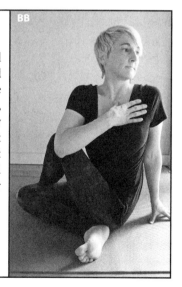

Description is for left spine twist. Reverse directions for right spine twist.

Start in a seated position with both legs extended. Bend the right knee, drawing the heel toward the buttock and flexing the toes. Take the opposite leg and cross over the bended leg, planting the sole of the foot on the ground and the knee stacked on top. Place the left hand on the ground behind you and, with the opposite hand of the upright knee, bend the elbow and place it on the outside of the vertical knee. Gently pull that elbow into the vertical knee, allowing the other hand that is placed on the ground to support patient. This will generate a pleasant twisting affect. Patient can get deeper into the twist by taking a deep breath and then applying more pressure in the elbow and rooted hand as patient exhales. Please take extra precaution if patient has any previous hip, spine, or disc problems.

Targets: Spine lengthening, spinal rotation

7.04.3 TAI CHI: TREATMENT DISCUSSION

Tai chi, as a traditional exercise regimen, has been practiced in China to improve balance and postural control. It is called a body-mind technique because the person uses his or her mind while accomplishing the exercise. Tai chi is a combination exercise involving weight-shifting, postural alignment, and slow coordinated movements with synchronized deep breathing. This combination involves many different mental and physical elements, such as calm concentration on the movement, following the instructor's example to achieve the proper form to improve muscle elasticity while tying the movement to deep breathing in order to enhance cardiac output and support the muscles with adequate blood flow. Tai chi differs from other forms of exercise such as running because the complex series of movements requires the individual to concentrate while performing each movement. Concentration during repetitive tasks aids in the learning process, especially in the damaged nervous system. In many patients with diabetes, the feet provide false (signal) information to the brain about ground reaction forces due to impaired sensory function. In tai chi, subjects move slowly, visualizing the movement while concentrating on how each movement feels; this helps people to become more aware of sensation (Alsubiheen, Petrofsky, Daher, Lohman, & Balbas, 2015).

There are five main styles of tai chi: Chen, Yang, Wu, Hao, and combination styles. These are briefly described here for reference.

1. *Chen*: Founded by the Chen clan in the 13th century, is characterized by alternating slow and explosive movements. The Chen style follows a variable tempo, moving from still positions to quick accelerating to full speed and power movements. Chen works primarily in large movements. It is more difficult for beginners, as it requires complex movements and physical coordination.

2. *Yang*: Founded by Yand Lu-ch'an, is the most popular style of tai chi. It is typically done with slow steady movements with emphasis on relaxation and feeling the flow of energy within the body. Yang works in medium to large movements and follows a steady tempo.

3. *Wu*: Second most popular form of tai chi, founded by Wu Quanyou in the late 19th century. This style emphasizes small circle hand techniques, pushing hands, and weapons training while emphasizing foot work and Horse Stance training with the feet closer together than Yang or Chen styles. Wu works generally in smaller movements and follows a steady tempo.

4. *Hao*: Founded by Wu Yu-hsiang in the 19th century, Hao is a distinctive style with small, subtle movements; highly focused on balance, sensitivity, and internal ch'i development. Ch'i is also known as life force or energy flow with breath work being a major part of tapping into the ch'i.

5. *Combination Styles*: Includes a unique mix of several styles of tai chi combined with moves from other martial arts.

Where's the Evidence?

Lee, Hui-Chan, and Tsang (2015) studied the effects of tai chi balance control and eye-hand coordination of older adults. Fifty-nine subjects from residential care facilities were assigned to a sitting tai chi group or mobilizing exercises group, the control group. The sitting tai chi group underwent 3 months of training with a total of 36 sessions. The tai chi practitioners showed significant improvement in their sequential weight-shifting while sitting, eye-hand coordination test, and in their maximum reaching distance from a sitting position. No such improvements were found in the control group. As traditional tai chi poses difficulties for older adults with poor standing balance, this pilot study showed that a 3-month sitting tai chi training program can improve sitting balance and accuracy in the finger pointing task in the older adults. Park and Song (2012) analyzed the effects of tai chi on fall-related risk factors through meta-analysis of randomized clinical trials published in English and Korean between 2000 and 2010. The authors found studies of randomized clinical trials indicate tai chi is effective in improving balance, flexibility, muscle strength, ADLs, and fear of falling when applied for 3 or 6 months. The findings provide the objective evidence to apply tai chi as a fall preventive intervention. Based on the of the effects of diabetes mellitus and peripheral neuropathy affecting the sensation in the feet and increasing fall risk, Alsubiheen et al, (2015) investigated the effect of 8 weeks of tai chi training combined with mental imagery on improving balance in people with diabetes and an age-matched control group. All subjects in both groups (healthy and diabetic) attended a Yang style of tai chi class using mental imagery strategies, two sessions a week for 8 weeks. All results showed an improvement in balance in the diabetic and the control groups. Since the diabetes mellitus group had more problems with balance impairment at baseline than the control, the diabetic group showed the most benefit from the tai chi exercise.

7.04.4 Tai Chi: Basic Maneuvers

The following maneuvers are done with body movements at incredibly slow speeds.

BREATHING EXERCISE:

Keep tip of tongue on roof of mouth while inhaling and exhaling through the nose. Work on long, continuous breaths without a pause between inhale and exhale. Breath is circular and should not stop. Breathe from the belly using diaphragmatic breathing. Relax eyes, chest, and jaw, and breath long and deep. This breathing technique continues throughout the tai chi workout (Beginners Tai Chi, 2016b).

HORSE STANCE/STANDING IN A NEUTRAL POSITION:

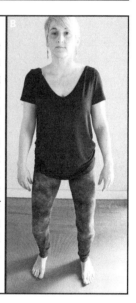

Standing in a neutral position with the hands at the sides is a common exercise to do before executing a tai chi set. This standing exercise is useful for identifying areas of tension within the body, even before the more difficult positions in a tai chi form. Patient begins by relaxing mind and body. Feet are parallel pointing forward, and hip-width apart, with weight distributed equally between feet. Knees are slightly bent, spine is lengthened, pulling tailbone so it points toward the floor, then relax into that position. Head is lifted away from shoulders with chin slightly tucked while hands are relaxed on lateral thighs, palms facing backward. Tongue tip is at the roof of the mouth as patient breathes as described above. Usually this is done for at least 5 minutes and progresses at 2- or 3-minute increments. The practice of tai chi standing isn't as easy as it may sound. Some would even say the practice of standing is not easy at all. It may immediately bring thoughts and sensations of aches or itches to the forefront, along with a list of other things one might be doing. The Chinese have a term for this and speak of the taming the "monkey mind." Holding a standing position can yield incredible benefits in terms of body and energy awareness, as well as better body alignments. It is also a way to develop strong roots and a sense of groundedness (Beginners Tai Chi, 2016c).

CIRCLING HANDS:

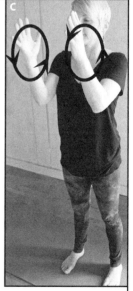

Tai chi is all about cycles and circles. It embodies the philosophy of cycles. In tai chi, all movements are circular. Expansion outward, including strikes and blows, is circular. Yielding, or retreating, also has a circular nature. The circling hands exercise is a simple way to practice the physical circles and energy cycles of tai chi. By isolating and repeating a simple circular movement, patients will be able to feel the energy cycles in the tai chi form better and movements will be smoother, fuller, and rounder.

Patient starts as if giving someone a standing applause. Palms are facing each other, but not touching, and hands are in front of the chest, fingers are oriented away from the body. The distance between the hands can be chosen and is the distance that will be used for the exercise. Instruct patient to feel the energy connection between the hands, but let the hands come in closer or spread further apart when making circles. Patient then starts making slow vertical circles with the hands. The hands move up and out away from the body, maintaining the same distance apart, then back down and inward. Someone watching from the side should see the hands tracing a circle in the air. As the hands move outward, instruct patient to expand them, feeling the hands and wrists growing as hands move away from the body, expanding the spaces between all of the bones in the hand and wrists. This expansion brings more blood and energy out to the hands and fingertips. As hands move inward, contract them, closing the joints and spaces back down again as hands come closer to the body. This will help to return the blood and energy back to the body. Once patient is comfortable with this, get the entire body involved by feeling this growing and shrinking throughout the entire body, from the feet, through the ankles, knees, and upward. Patient should feel the movement in the entire body. "One part moves, all parts move; one part stops, all parts stop," is one of the core principles of tai chi. Patient continues making the circles, growing and shrinking with the circles, keeping the size and position of the circle the same. Then, keeping the same circle in space, simply change the direction of the circle. Do the same number of backward circles as forward. Sometimes groups of tai chi practitioners have entire conversations while circling the hands. This is not too unusual in China. It is a useful and relaxing exercise (Beginner's Tai Chi, 2016a).

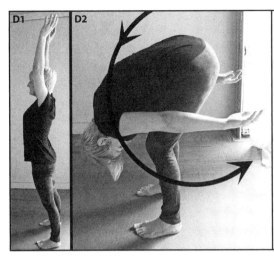

WINDMILL:

The windmill is a basic tai chi movement for promoting flexibility and opening up the spine. Patient stands with feet parallel, slightly wider than shoulder-width apart. Patient relaxes shoulders and lets the arms hang loosely, then brings hands in front of the body at level of pubic bone, fingers pointing down toward the floor. Patient inhales and raises arms up the center of the body and overhead, fingers pointing up, stretching toward the ceiling and arching spine slightly backward. Patient exhales and slowly bends forward to the floor, moving the hands down the center of the body, bending forward from the hip joints, allowing arms to hang loosely in front of them, then inhales and returns to starting posture (Halse, 2017).

KNEE ROLLS:

Knee rolls encourage mobility in the spine and knees and can help improve balance. Patient stands with feet a few inches apart, knees slightly bent, and places hands on the knees with the fingers pointing toward each other. Patient rotates the knees in a circle, rolling from the left, back, right, and front, as though tracing a large circle on the floor with the knees. Perform the circular motion in clockwise, then counter-clockwise, directions (Halse, 2017).

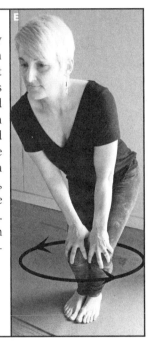

HAND EXERCISES:

The tai chi hand exercises help open up the hands and promote flexibility in shoulders, arms, and fingers. Patient stands with feet a bit wider than shoulder-width apart. Patient raises arms straight out in front of the palms, relaxed and hanging down parallel to the floor at shoulder height. Patient stretches hands as wide as possible, then begins rotating wrists in a clockwise, then counter-clockwise, direction (Halse, 2017).

HEAVY ARMS:

In *Horse Stance* (B), allow arms to be limp and swing front to back like a pendulum, allowing the shoulders to loosen (Avery et al., 2012).

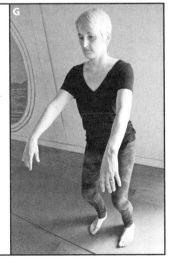

CRANE TAKES FLIGHT:

Starting in *Horse Stance* (B), patient bends knees while raises the arms out to the sides into shoulder abduction. Wrists are loose. Then, straightening the knees, the arms are lowered back to start. Palms are facing the thighs and torso remains straight (Avery et al., 2012).

BEAR ROOTING:

With elbows bent approximately 90 degrees and palms facing down, patient shifts weight entirely over one foot, allowing knee on stance leg to bend. Patient may lift the unweighted foot off the ground for an added challenge (Avery et al., 2012).

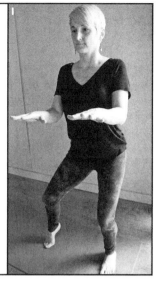

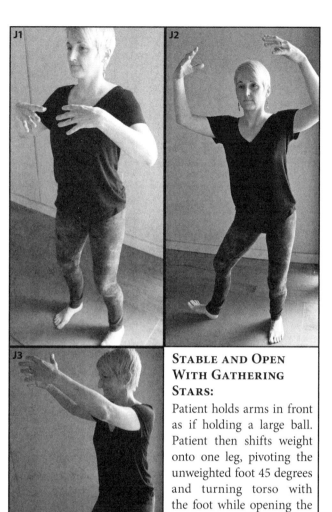

STABLE AND OPEN WITH GATHERING STARS:

Patient holds arms in front as if holding a large ball. Patient then shifts weight onto one leg, pivoting the unweighted foot 45 degrees and turning torso with the foot while opening the arms. Patient then returns the arms and foot back to center and repeats on the other side (Avery et al., 2012).

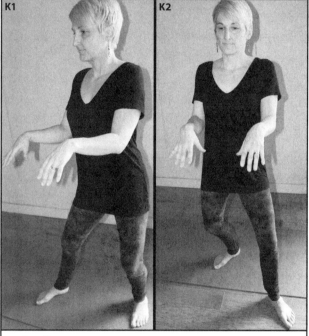

70/30 STANCE:

Starting in *Horse Stance* (B), patient shifts weight onto one leg, pivoting the unweighted foot 45 degrees and turning torso with the foot, then stepping onto pivoted foot heel first. Bringing the now-unweighted foot to step forward rotates the hips to facing forward with knees slightly bent and weight distributed over both feet. Knees stay aligned over feet (Avery et al., 2012).

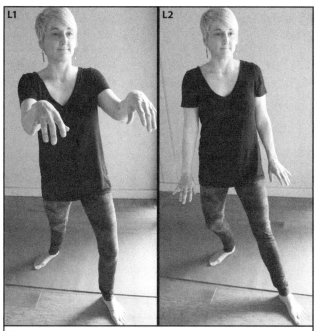

BEAR WALK:

Starting in *70/30 stance* (K), patient shifts weight to forward leg while lifting arms forward, palms down, then shifts weight to the back leg and lowers the arms back down (Avery et al., 2012).

BASIC BEAR:

Starting in *Horse Stance* (B), patient rotate the hips forward and to the side with shoulders following as in tai chi fold while slowly swinging the arms (Avery et al., 2012).

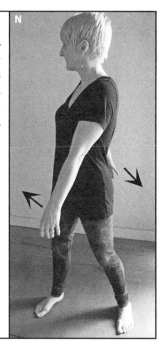

TAI CHI FOLD:

Starting in *Horse Stance* (B), patient shifts weight to one leg while rotating the hips forward and to the side with shoulders following hips (Avery et al., 2012).

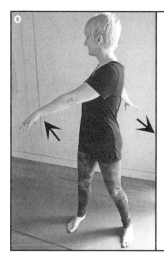

SKI MOVE:

This is the same as *Basic Bear* (N) with larger arm movements, bringing the arms higher (Avery et al., 2012).

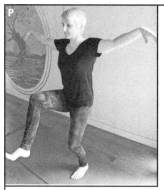

FLYING CRANE:

Beginning in *Horse Stance* (B) with feet diagonally outward, patient shifts weight entirely to one foot and then lifts unweighted knee directly in front of the hip as the arms rise to the side into shoulder abduction, followed by leg and arms lowering together. Patient may keep toes of unweighted foot in contact with the floor for added balance if needed (Avery et al., 2012).

DANCING CRANE:
Beginning in *Horse Stance* (B) with feet diagonally outward, patient shifts weight entirely to one foot and then lifts unweighted knee directly out to the side into hip abduction, opening arms as a dancer as shown, followed by leg and arms lowering together (Avery et al., 2012).

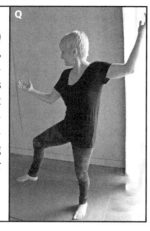

Patients should be focused on the breath, the positions and the movements, keeping the mind relaxed and focused on the present moment. Tai chi can be done every day and should be practiced on a set routine, such as every morning before breakfast or in the evenings before going to bed.

REFERENCES

Alsubiheen, A., Petrofsky, J., Daher, N., Lohman, E., & Balbas, E. (2015). Effect of Tai Chi exercise combined with mental imagery theory in improving balance in a diabetic and elderly population. *Medical Science Monitor: International Medical Journal of Experimental and Clinical Research, 21*, 3054-3061.

Amin, D. J., & Goodman, M. (2014). The effects of selected asanas in Iyengar yoga on flexibility: Pilot study. *Journal of Bodywork and Movement Therapies, 18*(3), 399-404.

Avery, C., Hutchison-Maravilla, K., Matsuda, S., Medow, T., Rietz, K., & Yu, T. (2012). T'ai Chi Fundamentals scientific evidence for innovative use of Tai Chi in rehabilitation, recovery, and wellness. Retrieved from http://files.abstractsonline.com/ctrl%5Ca4%5Cc9%5Ca1c%5Cb9%5Cb51%5Cc4cb%5Cc7ab%5Cce7b%5Caaf%5Cf00%5Cb3a%5Cd1%5Ca1534_1.pdf

Beginners Tai Chi. (2016a). A Tai Chi exercise: Circling hands. Retrieved from http://www.beginnerstaichi.com/tai-chi-exercise-circling-hands.html

Beginners Tai Chi. (2016b). Tai Chi breathing: Tips for beginners. Retrieved from http://www.beginnerstaichi.com/tai-chi-breathing.html

Beginners Tai Chi. (2016c). Tai Chi standing exercise. Retrieved from http://www.beginnerstaichi.com/tai-chi-standing.html

Chan, W., Immink, M. A., & Hillier, S. (2012). Yoga and exercise for symptoms of depression and anxiety in people with poststroke disability: A randomized, controlled pilot trial. *Alternative Therapies in Health and Medicine, 18*(3), 34-43.

Cramer, H. (2016). The efficacy and safety of yoga in managing hypertension. *Experimental and Clinical Endocrinology & Diabetes, 124*(2), 65-70.

Cramer, H., Lauche, R., Haller, H., & Dobos, G. (2013). A systematic review and meta-analysis of yoga for low back pain. *Clinical Journal of Pain, 29*(5), 450-460.

Cramer, H., Lauche, R., Haller, H., Steckhan, N., Michalsen, A., & Dobos, G. (2014). Effects of yoga on cardiovascular disease risk factors: A systematic review and meta-analysis. *International Journal of Cardiology, 173*(2), 170-183.

DiBenedetto, M., Innes, K. E., Taylor, A. G., Rodeheaver, P. F., Boxer, J. A., Wright, H. J., & Kerrigan, D. C. (2014). Effect of a gentle Iyengar yoga program on gait in the elderly: An exploratory study. *Archives of Physical Medicine and Rehabilitation, 86*(9), 1830-1837.

Farinatti, P. T., Rubini, E. C., Silva, E. B., & Vanfraechem, J. H. (2014). Flexibility of the elderly after one-year practice of yoga and calisthenics. *International Journal of Yoga Therapy, 24*, 71-77.

Halse, H. (2017). Tai Chi basic steps for beginners. Livestrong.com. Retrieved from http://www.livestrong.com/article/431042-tai-chi-basic-steps-for-beginners/

Lee, K. Y., Hui-Chan, C. W., & Tsang, W. W. (2015). The effects of practicing sitting Tai Chi on balance control and eye-hand coordination in the older adults: A randomized controlled trial. *Disability and Rehabilitation, 37*(9), 790-794.

Luu, K., & Hall, P. A. (2016). Hatha yoga and executive function: A systematic review. *Journal of Alternative and Complementary Medicine, 22*(2), 125-133.

Nejati, S., Zahiroddin, A., Afrookhteh, G., Rahmani, S., & Hoveida, S. (2015). Effect of group mindfulness-based stress-reduction program and conscious yoga on lifestyle, coping strategies, and systolic and diastolic blood pressures in patients with hypertension. *Journal of Tehran Heart Center, 10*(3), 140-148.

Ni, M., Mooney, K., Harriell, K., Balachandran, A., & Signorile, J. (2014). Core muscle function during specific yoga poses. *Complementary Therapies in Medicine, 22*(2), 235-243.

Ni, M., Signorile, J. F., Mooney, K., Balachandran, A., Potiaumpai, M., Luca, C., . . . Perry, A. C. (2016). Comparative effect of power training and high-speed yoga on motor function in older patients with Parkinson disease. *Archives of Physical Medicine and Rehabilitation, 97*(3), 345-354.e15.

Park, M., & Song, R. (2012). [Effects of Tai Chi on fall risk factors: A meta-analysis]. *Journal of Korea Academy of Nursing, 43*(3), 341-351.

Patel, N. K., Newstead, A. H., & Ferrer, R. L. (2012). The effects of yoga on physical functioning and health related quality of life in older adults: A systematic review and meta-analysis. *Journal of Alternative and Complementary Medicine, 18*(10), 902-917.

Posadzki, P., Cramer, H., Kuzdzal, A., Lee, M. S., & Ernst, E. (2014). Yoga for hypertension: A systematic review of randomized clinical trials. *Complementary Therapies in Medicine, 22*(3), 511-522.

Schmid, A. A., Miller, K. K., Van Puymbroeck, M., & DeBaun-Sprague, E. (2014). Yoga leads to multiple physical improvements after stroke, a pilot study. *Complementary Therapies in Medicine, 22*(6), 994-1000.

Sharan, D., Manjula, M., Urmi, D., & Ajeesh, P. (2014). Effect of yoga on the myofascial pain syndrome of neck. *International Journal of Yoga, 7*(1), 54-59.

Smith, C., Hancock, H., Blake-Mortimer, J., & Eckert, K. (2007). A randomised comparative trial of yoga and relaxation to reduce stress and anxiety. *Complementary Therapies in Medicine, 15*(2), 77-83.

Zettergren, K. K., Lubeski, J. M., & Viverito, J. M. (2011). Effects of a yoga program on postural control, mobility, and gait speed in community-living older adults: A pilot study. *Journal of Geriatric Physical Therapy, 34*(2), 88-94.

Chapter 8

THE ATHLETE

Bryan E. *The Comprehensive Manual of Therapeutic Exercises:*
Orthopedic and General Conditions (pp 545-562).

Section 8.01

Interval Sport Progression Training

Interval sport progression training utilizes a gradual progression of applied forces to lessen the chance of re-injury for patients wanting to sport. Patients must exhibit good dynamic stability, strength, and endurance before beginning the interval sport progression programs. All interval sport progression programs should include a proper warm-up and maintenance exercises, a graded progression of the sport activity, and constant monitoring of proper biomechanics to minimize the incidence of re-injury. If at any time during the activity sharp pain is experienced, particularly in the joint or point of injury, the athlete should cease all sport activity until the pain resolves. If pain persists, it is recommended the athlete be re-assessed.

8.01.1 Phase I and II Interval Throwing Progressions

Data-based interval throwing programs for baseball athletes are an integral training and conditioning element for both injured and uninjured athletes who are preparing for sports participation. Data-based age and level-of-play interval throwing programs for pitchers, catchers, infielders, and outfielders have been developed, tested, and implemented for more than 10 years. Progression is based on type and location of injury, symptoms in response to throwing, and pre-injury performance profile. Throwing programs are highly structured; however, therapists may modify them to meet the individual needs of athletes (Axe, Hurd, & Snyder-Mackler, 2009). An interval throwing program is used to gradually return baseball pitchers and positional players to competition. The interval throwing program is used for high school, college, and professional baseball players and is divided into two phases (Reinold, Wilk, Reed, Crenshaw, & Andrews, 2002). The interval throwing protocol should be implemented 3 days per week. Alternate days should focus on cardiovascular, core stabilization, stretching and LE, RC and scapular stabilization, and strengthening. The remaining seventh day is utilized for light ROM and stretching (Reinold et al., 2002).

Warm-Up

1. Aerobic: To increase blood flow and increase the muscular flexibility
   a. Jogging
   b. Biking
   c. Jumping rope
2. "Thrower's 10"
   a. One
      i. 5.14.6 Strengthen: Isotonic Wrist: All Planes
      ii. 5.12.12 Strengthen: Isotonic; Elbow Pronation and Supination With Hammer
   b. Two
      i. 5.12.16 Strengthen: Resistance Band, Elbow Extension, Overhead (or use cable machine or dumbbell).
      ii. 5.12.10 Strengthen: Isotonic; Elbow Flexion, Curls (1lbs)
   c. Three:
      i. 5.07.42 Strengthen: Isotonic; Resistance Band, Shoulder, Combination Movements PNF D1 and D2

   1. D2 Flexion: Unsheath your sword to Tada!
   2. D2 Extension: Tada! to sheath the sword
  d. Four
     i. 5.07.39 Strengthen: Isotonic: Resistance Band: Internal Rotation and Variations
     ii. 5.07.41 Strengthen: Isotonic: Resistance Band: External Rotation and Variations
     iii. 5.07.23 Strengthen: Isotonic; Shoulder External Rotation 90/90
  e. Five
     i. 5.07.11 Strengthen: Isotonic: Scaption; full can or empty can, empty can not recommended by this author
  f. Six
     i. 5.07.12 Strengthen: Isotonic: Shoulder Abduction to 90 degrees
  g. Seven:
     i. 5.07.24 Strengthen: Isotonic; Shoulder, Row (Prone)
  h. Eight
     i. 5.07.27 Strengthen: Isotonic: Posterior Cuff, 4-Way
  i. Nine
     i. 5.07.63 Strengthen: Closed Kinetic Chain: Scapular and Shoulder Depression
  j. Ten
     i. 5.07.62 Strengthen: Closed Kinetic Chain; Shoulder, Push-Up
3. Plyometrics
  a. 5.07.79 Plyometrics/Dynamic: Shoulder, Wall Dribbles5.07.80 Plyometrics/Dynamic: Ball Toss, Overhead
  b. 5.07.81 Plyometrics/Dynamic: Chest Pass
  c. 5.07.82 Plyometrics/Dynamic: Shoulder, Bench Press/Floor Throws
  d. 5.07.83 Plyometrics/Dynamic: Shoulder, Two-Handed Side Throw
  e. 5.07.84 Plyometrics/Dynamic: Shoulder, 90/90 Throw (start cautiously!)
  f. 5.07.85 Plyometrics/Dynamic: Shoulder, Multidirectional Catch/Throw
  g. 5.07.86 Plyometrics/Dynamic: Shoulder, Ball Toss, Overhead and Backwards
  h. 5.07.87 Plyometrics/Dynamic: Shoulder, Push-Up
  i. 5.07.88 Plyometrics/Dynamic: Shoulder, Slams
  j. 5.07.89 Plyometrics/Dynamic: Shoulder, Ball Squat, Push-Press
  k. 5.07.90 Plyometrics/Dynamic: Shoulder, Push-Offs

4. Neuromuscular control drills
  a. 5.07.91 Reactive Neuromuscular Training and Variations, Shoulder; move into sports positions.
5. Stretching ideas
  a. 2.02.3 Stretch: Self-Assisted Cervical Lateral Flexion Stretch
  b. 2.02.7 Stretch: Cervical Flexion and Rotation
  c. 5.06.2 Stretch: Shoulder Internal Rotation, "Chicken Wing", Active Assistive
  d. 5.06.4 Stretch: Shoulder Horizontal Abductors
  e. 5.06.5 Stretch: Shoulder Horizontal Adductors, Doorway
  f. 5.06.10 Stretch: Anterior Deltoid and Biceps Hand Clasp
  g. 5.11.7 Stretch: Biceps, Other Person Assist
  h. 5.11.5 Stretch: Biceps Using Table
  i. 5.11.4 Stretch: Biceps Using Wall
  j. 5.11.2 Stretch: Triceps
  k. 3.02.4 Thoracic Extension With Hands Clasped Behind Head, Using Wall
  l. 3.02.2 Stretch: Thoracic Flexion, "Child's Pose" or "Prayer Stretch", Add Side-Bend or Rotation
  m. 3.02.3 Thoracic With Hands On Bench/Chair/Ball, Using Foam Roll 3.03.7
  n. 5.05.12 Self-Joint Mobilization/Stretch: Anterosuperior Capsule
  o. 5.05.11 Self-Joint Mobilization/Stretch: Anterior Middle Capsule
  p. 5.05.10 Self-Joint Mobilization/Stretch: Anteroinferior Capsule

Interval Throwing Phase I

The program consists of throwing at each step, 2 to 3 times on separate days without pain or symptoms before progressing to the next step. Initially, the athlete will perform two sets of 25 throws at the specified distance. Positional athletes are instructed to progress through the entire interval throwing program before beginning position-specific drills.

All throws should be on an arc with a crow hop. A *crow hop* is a hop that outfielders use sometimes to gain momentum to add power and distance to their throws. The crow hop is done in two steps. As a right hander, once the baseball is in the athlete's glove securely, the athlete jumps off of left foot (which should still be in front of right foot) in the direction already traveling. While in the air, athlete turns body to the right to coil up for the throw. Athlete will then land on the right foot and is ready to throw the baseball. From this position, patient will be able to get the whole body into the throw.

Warm-up throws consist of 10 to 20 throws at approximately 30 feet.

See Table A (Reinold et al., 2002).

TABLE 8.01.1-A

45-FT PHASE	60-FT PHASE	90-FT PHASE	120-FT PHASE
Step 1: Warm-up throwing 45 ft, 25 throws Rest 5 to 10 min Warm-up throwing 45 ft, 25 throws	**Step 3**: Warm-up throwing 60 ft, 25 throws Rest 5 to 10 min Warm-up throwing 60 ft, 25 throws	**Step 5**: Warm-up throwing 90 ft, 25 throws Rest 5 to 10 min Warm-up throwing 90 ft, 25 throws	**Step 7**: Warm-up throwing 120 ft, 25 throws Rest 5 to 10 min Warm-up throwing 120 ft, 25 throws
Step 2: Warm-up throwing 45 ft, 25 throws Rest 5 to 10 min Warm-up throwing 45 ft, 25 throws Rest 5 to 10 min Warm-up throwing 45 ft, 25 throws	**Step 4**: Warm-up throwing 60 ft, 25 throws Rest 5 to 10 min Warm-up throwing 60 ft, 25 throws Rest 5 to 10 min Warm-up throwing 60 ft, 25 throws	**Step 6**: Warm-up throwing 90 ft, 25 throws Rest 5 to 10 min Warm-up throwing 90 ft, 25 throws Rest 5 to 10 min Warm-up throwing 90 ft, 25 throws	**Step 8**: Warm-up throwing 120 ft, 25 throws Rest 5 to 10 min Warm-up throwing 120 ft, 25 throws Rest 5 to 10 min Warm-up throwing 120 ft, 25 throws
150-FT PHASE	180-FT PHASE		FOR PITCHERS
Step 9: Warm-up throwing 150 ft, 25 throws Rest 5 to 10 min Warm-up throwing 150 ft, 25 throws	**Step 11**: Warm-up throwing 180 ft, 25 throws Rest 5 to 10 min Warm-up throwing 180 ft, 25 throws	**Step 13**: Warm-up throwing 180 ft, 25 throws Rest 5 to 10 min Warm-up throwing 180 ft, 25 throws Rest 5 to 10 min Warm-up throwing 180 ft, 20 throws Rest 5 to 10 min Warm-up throwing 15 throws, progressing from 90 to 120 ft	**Step 15**: Warm-up throwing 60 ft, 10 to 15 throws 90 ft, 10 throws 120 ft, 10 throws 60 ft (flat-ground) using pitching mechanics, 20 to 30 throws
Step 10: Warm-up throwing 150 ft, 25 throws Rest 5 to 10 min Warm-up throwing 150 ft, 25 throws Rest 5 to 10 min Warm-up throwing 150 ft, 25 throws	**Step 12**: Warm-up throwing 180 ft, 25 throws Rest 5 to 10 min Warm-up throwing 180 ft, 25 throws Rest 5 to 10 min Warm-up throwing 180 ft, 25 throws	**Step 14**: Return to respective position or progress to step 15 under "For Pitchers" if athlete is pitching.	**Step 16**: Warm-up throwing 60 ft, 10 to 15 throws 90 ft, 10 throws 120 ft, 10 throws 60 ft (flat-ground) using pitching mechanics, 20 to 30 throws 60 to 90 ft, 10 to 15 throws 60 ft (flat-ground) using pitching mechanics, 20 throws

Conversion to meters: 45 ft = 13.7 m; 60 ft = 18.3 m; 90 ft = 27.4 m; 120 ft = 36.6 m; 150 ft = 45.7 m; 180 ft = 54.8 m.

TABLE 8.01.1-B		
STAGE 1: FASTBALLS ONLY	*STAGE 2: FASTBALLS ONLY*	*STAGE 3*
Step 1: A) Interval throwing B) 15 throws, 50% **Step 2**: A) Interval throwing B) 30 throws, 50% **Step 3**: A) Interval throwing B) 45 throws, 50% **Step 4**: A) Interval throwing B) 60 throws, 50% **Step 5**: A) Interval throwing B) 70 throws, 50% **Step 6**: A) 45 throws, 50% B) 30 throws, 75% **Step 7**: A) 30 throws, 50% B) 45 throws, 75% **Step 8**: A) 10 throws, 50% B) 65 throws, 75%	**Step 9**: A) 60 throws, 75% B) 15 throws, batting practice **Step 10**: A) 50 to 60 throws, 75% B) 30 throws, batting practice **Step 11**: A) 45 to 50 throws, 75% B) 45 throws, batting practice	**Step 12**: A) 30 throws, 75% B) 15 throws, 50%, begin breaking balls C) 45 to 60 throws, batting practice, fastball only **Step 13**: A) 30 throws, 75% B) 30 breaking balls, 75% C) 30 throws, batting practice **Step 14**: A) 30 throws, 75% B) 60 to 90 throws, batting practice, gradually increase breaking balls **Step 15**: A) Simulated game: progressing by 15 throws per workout (pitch count)

Interval Throwing Phase II

Phase II is geared specifically toward pitchers and is implemented after the pitcher can perform Phase I without symptoms.

As the athlete progresses through Phase II, the number of pitches, as well as the percent effort of throwing, is gradually advanced until the athlete is allowed to pitch light batting practice. At this time, the athlete may start more stressful pitches such as breaking balls, as well as the initiation of simulated games (Reinold et al., 2002). Warm-up: Use interval throwing 120-feet (36.6-meters) phase as warm-up. All throwing off the mound should be done in the presence of a pitching coach or sport biomechanist to stress proper throwing mechanics.

Interval Throwing Little Leaguers

Olsen, Fleisig, Dun, Loftice, and Andrews (2006) and colleagues looked at 95 adolescent pitchers with shoulder or elbow surgery and 45 non-injured adolescent pitchers to identify pitching practices that increase risk for injury. They found that the injured group pitched significantly more months per year, games per year, innings per game,

pitches per game, pitches per year, and warm-up pitches before a game. These pitchers were more frequently starting pitchers, pitched in more showcases, pitched with higher velocity, and pitched more often with arm pain and fatigue. They also used anti-inflammatory drugs and ice more frequently to prevent an injury. Although the groups were age matched, the injured group was taller and heavier. There were no significant differences regarding private pitching instruction, coach's chief concern, pitcher's self-rating, exercise programs, stretching practices, relieving frequency, pitch type frequency, or age at which pitch types were first thrown. Adolescents with better pitching mechanics tend to generate lower humeral internal rotation torque, lower elbow valgus load, and are more efficient than do those with improper mechanics (Davis et al., 2009). Poor pitching mechanics also appear to contribute to injury risk. Existing research does not show a significant correlation between curveballs and injury. Adults should help youth pitchers avoid fatigue, overuse, and improper mechanics (Fleisig, Weber, Hassell, & Andrews, 2009). Based on their findings, Olsen et al. (2006) developed a new set of recommendations for adolescent pitchers. See Table C.

TABLE 8.01.1-C
SAFETY RECOMMENDATIONS FOR ADOLESCENT BASEBALL PITCHERS

1. Avoid pitching with arm fatigue.
2. Avoid pitching with arm pain.
3. Avoid pitching too much. Reasonable limits are as follows:
   ◦ Avoid pitching more than 80 pitches per game.
   ◦ Avoid pitching competitively more than 8 months per year.
   ◦ Avoid pitching more than 2500 pitches in competition per year.
4. Monitor pitchers with the following characteristics closely for injury:
   ◦ Pitchers who regularly use anti-inflammatory drugs or ice to "prevent" an injury
   ◦ Regularly starting pitchers
   ◦ Pitchers who throw with velocity > 85 mph
   ◦ Taller and heavier pitchers
   ◦ Pitchers who warm-up excessively
   ◦ Pitchers who participate in showcases

Alterations have been made to the interval throwing program for adolescent pitchers and throwing athletes based on the size of little league fields and the distance from home plate to the mound, compared to high school and adult playing situations. Similar warm-up and flexibility exercises have been incorporated. The Little League Interval Throwing program is provided here for your reference. See Table D (Reinold et al., 2002).

TABLE 8.01.1-D			
30-FT PHASE (9.1 M)	*45-FT PHASE (13.7 M)*	*60-FT PHASE (18.3 M)*	*90-FT PHASE (27.4 M)*
Step 1: Warm-up throwing 30 ft, 25 throws Rest 15 min Warm-up throwing 30 ft, 25 throws	**Step 3**: Warm-up throwing 45 ft, 25 throws Rest 15 min Warm-up throwing 45 ft, 25 throws	**Step 5**: Warm-up throwing 60 ft, 25 throws Rest 15 min Warm-up throwing 60 ft, 25 throws	**Step 7**: Warm-up throwing 90 ft, 25 throws Rest 15 min Warm-up throwing 90 ft, 25 throws
Step 2: Warm-up throwing 30 ft, 25 throws Rest 10 min Warm-up throwing 30 ft, 25 throws Rest 10 min Warm-up throwing 30 ft, 25 throws	**Step 4**: Warm-up throwing 45 ft, 25 throws Rest 10 min Warm-up throwing 45 ft, 25 throws Rest 10 min Warm-up throwing 45 ft, 25 throws	**Step 6**: Warm-up throwing 60 ft, 25 throws Rest 10 min Warm-up throwing 60 ft, 25 throws Rest 10 min Warm-up throwing 60 ft, 25 throws	**Step 8**: Warm-up throwing 90 ft, 20 throws Rest 10 min Warm-up throwing 60 ft, 20 throws Rest 10 min Warm-up throwing 45 ft, 20 throws Rest 10 min Warm-up throwing 45 ft, 15 throws

8.01.2 Interval Golf Program

Golf is considered a moderate-risk activity for sports injury; however, excessive time spent golfing and technical deficiencies lead to overuse injuries. Golf injuries originate either from overuse or from a traumatic origin and primarily affect the elbow, wrist, shoulder, and the low back. Professional and weekend golfers, although showing a similar overall anatomical distribution of injuries by body segment, tend to present differences in the ranking of injury occurrence by anatomical site; these differences can be explained by their playing habits and the biomechanical characteristics of their golf swing (Thériault & Lachance, 1998). Prospective, randomized studies have shown that focus on the TA and multifidi muscles is a necessary part of physical therapy for LBP. Some studies also suggest that the coaching of a "classic" golf swing and increasing trunk flexibility may provide additional benefit (Gluck, Bendo, & Spivak, 2008). Cole and Grimshaw (2008) studied muscle activation of the erector spinae and external oblique during golf drives and concluded reduced erector spinae activity demonstrated may be associated with a reduced capacity to protect the spine and its surrounding structures at the top of the backswing and at impact where the torsional loads are high. McHardy, Pollard, and Luo (2007) found that in a prospective study of 588 golfers, injury rate was 15 out of every 100 golfers and most likely sustained in the low back region as a result of the golf swing. They further identified that higher amounts of game play and an increased length of time since clubs were changed seemed to be significantly associated with risk of injury after adjusting for other risk factors. Additionally, carrying one's bag proved to be hazardous to the lower back, shoulder, and ankle (Gosheger, Liem, Ludwig, Greshake, & Winklemann, 2003). Many of these injuries can be prevented by a preseason and year-round sport-specific conditioning program, including strengthening, flexibility, and aerobic exercise components, as well as a short warm-up routine and the adjustment of an individual's golf swing to meet the physical capacities and limitations through properly supervised golf lessons (Thériault & Lachance, 1998). Only a small proportion of amateur golfers perform appropriate warm-up exercises. To improve on this, golfers should be educated about the possible benefits of warming up and be shown how to perform an appropriate warm-up routine (Fradkin, Finch, & Sherman, 2001).

Warm-Up Recommendations

1. 5 minutes: Putting from 20, 30, and 40 feet and from a variety of angles
2. 5 minutes: Putting 10 feet to 3 feet and 25 short putts uphill
3. 5 minutes: Chipping around the green with a tee as a target
4. 15 minutes: Full swing warm-up and stretching
   a. Stretching ideas
      i. 2.02.3 Stretch: Self-Assisted Cervical Lateral Flexion Stretch
      ii. 2.02.7 Stretch: Cervical Flexion and Rotation
      iii. 5.13.1 Stretch: Wrist Flexor Self-Assisted and Finger Flexor Variations Below
         ◦ Elbow extended
         ◦ Adding fingers
      iv. 5.13.3 Stretch: Wrist Extensor Self-Assisted and Finger Extensor Variation Below
         ◦ Elbow extended
         ◦ Add fingers
      v. 5.06.4 Stretch: Shoulder Horizontal Abductors
      vi. 5.06.10 Stretch: Anterior Deltoid and Biceps Hand Clasp
      vii. 5.10.7 Stretch: Biceps Other Person Assist
      viii. 5.10.2 Stretch: Triceps
      ix. 3.02.1 Stretch: Thoracic Flexion, "Child's Pose" or "Prayer Stretch"
      x. 3.02.9 Thoracic Rotation, Extended Triangle Pose (yoga)
      xi. 3.01.9 ROM: Thoracic Rotation, Active
      xii. 4.01.3 ROM: Lumbar Extension, Active
      xiii. 7.04.2 Yoga: Basic Poses For Clinicians
         ◦ Mountain pose
         ◦ Sun salutation
         ◦ "Rag doll"
         ◦ Flat back
      xiv. 6.03.3 Stretch: Hip Flexor, Standing Lunge
      xv. 6.08.1 Stretch: Quadriceps
         ◦ Standing Hand Assist Variation
      xvi. 6.08.3 Stretch: Hamstrings
         ◦ Standing foot on stool variation; prop foot on golf cart
   b. Full swing:
      i. 10 wedges
      ii. 5 to 10 each short irons, working up to the long irons and woods
      iii. Last few full swings should be with the club the individual intends to use on the first tee

The interval golf program follows a progression of approximately 5 weeks. The golfer is encouraged to begin using each club with a tee to avoid the deleterious forces that may be produced during a divot. Swings are initiated at partial effort and progressed to full effort as tolerated. The first week begins with light putting and chipping drills and progresses to light short-iron shots by the end of the week. Medium irons are initiated during week 2 while the number of shots is increased. Putting and chipping are performed throughout to allow for an active period of rest between sets of iron (Reinold et al., 2002). The interval golf program is provided here for your reference (Reinold et al., 2002).

TABLE 8.01.2			
WEEK	MONDAY	WEDNESDAY	FRIDAY
1	• 10 putts • 10 chips • Rest 5 minutes • 15 chips	• 15 putts • 15 chips • Rest 5 minutes • 25 chips	• 20 putts • 20 chips • Rest 5 minutes • 20 putts • 20 chips • Rest 5 minutes • 10 chips • 10 short irons
2	• 20 chips • 10 short irons • Rest 5 minutes • 10 short irons • 15 medium irons (5-iron off tee)	• 20 chips • 15 short irons • Rest 10 minutes • 15 short irons • 15 chips • Putting • 15 medium irons	• 15 short irons • 20 medium irons • Rest 10 minutes • 20 short irons • 15 chips
3	• 15 short irons • 20 medium irons • Rest 10 minutes • 15 short irons • 15 medium irons • 5 long irons • Rest 10 minutes • 20 chips	• 15 short irons • 15 medium irons • 10 long irons • Rest 10 minutes • 10 short irons • 10 medium irons • 5 long irons • 5 wood	• 15 short irons • 15 medium irons • 10 long irons • Rest 10 minutes • 10 short irons • 10 medium irons • 10 long irons • 10 wood
4	• 15 short irons • 15 medium irons • 10 long irons • 10 drives • Rest 15 minutes • Repeat	• Play 9 holes	• Play 9 holes
5	• Play 9 holes	• Play 9 holes	• Play 18 holes

Chips = pitching wedge
Short irons = wedge, 9-iron, 8-iron
Medium irons = 7-iron, 6-iron, 5-iron
Long irons = 4-iron, 3-iron, 2-iron
Woods = 3-wood, 5-wood
Drives = driver

8.01.3 INTERVAL TENNIS PROGRAM

Tennis is a popular sport with tens of millions of athletes participating worldwide. The volume of play, combined with the physical demands of the sport, can lead to injuries of the musculoskeletal system. Overall, injury incidence and prevalence in tennis has been reported with acute injuries, such as ankle sprains, more frequently in the lateral epicondylitis while chronic overuse injuries, such as lateral epicondylitis, are more common in the UE in the recreational athlete and shoulder pain more common in the high-level athlete (Abrams, Renstrom, & Safran, 2012). The shoulder is also at high risk for injury during overhead sports as well with recommendations for the prevention of recurrent injury and return to play after injury to include improving the glenohumeral internal-rotation deficit, commonly found in overhead throwers; improving RC strength, in particular the strength of the external rotators; and correction of scapular dyskinesis, in particular improving scapular position and strength (Cools, Johansson, Borms, & Maenhout, 2015).

The goal of the interval tennis program is to safely and efficiently transition from supervised rehabilitation to return to sport. Athlete should continue to be supervised by physician, physical therapist, and/or athletic trainer through each stage until able to return to unrestricted play. Any sharp pain or swelling requires adjustment of the program. Patient will have rest days between each interval tennis program day. During these rest days, athlete should be doing cardio, LE and core strengthening, and light RC and scapular stabilization/strengthening. Before advancing to the next step, athlete should be without pain, swelling, or excessive soreness. Repeat the same session or return to a previous session as appropriate if this occurs. With all activities, athlete should warm-up, maintain neutral stance, demonstrate good mechanics, follow through on swings, bend the knees, turn the body and stay on the balls of the feet. It is also not recommended to attempt heavy topspin or underspin to ground strokes until the later stages of the interval program (Ellenbecker, De Carlo, & DeRosa, 2009).

The basic interval tennis program is provided here for your reference (Reinold et al., 2002; Table A). An alternative interval tennis program is provided here as well, consisting of seven stages (Ellenbecker et al., 2009; Table B). Clinicians may use either of these programs as a guideline for gradually immersing the athlete back to competitive tennis.

	TABLE 8.01.3-A		
WEEK	MONDAY	WEDNESDAY	FRIDAY
1	• 12 FH • 8 BH • Rest 10 min • 13 FH • 7 BH	• 15 FH • 8 BH • Rest 10 min • 15 FH • 7 BH	• 15 FH • 10 BH • Rest 10 min • 15 FH • 10 BH
2	• 25 FH • 15 BH • Rest 10 min • 25 FH • 15 BH	• 30 FH • 20 BH • Rest 10 min • 30 FH • 20 BH	• 30 FH • 25 BH • Rest 10 min • 30 FH • 25 BH
3	• 30 FH • 25 BH • 10 SR • Rest 10 min • 30 FH • 25 BH • 10 SR	• 30 FH • 25 BH • 15 SR • Rest 10 min • 30 FH • 25 BH • 15 SR	• 30 FH • 30 BH • 15 SR • Rest 10 min • 30 FH • 15 SR • Rest 10 min • 30 FH • 30 BH • 15 SR *(continued)*

TABLE 8.01.3-A (CONTINUED)			
WEEK	MONDAY	WEDNESDAY	FRIDAY
4	• 30 FH • 30 BH • 10 SR • Rest 10 min • Play 3 games • 10 FH • 10 BH • 5 SR	• 30 FH • 30 BH • 10 SR • Rest 10 min • Play set • 10 FH • 10 BH • 5 SR	• 30 FH • 30 BH • 10 SR • Rest 10 min • Play 1.5 sets • 10 FH • 10 BH • 3 SR
SR = serves FH = forehand shots BH = backhand shots		During in-between days, athlete should be doing cardio, LE and core strengthening, and light RC and scapular stabilization/strengthening. On day 7, athlete performs only stretching.	

TABLE 8.01.3-B	
STAGE	INSTRUCTIONS
1: Low compression ball used	a. Have a partner feed 20 forehand ground strokes to you from the net. (Partner must use a slow, looping feed that results in a waist-high ball bounce.) b. Have a partner feed 20 backhand ground strokes as in 1a. c. Rest 5 minutes. d. Repeat 20 forehand and backhand feeds.
2: Standard tennis ball used	a. Begin as in Stage 1, with a partner feeding 10 forehands and 10 backhands from the net. b. Rally with a partner from the baseline, hitting controlled groundstrokes until you have hit 50 to 60 strokes. (Alternate between forehand and backhand, allowing 20 to 30 seconds rest after every two or three rallies.) c. Rest 5 minutes. d. Repeat 2b.
3	a. Rally ground strokes from the baseline for 15 minutes. b. Rest 5 minutes. c. Hit 10 forehand and 10 backhand volleys, emphasizing a contact point in front of the body. d. Rally ground strokes for 15 minutes from the baseline. e. Hit 10 forehand and 10 backhand volleys, as in 3c. *Pre-Serve Interval* Perform these tasks before Stage 4. ***(Note: This interval can be performed off court and is meant solely to determine readiness for progression into Stage 4 of the interval tennis program.)*** a. After stretching, with racket in hand, perform serving motion for 10 to 15 repetitions without a ball. b. Using a foam ball, hit 10 to 15 serves without concern for performance result (focusing only on form, contact point, and the presence or absence of symptoms).
4	a. Hit 20 minutes of ground strokes, mixing in volleys (70% ground strokes and 30% volleys). b. Perform 5 to 10 simulated serves without a ball. c. Perform 5 to 10 serves using a foam ball. d. Perform 10 to 15 serves using a standard tennis ball at approximately 75% effort. e. Finish with 5 to 10 minutes of ground strokes.

(continued)

TABLE 8.01.3-B (CONTINUED)	
STAGE	*INSTRUCTIONS*
5	a. Hit 30 minutes of ground strokes, mixing in volleys (70% ground strokes and 30% volleys). b. Perform 5 to 10 serves using a foam ball. c. Perform 10 to 15 serves using a standard tennis ball at approximately 75% effort. d. Rest 5 minutes. e. Perform 10 to 15 additional serves as in 5c. f. Finish with 15 to 20 minutes of ground strokes.
6	a. Repeat Stage 5, increasing the number of serves to 20 to 25 instead of 10 to 15. b. Before resting between serving sessions, have a partner feed easy, short lobs to attempt a controlled overhead smash.
7	a. Before attempting match play, complete Stages 1 to 6 without pain or excess fatigue in the UE. Continue to progress the amount of time rallying with ground strokes and volleys, in addition to increasing the number of serves per workout, until you can perform 60 to 80 overall serves interspersed throughout a workout. Remember that an average of up to 120 serves can be performed in a tennis match; therefore, be prepared to gradually increase the number of serves in the interval program before engaging in full competitive play.

During in-between days, athlete should be doing cardio, LE and core strengthening, and light RC and scapular stabilization/strengthening. On day 7, athlete performs only stretching.

8.01.4 RUNNING PROGRESSIONS

Absence from running due to an injury can substantially reduce VO^2 max and strength. Return to running after an injury must be done gradually with close monitoring of any recurrence or aggravation of injury or presentation of new injury. Novice runners who progressed their running distance by more than 30% over a 2-week period seem to be more vulnerable to distance-related injuries than runners who increase their running distance by less than 10% (Nielsen, Parner, et al., 2014). When running indoors on a treadmill, the lack of air resistance results in a lower energy cost compared with running outdoors at the same velocity. A slight incline of the treadmill gradient to 1% can be used to increase the energy cost in compensation (Jones & Doust, 1996). Obese individuals are at even greater risk of injury if they exceeded 3 km during the first week of their running program and should begin running training with an initial running distance of less than 3 km (1.9 miles) the first week of their running regime (Nielsen, Bertelsen et al., 2014). The rule is not to risk re-injury by going back too fast.

In looking at running speeds during slow and medium-paced running, stride length is increased by exerting larger support forces during ground contact, whereas in fast running and sprinting, stride frequency is increased by swinging the legs more rapidly through the air. Dorn, Schache and Pandy (2012) looked at experimental data to describe and explain the synergistic actions of the individual leg muscles over a wide range of running speeds. For speeds up to 7 m/s (15 mph), the ankle plantar flexors, soleus and gastrocnemius, contributed most significantly to vertical support forces and hence increases in stride length. At sprint speeds greater than 7 m/s (15 mph), these muscles shortened at relatively high velocities and had less time to generate the forces needed for support and used to increase running speed shifted to the goal of increasing stride frequency. The hip muscles, primarily the iliopsoas, gluteus maximus, and hamstrings, achieved this goal by accelerating the hip and knee joints more vigorously during swing.

For runners who want to return to long marathon or half marathon distance running, there are several factors to consider. Runners who run less than an average of 30 km/week (18 miles) had increased injury occurrence as compared with runners with an average weekly training volume of 30 to 60 km/week (18 to 37 miles), thus runners may be advised to run a minimum of 30 km/week before a marathon to reduce their risk of running-related injury (Rasmussen, Nielsen, Juul, & Rasmussen, 2013). Another study confirmed this; however, the training distance was a longer, with a training distance less than 40 km a week being a strong protective factor of future calf injuries. They also found regular interval training is a strong protective

TABLE 8.01.4-A

GENERAL RECOMMENDATIONS FOR RETURN TO RUNNING

1. Wear supportive running shoes.
2. Change running shoes every 300 to 500 miles (480 to 800 km).
3. Allow at least 1 day of rest per week.
4. Perform walk/run program and plyometrics every other day, 3 days per week.
5. Off days, cross train (biking, elliptical, swimming) and perform LE and core strengthening.
6. Start running program on flat surface, treadmill, or cushioned track.
7. Warm-up and cool-down 5 to 10 minutes each.
8. Stretch before and after running.
9. Increase run/walk distance, or time, by 10% each week until goal distance is achieved.
10. Avoid excessive downhill running.
11. Avoid excessive hard surface running.
12. General muscle soreness or slight stiffness that disappears within first 10 minutes of running is okay.
    - If soreness the day after running, take 1 day off. Do not advance to the next session.
    - If soreness disappears during warm-up, continue progression or stay at the same level.
    - If soreness continues during warm-up, drop back to the previous level of training, and take 2 days off.
13. Nocturnal pain, pain worsening as run progresses, or pain that changes stride pattern is not okay—rest and reassessment is indicated.

Adapted from combined protocols from Brigham and Women's Hospital, Department of Rehabilitation Physical Therapy (Wilcox, 2007) and the University of Delaware Physical Therapy Clinic (n.d.).

factor for knee injuries (Van Middelkoop, Kolkman, Van Ochten, Bierma-Zeinstra, & Koes, 2008). This was supported in another study of long-distance runners, which identified the incidence of LE running injuries ranging from 19.4% to 79.3%, with the predominant site of these injuries being the knee. They found strong evidence that a long training distance per week in male runners and a history of previous injuries were risk factors for injuries, and that an increase in training distance per week was a protective factor for knee injuries (van Gent et al., 2007). Wearing a knee brace with a patellar support ring may be effective in the prevention of anterior knee pain caused by running (Yeung & Yeung, 2001; Yeung, Yeung, & Gillespie, 2011). Custom-made biomechanical insoles may also be more effective than no insoles for reducing shin splints (medial tibial stress syndrome; Yeung et al., 2011).

Some general recommendations for returning to running are listed in Table A.

Patient should be able to walk, pain-free, aggressively (roughly 4.2 to 5.2 miles per hour), in a controlled environment, preferably on a treadmill, before beginning the plyometric and walk/jog program. Completion of a plyometric routine (Table B) that integrates 470-foot contacts per leg, would be equivalent to two-thirds of the foot contacts during a mile run. Successful completion of this would be a good indicator that an athlete is ready to attempt running a half to three-quarters of a mile distance (Wilcox, 2007). General treadmill (Table C) and track (Table D) running progressions are presented for reference (Developed by the University of Delaware Physical Therapy Clinic, n.d.). Alternatively, patient may utilize the walk/jog protocol provided here (Wilcox, 2007; Table E).

There are a multitude of running progression protocols available for short- and long-distance runners available. The protocols listed here are for distances of less than 3.2 miles (5 km).

Table 8.01.4-B

Plyometric routine: complete before beginning run/jog 3/4 to 1 mile (1.2 to 1.6 km)

EXERCISE	SETS	FOOT CONTACTS PER SET	TOTAL FOOT CONTACTS
Two-leg ankle hops: in place	3	30	90
Two-leg ankle hops: forward/backward	3	30	90
Two-leg ankle hops: side to side	3	30	90
One-leg ankle hops: in place	3	20	60
One-leg ankle hops: forward/backward	3	20	60
One-leg ankle hops: side to side	3	20	60
One-leg leg broad hop	4	5	20

Rest interval between sets: 90 seconds. Rest intervals between exercises: 3 minutes.

Table 8.01.4-C

BASIC TREADMILL RUNNING PROGRESSION

Level 1	0.1 miles walk and 0.1 miles jog: repeat 10 times
Level 2	Alternate 0.1 miles walk and 0.2 miles jog: 2 miles total
Level 3	Alternate 0.1 miles walk and 0.3 miles jog: 2 miles total
Level 4	Alternate 0.1 miles walk and 0.4 miles jog: 2 miles total
Level 5	Jog 2 full miles
Level 6	Increase workout to 2.5 miles
Level 7	Increase workout to 3 miles
Level 8	Alternate between running and jogging every 0.25 miles

Mandatory 2-day rest between workouts for the first 2 weeks.
Do not advance more than 2 levels per week.
2 days rest mandatory between levels 1, 2, and 3 workouts.
1 day rest mandatory between levels 4 to 8 workouts.

Table 8.01.4-D

BASIC TRACK RUNNING PROGRESSION

Level 1	Jog straights and walk curves: 2 miles total
Level 2	Jog straights and jog 1 curve every other lap: 2 miles total
Level 3	Jog straights and jog 1 curve every lap: 2 miles total
Level 4	Jog 1.75 laps and walk curves: 2 miles total
Level 5	Jog 2 miles
Level 6	Increase workout to 2.5 miles (4 km)
Level 7	Increase workout to 3 miles (4.8 km)
Level 8	Increase speed on straights and jog curves

Mandatory 2-day rest between workouts for the first 2 weeks.
Do not advance more than 2 levels per week.
2 days rest mandatory between levels 1, 2, and 3 workouts.
1 day rest mandatory between levels 4 to 8 workouts.

Table 8.01.4-E

WALK/JOG PROGRESSION

	WALK	JOG	REPETITIONS	TOTAL TIME
STAGE I	5 minutes	1 minute	5 times	30 minutes
STAGE II	4 minutes	2 minutes	5 times	30 minutes
STAGE III	3 minutes	3 minutes	5 times	30 minutes
STAGE IV	2 minutes	4 minutes	5 times	30 minutes
STAGE V	Jog every other day with a goal of reaching 30 consecutive minutes. Warm-up and cool down at a comfortable walking pace, 5 minutes each.			

8.01.5 Sprint Sequence

Once jogging and running are painless, sprinting can be initiated. Table 8.01.5 illustrates a progression for sprint sequence training (Bandy & Sanders, 2012).

Table 8.01.5
SPRINTING PROGRESSION STRAIGHT PLANES (FORWARD SPRINTS)
• Sprint half speed • Sprint 3/4 speed • Sprint full speed • Backward sprint 3/4 speed • Lateral spring 1/2 speed • Backward sprint full speed • Lateral sprint full speed • Add dribbling or high stepping for basketball athletes

8.01.6 Jump-Hop Sequence

Once jogging and running are painless, jump-hop activities can be initiated. Table 8.01.6 illustrates a progression for jump-hop sequence training (Bandy & Sanders, 2012).

Table 8.01.6		
JUMP-HOP SEQUENCE		
BILATERAL SUPPORT	Leg press Mini-squat	3 sets, 30 seconds Increase by 30 seconds until 2 minutes reached
UNILATERAL SUPPORT	One leg press One leg mini-squat	3 sets, 30 seconds Increase by 15 seconds until 1 minute reached
STRAIGHT PLANE, BILATERAL NONSUPPORT	Front-to-back jumps Side-to-side jumps Vertical jumps Horizontal jumps	Multiple sets at sport-specific duration at least 30 seconds
STRAIGHT PLANE, UNILATERAL, NONSUPPORT	Front-to-back hops Side-to-side hops Lateral stepping Lunges Vertical hops Horizontal hops	Multiple sets at sport-specific duration at least 30 seconds
MULTI-PLANE, BILATERAL NONSUPPORT	Diagonal jumps "V" jumps Five-dot drill	Multiple sets at sport-specific duration at least 30 seconds
MULTI-PLANE, UNILATERAL, NONSUPPORT	Diagonal hops "V" hops Five-dot drill	Multiple sets at sport-specific duration at least 30 seconds

8.01.7 CUTTING SEQUENCE-FIGURE 8 PROGRESSION

Once jogging and running are painless, sprinting can be initiated. Table 8.01.7 illustrates a progression for figure 8 and cutting sequence training (Bandy & Sanders, 2012).

TABLE 8.01.7						
DAY 1	*DAY 2*	*DAY 3*	*DAY 4*	*DAY 5*	*DAY 6*	*DAY 7*
40-yard figure 8's at jog pace	40-yard figure 8's at half-speed sprints	40-yard figure 8's at half-speed sprints	40-yard figure 8's at full-speed sprints	20-yard figure 8's at half-speed sprints	20-yard figure 8's at full-speed sprints	10-yard figure 8's at half-speed sprints
DAY 8	*DAY 9*	*DAY 10*	*DAY 11*	*DAY 12*	*DAY 13*	*DAY 14*
10-yard figure 8's at full-speed sprints	Off	45-degree straight cuts at set location half-speed sprint	45-degree straight cuts at set location full-speed sprint	45-degree straight cuts on command full-speed sprint	Off	60-degree straight cuts at set location half-speed sprint
DAY 15	*DAY 16*	*DAY 17*	*DAY 18*	*DAY 19*	*DAY 20*	*DAY 21*
60-degree straight cuts at set location full-speed sprint	60-degree straight cuts on command full-speed sprint	Off	90-degree straight cuts at set location half-speed sprint	90-degree straight cuts at set location full-speed sprint	90-degree straight cuts on command full-speed sprint	Off
Perform 2 sets of 10 repetitions of each.						

REFERENCES

Abrams, G. D., Renstrom, P. A., & Safran, M. R. (2012). Epidemiology of musculoskeletal injury in the tennis player. *British Journal of Sports Medicine, 46,* 492-498.

Axe, M., Hurd, W., & Snyder-Mackler, L. (2009). Data-based interval throwing programs for baseball players. *Sports Health, 1*(2), 145-153.

Bandy, W. D., & Sanders, B. (2012). *Therapeutic exercise for physical therapist assistants* (3rd ed.). Philadelphia, PA: Lippincott, Williams & Wilkins.

Cole, M. H., & Grimshaw, P. N. (2008). Electromyography of the trunk and abdominal muscles in golfers with and without low back pain. *Journal of Science and Medicine in Sport, 11*(2), 174-181.

Cools, A. M., Johansson, F. R., Borms, D., & Maenhout, A. (2015). Prevention of shoulder injuries in overhead athletes: A science-based approach. *Brazilian Journal of Physical Therapy, 19*(5), 331-339.

Davis, J. T., Limpisvasti, O., Fluhme, D., Mohr, K. J., Yocum, L. A., Elattrache, N. S., & Jobe, F. W. (2009). The effect of pitching biomechanics on the upper extremity in youth and adolescent baseball pitchers. *American Journal of Sports Medicine, 37*(8), 1484-1491.

Dorn, T. W., Schache, A. G., & Pandy, M. G. (2012). Muscular strategy shift in human running: Dependence of running speed on hip and ankle muscle performance. *Journal of Experimental Biology, 215*(Pt 11), 1944-1956.

Ellenbecker, T., De Carlo, M., & DeRosa, C. (2009). *Effective functional progressions in sport rehabilitation.* Champaign, IL: Human Kinetics.

Fleisig, G. S., Weber, A., Hassell, N., & Andrews, J. R. (2009). Prevention of elbow injuries in youth baseball pitchers. *Current Sports Medicine Reports, 8*(5), 250-254.

Fradkin, A. J., Finch, C. F., & Sherman, C. A. (2001). Warm-up practices of golfers: Are they adequate? *British Journal of Sports Medicine, 35*(2), 125-127.

Gluck, G. S., Bendo, J. A., & Spivak, J. M. (2008). The lumbar spine and low back pain in golf: A literature review of swing biomechanics and injury prevention. *Spine Journal, 8*(5), 778-788.

Gosheger, G., Liem, D., Ludwig, K., Greshake, O., & Winkelmann, W. (2003). Injuries and overuse syndromes in golf. *American Journal of Sports Medicine, 31*(3), 438-443.

Jones, A. M., & Doust, J. H. (1996). A 1% treadmill grade most accurately reflects the energetic cost of outdoor running. *Journal of Sports Sciences, 14*(4), 321-327.

McHardy, A., Pollard, H., & Luo, K. (2007). One-year follow-up study on golf injuries in Australian amateur golfers. *American Journal of Sports Medicine, 35*(8), 1354-1360.

Nielsen, R. O., Bertelsen, M. L., Parner, E. T., Sørensen, H., Lind, M., & Rasmussen, S. (2014). Running more than three kilometers during the first week of a running regimen may be associated with increased risk of injury in obese novice runners. *International Journal of Sports Physical Therapy, 9*(3), 338-345.

Nielsen, R. Ø., Parner, E. T., Nohr, E. A., Sørensen, H., Lind, M., & Rasmussen, S. (2014). Excessive progression in weekly running distance and risk of running-related injuries: An association which varies according to type of injury. *Journal of Orthopedic Sports Physical Therapy, 44*(10), 739-747.

Olsen, S. J., Fleisig, G. S., Dun, S., Loftice, J., & Andrews, J. R. (2006). Risk factors for shoulder and elbow injuries in adolescent baseball pitchers. *American Journal of Sports Medicine, 42*(8), 905-912.

Rasmussen, C. H., Nielsen, R. O., Juul, M. S., & Rasmussen, S. (2013). Weekly running volume and risk of running-related injuries among marathon runners. *International Journal of Sports Physical Therapy, 8*(2), 111-120.

Reinold, M. M., Wilk, K. E., Reed, J., Crenshaw, K., & Andrews, J. R. (2002). Interval sport programs: Guidelines for baseball, tennis, and golf. *Journal of Orthopedic and Sports Physical Therapy, 32*(6), 293-298.

Thériault, G., & Lachance, P. (1998). Golf injuries: An overview. *Sports Medicine,* 43-57.

University of Delaware Physical Therapy Clinic. (n.d.). Treadmill and track running progression. *Delaware Physical Therapy Clinic.* http://sites.udel.edu/ptclinic/files/2016/10/running_progression_2015-orf1zr.pdf

van Gent, R. N., Siem, D., van Middelkoop, M., van Os, A. G., Bierma-Zeinstra, S. M., & Koes, B. W. (2007). Incidence and determinants of lower extremity running injuries in long distance runners: A systematic review. *British Journal of Sports Medicine, 41*(8), 469-480.

Van Middelkoop, M., Kolkman, J., Van Ochten, J., Bierma-Zeinstra, S. M., & Koes, B. W. (2008). Risk factors for lower extremity injuries among male marathon runners. *Scandinavian Journal of Medicine and Science in Sports, 18*(6), 691-697.

Wilcox, R. (2007). Running injury prevention tips & return to running program. *Brigham and Women's Hospital.* http://www.brighamandwomens.org/Patients_Visitors/pcs/rehabilitationservices/Physical-Therapy-Standards-of-Care-and-Protocols/LE%20-%20Running%20Injury%20Prevention%20Tips%20&%20Return%20to%20Running%20Program.pdf

Yeung, E. W., & Yeung, S. S. (2001). A systematic review of interventions to prevent lower limb soft tissue running injuries. *British Journal of Sports Medicine, 35*(6), 383-389.

Yeung, S. S., Yeung, E. W., & Gillespie, L. D. (2011). Interventions for preventing lower limb soft-tissue running injuries. *The Cochrane Database of Systematic Reviews,* (7), CD001256.

Section 8.02

HOMEMADE EXERCISE EQUIPMENT

8.02.1 ICE MASSAGE

1. Using a Styrofoam coffee cup, fill with water and freeze. Peel top of Styrofoam off to reveal ice. Patient can hold the Styrofoam portion and perform ice massage at home.

8.02.2 GEL ICE PACK

With Rubbing Alcohol

1. Fill a plastic freezer bag with 1 cup of rubbing alcohol and 2 cups of water.
2. Try to get as much air out of the freezer bag before sealing it shut.
3. Place the bag and its contents inside a second freezer bag to prevent leakage.
4. Place bag in the freezer for at least 1 hour.

With Dish Soap or Corn Syrup

1. Fill a plastic freezer bag with dish soap or corn syrup.
2. Try to get as much air out of the freezer bag before sealing it shut.
3. Place the bag and its contents inside a second freezer bag to prevent leakage.
4. Place bag in the freezer for at least 1 hour.

With Dish Soap or Corn Syrup

1. Fill a plastic freezer bag with 2 tablespoons of salt and 2 cups of water.
2. Try to get as much air out of the freezer bag before sealing it shut.
3. Place the bag and its contents inside a second freezer bag to prevent leakage.
4. Place bag in the freezer overnight.

With Sponge

1. Soak a sponge with water.
2. Place sponge in the freezer overnight.

8.02.3 Warm Pack

1. Fill a cotton cloth bag (flannel is nice and soft) with one of the following and sew shut:
    a. Rice
    b. Wheat
    c. Feed corn
    d. Buckwheat hulls
    e. Barley
    f. Oatmeal
    g. Beans
    h. Flax seed
    i. Cherry pits

2. Microwave to desired warmth, and it is ready to use.
3. A sock can also work well in a pinch, as long as there are no synthetic materials in the sock.
4. Do *not* use oils or perfumes. These can be flammable when microwaved.
5. Do *not* use twist ties. They are made with metal, and plastic ties melt.

8.02.4 Cuff Weights

1. Fill two pairs of socks with one of the following:
    a. Rice
    b. Beans
    c. Sand (may want to put in plastic bag first)
    d. Small pebbles

2. Tie a knot in the end of each sock once shaped into a long, somewhat flattened oval.
3. Wrap sock around ankle or wrist and secure by tying a long piece of material around the sock.
4. These also can be held in the hands for UE resistance.

8.02.5 Other Items Around the House That Can Be Used as Weights

1. 1 pounder:
    a. Cans of food (16-oz can = 1 lb of weight resistance)
    b. Salad dressing
    c. Spoons looped together with rubber bands
2. 2 pounder:
    a. 32-oz food cans
    b. 32-oz small cartons of soy milk
    c. Small bags of rice
3. 3 pounder: (check weight)
    a. Produce bag of apples, onions, or oranges

4. 4 pounder:
    a. Large ketchup (full)
    b. Small bags of pet food
5. 5 pounder:
    a. Bag of potatoes
    b. Standard bag of flour
6. 8 pounder:
    a. Gallon of water
7. 10 pounder:
    a. Large bottle of laundry detergent

INDEX